# Surgery of
# THE SHOULDER

# Surgery of
# THE SHOULDER

Anthony F. *rederick* DePalma, M.D.

*Professor of Orthopaedic Surgery and Chairman of the
Division of Orthopaedic Surgery, New Jersey College of
Medicine and Dentistry, Newark, N.J.*

*Emeritus Professor of Orthopaedic Surgery,
Jefferson Medical College, Philadelphia*

## SECOND EDITION

*476 Figures*

# J. B. Lippincott Company

Philadelphia · Toronto

Library of Congress Catalog Card Number 72-6346

ISBN 0-397-50301-6

Printed in the United States of America
6    5    4    3    2    1

**Library of Congress Cataloging in Publication Data**

De Palma, Anthony F
  Surgery of the shoulder.

  Includes bibliographies.
  1.  Shoulder—Surgery.  I.  Title.  [DNLM:  1.  Shoulder—
Surgery—Surgery. WE810 D419s 1972]
RD557.D35 1972   617'.572   72-6346
ISBN 0-397-50301-6

*I Dedicate This Second Edition To*
## MY WIFE, TRUDY

# Foreword

The Surgery of the Shoulder begins with chapters on comparative anatomy, embryology, normal anatomy and variations, biomechanics and changes induced by aging as well as congenital anomalies.

This introductory approach to problems of afflictions of the shoulder and its surgical treatment is very valuable in view of the presently increasing tendency in teaching programs of the medical schools to reduce—to the point of elimination—courses of anatomy based on dissection.

It is especially rewarding to find in this text the important section on anatomical variations. In the diagnosis of many diseases, as well as in cases of trauma and, also, in the technique of surgical approaches, the knowledge and comprehension of the variations is of essential importance.

Functional morphology based on principles of kinesiology, biomechanics and changes connected with growth and aging also enhance the value of the introductory chapters.

The chapters that follow include a comprehensive and clear description of the multiple entities of systemic, neoplastic, traumatic and congenital conditions which are of importance to the orthopaedic surgeon of any period of clinical development. The various methods of surgical treatment are considered in the light of the author's experience. The conclusive chapter deals separately with the complex problem of pain in the shoulder and arm, based on mesodermal, neurogenic and vascular etiology. This section has special merit as a subject rarely sufficiently elucidated.

The extensive clinical experience of the author enhanced by personal research work, and long years of teaching are reflected throughout the text. Simplicity, practical precision, ways to avoid errors and proper evaluation of methods of surgical approaches and treatment are presented.

This is the result of many years spent in devotion to the art and science of surgery and in sharing the acquired experience and knowledge.

EMANUEL KAPLAN, M.D.

# Preface to the Second Edition

Since the publication of the first edition, the shoulder region has continued to be an area of major interest to those concerned with lesions of the musculoskeletal system. No other area in the field of sports-medicine occupies a role of greater importance. Within the past two decades many workers have concentrated their efforts on lesions of the "throwing arm" with the result that many new concepts related to mechanisms of injuries have evolved. Comprehension of these new concepts permits management of the lesions to be based on a more rational and scientific basis. In addition, new roentgenographic techniques and the arthrogram of the glenohumeral joint have increased the diagnostic acumen of lesions of the shoulder. My sustained interest in lesions of the shoulder and my accumulated experience in their management during the past twenty years force me to stand firm on some of my convictions recorded in the first edition; but, also, this interest and experience force me to revise or even discard others. For the reasons mentioned above and many others, I present this second edition with the hope that the revised old material and the addition of the new will up-date the saga of the shoulder joint.

Much of the material in this edition is new, such as the chapter "Prenatal Development of the Human Shoulder". In the chapter "Biomechanics of the Shoulder" I present a new method of measuring the movements of the arm; and in the chapter "Normal, Regional and Variational Anatomy of the Shoulder," both in the text and by new drawings, I place special emphasis on the surgical anatomy of the region under discussion.

An important new addition is the material dealing with the degenerative changes in the acromioclavicular and sternoclavicular joints with aging and the role these changes play in lesions of these articulations. This study parallels the study recorded in the first edition on degenerative changes in the glenohumeral joint.

The material in the chapter "The Unstable Shoulder" is also new and is based on: (1) an extensive study made on anatomical specimens of the shoulder and (2) the correlation of the observations made in the dissected specimens with the pathology found at the operating table on shoulders with recurrent dislocation.

The current concepts of lesions of neurogenic and vascular origin capable of producing shoulder, arm and hand pain are recorded in the chapter "Shoulder-Arm-Hand Pain of Neurogenic and Vascular Origin". In this chapter I stress the important role lesions of the cervical spine (both traumatic and degenerative) play in the production of symptoms.

In the chapter "Surgical Approaches and Procedures" I group together all the useful and currently used operations on the shoulder region. By so doing, the material, in a simplified manner, is readily accessible to the reader. All the illustrations in this chapter are new and the operative procedures are depicted step by step from incision to closure of the wound.

Of the 476 illustrations in this edition, approximately 85 per cent of them are new or revised.

I make the following acknowledgments with a deep feeling of humility and gratitude: to my resident staff at the Jefferson College of Medicine and to the resident staff at the Martland Medical Center of the New Jersey School of Medicine and Dentistry; these young men helped to collect much of the material presented in this volume; to Dr. P. Hodes and Dr. J. Edeikin, Professors of Radiology, Jefferson Medical College, who not only permitted me to use their facilities but conveyed freely much valuable information in the discussions of many of the clinical entities presented in this edition; to Barbara Finneson, the artist, who with great skill and talent made all the new drawings and revised all the old ones; to Dr. J.W. King, who provided many of the illustrations in the chapter "Injuries of the Shoulder in Sports"; to Dr. R.H. Freiberger, who so generously provided me with illustrations of arthrograms of the different lesions of the glenohumeral joint. A special acknowledgment with gratitude is due to my wife, Trudy, who conscientiously typed and edited the many drafts of the manuscript; and, finally, to Walter Kahoe of the J.B. Lippincott Company for his encouragement to produce this volume.

A.F. DePALMA

# Preface to the First Edition

Before any work is contemplated on the shoulder, tribute must be paid to Dr. E.A. Codman, whose meticulous and comprehensive investigation recorded in his book, The Shoulder, has laid down the foundation for all further study in this region. No one has done more to extract from the vague symptom complex "the painful and stiff shoulder" the numerous heterogenous entities which it comprises. His observations relative to the pathology and the management of lesions of the musculotendinous cuff, subacromial bursa and his concept of the mechanism of dislocation and fracture of the upper end of the humerus have stood up under the critical assessment of many workers and now have been generally accepted. His work has provided the stimulus for much painstaking research which has resulted in valuable contributions to our stock of knowledge on the shoulder. A few of the more recent and outstanding contributions are the work of Inman, Saunders and Abbott on the functional mechanism of the shoulder, the study of McLaughlin and D. Bosworth on lesions of the musculotendinous cuff and that of Hitchcock and Bechtol and of Lippmann on lesions of the tendon of the long head of the biceps brachii muscle.

The writing of this book has been prompted by the desire to assemble under one cover the accumulated knowledge on the anatomy and the physiology of the shoulder and some of the more common entities responsible for dysfunction of the shoulder; also, to record the observations made referable to the variational anatomy and the degenerative lesions of the inner side of the scapulohumeral joint noted in successive decades. Knowledge of these alterations enables one to formulate the norm for the different age periods and facilitates comprehension of the many pathologic processes implicating the musculotendinous cuff and the biceps tendon which may result in impairment of function.

An attempt has been made to interpret the clinical significance of the degenerative abnormalities observed in shoulders of individuals in different decenniums. For example, as will be shown in the text, wear and tear and senescence are responsible for pulling away of the labrum glenoidale from its bony attachment on the glenoid brim; this lesion increases in severity in each successive decade. In the light of this information it becomes apparent that the labrum glenoidale is in no way associated with the stability of the glenohumeral joint. The operations designed to restore the normal relationship of the labrum, with the hope that a cure for recurrent dislocations of the shoulder will be affected, are based on an erroneous premise. On the other hand, this same study on degenerative lesions provides an explanation of the success of some and the failure of other procedures.

The observations made on a series of shoulder joints obtained postmortem from individuals on whom an examination of the extremities was made prior to their deaths are of particular clinical importance and therefore should be reported. It was noted that large defects in the cuff are compatible with good function. This information demands that we revise our concept of the size of a rupture of the cuff, which may cause impairment of function, and our present-day management of these lesions. However, one is well aware that the aforementioned degenerative lesions differ from traumatic rupture sustained suddenly. In the former, nature has ample time to rearrange the mechanics of the shoulder joint so that dysfunction does not ensue; in the latter, this readjustment is lacking; hence, marked impairment of function results. However, if given time, nature in many instances will make the necessary alterations to restore function.

Many readers may believe that the manner in which the material was obtained for the investigation on "Degenerative Lesions Compatible with Good Function" was unorthodox. That the method was such is true; nevertheless, in no other way can such material be obtained in sufficient quantities to allow adequate evaluation from a clinical viewpoint of the lesions found. One is forced to admit that the significance of the observations justified the method.

The chapter dealing with frozen shoulder and bicipital tenosynovitis emphasizes that although these are two distinct entities they are closely related. Many workers do not agree with this concept; however, gross and microscopic studies made on many anatomic and postmortem specimens and on subjects at the operating table support this belief. Whether the pathology, the pathogenesis and the management recorded of the above lesions is or is not accepted, it is hoped that sufficient interest will be aroused to stimulate further investigation which will either support or disprove the interpretation of the observations made in this chapter.

The theory of the pathogenesis of recurrent dislocation of the shoulder is not an original one. Magnuson, in describing his operation for recurrent dislocation of the shoulder, referred to muscular imbalance about the shoulder as the causative factor responsible for the malady. This observer and many others believe that any method that will limit external rotation of the shoulder will effect a cure. With this concept the author is in complete agreement and makes a plea that the most simple operative procedure which will achieve restriction of external rotation of the extremity be adopted.

It has been necessary to draw heavily from numerous sources in order to compile all the material deemed essential in this book. Every effort possible has been made to give full credit to the authors of the material used; however, it may be possible that some omissions have occurred unknowingly. In such instances, the author begs to offer his apologies and express his regret.

It is hoped that the practitioner and the surgeon will find this book a valuable source of information in the more common pathologic conditions affecting the shoulder region. In addition it is hoped that the studies recorded herein will result in more adequate comprehension of the pathogenesis of these lesions, increased acumen in diagnosis and more effective methods of management.

The author makes the following acknowledgments with a deep feeling of gratitude: first, to Dr. G.A. Bennett, Director of the Department of Anatomy of the Jefferson Medical College, who, together with Dr. G. Callery and the author, conducted the investigation on Variational Anatomy and Degenerative Lesions of the Shoulder Joint recorded in Part I of Chapter 3. Dr. Bennett was more than a collaborator in this study. He provided the stimulus necessary to guide the work to a successful termination. His profound knowledge of anatomy and its practical application, together with his keen powers of observation, made possible the many significant findings noted. The author is deeply indebted to

Dr. Bennett for the many hours of detailed instruction in the manner of approach and conduction of a problem in research; also for the use of the anatomic specimens which were employed in subsequent studies in the shoulder and for the advice, guidance and encouragement that he readily gave. All of the illustrations on the glenoid side of the scapulohumeral joint used in this book were obtained from the investigation conducted together with Dr. Bennett and Dr. Callery.

Acknowledgment is also due to: Dr. P.C. Swenson, Professor of Radiology, Jefferson Medical College, who so kindly permitted us to use all the facilities of his department; Dr. R.L. Breckenridge, who gave valuable aid in the interpretation of the microscopic sections; Dr. J.B. White, who faithfully assisted in the study on the Lesions of the Shoulder Joint Compatible with Good Function; Dr. G. Diebert, Dr. J. Gartland and Dr. T. Armstrong, who helped collect the gross specimens and the case histories used in this work; Dr. M. Blaker and Dr. I. Kaplan, who gathered much material and prepared the bibliography and the index; Mrs. M. Gross, who so carefully edited the manuscript; my able office staff, Miss T. Everett and Miss V. Quick, for their painstaking work on the many drafts of the manuscript and the arrangement of the illustrations; Mr. A. Hancock, the photographer for the Jefferson Hospital, for his conscientious and meticulous work; the editor and publishers of the Instructional Course Lectures, for the privilege of using material which appeared previously in this publication; Mr. C. Brill, the artist, who painstakingly made all the original drawings in this work; and, finally, the J.B. Lippincott Company for their guidance and many suggestions in the production of this book.

A.F. DePALMA

# Contents

# Surgery of
# THE SHOULDER

# 1

# Origin and Comparative Anatomy of the Pectoral Limb

## ORIGIN OF PAIRED APPENDAGES

The origin of paired appendages has been the source of considerable controversy among morphologists. The lateral-fin theory has supplanted the gill-arch theory of Gegenbaur and is now accepted as the most plausible explanation of the beginning of these appendages.

According to the lateral-fin theory, paired limbs are derived from longitudinal lateral folds of epidermis extending backward along the body from just behind the gills to the anus. By accentuation of the anterior and the posterior and suppression and reduction of the intermediate portions of the folds the pectoral and the pelvic fins were formed (Fig. 1-1). Into these folds muscle buds migrated from the ventral border of the adjoining myotomes, giving rise to radial muscles which motivated the fins and were the forerunners of the intrinsic muscles of the hand (Boyes). The muscle buds disclosed a metameric arrangement and derived their nerve supply from ventral roots of the spinal nerves.

Peripheral nerve fibers in the base of the fin divide repeatedly, giving rise to a complex plexus. The number of myotomes which comprise the muscular apparatus of the fin is disclosed by the number of spinal nerves which contribute to the plexus. In ontogeny, motor nerves always supply the muscles for which they were designed originally. Muscles exhibiting a nerve supply from more than one spinal nerve denote combining of muscle tissue of several seg-

ments. Next in the process of evolution of the appendages was the appearance of radials (cartilage rays) between the muscle buds; these provided more strength and support to the fins (Fig. 1-2).

Concentration and fusion of the proximal (basal) ends of the radials in the fin gave rise to the basilia (basal cartilages) which extended inward into the body wall to form the most primitive girdle (Fig. 1-3). In order to meet the requirements of a freely movable fin an articulation appeared in the basal plates. Further evolution of the girdle included fusion of the basilia of either side in the midline to form a ventral bar; also included is a dorsal extension of the arch above the level of the articulation to join the axial skeleton. Thus a complete girdle is formed around the body. The above steps in the ontogeny of the girdle have been noted in the Selachii (elasmobranchs) and also in Chondrostei and Teleostei.

## EVOLUTION OF THE PECTORAL GIRDLE

### Fishes

In its basic pattern the girdle is an inverted arch spanning the ventral surface of the body and extending dorsally on either side above the level of the articulation. Both the girdle and the limb are free. Each girdle comprises a ventral segment (coracoid) and a dorsal segment (scapula). These at the point of conjuncture form the glenoid fossa, which articulates with the basal com-

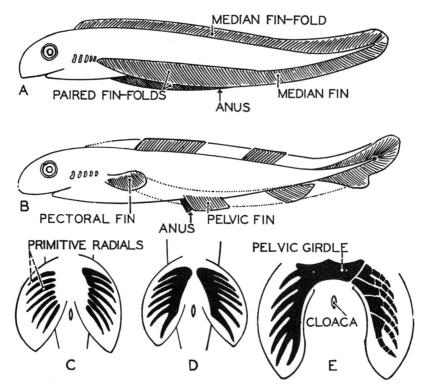

FIG. 1-1. Hypothetical evolution of paired fins and their skeletal supports. (A) Primitive stage, characterized by continuous fin folds; the dorsal and ventral fins posterior to the anus are median and unpaired. (B) Elasmobranch stage; paired fin-folds persist only in the region of the pectoral and pelvic fins; median fins have become discontinuous. (C-E) Hypothetical stages in the evolution of the skeleton of the pelvic fins of elasmobranch fishes. The right side of C and E represent a later stage in the phylogenesis than the left. E represents the differentiated skeletons of the girdle and the extremity. (After Wiedersheim) (Neal, H. V., and Rand, H. W.: Chordate Anatomy. New York, Blakiston Div. McGraw-Hill, 1936)

ponent of the skeleton of the limb. Further segmentation of the scapula gives rise to the suprascapula, which may become attached to the axial skeleton (as in skates). All the above elements have separate centers of chondrification (Fig. 1-4).

Further in the scale of evolution of the pectoral girdle is the appearance of a girdle of membranous bones derived from the skin. It encircles the head, starting from behind the gills. The elements of either half of the girdle join and fuse in the midline on the ventral surface of the body through the medium of the interclavicle. Each half of this membranous circle consists of 4 membranous bones: (1) post-temporal, which is jointed with the skull, (2) supracleithrum, (3) cleithrum and (4) clavicle.

The interclavicle, which unites the girdle ventrally, is an unpaired bone. The basal girdle and the membranous girdle eventually became attached to one another. Such is the basic plan of the pectoral girdle as noted in two genera (Eusthenopteron and Sauropterus of the upper Devonian crossopterygians). These are considered the ancestors of the amphibia whose appendages possessed the pattern which made the evolution of the tetrapod limb possible (Fig. 1-5).

## Amphibia

With the attainment of terrestrial habits most of the elements of the membranous girdle (post-temporal and supracleithrum) decreased in size and disappeared, while the cartilaginous girdle began to assume a more significant role. The skull was freed of all attachment to the girdle. In urodeles all vestiges of the membranous girdle have disappeared.

In the amphibia the tripartite type of pectoral girdle made its first appearnce; the coracoid represented by the ventral bar in the fishes became segmented into the anterior procoracoid and posterior coracoid, while the clavicle came in relation to the procoracoid. No significant alterations occur in the suprascapula and the scapula. A noteworthy observation in the pectoral girdle of large amphibia (Rhachitomi) is the direction of the glenoid fossa. It faces laterally, indicating that the humerus extended away from the trunk in the coronal plane horizontal to the ground. Its articular surface was "screw shaped" (Howell), indicative of clumsy arm movement.

## Reptiles

Whereas in the amphibia the pectoral girdle is just behind the head, in the reptile it has migrated a considerable distance from this position. Essentially, the girdle comprises a scapula, a procoracoid and a coracoid. In general, the clavicle replaces the procoracoid, as evidenced by the latter's reduction in size. However, in some reptiles the clavicle is absent (Crocodilia and Chamaeleonidae). Some reptiles lost their limbs, and the girdles either are greatly reduced or have disappeared (Amphisbaenides, Ophidia).

## Birds

Elements of the girdle of the reptiles were modified in birds to permit flight. The clavicles exhibit a marked degree of development, their ventral ends fusing to form the wishbone (furcula). The scapula is small,

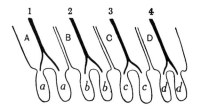

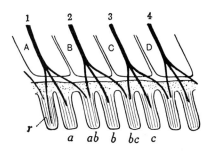

FIG. 1-2. Formation of adult radial muscles from embryonic muscle buds, and their motor nerve supply. (*Above*) Embryonic stage with a pair of buds to each segment. (*Below*) Adult stage with radial muscles compounded of material from adjacent buds. 1-4, Four spinal nerves; A-D, four myomeres; *a-d*, muscle buds; *r*, radial muscle. (Goodrich, E. S.: Studies on the Structure and Development of Vertebrates. p. 134. London, Macmillan, 1930.)

curved and narrow, extending backward. The coracoid is large and strong, one end together with the scapula forming the glenoid fossa, while the other unites with the sternum. The keeled sternum provides attachment for the strong pectoral muscles used in flight. In some cursorial birds the clavicles are greatly reduced (emu), and in others they are absent.

## Mammals

In monotremes, the lowest order of mammals, large coracoids are found between the sternum and the glenoid fossa. In all other mammals, the coracoid tends to be greatly reduced, forming an insignificant process on the scapula. The only other vestige of the bone is the coracoid ligament,

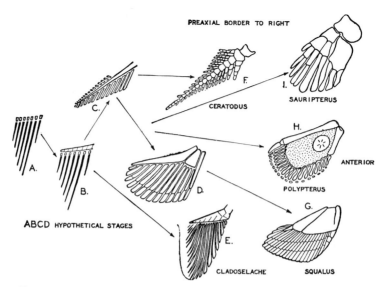

FIG. 1-3. Diagrams illustrating hypothetical evolution of the extremities of diapnoan (I), ganoid (H) and elasmobranch (G) from a fin fold supported by a series of similar radial cartilages. By fusion of radial cartilages basilia (basal cartilages) are formed. Skeletal supports of the fins eventually differ in relation of the basal elements to the radialia. (Redrawn from A. Brazier Howell) (Neal, H. V., and Rand, H. W.: Chordate Anatomy. New York, Blakiston Div. McGraw-Hill, 1936)

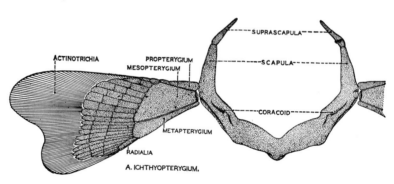

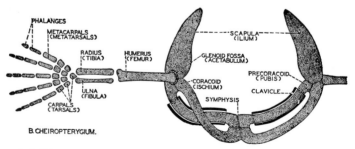

FIG. 1-4. Diagrams illustrating scheme of pectoral appendages of lower vertebrates (*top*) and higher vertebrates (*bottom*). Names of corresponding parts of pelvic appendages are shown in parentheses. (Neal, H. V., and Rand, H. W.: Chordate Anatomy. New York, Blakiston Div. McGraw-Hill, 1936)

extending from the coracoid process to the bone, in which may be found isolated masses of cartilage. The coracoid has a separate center of ossification. This arrangement frees the scapula from any bony attachment to the skeleton. In mammals without clavicles the scapula has no bony attachments whatsoever. It becomes the sole support for the limb and provides attachment for muscles necessary for a freely movable extremity. New functional demands on the girdle resulted in the development of a projection of bone on the dorsal surface of the scapula (spina scapulae) which extends downward and ends in the acromion (Fig. 1-6).

Generally, the clavicle articulates with the acromion and the sternum, its only connection to the coracoid process being by the coracoclavicular ligaments (conoid, trapezoid). In mammals that have acquired freedom of the forelimb to a marked degree, such as insectivores, primates and some marsupials and rodents, the clavicle is usually well developed. In others, including ungulates, carnivores, cetaceans and some rodents, edentates and marsupials, it is absent or rudimentary.

## EVOLUTION OF THE UPPER EXTREMITIES

There has been considerable controversy as to the derivation of the cheiropterygium (tetrapod limb, also called the pentadactyl limb) from the icthyopterygium (paired fins of fishes). As noted above, in the evolution of the free paired appendages the proximal or basal ends of the radials (cartilage rays) fused to form basilia, and later, with the demand of greater movability of the fin, a joint appeared between the radials and the basilia, several of which in turn articulated with the girdle. Such a scheme is discernible in the paired fins of the elasmobranchs, which possess three basilia (propterygium, mesopterygium and metapterygium) located between the girdle and the radials of the fin (see Fig. 1-4).

In the pectoral girdles and the fins of the crossopts Eusthenopteron and Sauropterus (fossils from upper Devonian) is found an arrangement of the skeletal elements, generally accepted as a link between paired fins of fishes and tetrapod limb (see Fig. 1-5). These two genera of crossopterygian fishes are considered close to the forms

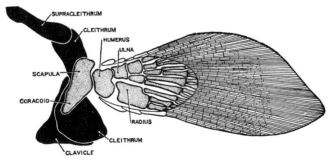

FIG. 1-5. Diagram of reconstructed pectoral girdle and fin of Sauropterus, an upper Devonian crossopterygian fish. It exhibits a close similarity of relations of proximal elements of the extremity to those found in the pectoral extremity of tetrapods. (Redrawn from Brown) (Neal, H. V., and Rand, H. W.: Chordate Anatomy. New York, Blakiston Div. McGraw-Hill, 1936)

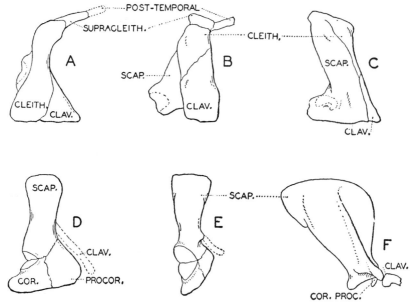

FIG. 1-6. Phylogenesis of the pectoral girdle. (A) Sauropterus (Devonian crossopterygian lung fish). (B) Eogyrinus (Carboniferous embolomerous amphibian). (C) Eryops (Permian rhachitomous amphibian). (D) Moschops (Permian dinocephalian reptile). (E) Cynognathus (Triassic theriodont reptile). (F) Macaca (an Old-World Recent monkey). (Howell, A. B.: Speed in Animals. p. 138. Chicago, University of Chicago Press, 1944)

from which the amphibia evolved. The basic pattern of their pectoral limb comprised a proximal segment which was joined to two middle segments, which in turn articulated with several distal elements. The proximal element was destined to become the humerus, the middle elements the radius and the ulna, the distal elements the carpus and the digits.

The change from an aqueous to a terrestrial existence was accompanied by pronounced alterations in the skeletal elements of the pectoral fin which must now be used for support and locomotion. Therefore, in the amphibia, the first animals to adopt terrestrial habits, the pentadactyl limb evolved from the paired fins. From the distal element arose the carpus, the metacarpus and the phalanges. The principal element on the radial side became the thumb, and those on the ulnar side the other four digits. In all stages of evolution up to and including man the basic plan of the pentadactyl limb has been maintained.

## Scapula

The scapula, more than any other bone of the shoulder girdle, reflects momentous alterations brought about, during the evolution of the upper extremity, by increased functional demands of a prehensile limb. Changes in posture provided the stimulus that initiated the numerous morphological changes. In the amphibia the scapula was high in the cervical region but was freed from the skull. Rhachitomous amphibians possessed massive scapulae with the glenoid cavity pointing laterally. The articulating surface was screw shaped, and the limbs were held in the coronal plane horizontal to the ground.

In the Reptilia the scapula, with the entire girdle, migrated a great distance from the skull in order to permit a more efficient mode of locomotion. The scapula was still broad and massive in the primitive forms. Later, however, with increased efficiency in locomotion, there was a trend toward re-

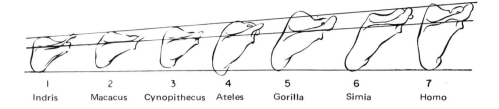

| 1 | 2 | 3 | 4 | 5 | 6 | 7 |
| Indris | Macacus | Cynopithecus | Ateles | Gorilla | Simia | Homo |

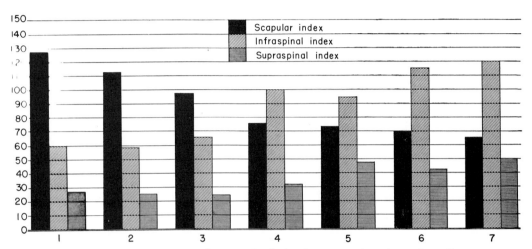

FIG. 1-7. Progressive decrease in scapular index in successive stages from the prono-grade to the orthograde. (Redrawn from Inman, V. T., Saunders, J. B. DeC., and Abbott, L. C.: J. Bone & Joint Surg., *26*:2, 1944)

duction of this bone, the glenoid cavity shifting from a position directed laterally to one directed posteriorly and inferiorly. As a result of the change in posture, the coracoid's function decreased. Hence, a gradual reduction in its size is noted in this group. Up to this stage in evolution of the pectoral girdle no evidence of a spine on the dorsal surface of the scapula is found except in the Therapsida, whose posture is not unlike that of the mammals.

Posture was responsible for the development of the scapular spine which is found in all mammals except the very primitive forms, the Monotremata. With rearrangement of some and disappearance of other muscles, the need of a procoracoid and a coracoid no longer existed. Therefore, the former element disappeared entirely, while the latter was reduced to the coracoid process.

The shape of the scapula is dependent upon posture and the functional requirements of the muscles attached. The scapula is broad and massive in forms that need large powerful serratus anticus muscles to support heavy bodies in a quadruped position. In mammals that have partially or completely freed the pectoral limbs, the shape of the scapula exhibits a trend toward the pattern found in man. These alterations are brought about by change in posture from the pronograde to the orthograde and highly specialized functional requirements of a prehensile limb. The most significant scapular change is in the relation of length to breadth of the bone. Pronograde forms disclose a long narrow scapula, while in the ascent toward man it becomes broader. This morphological change is most obvious in the primates. That portion of the scapula below the spine demonstrates the most pro-

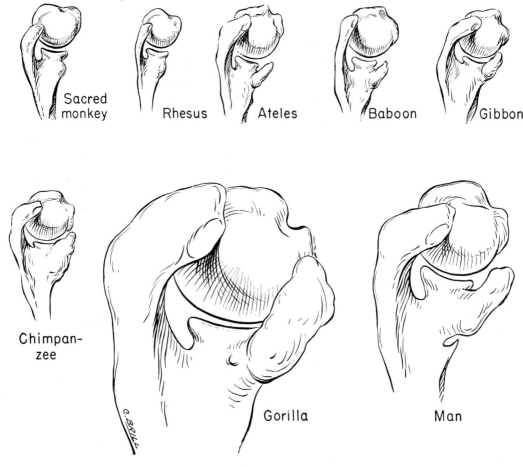

FIG. 1-8. Gradual increase in spine of the scapula and the acromion process during development from the pronograde to the orthograde. This change reflects the increasing importance of the deltoid muscle. Also note the increase in size of the coracoid process, the inequality of the two tuberosities of the head of the humerus and the inner displacement of the intertubercular sulcus in successive stages of development.

nounced alterations, those in the region above the spine being insignificant.

Morphological modifications in the scapula can be expressed by a scapular index, a ratio of the breadth (measured along the base of the spine) to the length (measured from the superior to the inferior angle). The scapular index is high in the pronograde in which the scapula is long, narrow and slender. The index progressively decreases in the successive stages of development approaching man (orthograde). This is the result of a gradual increase in the breadth of the scapula and elongation of the bone be-

low the level of the spine, giving rise to a progressive increase in the "infraspinous index" (Fig. 1-7). Inman, Saunders and Abbott, in their comprehensive study of the function of the shoulder joint, observed that lengthening of the scapula below the spine changed the relation of the axillary border of the scapula to the glenoid fossa, thereby altering the angle of pull of the muscles attached to this region, a feature of great significance in the mechanism of the shoulder.

In the primates, as one approaches man, the increasing importance of the role of the deltoid muscle is reflected in the promi-

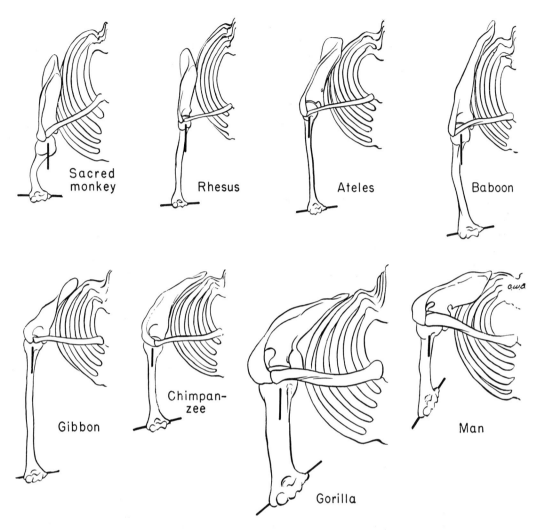

FIG. 1-9. Changes in the thoracic cage, the scapula and the humerus, in successive stages from the pronograde to the orthograde. The thoracic cage shows flattening in the anteroposterior plane, and the scapula migrates to a dorsal position so that the glenoid cavity is directed laterally. The humerus shows a progressive increase in the torsion angle.

nence of the outer end of the spine, the acromion process. Whereas in pronograde forms the acromion process is insignificant, in orthogrades it is a massive structure overlying the humeral head (Fig. 1-8).

## Humerus

During evolution of a prehensile extremity, profound morphological modifications occurred in the humerus. In rhachitomous amphibians the humerus was a massive bone flattened at either end, the distal end being larger than the proximal to provide attachment for large forearm muscles. In reptiles with free motion in the forelimb the upper extremity was brought beneath the body, and the humerus became less massive. Two nodules appeared at the proximal end, which evolved into the tuberosities of the mammalian humerus. The anterior became the greater, and the posterior the lesser tuberosity.

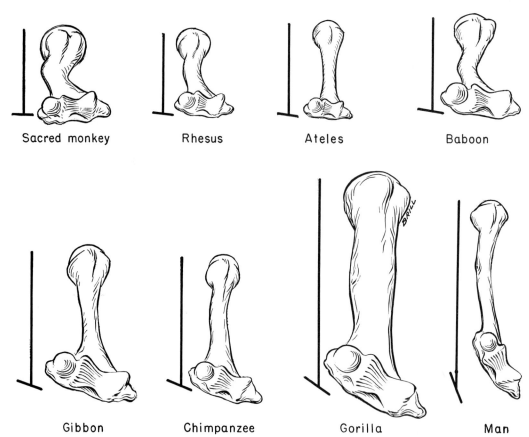

Sacred monkey     Rhesus     Ateles     Baboon

Gibbon     Chimpanzee     Gorilla     Man

FIG. 1-10. Progressive increase in torsion in shaft of the humerus, resulting in inward rotation of the bicipital groove. The articular surfaces at either end of the humerus rotate in opposite directions.

Generally speaking, in mammals adapted for running (ungulates — horse) the articular surfaces of both ends of the humerus function in the same plane (sagittal plane); a line passing through the long axis of the head of the humerus is directed forward and one through the distal articular surface is directed transversely. Meeting of these two axes describes a torsion angle of 90°. In primates, as the orthograde form is approached, the torsion angle increases. Man discloses some variation in the torsion angle; Australian aborigines exhibit an angle of 134°, and the French and the Swiss 164° (Martin, 1928).

Several factors are responsible for the changing relationship of the articular surfaces of the humerus. Development of the orthograde forms was accompanied by anteroposterior flattening of the thoracic cage and dorsal displacement of the scapula. The glenoid fossa is now directed laterally (Fig. 1-9). Prehensile requirements, however, demand that the extremity as a whole function anterior to the body and that the elbow be maintained in the parasagittal plane. To meet these specifications, the humeral shaft has twisted inwardly, while the articular surfaces at either end were rotated in the opposite directions (Fig. 1-10). The dominant role acquired by the deltoid in the higher primates is demonstrated further by the progressive shift of the deltoid insertion on the humerus to a more distal position. This feature, together with increase in size of the acromion, greatly increases

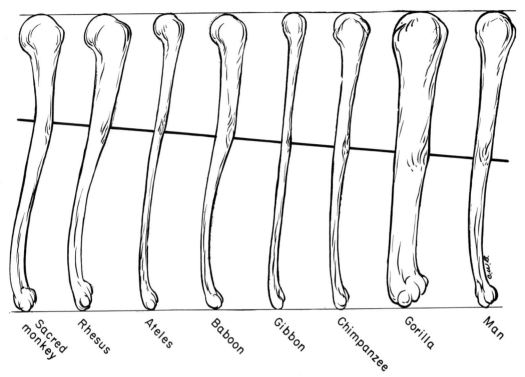

Sacred monkey    Rhesus    Ateles    Baboon    Gibbon    Chimpanzee    Gorilla    Man

FIG. 1-11. Deltoid insertion migrates progressively to a lower level on the shaft of the humerus, indicating the significant role played by the deltoid in higher primates.

the leverage of the deltoid muscle (Fig. 1-11).

Other significant morphological alterations were recession of the lesser tuberosity and medial displacement of the bicipital groove. Pronograde forms disclose the biceps tendon passing over the center of the head of the humerus and entering the groove in the same plane. In this postion it acts as a strong elevator of the arm. Both tuberosities in these forms are approximately the same size.

A different relationship is found in orthogrades. In these forms, the bicipital groove has been rotated medially by torsion of the humerus so that a line passing through the center of the head of the humerus in man makes an angle of 30° with one passing through the plane of the groove (Inman, Saunders and Abbott). Marked reduction in the size of the lesser tuberosity is a characteristic feature in the higher primates.

From the above observations it is obvious that the biceps tendon (long head) functions at a great mechanical disadvantage, further increased by using the arm in a position of internal rotation. In this position the biceps tendon plays over the medial wall of the groove, and the lesser tuberosity now really functions as a trochlea.

## Muscles

Changes in posture and functional requirements of a prehensile extremity were responsible for alterations in the topography and the morphology of muscles about the shoulder. Such changes were primarily responsible for the skeletal modifications previously indicated. The extent of the change in any individual muscle becomes apparent when its relative mass is compared with the total mass of the group to which it belongs. Following the scheme of Inman,

Saunders and Abbott, the muscles that partake in shoulder mechanism can be categorized into three topographical units: (1) scapulohumeral group; (2) axiohumeral group, and (3) axioscapular group.

The study made on the functional mechanism of the shoulder by the aforementioned workers is so complete, comprehensive and logical that one is forced to draw heavily from this source of information when discussing this topic. Many of their observations are noted in the subsequent section.

**The Scapulohumeral Group.** These connect the scapula to the humerus and consist of the supraspinatus, infraspinatus, teres minor, subscapularis and deltoid muscles. Concurrently with acquisition of a free limb, the relative deltoid mass increases, while the relative mass of the supraspinatus decreases. Forty-one percent of the total mass of this unit in man is made up by the deltoid muscle.

Comparative anatomy further discloses that the teres minor muscle is wanting in early mammals and that it evolved from the deltoid to form a separate muscle passing from the inferior angle of the scapula to the humerus. With elongation of the infraspinatus portion of the scapula, the relative mass of this muscle progressively increased until, in man, it makes up 5 percent of the total mass. Although it is a morphological component of the deltoid, the teres minor, because of topographic changes, plays an entirely different role in the mechanism of the shoulder from that of the deltoid.

The subscapularis muscle is little affected by morphological alterations from the primitive to the higher primates. It makes up 20 percent of the mass of the scapulohumeral group. The only significant alteration is an increase in number of fasciculi of origin. This is the result of elongation of the scapula. The same skeletal change brought about an increase in the area of attachment of the infraspinatus, which constitutes approximately 16 percent of the total mass.

According to Inman, Saunders and Ab-

bott, the subscapularis, teres minor and infraspinatus, by reason of alterations in the morphology and the topography of the group and the elongation of the scapula, function as a unit. They are both rotators and depressors of the head of the humerus.

**The axioscapular group,** chiefly concerned with the mechanism of the shoulder, comprises (1) serratus anterior, (2) rhomboids, (3) levator scapulae and (4) trapezius muscles. Serratus anterior, the rhomboids, and levator scapulae originated from one complex of muscle fibers arising from the ribs (first 8 or 10) and their homologues (transverse processes of the cervical vertebrae) in the cervical region and inserting into the vertebral border of the scapula. In primitive forms the dominant function of this group was to control the movements of the vertebral border of the scapula.

In general, those fibers concerned with dorsal motion of the scapula became the rhomboid muscles; those with ventral motion, the serratus muscle; and those with cranial displacement of the scapula, the levator scapulae. Function and posture were responsible for evolution of the individual muscles as they exist in the higher primates. The serratus anterior formed the basal unit for all three muscles. Concentration of the proximal and distal fibers and progressive reduction of the intermediate fibers gave origin to two distinct muscles, the levator scapulae and the serratus anterior.

Further morphological alterations in the serratus anterior comprise grouping of its proximal and distal fibers, progressive reduction in size of its intermediate fibers, and insertion of the dominant upper and lower portions of the muscle into the superomedial and inferior angles of the scapula.

The trapezius, like the sternocleidomastoid muscle, evolved from a muscle sheet passing from the last gill arch to the membranous girdle. In terrestrial forms it attained a position from the occipital region to the trunk; in tetrapods it arises from the occiput, and the mid-dorsum of neck and thorax, and inserts into the spine of the scapula, the acromion and the scapula. Little change has occurred in the trapezius in the evolution of the primates. There has been, however, some concentration of its proximal and distal muscle components and reduction in mass and efficiency of its middle components.

**The axiohumeral group** is made up of the pectoralis major, the pectoralis minor and the latissimus dorsi muscles and extends from the trunk to the humerus. The pectoral group evolved from a primitive muscle sheet that connected the coracoid with the humerus. Change in posture and increased functional demands made on the limb were responsible in the later reptilian and early mammalian forms for displacement of part of this muscle sheet dorsally to gain attachment to the scapula, which later gave rise to the supraspinatus, the infraspinatus and the anterior part of the subscapularis. All other components of the muscle migrated from the procoracoid to the sternum and gave rise to the pectoralis major.

Further morphological modification in the pectoralis major resulted in a division of this mass into a superficial and a deep layer. Part of the sternal attachment of the superficial fibers shifted forward and gained attachment to the clavicle (clavicular head of the pectoralis major). From the deep layer evolved the pectoralis minor muscle which, in higher primates, discloses its humeral attachment in primitive forms to have migrated to the coracoid process.

The latissimus dorsi and teres major muscles originate from a single basic muscle sheet extending from the trunk, caudal to the scapula, to the humerus. They demonstrate in the higher primates no significant morphological or topographic alterations except that they are unusually well developed in forms specializing in climbing.

**Biceps Brachii and Triceps Muscles.** Both of these muscles evolved from ventral and dorsal brachial muscle elements which were concerned primarily with motion in the more distal joints, the elbow and the wrist. From the ventral brachial elements arose the biceps muscle by proximal migration along a fascial plane of brachial components to reach the scapula (Howell). In mammals other than primates, it is a single muscle. Cursorial forms (horse) disclose powerful biceps which together with the supraspinatus act as a single functional unit to elevate the foreleg.

Primates exhibit two heads of origin: one from the supraglenoid tubercle and the other from the coracoid process. Medial displacement of the bicipital groove resulting from torsion of the humeral shaft places the long head at a mechanical disadvantage, thereby losing its efficiency as an elevator of the arm which it possesses in other forms. However, the biceps can be made to function as an abductor of the extremity if the arm is rotated externally, hence, restoring the tendon to the top and the center of the humeral head. This maneuver is not infrequently utilized by individuals with paralyzed abductors of the arm.

The triceps originated from a dorsal brachial muscle element. Like the biceps, its three heads migrated proximally. The scapular or long head gained attachment to the infraglenoid tubercle, the medial head to the upper and posteromedial surface of the humerus, and the lateral head to the upper posterolateral surface. No significant morphological or topographic alterations have occurred in this muscle. It functions as a powerful extensor (dorsiflexor) of the arm.

## BIBLIOGRAPHY

Ashley Montagu, F. M.: An Introduction to Physical Anthropology. Springfield, Ill., Charles C Thomas, 1947.
Bardeen, C. R., and Lewis, W. H.: Development of limbs, body wall and back. Am. J. Anat., *1*:1-36, 1901.
Boyes, J. H.: Bunnell's Surgery of the Hand. ed. 5. Philadelphia, J. B. Lippincott, 1970.
Goodrich, E. S.: Studies on the Structure and Development of Vertebrates. London, Macmillan, 1930.

Gregory, W. K.: Present status of the problem of the origin of the tetrapod with special reference to the skull and paired limbs. Ann. N. Y. Acad. Sci., *26*:317-383, 1915.

————: Further observations on the pectoral girdle and fin of Sauripterus Taylori Hall, a crossopterygian fish from the upper Devonian of Pennsylvania; with special reference to the origin of the pentadactylate extremities of tetrapods. Proc. Am. Philosoph. Soc., *75*: 673, 1935.

Howell, A. B.: Speed in Animals. Chicago, Univ. Chicago Press, 1944.

Huxley, T. H.: Anatomy of the Vertebrates. New York, D. Appleton & Co., 1881.

Inman, V. T., Saunders, J. B. deC. M., and Abbott, L. C.: Observations on the function of the shoulder joint. J. Bone & Joint Surg., *26*: 1-30, 1944.

Jones, F. W.: Attainment of upright position of man. Nature (Lond.), *146*:26-27, 1940.

Kingsley, J. S.: Comparative Anatomy of the Vertebrates. Philadelphia, Blakiston, 1917.

Lewis, W. H.: The development of the arm in man. Am. J. Anat., *145*:184, 1902.

Minor, R. W.: The pectoral limb of Eryop and other primitive tetrapods. Bull. Am. Museum Nat. Hist., *51*:145, 1924-1925.

Neal, H. V., and Rand, H. W.: Chordate Anatomy. Philadelphia, Blakiston, 1936.

# 2

# Prenatal Development of the Human Shoulder Joint

Much of the information on the developmental process of the upper and lower limbs was provided by the work of C. R. Bardeen and W. H. Lewis. In the past two decades, studies by E. Gardner shed more light on the development and physiology of synovial joints including the shoulder joint. For the orthopaedic surgeon comprehension of these processes is most essential. It provides understanding of the origin of the numerous skeletal, muscular, neurogenic or vascular congenital abnormalities which occur in the region of the shoulder, and permits an intelligent approach to the management of both congenital and acquired disorders in this region.

## STAGES OF THE DEVELOPMENTAL PROCESS

The most striking feature of the developmental process is the precise timing of the many events occurring in rapid and orderly sequence. The total process is divided into two stages, the embryonic stage and the fetal stage. The 7 to 8 weeks after fertilization comprise the embryonic period. At this stage the embryo is 28 to 30 mm. in crown-rump length. Termination of this period coincides with almost complete differentiation of the many components of the limb and of the various tissues and organs; the embryo assumes the anatomical characteristics of a miniature adult. The fetal period begins with the termination of differentiation and ends at term. During this period the final adult conditions are approached by an increase in size and complexity of the various tissues and organs, and migration or shifting of parts to their adult position.

Streeter has given us a time table for the various stages of development during the embryonic period. He divided the embryonic period into 23 stages. Each stage is identified by the size and shape of the embryo and by the level of differentiation of the various tissues and organs. No such time table exists for the fetal period. Development during this period is generally related to crown-rump length or to age in menstrual weeks.

## EMBRYONIC PERIOD

No indications of the upper extremity are demonstrable in a developing embryo until the fourth week after fertilization. At this time a minute swelling appears on the anterior aspect of the wolffian ridge and rapidly increases in size so that, at the end of the fourth week, when the embryo measures 4 to 5 mm., its base occupies a position opposite the spinal segments C-4 to T-1. At this time, the arm bud comprises closely packed undifferentiated mesenchymal tissue. No nerves enter the limb bud and although it contains cells destined to become muscles and skeletal elements no evidence of these structures is discernible (Fig. 2-1).

During the fifth week the central core of the blastema evidences chondrification pro-

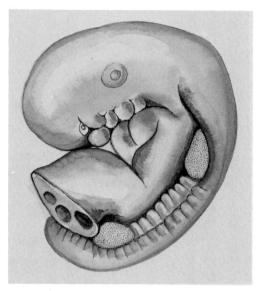

FIG. 2-1. Embryo, age 4 weeks, vertex-breech length 6 mm. The arm bud projects caudally and its base is opposite the fifth to the eighth cervical and the first thoracic myotomes.

ceeding rapidly from the caudal area distally; the proximal portions chondrify before the distal portions. The outer portions of the central core develop into recognizable muscle masses and the nerves invade the base of the arm and unite to form the beginnings of the cervicobrachial plexus. During the sixth week the nerves extend into the premuscle sheaths and encircle the central skeletal core.

With termination of the sixth menstrual week the central skeletal core has differentiated into many skeletal elements, three of which—the humerus, the radius and the ulna—exhibit advanced chondrification. With this event the first indication of a shoulder joint appears, followed by chondrification of the remaining skeletal components of the shoulder joint. By the end of the seventh week the humeral head has assumed a rounded configuration and exhibits a neck and a greater and a lesser tubercle. The scapula is clearly delineated, with coracoid and acromion processes and

a spine. Gardner noted that at 6½ weeks initial bone formation is demonstrable in the form of a periosteal collar around the humerus. With the end of the embryonic period all the skeletal components of the upper limb, including the clavicle, are in evidence and showing advanced chondrification. The clavicle appears during the sixth week, as a condensation of tissue projecting from the acromion toward the first rib and spanning about one third of this distance. From it an ill defined mass extends to the coracoid process and represents the coracoclavicular ligament. During the seventh week the clavicle, consisting of dense tissue, extends to the first rib where it blends with the half sternal anlage. At the end of the embryonic period, the clavicle is completely chondrified and is linked with the sternum and the acromion by condensed tissue.

It was noted previously that differentiation of muscles occurs during the fifth week; this is rapidly followed by differentiation of tendons, exhibited by areas of cellular condensation. The long head of the biceps tendon is discernible at about 5½ weeks. At the end of the embryonic period all muscles can be recognized. All tendons and ligaments in the region of the shoulder are well developed.

## Development of the Synovial Joint Space, Ligaments and Bursae

The formation of the joint space of the glenohumeral joint is similar to the formation of other synovial joint spaces. According to Gardner, two basic processes are involved—the formation of interzones, and the creation of cavities, the latter being most likely the result of some enzymatic action. First, minute limb buds appear which consist of undifferentiated mesenchymal cells; this is soon followed by rapid proliferation and rearrangement of the cells to form a central longitudinal core designated the blastema. The central portion of the core soon becomes cartilage and produces the skeleton. That portion of the blastema left between the cartilaginous elements comprises homogenous cellular areas termed interzones which often comprise three discernible layers, a chondrogenic layer on either side of a looser layer of cells. The joint capsule and many of the interarticular structures such as the synovial membrane, the ligaments, the menisci and the bursae differentiate in situ from the vascular mesencyhmal tissue surrounding the joint.

With completion of the articular form, vascularization begins in the surrounding mesenchymal tissue and the middle layer of the interzone. Extension of this process and coalescence of the resulting spaces form the joint cavity. The total developmental process, from undifferentiated mesenchymal cells of blastema, through the period of differentiation, to structures of adult configuration, requires a relatively short period of time—approximately from four and one-half weeks to seven weeks after fertilization. As previously noted the events occur rapidly and in a precise order.

By the end of the embryonic period and the beginning of the fetal period many bursae and synovial sheaths are discernible, but some bursae are not formed until late in the fetal period.

## Development of the Glenohumeral Joint

The glenohumeral joint follows the general pattern of development of the synovial joint outlined above. At approximately 5 weeks the central core of the humerus begins to chondrify but a homogenous interzone remains between the humerus and the scapula (Fig. 2-2). By 6 weeks considerable condensation occurs around the glenoid, forming the glenoid lip, and the interzone assumes a 3-layered configuration (Fig. 2-3). Also, condensation of tissue from the base of the coracoid to the humerus indicates the formation of the long head of the biceps tendon.

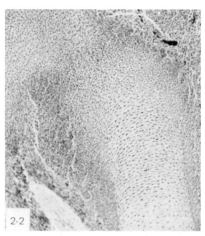

FIG. 2-2. At approximately 5 weeks (12 mm.). The central core of the humerus begins to chondrify but a homogenous interzone remains between the scapula and the humerus. (Gardner, E., and Gray, D. J.: Prenatal development of the human shoulder and acromioclavicular joints. Am. J. Anat., 92:219, 1953)

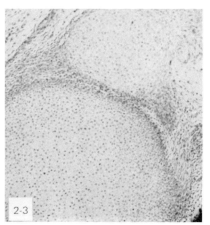

FIG. 2-3. Three layered interzone at 21 mm. (approximately 6 weeks). Note the condensation around the glenoid to form the glenoid lip; the interzone assumes a 3-layered configuration. (Gardner, E., and Gray, D. J.: Prenatal development of the human shoulder and acromioclavicular joints. Am. J. Anat., 92:219, 1953)

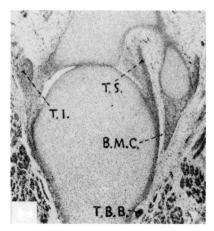

FIG. 2-4. At approximately 7 weeks (27 mm.). The joint is well formed: the humeral head is spherical and is delineated from the shaft of the humerus. The scapula shows advanced chondrification. The tendons of the infraspinatus (T.I.), subscapularis (T.S.) and the biceps (T.B.B.) are clearly seen, as is the bursa of the coracobrachialis muscle (B.M.C.). (Gardner, E., and Gray, D. J.: Prenatal development of the human shoulder and acromioclavicular joints. Am. J. Anat., 92:219, 1953)

Chondrification in the humerus and scapula continues at a rapid pace. The humeral head increases considerably in size, assuming a spherical configuration; the greater and the lesser tubercles appear and the head is delineated from the humeral shaft by the neck of the humerus. Concurrently the scapula exhibits rapid chondrification and increases in size with formation and enlargement of the spine, the acromion and the coracoid process. Also at this time, by proliferation and condensation of the cellular elements, the outline of the fibrous capsule and most of the ligaments appear, including the superior glenohumeral ligament.

By 6 or 7 weeks the middle zone of the three layered interzone becomes less dense and in it small cavities appear which, by extension and coalescence, soon produce a space between the humerus and the scapula. Concurrently cavitation occurs in the mesenchymal tissue surrounding the articular forms. Finally, a complete joint cavity is formed and lined by a smooth thin membrane—the synovial membrane, which at this time lacks a subjacent vascular stratum. Most bursae are not formed during this period; however, the infraspinatus and the coracobrachial bursa may be present. With termination of the embryonic period the shoulder joint exhibits the features of the adult joint (Fig. 2-4).

## Further Changes in the Embryonic Period

During the embryonic period, particularly during the stage of differentiation, other events must occur before the limb assumes its normal adult configuration and its normal anatomical position in relation to the rest of the body. Essentially these changes are migration caudally of the whole arm, migration or extension caudally of certain muscles of the arm to the trunk and migration caudally of other muscles from a cervical position to a position in closer relation to the shoulder girdle and thorax.

### Migration of Scapula and Whole Arm

The normal position of the scapula and the inclination of the brachial plexus indicate the degree of downward displacement of the whole arm from its original cervical position. At 4½ weeks the scapula occupies a position in relation to the fourth and the fifth cervical vertebrae, and the nerves of the brachial plexus enter the base of the arm at right angles without any downward inclination (Fig. 2-5). At 6 weeks the scapula exhibits marked enlargement, extending from the fourth cervical to the first thoracic vertebra. Its center has shifted downward slightly, and the brachial plexus discloses a slight downward inclination. By the end of the seventh week the greater portion of the scapula is located below the level of the first rib and its inferior border is opposite the level of the

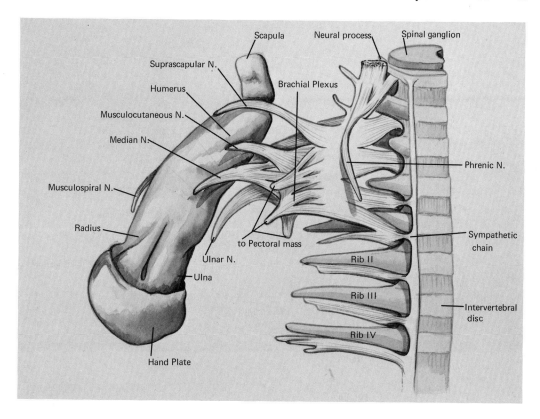

FIG. 2-5. At 4½ weeks (embryo 9 mm.). The nerves of the brachial plexus enter the base of the arm at right angles without any downward inclination. (Redrawn from Lewis, W. H.: The development of the arm in man. Am. J. Anat., 1:156, 1901-1902)

fifth rib. During the descent of the scapula the muscles attached to it pull their nerves downward so that now the brachial plexus exhibits a decided caudal inclination (Fig. 2-6). At the end of the embryonic period (the end of the eighth week) only a small portion of the scapula lies above the first rib and its inferior angle is in relation to the fifth intercostal space. At this time, the brachial plexus reveals a pronounced caudal inclination and is bent over the first rib. The final few degrees of downward displacement of the scapula occurs when the anterior rib cage drops obliquely downward. During the above stages the ribs still occupy a horizontal position, being on the same plane as the vertebra from which they originate.

Comprehension of the excursion of the scapula during the embryonic period, from a cervical to a thoracic position, provides understanding and appreciation of some of the bizarre congenital abnormalities involving the scapula and the cervical spine, which are occasionally encountered in the cervical and upper thoracic regions. Essentially these comprise adult abnormalities of the scapula's failure of descent, in varying degrees, from its original cervical position. In these incidents, the whole arm occupies a position on the trunk more cephalic than the normal extremity; the shoulder girdle is usually smaller than normal and invariably the anomaly is associated with some errors of development in the cervical spine.

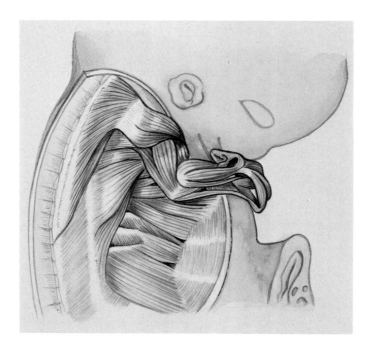

FIG. 2-6. At the end of the 7th week (embryo 20 mm.). The greater part of the scapula lies below the level of the first rib and the arm assumes a downward inclination, pulling the brachial plexus downward. (Redrawn from Bardeen, C. R., and Lewis, W. H.: Am. J. Anat., 1:1, 1901)

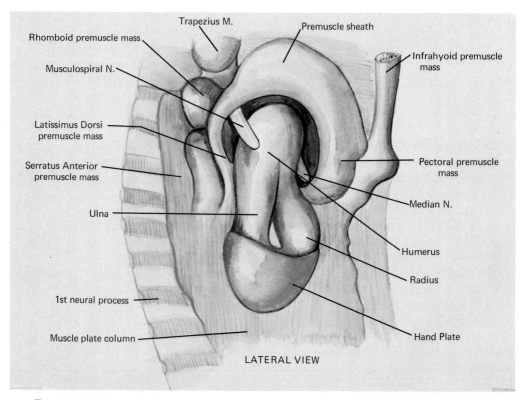

LATERAL VIEW

FIG. 2-7. At 4½ weeks (embryo 9 mm.), lateral view, showing muscle masses. (Redrawn from Lewis, W. H.: The development of the arm in man. Am. J. Anat., 1:156, 1901-1902)

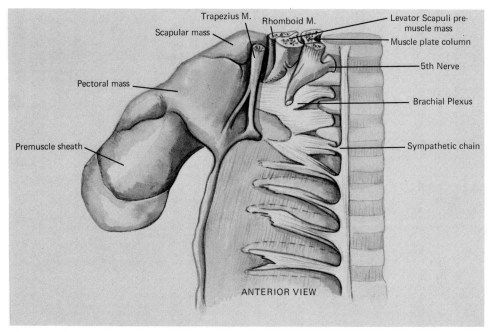

FIG. 2-8. Same embryo shown in Figure 2-7, ventral view. (Redrawn from Lewis, W. H.: The development of the arm in man. Am. J. Anat., *1*:157, 1901-1902)

## Migration of Muscle Masses

Like the skeletal elements, development of premuscle masses to individual muscles follows a precise sequence. From the earliest period of differentiation (4½ to 5 weeks) until the end of the embryonic period (7½ to 8 weeks), development of the premuscle masses most closely associated with the trunk presents the greatest advances; next advanced are those connecting the arm with the trunk, and the least advanced is the premuscle mass of the arm. As early as 5 to 5½ weeks, certain premuscle masses are discernible, and, although as yet they contain no muscle fibers, they already have been invaded by the nerves that supply the muscles that evolve from them. The premuscle masses are five: one for the trapezius and the sternocleidomastoid muscle, one for the levator scapulae and the serratus anterior, one for the latissimus dorsi and the teres major, one for the pectoral muscles and one for the rhomboid muscles. At this time no demarcation of muscles masses is present in the arm, the skeletal core being surrounded only by a diffuse mass of mesenchymal tissue showing no evidence of splitting into separate areas (Figs. 2-7 and 2-8).

**Trapezius and Sternocleidomastoid Muscles.** These two muscles evolve from a single muscle sheath which originates high in the head and cervical areas opposite the first four cervical vertebrae. The premuscle mass splits so that its dorsal portion evolves into the trapezius, and the ventral portion into the sternocleidomastoid muscle. At 5½ weeks, the distal end of the trapezius is at the level of the fourth cervical vertebra. It then begins to migrate and extend caudally so that at the seventh week it lies at the level of the fifth thoracic vertebra and at this time gains attachment to the scapula and the clavicle. At 8 weeks it reaches the level of the sixth thoracic vertebra. Its high cervical origin accounts for its cranial nerve supply; the accessory nerve penetrates the muscle mass as early as the sixth week and is dragged caudally as the muscle migrates in that direction (Fig. 2-9).

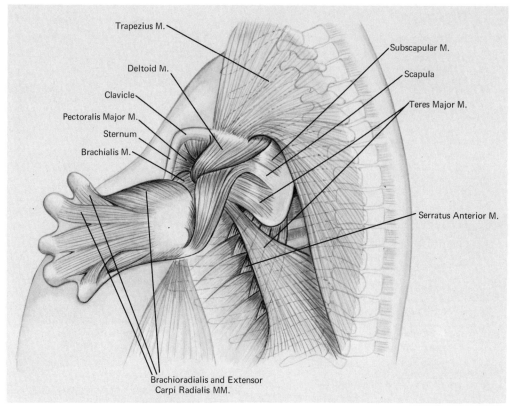

FIG. 2-9. At 6½ to 7 weeks (embryo 14 mm.). The trapezius has descended and gained attachment to the clavicle and the scapula; it extends from the occiput to the fifth rib. (Redrawn from Lewis, W. H.: The development of the arm in man. Am. J. Anat., *1*:184, 1901-1902)

The sternocleidomastoid muscle originates from the same premuscle mass giving origin to the trapezius, its origin being high in the cervical region. It migrates and extends caudally and ventrally and, at 7 weeks, gains attachment to the sternum and the clavicle. Like the trapezius, it is penetrated by fibers of the accessory nerve as early as the sixth week.

**Levator Scapulae and Serratus Anterior.** These two muscles evolve from the same premuscle mass, which originates in the upper cervical region and is discernible as early as 5½ weeks. At 6 weeks the mass shows advanced differentiation and now extends from the first cervical vertebra to the ninth rib and is penetrated by branches from the cervical nerves (second to seventh). No attachment to the scapula exists. Marked

alterations are noted at the seventh week; the serratus anterior is now a broad thin sheet of muscle extending from the dorsal border of the scapula and the first nine ribs, being attached by a digitation to each rib. The levator scapulae is not completely separated at this time. By the eighth week the separation of the two muscles is complete except near the attachment of the serratus anterior to the scapula (Fig. 2-9).

**Latissimus Dorsi and Teres Major.** Both of these muscles evolve from a single premuscle mass first noted at 5 weeks. It lies dorsal to the brachial plexus and extends upward, blending with the arm premuscle sheath at the upper end of the humerus and with that about the scapula. At 6 weeks it joins the sternocleidomastoid at the level of the second cervical vertebra, the latter muscle having ascended from a more ventral position in the neck. Distally, the muscle lies in relation to the lateral surface of the body and has descended as far as the second thoracic vertebra. It has received its adult nerve supply. By the seventh week the latissimus dorsi is a broad, thin sheet of muscle tissue and now is connected to the lower thoracic and lumbar neural processes. Its humeral insertion is closely connected to that of the teres major. At this time the teres major has attained its adult configuration and anatomical position. At the end of the eighth week the distal muscle fibers of the latissimus dorsi extend to the ninth rib and they blend with ill defined fascia that extends to the lower thoracic and the upper three lumbar neural processes. Its proximal tendon of insertion is separated from that of the teres major, around which it twists to insert into the humerus.

At this stage, the teres major extends from the lower angle of the scapula to the proximal end of the humerus. As these muscles descend from their cephalic position of origin each drags its nerve with it (Fig. 2-9).

**Pectoral Muscles.** At the fifth week the pectoral premuscle mass lies opposite the premuscle mass of the latissimus dorsi and teres major on the ventral side of the brachial plexus and, with the arm premuscle sheath, lies at the level of the upper end of the humerus. By the sixth week the muscle mass extends from the level of the second rib to the upper end of the humerus and is attached to the clavicle. Most of the fibers are proximal to the first rib. The medial side of the mass projects slightly toward the coracoid process; this portion eventually becomes the pectoralis minor. At this point in development, the mass has already received its nerve supply from the fifth, sixth and seventh cervical nerves. By the seventh week the pectoral mass has developed into a broad thin sheet and has separated into the major and minor components. A distinct interval is noted between the clavicular and the sternocostal portions of the pec-

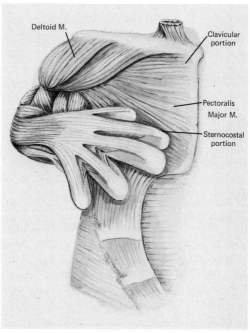

FIG. 2-10. At 7 weeks (embryo 20 mm.). The pectoral mass has divided into its clavicular and sternocostal portions. (Redrawn from Bardeen, C. R., and Lewis, W. H.: Am. J. Anat., 1:1, 1901-1902)

toralis major. The clavicular fibers on their way to their insertion into the humerus overlap the fibers of insertion of the sternocostal portion which arises from the first six ribs and the sternal anlage. The pectoralis minor is now a distinct muscle extending from the second, third and fourth ribs to the coracoid process (Fig. 2-10).

**Rhomboid Muscle.** The premuscle mass of the rhomboid muscle is discernible at 5 to 5½ weeks. At this time it is at the level of the fifth cervical vertebra and it has received a branch from the fifth cervical nerve. It proceeds caudally so that at 7 weeks it is at the level of the sixth cervical vertebra. At 8 weeks it extends from the seventh cervical to the fourth thoracic vertebra and exhibits its final attachment along the dorsal border of the scapula.

**Deltoid Muscle and Muscles Comprising the Rotator Cuff.** Development of this group lags a little behind the groups previously described. It is first clearly discernible about 5½ to 6 weeks. The deltoid appears as a bulging mass extending from acromion and clavicle to the humerus and lies over the fascia of the infraspinatus, with which it blends. At this period the two muscles are essentially one mass and can be distinguished from each other only by the difference in nerve supply. Teres minor also is part of this mass and it, too, can be identified only by its nerve supply. The supraspinatus, which is more cephalad, also is included in the deltoid-infraspinatus mass. The only other distinguishing feature identifying the deltoid from the supraspinatus and infraspinatus muscles is its attachment to the acromion and the clavicle. At this time, the deltoid is connected by dense mesenchymal tissue to the triceps and pectoral muscles. The circumflex nerve is seen entering the deltoid and also sending a branch to the lower portion of the total deltoid-spinati mass, which portion is destined to become the teres minor.

Although the deltoid and the spinati muscles are indistinguishable in the region of the humerus just beyond the acromion, they are separated and recognizable at more cephalic points. That portion of the infraspinatus located on the lateral surface of the scapula is readily identified. This is also true of the portion of the supraspinatus lying on the upper and median surfaces of the scapula. The suprascapular nerve is seen penetrating both the supraspinatus and the infraspinatus.

At this point of development, the subscapularis mass is present on the distal half of the median surface of the scapula and continues to the humerus, passing under the coracoid process. Although the circumflex nerve passes between the subscapularis and the teres major, the two muscles are closely connected in the scapular region.

By the seventh week the deltoid has assumed its adult configuration and attachments; the supraspinatus arises from the thickened proximal border of the scapula and proceeds to its insertion in the greater tuberosity of the humerus; also the infraspinatus is readily identified as it arises from the upper portion of the lateral aspect of the scapula and passes to its insertion in the greater tuberosity. The subscapularis is clearly recognized as it arises from the central area of the médian surface of the scapula and extends to the lesser tuberosity of the humerus. It is completely free of the teres major (Figs. 2-9 and 2-10).

At the end of the embryonic period (8 weeks) the deltoid is large, well developed and clearly demarcated. The supraspinatus is seen to arise from the thickened superior border of the scapula, overlapping onto both the medial and the lateral surfaces of the scapula. The infraspinatus now occupies the central portion of the lateral surface of the scapula, passing beneath the deltoid to the greater tuberosity of the humerus. By now the greater portion of the median surface of the scapula is taken up by the subscapularis muscle. It inserts into the lesser tuberosity by a wide, thin tendon that blends with the capsule of the joint.

**Biceps, Coracobrachialis and Triceps Muscles.** This group of muscles lags in development more than the group of the deltoid and spinati muscles. At 5 weeks the premuscle masses of these muscles as yet are not present. The skeletal core is surrounded by undifferentiated mesenchymal tissue showing no indication of splitting into specific areas. However, along the medial aspect of the humerus, the tissue is invaded by brachial plexus, nerves and blood vessels. By the sixth week the biceps and coracobrachialis muscles on the medial side of the humerus are seen extending from the coracoid process to the radius. The two heads of the biceps are identifiable but are closely united up to their sites of insertion. A portion of the coracoid process from which the long head of the biceps arises ultimately evolves into the upper portion of the head of the scapula. Distally the coracobrachialis joins the humerus by dense

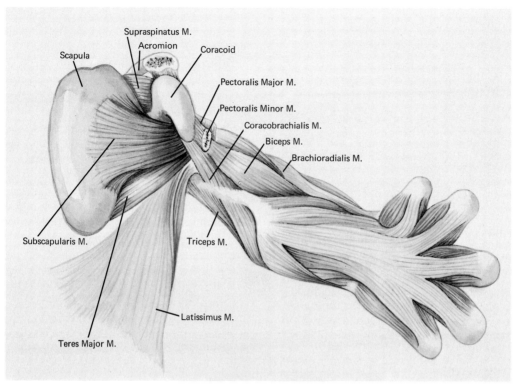

FIG. 2-11. At 7 weeks (embryo 20 mm.). The triceps has elongated and its heads are distinguishable. The biceps has also elongated and its two heads are separating; the short head is closely associated with the coracobrachialis. (Redrawn from Lewis, W. H.: The development of the arm in man. Am. J. Anat., *1*:145, 1901-1902)

tissue, and the biceps joins the radius in like manner. The mass is penetrated by the musculocutaneous nerve.

The triceps occupies a position on the posterolateral aspect of the humerus, spanning the interval from the scapula to the ulna. Although its three heads are recognizable, as yet they have not separated.

At 7 weeks the biceps has gained length. Its two heads are separating and the long head is still in close proximity to the base of the coracoid process. The short head is closely associated with the insertion of the coracobrachialis on the tip of the coracoid process. The triceps also is more elongated and its three heads are recognized more readily (Fig. 2-11).

By 8 weeks the adult form of these muscles has been reached. The long head of the biceps now originates at the junction of the coracoid process and the head of the scapula and passes through the bicipital groove of the humerus. The short head of the biceps and the coracobrachialis are closely joined throughout their entire length. All three heads of the triceps are separated from one another; distally the triceps is continuous with the anconeus muscle and inserts into the ulna.

## FETAL PERIOD

As previously noted, at the end of the embryonic period the components of the shoulder region are adult in configuration but miniature in size. During the fetal period the structures undergo further maturation and enlargement, collagenous fibers increase in size and the synovial cavities, including the joint cavity, increase in size and the lining proliferates actively.

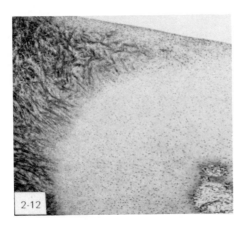

FIG. 2-12. A fetus 366 mm. (at term). The labrum, a dense fibrous structure, is clearly delineated from the hyaline cartilage. The area next to the scapula consists of cellular elements suggesting fibrocartilage. (Gardner, E., and Gray, D. J.: Prenatal development of the human shoulder and acromioclavicular joints. Am. J. Anat., 92:219, 1953)

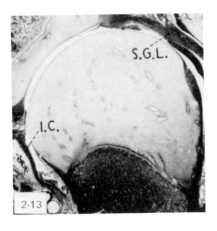

FIG. 2-13. A fetus 348 mm. (at term). The superior glenohumeral ligament (S.G.L.) and the inferior capsule (I.C.) are clearly seen. (Gardner, E., and Gray, D. J.: Prenatal development of the human shoulder and acromioclavicular joints. Am. J. Anat., 92:219, 1953)

The tendons and ligaments are invaded by a vascular network and early in the fetal period the epiphyses show evidence of vas-cular penetration. The glenoid lip assumes a triangular configuration and its fibrous elements increase, but no evidence of fibrocartilage is noted. However, a transitional zone of fibrocartilage between glenoid lip and the hyaline cartilage of the glenoid fossa was noted by Gardner, Moseley and Overgaard. This observation disproves the conception previously held by most, including the author — namely, that the labrum consisted of fibrocartilage.

At term the labrum consists of dense fibrous tissue and some elastic fibers. It is continuous on the inner side with the hyaline cartilage of the glenoid fossa via the intermediate zone of fibrocartilage; on the outer side it is continuous with the fibrous capsule attached to the scapula (Fig. 2-12). On the anterior aspect of the joint, by proliferation of the fibrous elements, the glenohumeral ligaments attain their ultimate adult configuration. As in the adult shoulders, the anatomical arrangement of the glenohumeral ligaments in regard to size, shape and relation to the bursae varies greatly. Also at term the fibrous capsule is intimately attached to the humerus along the edge of the articular hyaline cartilage of the head of the humerus except on the inferior aspect. Here the capsule is attached lower down on the neck so that part of the metaphysis becomes intracapsular (Fig. 2-13).

Not all the bursae are present or fully developed at the end of the embryonic period. The subdeltoid bursa may appear as a small space in the early fetal period; by term it increases markedly and extends as far as the subacromial region. The subcoracoid bursa may or may not be present in the early stages of the fetal period; however, by term it is always present and in some instances communicates with the joint cavity. The subscapular bursa develops independently but soon communicates with the joint cavity via the subscapular recess, whose location in relation to the superior and inferior glenohumeral ligaments shows considerable variation.

Fig. 2-14. Ossification of the upper epiphysis is accomplished by 3 centers: one for the head, which appears between the 4th and 6th months; one for the greater tuberosity, appearing usually during the 3rd year; and one for the lesser tuberosity, appearing about the 5th year. The epiphyses of the tuberosities fuse into one mass at about the 5th year, and this, in turn, unites with the epiphysis of the head about the 7th year. The head and the shaft of the humerus unite at about the 19th year.

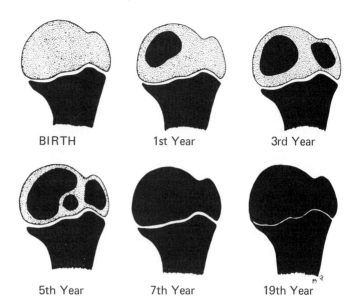

BIRTH        1st Year        3rd Year

5th Year        7th Year        19th Year

## POSTNATAL DEVELOPMENT OF THE SHOULDER JOINT

During this period the soft tissue elements reveal no change except increase in size, ultimately attaining their adult proportion. However, the skeletal elements do exhibit changes, namely, the appearance of centers of ossification, or epiphyses, and the fusion of these centers with the rest of the skeletal element. Growth of these centers determines the ultimate size and shape of the adult bone, and frequently errors of development are responsible for some of the congenital anomalies encountered in the shoulder region.

### Humerus

At birth the proximal epiphysis consists of a rounded mass of cartilage with its greater and lesser prominences. In rare instances, an ovoid bony nucleus in the head is noted at the time of birth. Ossification of the upper epiphysis is accomplished by three centers: one for the head, which generally appears between the fourth and the sixth month; one for the greater tuberosity, appearing before the third year (usually during the second year), and one for the lesser tuberosity, appearing before the fifth year or, as a rule, during the fifth year. The epiphyses of the tuberosities fuse into one mass usually about the fifth year, and this, in turn, unites with the epiphysis the head of the humerus before the seventh year; however, this union may occur as late as the fourteenth year. Union between the head and shaft of the humerus occurs during the nineteenth year (Fig. 2-14).

From the time schedule for the appearance of the centers of ossification for the head of the humerus as presented above it is apparent that at birth the upper end of the humerus cannot be demonstrated (except in rare cases) by roentgeograms. This makes early diagnosis of birth injuries to this region difficult and sometimes impossible.

It also should be noted that the upper end of the diaphysis is shaped like an asymmetrical cone. That portion of the epiphysis comprising the head and the lesser tuberosity lies on the medial side of the cone while the greater tuberosity rests on the lateral side. This configuration places the epiphyseal plate high above the surgical neck and the epiphyseal plate also digs into the medial aspect of the head so that the

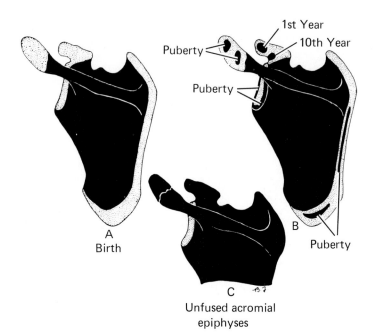

1st Year

10th Year

Puberty

Puberty

A
Birth

B

Puberty

C
Unfused acromial
epiphyses

FIG. 2-15. Date of appearance of the ossification centers of scapula, coracoid, acromion and glenoid fossa.

medial aspect of the plate actually lies within the joint cavity.

**Scapula**

At birth, only the body of the scapula shows advanced ossification; the acromion, the coracoid, the vertebral border of the scapula and the inferior angle of the scapula are cartilaginous. During the first year an ossific center appears in the center of the coracoid. At 10 years one appears at the base of the coracoid, contributing also to the formation of the upper end of the glenoid cavity. These centers unite with the scapula during the fifteenth year. A waferlike ossific center appears at puberty at the tip of the coracoid; this center occasionally fails to fuse with the rest of the coracoid.

The acromion has two — and occasionally three — centers of ossification. They make their appearance around puberty and fuse about the twenty-second year. Failure of fusion of these two centers may be erroneously interpreted as a fracture through the end of the acromion.

Two centers appear for the glenoid: One appears during the tenth year and contributes to the formation of the base of the

coracoid and the upper end of the glenoid. It fuses to the scapula during the fifteenth year. The second is a horseshoe-shaped ossific center appearing about puberty. It contributes to the formation of the lower portion of the glenoid.

The vertebral border and the inferior angle of the scapula each have one ossific center. These appear about puberty and fuse before the twenty-second year (Fig. 2-15).

**The Clavicle (Fig. 2-16)**

The clavicle is one of the first bones in the body to ossify. Chondrification of the dense bar of mesenchymal tissue comprising the early clavicle is completed by the end of the embryonic period. Chondrification begins in two centers close to one another at the juncture of the outer third and inner two thirds of the primitive core. When chondrification is completed the centers unite and ossification begins; it extends in two directions, laterally toward the acromion and medially toward the sternum. The clavicle also has a thin ossific center covering its sternal end; it begins to ossify about the eighteenth year and fuses to the main bone about the twenty-second year.

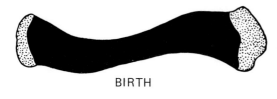

BIRTH

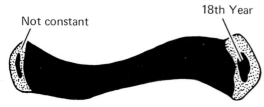

Not constant

18th Year

FIG. 2-16. Date of appearance of ossification centers of the clavicle.

Occasionally a scalelike epiphysis may appear at the acromial end. The development of the clavicle provides an explanation for the types of congenital anomalies that are encountered in this region. These anomalies are discussed under congenital abnormalites of the neck-shoulder region.

## BIBLIOGRAPHY

Bardeen, C. R., and Lewis, W. H.: Development of the limbs, body-wall and back in man. Am. J. Anat., *1*:1-26, 1901.

Gardner, E.: The innervation of the shoulder joint. Anat. Rec., *102*:1-18, 1948.

Gardner, E., and Gray, D. J.: Prenatal development of the human shoulder and acromioclavicular joints. Am. J. Anat., *92*:219-276, 1953.

———: Prenatal development of the human hip joint. Am. J. Anat., *87*:163-212, 1950.

Gray, D. J., and Gardner, E. D.: The human sternochondral joints. Anat. Rec., *87*:235-253, 1943.

———: Prenatal development of the human knee and superior tibiofibular joints. Am. J. Anat., *86*:235-288, 1950.

———: Prenatal development of the human elbow joint. Am. J. Anat., *88*:429-470, 1951.

Lewis, W. H.: The development of the arm in man. Am. J. Anat., *1*:145-184, 1901.

Moseley, H. P., and Overgaard, B.: The anterior capsular mechanism in recurrent anterior dislocation of the shoulder. J. Bone & Joint Surg., *44-B*:913-927, 1962.

Streeter, G. L.: Weight, sitting height, head size, foot length and menstrual age of the human embryo. Contrib. Embryol., *11(55)*:143-170, 1920. (Pub. No. 274, Carnegie Inst., Washington, D.C.)

———: Developmental horizons in human embryos. Description of age group XI, 13 to 20 somites, and age group XII, 21 to 29 somites. Contrib. Embryol., *30(197)*:211-245, 1942. (Pub. No. 541, Carnegie Inst., Washington, D.C.)

———:Development horizons in human embryos. Descriptions of age group XIII, embryos about 4 or 5 millimeters long, and age group XIV, period of indentation of the lens vesicle. Contrib. Embryol., *31(199)*:27-63, 1945. (Pub. No. 557, Carnegie Inst., Washington, D.C.)

———: Developmental horizons in human embryos. Descriptions of age groups XV, XVI, XVII, XVIII, being the third issue of a survey of the Carnegie Collection. Contrib. Embryol., *32(211)*:133-203, 1948. (Pub. No. 575, Carnegie Inst., Washington, D.C.)

———: Developmental horizons in human embryos (fourth issue). A review of the histogenesis of cartilage and bone. Contrib. Embryol. *33(220)*:149-167, 1949. (Pub. No. 583, Carnegie Inst., Washington, D.C.)

———: Developmental horizons in human embryos. Description of age groups XIX, XX, XXI, XXII, and XXIII, being the fifth issue of a survey of the Carnegie Collection. Contrib. Embryol., *34(230)*:165-196, 1951. (Pub. No. 592, Carnegie Inst. Washington, D.C.)

# 3

# Congenital Abnormalities of the Neck-Shoulder Region

Some rather bizarre developmental errors are encountered in the interval between the occiput and the base of the shoulder. Fortunately, their frequency is low, being greater in the more distal part of the upper extremity. The course of prenatal development and migration of the upper extremity from an occiput-cervical position to a position opposite the thoracic cage indicates that these abnormalities occur during the embryonal period. In most instances the error is not confined to one skeletal element; rather, a number of them may be implicated, such as the scapula, cervical spine, clavicle and thoracic cage. Abnormalities may involve not only the skeletal elements but also adjacent muscle groups. These may be absent or poorly developed or in an abnormal anatomical position. The abnormality most frequently encountered is failure of the scapula to descend from its high cervical position during the embryonic period.

## CONGENITAL ELEVATION OF THE SCAPULA (SPRENGEL'S DEFORMITY)

This anomaly, also referred to as undescended scapula or elevated scapula, is by far the most frequently encountered of congenital deformities of the shoulder girdle. In this condition, the scapula, which arises as a cervical appendage, fails to migrate caudally to its normal postion on the thorax during early embryonic development.

Normally, the scapula meets the upper portion of the thorax by the end of the third month. Occasionally, however, the scapula fails to free itself from the cervical vertebrae and remains attached to the cervical spine by its vertebral border or by a fibrous or bony structure varying in size from a thin strip to a large bony plate, the suprascapula. This extends from the angle formed by the superior and the inferior vertebral borders to the lower cervical or first thoracic spine. The scapula may be normal in size and shape or smaller than normal with an altered configuration, the breadth being increased and the length decreased. Occasionally, the deformity is bilateral. The portion above the spine may be angulated sharply forward to conform to the contour of the upper portions of the thoracic cage (Figs. 3-1, 3-2 and 3-3).

Elevation of the scapula usually is combined with other congenital anomalies, such as failure of fusion in the midline of the laminae of some cervical vertebrae, cranium bifidum, defects in the upper dorsal vertebrae, and with developmental anomalies of the thoracic outlet such as cervical ribs and abnormal first thoracic ribs, hemivertebrae, congenital scoliosis, fusion of ribs and irregular vertebral segmentation. Developmental defects of the shoulder musculature may exist. All or part of the trapezius may be absent, and the levator scapulae and the rhomboidei may exist as strips of fibrous or cartilaginous tissue running from the base of the occuput or spine to the vertebral border of the scapula. Torticollis may be a concomitant deformity.

When the arm is elevated the scapula fails to shift laterally and its lower angle

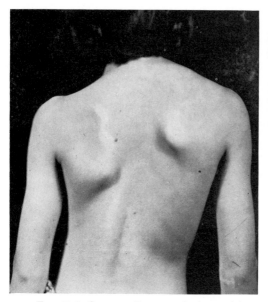

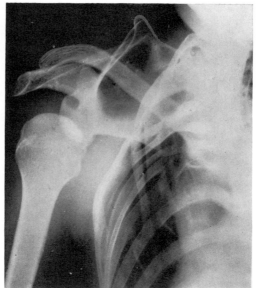

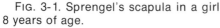

FIG. 3-1. Sprengel's scapula in a girl 8 years of age.

(*Top*) FIG. 3-2. Congenital elevation of the scapula. Observe that the scapula is placed high on the thoracic cage; its breadth is increased and its length decreased. It is rotated outward and forward on its vertical axis, and it possesses a suprascapular bone. Note the congenital malformation of the upper thoracic cage and the presence of long cervical ribs. (H. Ostrum: Philadelphia General Hospital)

(*Bottom*) FIG. 3-3. Congenital elevation of the scapula with an omovertebral bone. (H. Ostrum)

does not rotate outward when the extremity is brought above the horizontal. Little or no dysfunction of the shoulder exists when the deformity is mild. In these instances, slight restriction of elevation of the extremity in the coronal and sagittal plane usually exists; other movements are not affected. The overall functional efficiency of the shoulder girdle is good. When the deformity is severe and associated with other deformities of the cervical spine and upper thorax, motion in the shoulder girdle may be severely impaired.

The undesirable cosmetic appearance of the shoulders rather than dysfunction forces the parents to seek medical advice. Surgery, in most instances, does not yield good results, and one wonders whether the operations performed to correct this deformity are justifiable in the face of so many disappointing results. Nevertheless, operation may improve the appearance of the patient slightly and increase the range of motion of the scapula on the thorax. This is particularly true if surgery is performed in the early years of life (rarely before the age of

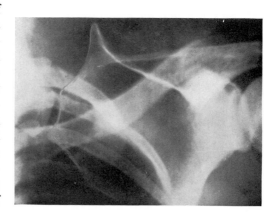

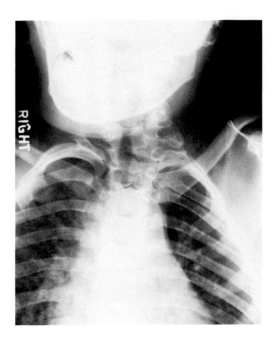

FIG. 3-4. Cervical anomalies associated with elevation of the scapula. A hemivertebra on the left produces torticollis. Note the failure of fusion of the posterior elements of the first thoracic vertebra.

3) before marked adaptative structural changes have occurred which preclude any correction or increase in function of the extremity. After the age of 6 years, surgery should be restricted to the improving of the cosmetic appearance only, for appreciable improvement in function is rarely achieved. The surgical management of this deformity is discussed on page 245.

## CONGENITAL ABNORMALITIES OF THE CERVICAL SPINE

### Fusion and Absence of Cervical Elements

Although many abnormalities of the cervical region are associated with elevation of the scapula, occasionally they may exist as isolated lesions.

Failure of segmentation of a portion of the primitive mesenchymal core destined to form the cervical segments may result in fusion of one or more vertebral bodies or the absence of one or more bodies. If there is failure of segmentation without de-crease in the number of vertebrae, the anomaly gives rise to no clinical manifestations and is discovered accidentally by roentgenograms of the area. If there is a reduction in size, the patient will exhibit some shortening of the neck. The amount of limitation of motion present is governed by the number of segments involved. Fusion of the posterior elements may be associated with fusion of the bodies or it may exist independently.

### Hemivertebra

Failure of development of one half of a cervical vertebra results in the formation of a wedge-shaped body on the opposite side of the cervical column. With growth, a curvature of the cervical spine results (Fig. 3-4). Frequently, a number of vertebrae are implicated and there may be failure of fusion of some of the posterior elements, producing a spina bifida. The extent of the deformity depends on the number of vertebrae involved. When several vertebrae are involved, the deformity may be marked, causing tilting of the head such as occurs in torticollis. There may be a compensating curve in the upper thoracic region. Generally, except for the cosmetic effect, no clinical manifestations appear in early life. However, later in life because of secondary degenerative changes in the cervical column, local and radiating pain may develop.

In the early years no form of therapy is indicated except that the patient should try to retain as free a range of motion as possible by exercises. If symptoms are present, conservative measures such as wearing of of a cervical collar and mild traction may give relief. Surgical intervention is rarely indicated except in cases of severe symptoms, in which fusion of the affected elements should give relief.

## Klippel-Feil Syndrome

In this disorder there is widespread fusion of the cervical elements, implicating not only the bodies but also the posterior elements and causing marked shortening of the cervical column (Fig. 3-5). There may be marked distortion of the thoracic outlet, and cervical ribs in various stages of development may be present. In severe cases the head appears to sit directly on the trunk. Motion is severely restricted in all arcs. Frequently, prominent skin folds extend from the mastoid processes to the top of the shoulders, producing a rather grotesque appearance. As a rule, the only complaint is the unacceptable cosmetic effect. Some improvement in appearance is attainable by plastic procedures.

## CONGENITAL ABNORMALITIES OF THE CLAVICLE

Developmental errors implicating the clavicle produce a group of interesting abnormalities. The lesion may be local or it may be part of a generalized defective developmental process involving many bones. Generally, the deformities give rise to no serious impairment of function. Occasion-

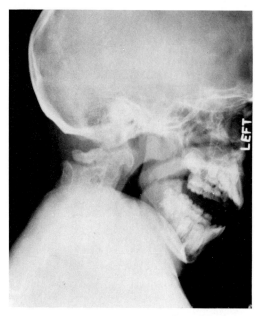

FIG. 3-5. Note the failure of segmentation of the cervical spine below the level of the atlas (Klippel-Feil Syndrome).

ally, the child complains of pain and weakness in the shoulder girdle.

## Cleidocranial Dysostosis

This is an exceedingly rare congenital abnormality, and hereditary transmission exists in most instances (Fig. 3-6). Occasionally, however, heredity plays no part. The characteristic features are:
  1. Aplasia of the clavicles
  2. Delay in closure of the cranial suture
  3. Excessive enlargement of the transverse diameter of the cranium while the base of the skull and the face remain relatively small.

Cases have been reported in which this lesion was associated with other congenital defects such as achondroplasia, defective development of the small bones of the hands and the feet, malformation of the vertebral column, the pelvis and the femora, and disturbance of normal dentition. Bones of both membranous and endochondral derivation may be affected.

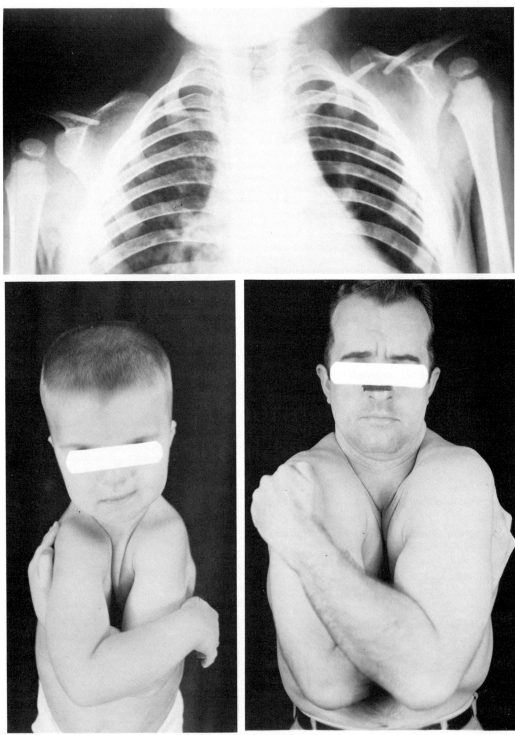

FIG. 3-6. (*Top*) Note the incomplete development of the clavicles in a child with cleido-cranial dysostosis. (*Bottom, left*) Another example of cleidocranial dysostosis. This child can bring the tips of the shoulders almost to the midline anteriorly. (*Bottom, right*) Father of the child shown in bottom, left.

Varying degrees of aplasia of the clavicles may be caused by developmental failures, ranging from aplasia of only a small portion, usually the acromial end, to absence of the entire clavicle. There may also be abnormal development of the large shoulder girdle muscles, particularly the pectoralis major, the deltoid and the trapezius. The clavicular portion of the trapezius and the deltoid muscles may be deficient or absent (Fig. 3-6).

As a rule, the condtion causes no shoulder dysfunction. The excessive mobility of the girdles does not impair the efficiency of the extremities. Individuals so afflicted can readily bring together the tips of their shoulders in the midline beneath their chins. Rarely is any form of therapy indicated. Occasionally, however, one of the free ends of the clavicle presses on the subclavian structures, and in such instances, resection of the part is justified.

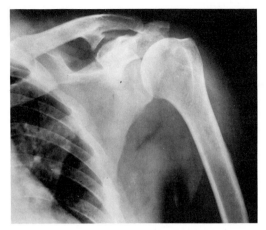

Fig. 3-7. Congenital anomalies in the coracoclavicular region; a bony process on the inferior aspect of the clavicle articulates with a similar bony prominence arising from the coracoid process.

## Local Developmental Abnormalities of the Clavicle

The variety of the lesion found is dependent entirely upon the portion of the primitive mesenchymal core of the clavicle that is affected during chondrification and ossification. It was previously noted that two centers of chondrification appear at the juncture of the middle and outer thirds of the clavicle and that ossification starts at these points and proceeds medially toward the sternum and laterally toward the acromion. One or both of these centers may be involved; hence, in the adult the inner two thirds of the clavicle may be absent or the inner third may be deficient or the entire clavicle may not appear; also there may be a defect in the middle of the clavicle.

When the entire clavicle or either the outer or the inner portions of it are absent, serious symptoms do not arise although there may be some slight weakness of the girdle, owing to abnormal muscle attachments. However, defects in the middle of the clavicle are very likely to produce local

pain and disturbing weakness of the girdle. Severe symptoms may be relieved by spanning the defect with a bone graft. The surgical management of these lesions is described on page 211.

## Coracoclavicular Abnormalities

During normal development of this region the primitive mesenchymal tissue between the rudiments of the clavicle and the coracoid evolves into the coracoclavicular ligament (the conoid and trapezoid ligaments). Defective development may result in one of several abnormalities:

1. A solid bony strut connects the coracoid with the clavicle.

2. A bony process on the inferior aspect of the outer third of the clavicle articulates with a similar process arising from the coracoid process (Fig. 3-7).

3. The bone bar may be incompete; only a bony spur projects from the inferior surface of the clavicle.

Rarely do these lesions produce symptoms. In the event that serious symptoms do arise, the bar or false joint should be resected.

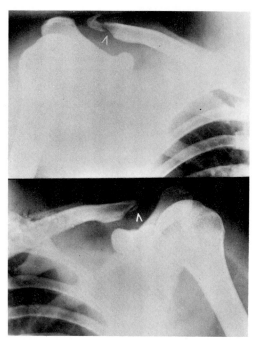

FIG. 3-8. Bilateral congenital anomalies of the acromioclavicular joints. These joints are lax and unstable but produce no symptoms or dysfunction.

## Congenital Abnormality of the Acromioclavicular Joint

Congenital subluxation of this joint is a relatively rare lesion and usually is bilateral (Fig. 3-8). The distal end of the clavicle rides above the level of the superior surface of the acromion and is very loosely attached to the capsular and ligamentous tissues. The lesion is believed to be the result of some abnormal development of the outer end either of the clavicle or of the acromion. Although it gives rise to no symptoms, it creates an unfavorable cosmetic effect. Often the appearance is such that correction is justifiable. The subluxation can be corrected by the same procedures employed for traumatic dislocations of the joint.

## ABNORMAL DEVELOPMENT OF THE GLENOID FOSSA

Although rare, abnormal development of the glenoid does occur and may result in a true congenital dislocation of the joint (Fig. 3-9). It is now firmly established that traumatic dislocation at birth is indeed a rare lesion and some authorities doubt that it ever occurs. The lesions most likely to occur at birth are traumatic separation of the humeral epiphysis and injury to the cervicobrachial plexus. In the latter instance, the ensuing muscle paralysis may result in a secondary dislocation of the joint; this, of course, is not a true congenital dislocation.

Several developmental deformities of the glenoid are encountered. In one there is faulty development of the upper epiphysis of the glenoid, which also forms the base of the coracoid; the portion of the inferior glenoid that develops from the scapula is not primarily affected. In this instance, the upper portion of the glenoid is rotated posteriorly so that its articular surface tends to face backward. The coracoid extends laterally and is bent in front of the humerus; the acromion is distorted and also is bent downward in front of the head. The head of the humerus assumes a posterior position and only its inferior surface makes contact with the lower portion of the glenoid. Therefore, the dislocation is not complete; rather, the joint develops in a posterior position. In these instances, the arm is in an internal position and the forearm is flexed slightly; all movements are restricted, particularly elevation and external rotation.

Another deformity of the glenoid essentially comprises aplasia of the entire glenoid. The underdeveloped glenoid faces anteriorly and the head finds a posterior position. In this instance the dislocation is complete.

Two other congenital abnormalities are encountered. In one, the glenoid cavity is replaced by a convex protuberance that articulates with a concave articular surface on the medial aspect of the head of the humerus. In the other, the glenoid fossa is flattened (Fig. 3-10). This is due to failure of development of the epiphysis of the lower rim of the glenoid cavity. Usually the defect is bilateral.

FIG. 3-9. A true congenital dislocation of the right shoulder. Note the malformation of the glenoid. The child had an excellent range of motion and normal function of all muscle groups of the shoulder girdle.

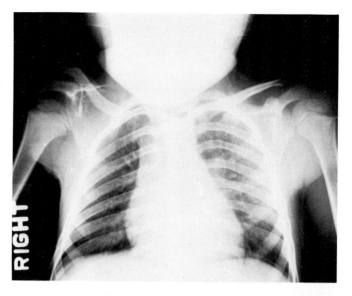

## CONGENITAL ABNORMALITIES OF THE UPPER END OF THE HUMERUS

Although rare, errors in development of the upper end of the humerus do occur. Congenital absence of the upper end of the humerus occasionally is encountered, as are various degrees of aplasia. Of interest are deformities discussed in the following sections.

### Humerus Varus

The angle of the head of the humerus is smaller during fetal development than that existing in the adult state. But, occasionally this fetal-type relationship of the head to the shaft of the humerus is found in adults; it is then designated humerus varus (Fig. 3-11).

In the normal humerus the head is directed upward, making an angle of 130° to 140° with the shaft, whereas in humerus varus the head is directed sideways at an angle of 100° or less. Usually the affection is bilateral.

There is disagreement as to the true cause of this deformity. Some workers contend that it is a developmental defect; others maintain that it may be the result of stress applied to soft demineralized bone during the acute phases of diseases such as rickets,

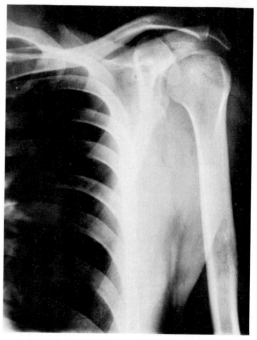

FIG. 3-10. Congenital flattening of the glenoid fossa, due to failure of development of the epiphysis of the lower rim of the glenoid cavity.

scurvy and hypothyroidism, producing a varus deformity of the humerus similar to that of coxa vara. Cases are on record in which the defect was observed in normal individuals.

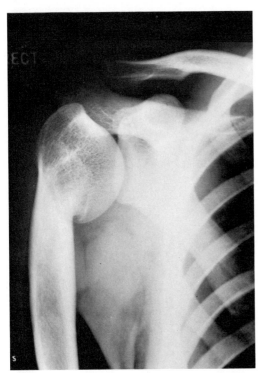

FIG. 3-11. Congenital deformity of the upper end of the humerus (humerus varus).

### Concave Humeral Head

This lesion has been described above in association with maldevelopment of the glenoid, the articular surface of which is convex instead of being concave. The humeral deformity is most likely secondary to the primary developmental error in the glenoid.

### Abnormal Development of the Bicipital Groove

The bicipital groove in the humerus in adult specimens reveals many variations in size, shape and depth. This is significant because the groove contains the tendon of the long head of the biceps. Abnormal variations may lead to subluxation or dislocation of the tendon and in older individuals to attrition and rupture of the tendon. The lesions of this area are discussed fully in Chapter 4.

## CONGENITAL ABNORMALITIES OF MUSCLES

Some interesting developmental defects occur involving the muscles of the shoulder region. These are rare deformities and may occur as isolated abnormalities or in association with skeletal deformities of the cervicothoracic region. The latter have been mentioned previously in the discussions on the skeletal anomalies of this region.

### Congenital Abnormalities of the Pectoral Muscles

**Absence of the Sternocostal Portion of the Pectoralis Major.** This abnormality of the

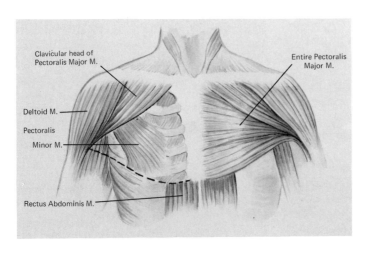

FIG. 3-12. Congenital absence of the sternocostal portion of the pectoralis major.

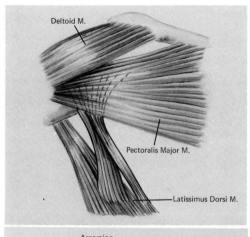

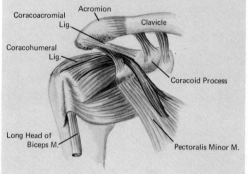

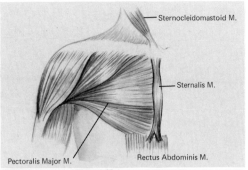

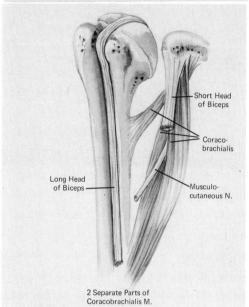

(*Top*) FIG. 3-13. Congenital anomaly of the pectoralis major; an extension of the deep portion of the muscle passes across the axilla and becomes continuous with the latissimus dorsi.

(*Bottom*) FIG. 3-14. Abnormal insertion of the pectoralis minor into the humeral head in the region of the coracohumeral ligament.

(*Top*) FIG. 3-15. Sternalis muscle — an accessory muscle.

(*Bottom*) FIG. 3-16. Congenital anomaly of the coracobrachialis: it may have two or three bellies.

pectoral group is the one most commonly found in isolation. It frequently is associated with hypertrophy of the latissimus dorsi. Function of the girdle is not impaired but there is asymmetry of the shoulder girdle anteriorly (Fig. 3-12).

**Axillary Arch.** This is formed by an extension of the deep portion of the pectoralis major across the base of the axilla, which then becomes continuous with the latissimus dorsi (Fig. 3-13).

**Abnormal Insertion of the Pectoralis Minor.** The pectoralis minor inserts into the humerus in the region of the coraco-

humeral ligament. Its tendon passes over the coracoid process and proceeds to its insertion, passing between the two limbs of the coracoacromial ligament. Grant notes this anomaly in 15 percent of upper extremities (Fig. 3-14).

### Accessory Muscles

**Sternalis Muscle.** This is a long thin muscle on the lateral aspect of the sternum. It extends from the sternocleidomastoid to the rectus abdominis (Fig. 3-15).

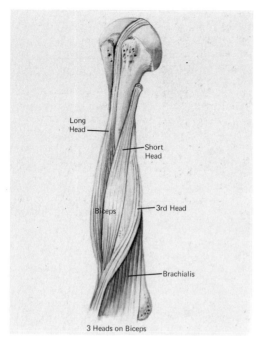

FIG. 3-17. The long head of the biceps may end in two or three tendons.

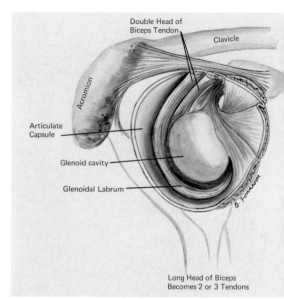

FIG. 3-18. The biceps may have three bellies.

## Splitting of the Coracobrachialis

The coracobrachialis exists as two separate bellies, with the musculocutaneous nerve passing between them. Occasionally a third belly is present (Fig. 3-16).

## Abnormalities of the Biceps Brachii Muscle

The long head may end in two or even three tendons inserting into the superior region of the glenoid. Occasionally a third belly is present (Figs. 3-17 and 3-18).

## BIRTH INJURIES TO THE SHOULDER JOINT

### Separation of the Proximal Epiphysis of the Humerus (Birth Injury)

This is the most common of traumatic lesions of the shoulder region encountered at birth. The line of union between the upper epiphysis and the metaphysis is the weakest area at this time and is the region most likely to give under abnormal stresses. This is not a dislocation but because the upper end of the humerus is entirely cartilaginous and not visible on roentgenograms, the diagnosis is difficult to make. Awareness of the lesion and clinical manifestations of trauma to the area help in establishing the diagnosis. This lesion may be associated with birth injury to the brachial plexus. In these instances, it may not be recognized until later when the child presents a posterior subluxation of the joint. The injury is discussed more fully in the section on "Obstetric Paralysis."

Treatment consists in restoring anatomical alignment of the epiphysis in relation to the shaft and fixing the arm to the side for from 10 to 14 days. Minor displacement can be accepted because with healing remodeling occurs, correcting the malposition.

### Fracture of the Clavicle (Birth Injury)

This lesion is relatively common and, in most instances, is an isolated lesion. The diagnosis can be made readily by the presence of a deformity involving the clavicle and the visualization of the fracture by roentgenograms. Treatment requires nothing more than fixing the arm to the side for 10 to 14 days. No reduction is necessary. With healing and remodeling the normal configuration of the clavicle will be restored.

## Obstetrical Paralysis

Injuries to the cervicobrachial plexus are relatively frequent. These may or may not be associated with dislocation of the glenohumeral joint. If a dislocation does occur it is the result of muscular paralysis and is not a primary lesion. C5 and C6 are the nerve roots most frequently implicated. At first, loss of muscle tone favors subluxation; this is followed by dislocation. Contracture of tissues and muscle imbalance fix the head in the abnormal position. Paralytic dislocations are discussed more fully in Chapter 12.

## BIBLIOGRAPHY

Bonola, A.: Surgical treatment of the Klippel-Feil syndrome. J. Bone & Joint Surg., 38-B: 440, 1956.

Green, W. T.: The surgical correction of congenital elevation of the scapula (Sprengel's deformity). Proc. Am. Orthopaedic Ass., June 24-27, 1957. J. Bone & Joint Surg., 39-A:1439, 1957.

———: The surgical correction of congenital elevation of the scapula. Personal communication. 1962.

Greville, N. R., and Coventry, M. B.: Congenital high scapula (Sprengel's) deformity. Proc. Staff Meet. Mayo Clin., 31:465, 1956.

Horwitz, A. E.: Congenital elevation of the scapula—Sprengel's deformity. Am. J. Orthop. Surg., 6:260, 1908.

Huc, G.: De l'adaptation de la ceinture scapulaire au thorax; essai d'anatomie, de physiologie, de pathologie et de therapeutique. Paris, Viellemard Imp., 1924.

Inclan, A.: Congenital elevation of the scapula or Sprengel's deformity; two clinical cases treated with Ober's operation. Cir. ortop. y traumatol., 15:1, 1949.

Jeannopoulos, C. L.: Congenital elevation of the scapula. J. Bone & Joint Surg., 34-A:883, 1952.

Koenig, F.: Eine neue Operation des angeborenen Schulterblatthochstandes. Beitr. klin. Chir., 94:1914. (Cited in Lange, Max: Orthopädisch-Chirurgische Operationslehre, p. 240. München, J. E. Bergmann, 1951.

Lange, Max: Orthopädisch-Chirurgische Operationslehre. München, J. F. Bergmann, 1951.

McFarland, B.: Congenital deformities of the spine and limbs. In: Platt, Sir Harry, (ed.): Modern trends in orthopaedics. New York, Paul B. Hoeber, 1950.

Schrock, R. D.: Congenital elevation of the scapula. J. Bone & Joint Surg., 8:207, 1926.

———: Congenital elevation of the scapula. In: Nelson's new loose leaf surgery, vol. III, p. 179 M. New York, Thomas Nelson & Sons, 1935.

Smith, A. D.: Congenital elevation of the scapula. Arch. Surg., 42:529, 1941.

Whitman, A.: Congenital elevation of scapula and paralysis of serratus magnus muscle. JAMA, 99:1332, 1932.

Woodward, J. W.: Congenital elevation of the scapula. Correction by release and transplantation of muscle origins. A preliminary report. J. Bone & Joint Surg., 43-A:219, 1961.

# 4

# Normal Regional and Variational Anatomy of the Shoulder

The term "shoulder joint" needs clarification because of the intricacies of the arm-trunk mechanism. This is a complex system, the components of which function synchronously to produce precise, coordinated movements, which, in turn, permits man to use the prehensile extremity at a maximum level of efficiency. This complex comprises four distinct articulations: (1) the scapulohumeral, (2) the sternoclavicular, (3) the acromioclavicular, and (4) the scapulothoracic. Although the last structure is not a true joint anatomically, it must be considered as such functionally.

In considering the functional characteristics of the arm-trunk mechanism comprehension of the regional anatomy of the shoulder region is essential. This knowledge not only facilitates understanding of the systems providing stability and movements of the shoulder girdle but also provides the information necessary in designing surgical procedures in this region. The bony configuration of the pectoral girdle is such that it permits the total areas concerned to be divided into distinct regions, all of which contain anatomical structures of great importance. These bony boundaries must be regarded as artificial because the regions are intricately related functionally —for example, the root of the neck and the contents of the posterior triangle are as important to the total performance of the arm-trunk mechanism as are the contents of the axilla.

The clavicle anteriorly and the spine of the scapula posteriorly permit the shoulder region to be divided into the infraclavicular region, the root of the neck and the posterior triangle, and the infraspinous and subdeltoid regions. The acromion and the coracoacromial arch (formed by the coracoacromial ligament spanning the interval between the acromion and the coracoid process) delineate the subacromial and anterolateral subdeltoid region. Finally, the thoracic cage medially and the upper end of the humerus laterally form two of the boundaries of the axilla.

## INFRACLAVICULAR REGION

This region extends from the sternoclavicular joint medially to the acromioclavicular joint laterally. It encompasses the clavicle, the sternoclavicular joint, the acromioclavicular joint, the coracoclavicular ligaments, the pectoralis major and pectoralis minor muscles, the deltoid muscle (anterior portion), the clavipectoral fascia, and the coracoid process and adjacent structures.

### Clavicle

The clavicle is interposed between the acromion process and the sternum. It exhibits a double curve, being thick and cylindrical at the inner end and broad and flat at the outer end. It is generally believed to form a strut between the scapula and the axial skeleton, holding the upper extremity away from the body so that it can perform in the parasagittal plane. Nevertheless, it has been demonstrated clinically that re-

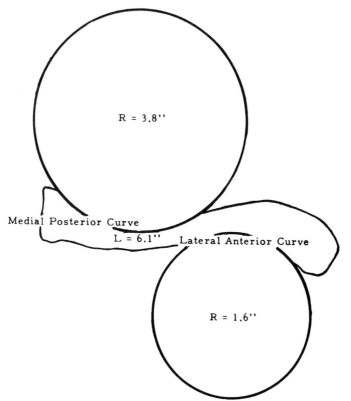

R = 3.8''

Medial Posterior Curve

L = 6.1''     Lateral Anterior Curve

R = 1.6''

$$\frac{\text{Radius Lateral Anterior + Radius Medial Posterior}}{\text{Length of Clavicle}} = \frac{(1.6 + 3.8)}{6.1} = .88 = \text{Index}$$

i.e. $\dfrac{\text{Sum of Radii}}{\text{Length}}$ = Index

FIG. 4-1. Method of determining the clavicular index. The sum of the radii is divided into the length of the clavicle. (DePalma, A. F.: Degenerative Changes in the Sternoclavicular and Acromioclavicular Joints in Various Decades. P. 116. Springfield, Ill., Charles C Thomas, 1957)

section of part or all of the clavicle does not allow a forward droop of the scapula.

One is forced to conclude that the axioscapular group of muscles are capable of maintaining the scapula in its normal dorsal position without the anterior bony strut. Through the joints at either end, the clavicle is capable of a wide range of motion, which is essential to achieve complete elevation of the arm. The clavicle is bound to the coracoid process by the coracoclavicular ligaments, whose fibers permit considerable rotation in its long axis. It provides attachment to the upper digitations of the trapezius, which elevates and supports the shoulder, and to the deltoid and the pectoralis major (clavicular head), which participate in elevation of the arm.

The medial end of the clavicle is moored to the first rib by the intra-articular fibrocartilage of the sternoclavicular joint, which acts as a ligament; it holds the upper margins of the articular surface of the clavicle firmly to the first rib. Stability of the sternal end of the clavicle is further enhanced by the oblique fibers of the costoclavicular ligaments and to a lesser degree by the subclavius muscle. Most of the stresses traveling along the length of the clavicle are transmitted through its medial two thirds,

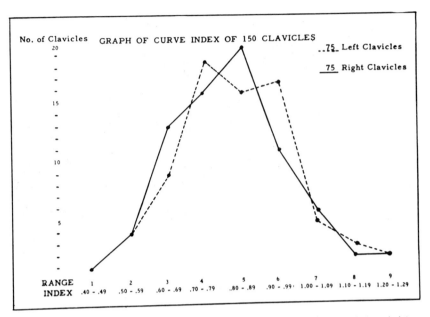

FIG. 4-2. Note that the graphs, described by the indices of the right clavicles and those of the left clavicles, are essentially the same. (DePalma, A. F.: Degenerative Changes in the Sternoclavicular and Acromioclavicular Joints in Various Decades. P. 117. Springfield, Ill., Charles C Thomas, 1957)

which provides an explanation for its massiveness as compared to the outer one third. The S-shaped configuration of the clavicle allows stresses traveling the length of the bone to be concentrated at its weakest point, the junction of the outer and middle thirds. When the stresses are severe, fractures of the clavicle occur at this site.

A study of 150 clavicles (75 right and 75 left clavicles) was conducted by the author. Marked variations were found in clavicles from different individuals; no two clavicles presented the same configuration in all details. Fich reported that the right clavicles of right-handed persons possessed more pronounced curves than the left clavicles. This implies that the curves of the right clavicles are more marked than those of the left clavicles. This impression was not confirmed in my study. However, a definite relationship was observed between the severity of the curves and the length of the bone.

The medial and lateral curves form arcs of almost perfect circles. The sum of the radii of the two circles was divided into the length of the clavicle (measured in inches); this provided an index for each clavicle (Fig. 4-1). The index of each of the 150 clavicles fell into one of nine categories, each category establishing a specific configuration relative to the type of the curves and the length of the clavicle. The indices ranged from 0.40 to 1.29; nine groups were derived from this range. They were: (1) 0.40 to 0.49, (2) 0.5 to 0.59, (3) 0.6 to 0.69, (4) 0.7 to 0.79, (5) 0.8 to 0.89, (6) 0.9 to 0.99, (7) 1.0 to 1.09, (8) 1.10 to 1.19 and (9) 1.20 to 1.29. The great majority of the clavicles fell in the third, fourth, fifth and sixth groups. In Figure 4-2 the graphs described by the indices of the right and those of the left clavicles are in all important aspects similar, contrary to Fich's report that the curves of the right clavicles are more pronounced than those of the left clavicles. A representative right and left bone for each group is depicted in Figure 4-3; note the similarity of the right and the left bone in each index range.

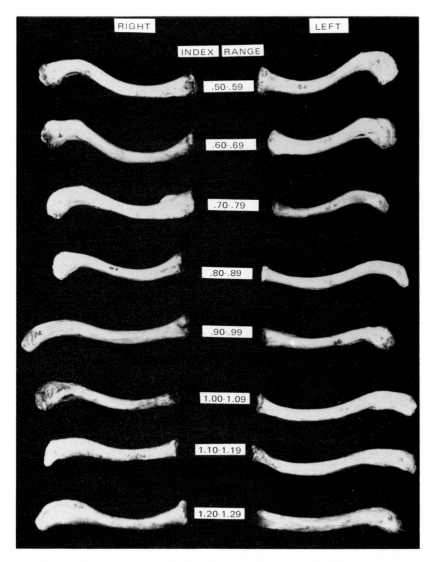

FIG. 4-3. Representative clavicles, a right and a left, for each index are depicted. Observe the similarity between the right and the left bone for each index. (DePalma, A. F.: Degenerative Changes in the Sternoclavicular and Acromioclavicular Joints in Various Decades. P. 118. Springfield, Ill., Charles C Thomas, 1957)

Of more significance was the observation that the lateral one third of the clavicles exhibits varying degrees of anterior torsion. This is readily noted if the clavicle is observed with the sternoclavicular and acromioclavicular joints intact, and if the sternum is placed in a vertical position (Fig. 4-4). Sixty-six such specimens obtained from cadavers were studied; the clavicles fell into one of three types, each of which exhibited specific features (Fig. 4-5).

**Type 1.** In this group the clavicles show the greatest amount of anterior torsion of their lateral thirds. The acromial end is flat and thin and possesses a small articular surface; the plane of the acromioclavicular

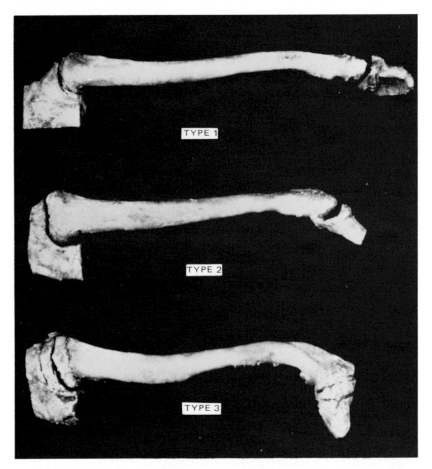

Fig. 4-4. Note the degrees of anterior torsion of the outer third of the clavicle in the three types. (DePalma, A. F.: Degenerative Changes in the Sternoclavicular and Acromioclavicular Joints in Various Decades. P. 119. Springfield, Ill., Charles C Thomas, 1957)

joint is directed downward and inward, the angle ranging from 10° to 22°, the average being 16°. At the sternal end of the clavicle the plane of the sternoclavicular joint is not far from the vertical and is directed downward and outward. The angle ranges from 0 to 10°, the average angle being 7.5° (Fig. 4-5).

**Type 2.** The anterior torsion of the lateral one third of the clavicles of this category is less than that noted in Type 1. Also the acromial end is stouter and slightly more rounded. The plane of the acromioclavicular joint forms a greater angle with the vertical than that noted in Type 1, the average

angle being 26.1°. Of interest is the configuration of the lateral curve of the clavicle: it describes an arc of a circle smaller than the circle of the arc of the lateral curve in Type 1. The angle of the plane of the sternoclavicular joint is slightly greater, the average angle measuring 10.9° (Fig. 4-5).

**Type 3.** In this group the outer third of the clavicle has the least amount of anterior torsion. Its acromial end is stout and rounded, presenting almost a complete circular articular surface. The arc of the lateral curve is of a circle smaller than the circles of the arcs noted in Type 1 and Type 2. The

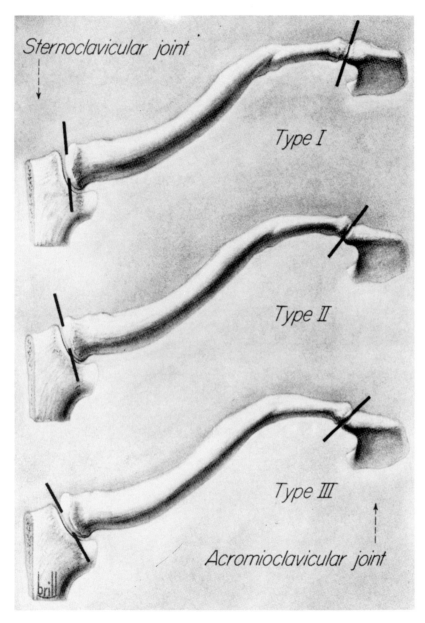

Sternoclavicular joint

Type I

Type II

Type III

Acromioclavicular joint

FIG. 4-5. The degree of anterior torsion of the clavicle determines the inclination of the articular surfaces of the sternal and acromial ends of the clavicle, permitting the joints to be grouped into one of three categories or types. (DePalma, A. F.: Degenerative Changes in the Sternoclavicular and Acromioclavicular Joints in Various Decades. P. 120. Springfield, Ill., Charles C Thomas, 1957)

plane of the acromioclavicular joint is not far from the horizontal, the average angle being 36.1°; on the other hand, the plane of the sternoclavicular joint forms an average

angle of 13.9° with the vertical (Fig. 4-5).

From this study it is clear that from Type 1 to Type 3 the angles of the planes of both the acromioclavicular and the sternoclavic-

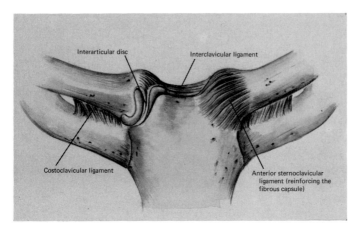

FIG. 4-6. The ligaments of the sternoclavicular joint. Note that the interarticular disc is convex-concave and divides the joint into two compartments: the discosternal, and the discoclavicular compartment.

ular joints increase progressively, whereas the size of the circles of the arcs of the lateral curves diminishes. Of the 66 specimens studied, 27 (41%) were Type 1, 32 (48%) were Type 2 and seven (11%) were Type 3. That these observations have significant clinical application was shown in a clinical study of the relationship between painful acromioclavicular joints due to de-

generative changes and the three aforementioned types of clavicles; it was found that the great majority of the patients possessed clavicles classified as Type 1. It appears that in Type 1 the plane of the joint is such that during motion more shearing forces act on the articular surfaces than act on the articular surfaces of the other two types of clavicles. Moreover, the articular

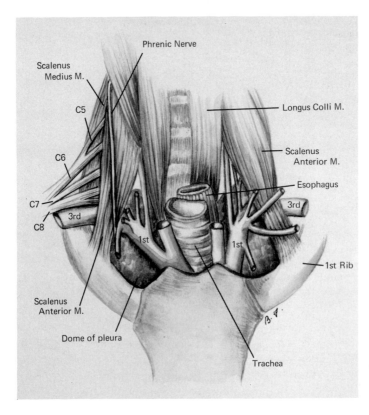

FIG. 4-7. Important structures occupying the region immediately behind the sternoclavicular joint.

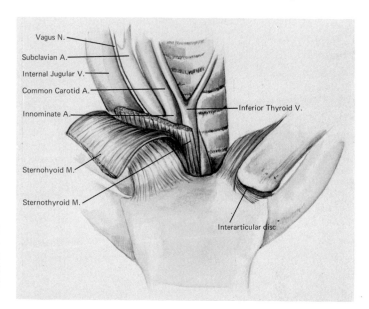

Vagus N.

Subclavian A.

Internal Jugular V.

Common Carotid A.

Innominate A.

Inferior Thyroid V.

Sternohyoid M.

Sternothyroid M.

Interarticular disc

FIG. 4-8. Note that the sternothyroid and the sternohyoid lie between the posterior capsule of the joint and the great vessels of the neck.

## Sternoclavicular Joint

This articulation is formed by the mesial end of the clavicle and the facet on the posterolateral aspect of the manubrium sterni and the cartilage of the first rib. The sternal end of the clavicle is roughly prismatic in configuration and is larger than the articular surface of the sternum so that it protrudes a considerable distance above the slanting articular surface of the sternum. The components of this joint exhibit striking structural irregularities; this is particularly true of the clavicular element. For this reason, a pronounced lack of congruence exists between the articular surfaces of the bony portions of the joint. However, nature has compensated for this lack of congruence by interposing between the articular surfaces a stout fibrocartilaginous disc, whose internal structural arrangement makes it an effective buffer to stresses and strains incident to function (Fig. 4-6).

The interarticular disc is convex-concave; its circumference is slightly thicker than

its center and the superior portion is thicker than the inferior. It is attached to the upper and posterior aspect of the clavicle over a broad, roughly circular area, and, below, it fuses with the cartilage of the first rib at its juncture with the sternum. This arrangement makes the interarticular disc the chief stabilizing element of the sternal end of the clavicle, preventing abnormal elevation of the clavicle. The disc divides the joint cavity into two compartments, the disco-sternal and the disco-clavicular compartment. A study of this joint by the author revealed that in 2.6 percent of the joints investigated the disc showed a developmental defect in its inferior portion which permitted direct communication of the two compartments. In the late decades of life many discs exhibit advanced degenerative changes and even perforations of the central portions.

The articular surfaces of the joint are enclosed in an articular fibrous capsule which is also attached to the edges of the disc. Both anterior and posterior surfaces of the capsule are reinforced by the strong, oblique fibrous bands of the anterior and posterior sternoclavicular ligaments. In addition to the aforementioned structures, stability of the joint is further reinforced by inter-

surfaces of the joints in Type 1 are smaller than those of the other two types. This may be another factor predisposing the articular cartilage to degenerative alterations.

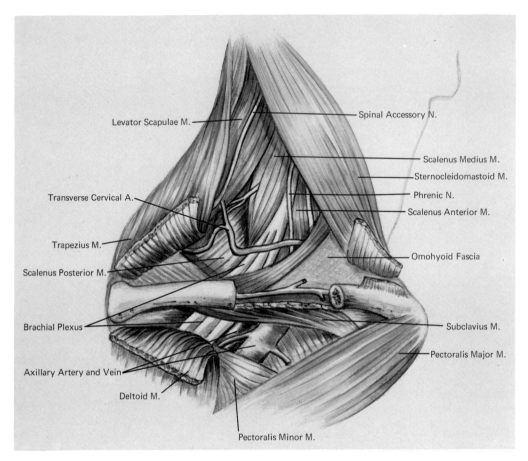

FIG. 4-9. Note the myofascial layer between the clavicle and the great vessels and nerves as they run distally to enter the axilla. The myofascial layer consists of the omohyoid fascia, enclosing the omohyoid muscle, and the clavipectoral fascia, enclosing subclavius and pectoralis minor.

clavicular and costoclavicular ligaments; the latter structure lies outside the sternoclavicular joint. It comprises oblique, spiral fibers directed upward and outward between the first costal cartilage and the undersurface of the proximal end of the clavicle. When the shoulder is brought upward, these fibers unwind; also, they prevent abnormal elevation of the clavicle and, hence, of the scapula (Fig. 4-6).

It will be shown subsequently that the sternoclavicular joint, which is the only joint between the trunk and the upper extremity, plays an important role in the arm-trunk mechanism. Integrity of this joint must be maintained in order to attain total

shoulder movement and disorders of this articulation are reflected in definite impairment of shoulder function.

Although rarely, this joint may be affected by mechanical disorders and other pathological conditions necessitating surgical intervention. Therefore, it is essential that the surgeon be familiar with the structures lying immediately behind the joint. In this region are found the main vessels of the neck, the dome of the pleura, and the trachea and esophagus (Fig. 4-7). Immediately behind the joint and in close proximity to the posterior capsule are the sternothyroid and the sternohyoid muscles which provide an effective barrier, providing protection for

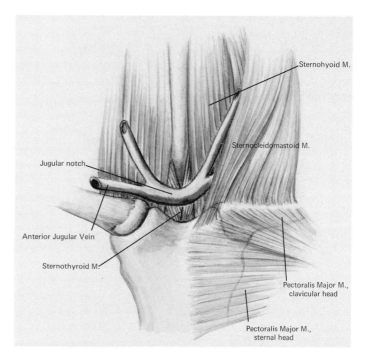

FIG. 4-10. The sterno-cleidomastoid lies in front and the sternohyoid and sternothyroid behind the sternoclavicular joint. The two heads of pectoralis major meet at the sterno-clavicular joint.

the great vessels of the neck. This is especially true on the right side of the neck (Fig. 4-8). In addition, the vessels are protected by a myofascial layer which lies in front of the vessels as they continue downward from the root of the neck to the axilla. Essentially this sheath comprises the omohyoid fascia enclosing the omohyoid muscle and the clavipectoral fascia enclosing the subclavius and the pectoralis minor muscles (Fig. 4-9). In extraperiosteal removal of the clavicle preservation of this layer ensures protection to the vital structures beneath it.

At this point, mention must be made of the important muscle attachments in the region of the sternoclavicular joint. The sternocleidomastoid lies in front and the sternohyoid and sternothyroid muscles lie behind the joint. The two heads (sternal and clavicular) of the pectoralis major meet at the sternoclavicular joint (Fig. 4-10).

## Acromioclavicular Joint

Essentially the acromioclavicular articulation is a plane joint formed by the outer end of the clavicle and the acromion. In the adult, the joint contains an intra-articular disc which is meniscoid in shape. The articular surfaces permit motion in all directions, including rotation of the clavicle; they vary in size, as does their plane of contact. The ends of the bones are enveloped in a weak, relaxed capsule, which is reinforced above by the superior acromioclavicular ligament and below by the inferior acromioclavicular ligament; the former is the stronger structure (Fig. 4-11).

A very important extra-articular component of this articulation is the coracoclavicular ligament, which binds the scapula to the clavicle. It comprises two tough fasciculi, the trapezoid and conoid ligaments, which are directed upward and laterally to insert into the trapezoid line and the conoid tubercle on the undersurface of the clavicle just where it curves posteriorly on its outer third. This manner of attachment provides a mechanism capable of producing further outward rotation of the scapula. As the scapula rotates during abduction of the arm, the coracoid process is displaced downward. Through the action of the coracoclavicular ligaments on the

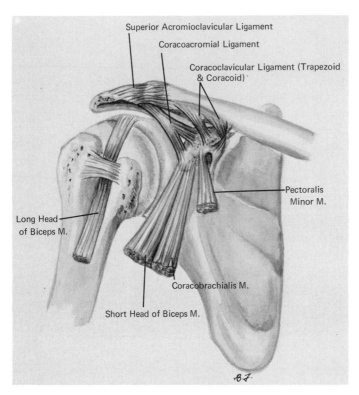

Superior Acromioclavicular Ligament

Coracoacromial Ligament

Coracoclavicular Ligament (Trapezoid
& Coracoid)

Pectoralis
Minor M.

Long Head
of Biceps M.

Coracobrachialis M.

Short Head of Biceps M.

FIG. 4-11. Note the ligaments binding the coracoid to the clavicle and the acromion, and the relation of the three muscles inserting into the coracoid.

posterior curvature of the clavicle, the clavicle now rotates on its long axis. Without this cranklike action of the clavicle, made possible by its S-shaped curve, abduction of the arm would be restricted.

The mechanism described above is undoubtedly the most important function of the coracoclavicular ligaments. Too much emphasis has been placed on the stabilizing influence of this ligament on the acromioclavicular joint and its function as a suspensory ligament of the shoulder girdle. It has been demonstrated that severance of this ligament in an intact joint does not produce subluxation or luxation of the acromioclavicular joint. These conditions occur only when, in addition to severance of the coracoclavicular ligaments, the superior acromioclavicular ligament is divided. This observation has significant clinical application: following a traumatic subluxation or luxation of the acromioclavicular joint, stability can be readily achieved by repairing the superior acromioclavicular ligament and reefing the aponeurotic attachments of

the deltoid and trapezius muscles one on the other; this last step restores muscle balance between the deltoid and trapezius over the outer third of the clavicle. It is not necessary to repair or reconstruct the acromioclavicular ligaments in order to restore normal aligment of the articular surfaces of this joint.

As will be shown subsequently, the acromioclavicular joint exhibits rapid and extensive degenerative changes beginning as early as the second decade. The intra-articular disc provides no protection to the articular surfaces of the joint. Fortunately these changes do not necessarily produce symptoms, but they do render the joint vulnerable to even minor injuries and to excessive stress and strains incident to function.

## Coracoid Process and Adjacent Structures

The coracoid process is an important landmark in the infraclavicular region. It

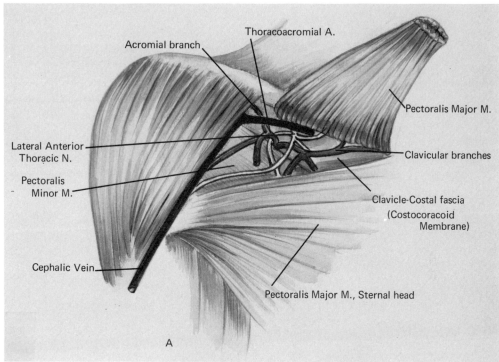

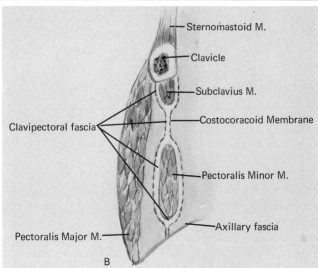

FIG. 4-12. (A) Neurovascular structures piercing and overlying the clavipectoral fascia. (B) Schematic drawing of the clavipectoral fascia.

is readily palpable just below the clavicle under the medial border of the deltoid muscle. It is a signal post for surgeons working in this area, drawing their attention to the important and vital structures in its vicinity. It is a crooked, curved, stubby bony process arising from the neck of the scapula just

behind and to the inner side of the glenoid fossa. It is directed forward, outward and downward, overhanging the humeral head anteriorly as the acromion does posteriorly. Just above the coracoid process lies the outer third of the clavicle, to which the coracoid is attached by the coracoclavicu-

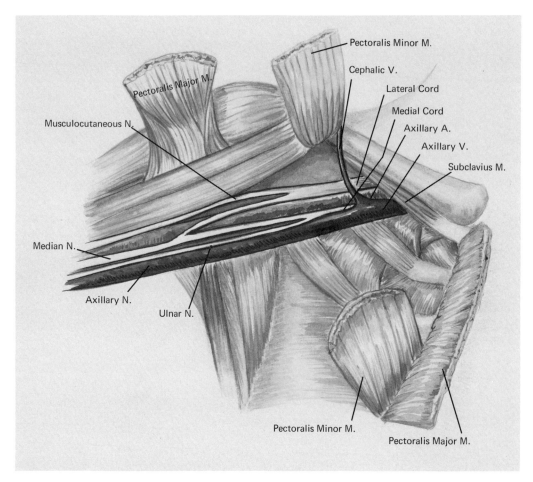

FIG. 4-13. Immediately behind the pectoralis minor and a finger's breadth below the coracoid process lie the axillary artery and vein, the latter medial to the artery. At this point the medial cord lies medial to the artery and the lateral cord lateral to it.

lar ligament; its outer surface provides attachment for the inner end of the coracoacromial ligament. The pectoralis minor inserts into its medial aspect and the short head of the biceps and coracobrachialis into its tip (Fig. 4-11).

The important structure first encountered is the clavipectoral fascia, which is an offshoot of the axillary fascia; this structure first envelops the pectoralis minor and then continues upward as the costocoracoid membrane, embracing first the subclavius and then the clavicle (Fig. 4-12). Just above the margin of the pectoralis minor the costo-

coracoid membrane is pierced by the lateral pectoral nerve and the thoracoacromial artery; the latter promptly divides into pectoral, acromial, clavicular and deltoid branches. Below and medial to the exit of the lateral pectoral nerve, the medial pectoral nerve pierces the pectoralis minor and the overlying fascia. The cephalic vein pierces the costocoracoid membrane just beneath the clavicular origin of the pectoralis major (Fig. 4-12).

Beneath the clavipectoral (costocoracoid) membrane lie the pectoralis minor muscle and the vital structures beneath it. A finger's

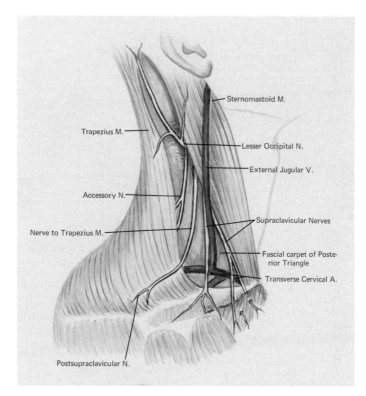

FIG. 4-14. Boundaries and contents of the posterior triangle of the neck (superficial compartment).

breadth from the tip of the coracoid process and behind the pectoralis minor muscle lie the axillary artery and vein, the latter being medial to the artery. Also in this location the medial cord of the brachial plexus lies medial to the artery and the lateral cord lies lateral to it (Fig. 4-13).

It was previously noted that all the above vital structures lie beneath a myofascial layer, the clavipectoral fascia, of which the costocoracoid membrane is a part; this structure is continuous with the axillary fascia. It becomes apparent that changes in this myofascial layer producing thickening or shortening of the structure may make abnormal pressure on the neurovascular bundle. Also certain movements of the arm, particularly abduction and external rotation, may squeeze the neurovascular bundle between the head of the humerus and the myofascial layer (see Fig. 4-9). Also, forcing the limb downward and backward may cause compression of great vessels between the clavicle and the first rib.

## Large Muscles in Infraclavicular Region

The two important muscles in this region are the clavicular origin of the deltoid muscle and the clavicular origin of the pectoralis major. Just beneath the clavicle they form the deltopectoral triangle which is traversed by the cephalic vein. By visualizing the cephalic vein and following it proximally, its exit from the costocoracoid membrane is readily located. Beyond this it promptly empties into the axillary vein. Therefore, it is a handy guide to the large vessels in the axilla.

## ROOT OF THE NECK

This area lies between the clavicle anteriorly and the spine of the scapula posteriorly. It contains the posterior triangle whose lower part contains structures most vital to the function of the shoulder. Also,

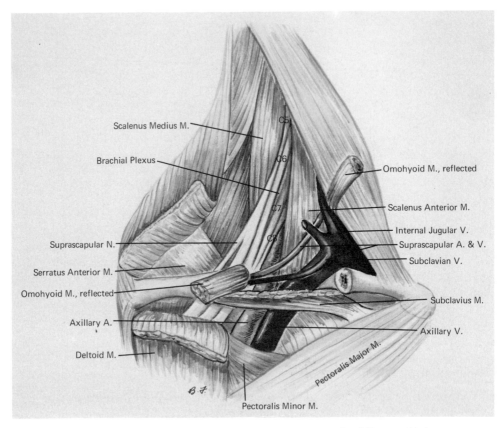

Scalenus Medius M.

Brachial Plexus

C5

C6

C7

C8

Omohyoid M., reflected

Scalenus Anterior M.

Internal Jugular V.

Suprascapular A. & V.

Subclavian V.

Suprascapular N.

Serratus Anterior M.

Omohyoid M., reflected

Axillary A.

Deltoid M.

Subclavius M.

Axillary V.

Pectoralis Major M.

Pectoralis Minor M.

FIG. 4-15. Structures in the deep compartment of the posterior triangle of the neck; the scaleni form its floor. Note the brachial plexus exiting from between scalenus medius and scalenus anterior, and the scalenus anterior lying between the artery and the vein.

in the root of the neck lies the suprascapular region in which are found important structures, comprehension of which is necessary to perform surgical procedures in this area safely.

## Posterior Triangle of the Neck

This region lies in the interval bounded anteriorly by the sternomastoid muscle, posteriorly by the edge of the trapezius muscle and inferiorly by the middle third of the clavicle. It is divided into a superficial and a deep compartment by a "fascial carpet" which covers the deep muscular floor.

In the superficial compartment lies (1)

the accessory nerve after it has pierced the fascial layer and then descends and disappears under the anterior margin of the trapezius; (2) the supraclavicular nerves, and (3) the external jugular vein, which runs vertically downward from behind the angle of the jaw, crossing the sternomastoid muscle and then, one and one half fingersbreadth above the clavicle, piercing the deep fascia (Fig. 4-14).

The floor of the lower part of the posterior triangle is formed by the scaleni muscles (the posterior, medius and anterior) and the serratus anterior muscle. The brachial plexus and subclavian artery emerge from between the scalenus medius muscle and the scalenus anterior muscle. The artery is below the plexus; the scalenus

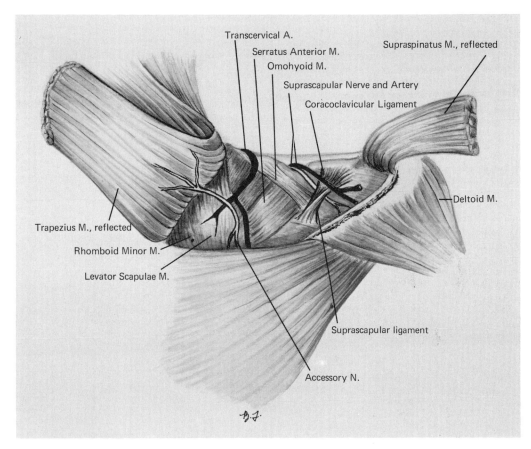

FIG. 4-16. Structures in the suprascapular region. Note the course of the accessory nerve and transcervical artery, and observe that the suprascapular nerve runs under the suprascapular ligament whereas the artery runs over it.

anterior muscle lies between the subclavian artery and the subclavian vein. The suprascapular nerve can be seen leaving the lateral border of the brachial plexus. Overlying the floor of the triangle and its contents, just anterior to the clavicle, is the omohyoid muscle, and inferior to the clavicle is the subclavius muscle. When the limb is pulled downward and backward these two muscles and their ensheathing fascia, together with the clavicle, are capable of compressing the subclavian vessels against the first rib (Fig. 4-15).

## Suprascapular Region

This region lies directly under the fibers of the trapezius muscle and above the level of the crest of the spine of the scapula. Under this muscular flap lie the rhomboid minor and levator scapulae muscles medially, the serratus anterior and omohyoid muscles centrally, and the supraspinatus traversing the supraspinous fossa. The important nerves in this region are the accessory nerve, which courses the superior angle of the scapula, and the suprascapular nerve, which traverses the interval obliquely from above downward under the suprascapular ligament. Two important arteries occupy this space — the transcervical artery, a branch of which follows the course of the accessory nerve, and the suprascapular artery, which follows the course of the suprascapular nerve, except that it runs over the suprascapular ligament (Fig. 4-16).

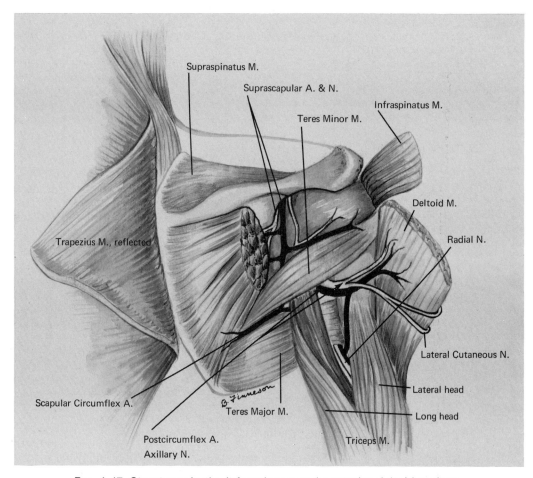

Supraspinatus M.

Suprascapular A. & N.

Infraspinatus M.

Teres Minor M.

Deltoid M.

Radial N.

Trapezius M., reflected

Lateral Cutaneous N.

Lateral head

Scapular Circumflex A.

Long head

B. Finneson

Teres Major M.

Postcircumflex A.

Triceps M.

Axillary N.

FIG. 4-17. Structures in the infraspinous and posterior deltoid regions.

## INFRASPINOUS AND POSTERIOR SUBDELTOID REGION

This region lies under the oblique fibers of the trapezius muscle, below their line of insertion into the spine of the scapula, and under the posterior portion of the deltoid muscle. The course of the nerves and arteries found in this region has important clinical and surgical significance. In the upper and lateral aspect of the area and under the infraspinatus muscle the suprascapular nerve and artery appear as they wind around the spine to reach the infraspinous fossa. Here the suprascapular nerve supplies branches to the infraspinatus muscle and to the capsular ligaments of the shoulder joint and scapula. This nerve also supplies the supraspinatus muscle (Fig. 4-17).

The quadrangular space is another important area of this region. It is formed by the teres minor muscle above, the teres major muscle below, the long head of the triceps muscle medially and the inner aspect of the upper end of the humerus laterally. This space is traversed by the axillary nerve and posterior humeral circumflex artery. Together they pass through the space and thence wind around the surgical neck of the humerus and, under cover of the deltoid, reach the anterior aspect of the shoulder. At its exit from the space, the nerve divides into anterior and posterior branches, the posterior branch innervating the teres minor and the posterior portion of the deltoid. It then continues laterally as the lateral brachial cutaneous nerve supplying the skin over the lower posterior and lateral portions of the deltoid.

The anterior branch, together with the posterior humeral circumflex artery, winds around the surgical neck of the humerus, giving off branches which pass vertically upward into the substance of the deltoid muscle; as it approaches the anterior border of the deltoid it diminishes progressively in size. Throughout its entire course, from its origin posteriorly to its termination anteriorly, the anterior division runs a horizontal course roughly 2 inches below the lateral border of the acromion process. This feature establishes a zone of safety between the line of origin of the deltoid and the course of the nerve which can be invaded in surgical approaches to the subacromial region and to the glenohumeral joint (Fig. 4-17).

## SUBACROMIAL AND ANTEROLATERAL SUBDELTOID REGION

This region extends from the deltopectoral groove anteriorly to the posterior tip of the acromion process posteriorly. It overlaps slightly the infraclavicular region previously described. The area is entirely under cover of the deltoid muscle, which at this point deserves more detailed consideration.

### Deltoid Muscle

The deltoid, which forms the outer of the two muscle sleeves, is a massive triangular muscle that drapes itself around the anterior, lateral and posterior aspects of the outer third of the clavicle, the lateral border of the acromion process and the lower border of the spine of the scapula. Its fleshy fibers converge distally to form a stout short tendon which inserts into the deltoid tubercle. The arrangement of the

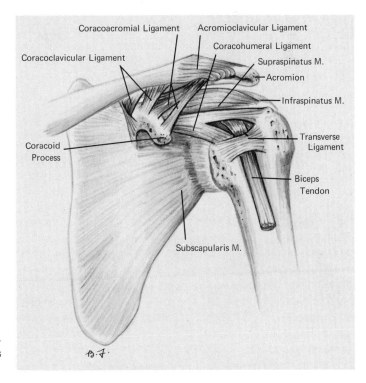

FIG. 4-18. The coracoacromial arch and the structures immediately under it.

anterior and posterior fibers of the deltoid, which arise from the clavicle and the spine of the scapula respectively, differs from that of the central fibers, which arise from the acromion.

The central muscle mass consists of oblique fibers that arise pinnate fashion from either side of 4 or 5 tendinous bands whose proximal ends are attached to the acromion. These fibrous septa proceed distally and parallel to one another and become lost in the muscle substance. From the tendinous insertion of the deltoid 3 or 4 similar tendinous strands pass upward into the muscle substance, alternating with those passing downward. The oblique fibers arising from the descending septa insert into the ascending septa. Such a complex scheme does not exist in the anterior and posterior portions of the deltoid muscle (see Fig. 5-16). Between the adjacent borders of the deltoid and the pectoralis major muscles is a distinct interval which widens at its proximal end to form the inferior clavicular fossa or deltopectoral triangle.

The origin of the deltoid muscle is of practical significance. It originates on the clavicle, the acromion and the spine of the scapula and consists of tendinous fibers that blend with the periosteum of these bony structures. Part or all of the origin of the muscle may be detached subperiosteally and enough sturdy tissue still remains to effect firm reattachment of the muscle on either side of the line of division.

## CEPHALIC VEIN

The cephalic vein traverses the deltopectoral groove, picking up tributaries as it proceeds cephalad. It occupies progressively a deeper level as it ascends until it lies on the clavipectoral fascia; below the clavicle it perforates the costocoracoid fascia, passes anterior to the axillary artery and empties into the axillary vein. The cephalic vein is a landmark in surgical procedures in this region; it points to the structures at a lower level. The axillary vessels

are readily identified by tracing the cephalic vein upward.

## CORACOACROMIAL ARCH

Directly beneath the insertion of the deltoid lies the important coracoacromial arch which consists of the acromion process and the coracoacromial ligament spanning the interval between the coracoid process and the acromion process. These structures have particular surgical and functional significance and, therefore, require detailed consideration. The coracoid process has been described previously.

### Acromion Process

The spine of the scapula terminates in the acromion process, a prominent, massive, flat, bony projection that overhangs the humeral head from behind. Its superior flat surface slants outward, backward and downward. The acromion articulates with the clavicle by means of an oval elongated articular facet facing obliquely upward. Anterior to the articular facet, the acromion receives the outer end of the coracoacromial ligament (Fig. 4-18).

The acromion forms the outer bony component of the coracoacromial arch. It is important to visualize the topographic anatomy of this bony process. As will be shown later, it plays a major role in the mechanism of shoulder movements, traumatic and degenerative lesions of the head of the humerus and the musculotendinous cuff and lesions of the subacromial bursa. Moreover, it protects the humeral head from impacts from behind and above.

In elevation of the arm the humeral head and tuberosities pass beneath the acromion. It is impossible to traumatize the humeral head directly unless a blow is directed to the front and the top of the shoulder while the arm is at the side and the elbow pulled backward (position of backward extension).

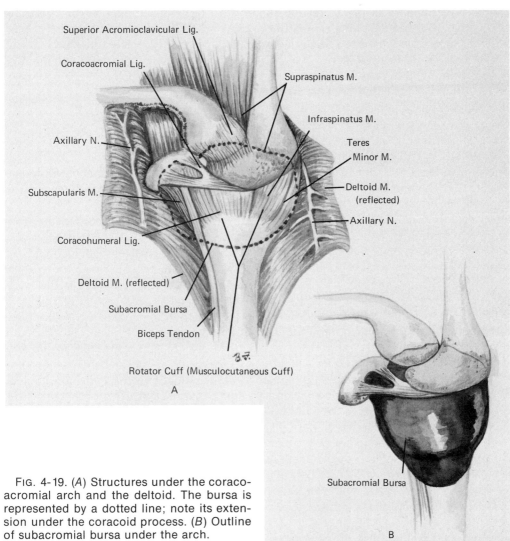

FIG. 4-19. (A) Structures under the coraco-acromial arch and the deltoid. The bursa is represented by a dotted line; note its extension under the coracoid process. (B) Outline of subacromial bursa under the arch.

## Coracoacromial Ligament

This triangular structure forms a strong arch across the coracoid and the acromion. It arises with a wide base from the outer edge of the coracoid and tapers to a narrow band to insert into the inner border of the acromion just in front of the acromioclavicular joint. Its central fibers are very thin and often wanting, forming essentially two strong limbs, an anterior and a posterior limb, which join at their point of insertion into the acromion (Fig. 4-18).

Considerable significance is attached to the coracoacromial ligament. It separates the subacromial bursa from the acromioclavicular joint, and its undersurface forms the roof of the posterior part of the subacromial bursa. In elevation of the limb, the tuberosities pass beneath the arch. Codman believed that in elevation of the arm this structure guided the head of the humerus and prevented it from gaining a fulcrum on the acromioclavicular joint. On the contrary, it has been demonstrated that the integrity of this structure may be sacrificed without noticeable effect on the functional mechanism of the joint, provided that the muscular apparatus is intact. The ligament or segments of it are often severed or removed without unfavorable sequelae.

The coracoacromial arch, with the underlying subacromial bursa and loose areolar tissue, provides a gliding mechanism between the deep and the superficial muscle strata. Thus it becomes clear why either lesions disturbing this mechanism or impingement of the tuberosities or of a hypertrophied subacromial bursa against the coracoacromial arch interfere with the smooth rhythmic elevation of the arm. Such lesions are discussed in the appropriate chapters.

## SUBACROMIAL BURSA

This is the next structure of importance encountered directly under the deltoid muscle. The muscles that overlie the scapulohumeral joint are complex in arrangement and comprise two muscle sleeves: an inner sleeve, made up of the short rotator muscles, and an outer sleeve composed of the deltoid and the teres major muscles. These muscle sleeves operate one within the other—a performance made possible by an efficient gliding mechanism between the two strata. Fine, filmy, areolar tissue and the subacromial bursa constitute the gliding mechanism. So efficiently does this arrangement function that often it is referred to as a secondary scapulohumeral joint.

The subacromial bursa adheres firmly by its base to the upper and outer portions of the greater tuberosity and to the outer surface of the musculotendinous cuff. Its roof is adherent to the undersurface of the acromion and the undersurface of the coracoacromial ligament. Its lateral walls are prolonged loosely downward under the deltoid muscle, backward and outward under the acromion and mesially under the coracoid process.

It is apparent that the bursa in the subcoracoid area is part of the subacromial bursa. The subacromial bursa communicates with the joint cavity only if a tear, involving the complete thickness of the musculotendinous cuff, opens into the floor of the bursa (Fig. 4-19).

## ROTATOR CUFF (MUSCULOTENDINOUS CUFF)

Immediately under the bursa lies the rotator cuff, a structure that plays an important role in the functional mechanism of the shoulder joint. All four short rotator muscles (supraspinatus, infraspinatus, teres minor and subscapularis) comprise this structure. The muscles end in broad flat tendons whose fibers fuse with those of the fibrous capsule. So complete is the interlacing of tendon and capsular fibers that it is impossible to separate the two structures by sharp dissection. The musculotendinous cuff inserts into the upper half of the anatomical neck of the humerus, completely filling the sulcus. In this position it is apparent that this structure functions as a suspensory ligament for the humeral head (Fig. 4-19).

### Coracohumeral Ligament

An important component of the rotator cuff is the coracohumeral ligament. This ligament originates in the outer border of the horizontal limb of the coracoid process and passes forward and downward in the interval between the supraspinatus and the subscapularis muscles. Here its fibers interlace with those of the fibrous capsule and insert with the capsule into both tuberosities bridging the bicipital groove. In this position it acts as a suspensory ligament of the humeral head. Its most proximal fibers are so arranged that they unwind and elongate upon external rotation of the shaft of the humerus, functioning as a checkrein to external rotation. The ligament shortens upon internal rotation. This fiber arrangement is significant in the frozen shoulder. In this lesion, as the result of a diffuse in-

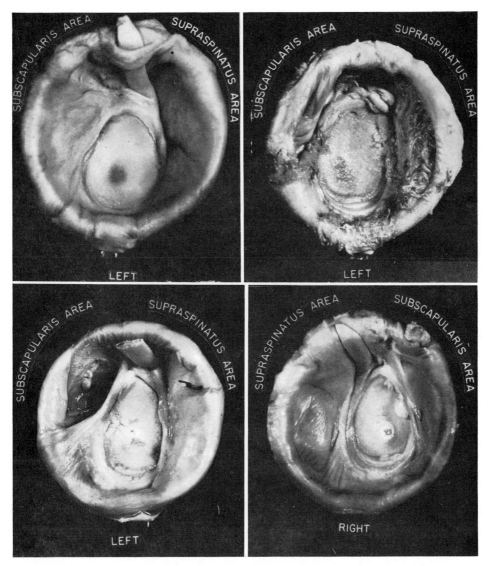

FIG. 4-20. Abnormal development of the biceps tendon. (*Top, left*) Note that a portion of the biceps tendon is still extrasynovial, lying in a tunnel within the fibrous capsule. Circular area in this specimen is well defined.

flammatory process, the fibers become fixed in the shortened position and help freeze the head in a position of internal rotation.

Occasionally, the ligament is continuous with the tendon of the pectoralis minor, running between the two limbs of the coracoacromial ligament to reach the fibrous capsule of the glenohumeral joint (Figs. 4-18 and 4-19).

The break in the continuity of the cuff between the supraspinatus and the subscapularis tendon, created by the coracohumeral ligament, provides an excellent surgical approach to the inside of the glenohumeral joint. The exposure is attained by dividing the capsule in the interval just described, parallel with the fibers of the coracohumeral ligament. The incision can be extended readily as far as the brim of the glenoid cavity.

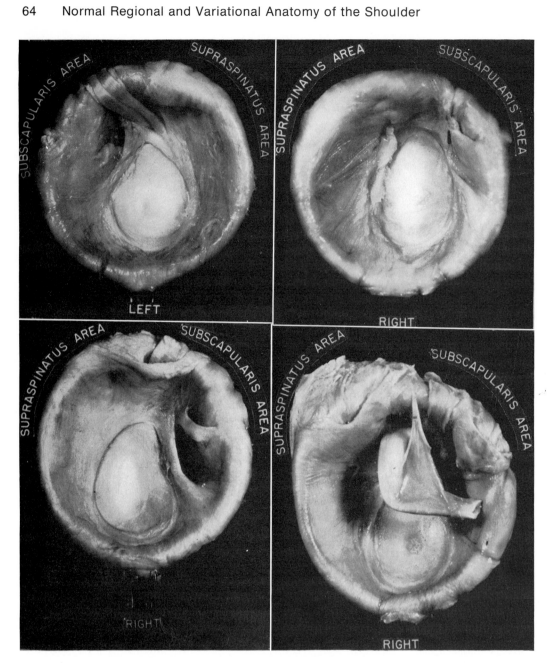

FIG. 4-21. Abnormal development of the biceps tendon. (*Top, left*) A double biceps tendon. (*Top, right*) Absence of the biceps tendon. (*Bottom, left*) The biceps tendon is entirely extrasynovial, lying within the fibrous capsule. This structure has failed to migrate to an intracapsular position. (*Bottom, right*) A well-formed mesentery of the biceps tendon.

## HEAD OF THE HUMERUS

The head of the humerus is the globular massive bony structure directly under the coracoacromial arch and the acromion. The spherical head of the humerus rests on the shaft at an angle, its articular surface directed backward, medially and upward. Only a small portion of the head is in contact with the glenoid fossa at any moment during motion or at rest. Inward torsion of the shaft of the humerus has displaced the tuberosities and the bicipital groove medially. The humeral torsion angle varies from 134° to 160°. The bicipital groove is displaced medially 30° from a line passing through the center of the head of the humerus. The greater tuberosity is directed externally, forming the outer wall of the bicipital groove. Between the tuberosities and the edge of the articular surface of the anatomical head is a broad sulcus called the anatomical neck of the humerus.

In living subjects the sulcus is obliterated by the musculotendinous cuff which completely fills this groove. It is very much in evidence in humeri stripped of all soft tissue structures. The musculotendinous cuff gradually recedes from its line of insertion in shoulders of persons past middle life. It is not uncommon to see in these shoulders (when viewed from the inside of the joint) bare portions of the anatomical neck between the edge of the articular cartilage of the humeral head and the receding cuff. Such lesions were designated "rim rents" by Codman.

During elevation of the arm, the greater tuberosity glides under the acromion or coracoacromial arch with ease. However, in lesions that produce hypertrophy of this bony process, the tuberosity impinges on the acromion or the coracoacromial arch, thereby restricting the range of motion or causing a painful jog as it passes beneath the overlying structures. As will be shown in the discussion on motion at the shoulder, complete elevation can be achieved only in the frontal plane with the arm in internal rotation and in the coronal plane with the arm in external rotation.

## BICEPS TENDON

The intracapsular portion of the biceps tendon is continuous with the fibers of the superior posterior portion of the labrum. Its relation to the glenohumeral ligaments varies; in most specimens it blends with the superior ligament; in some it is continuous with the middle ligament and in a few

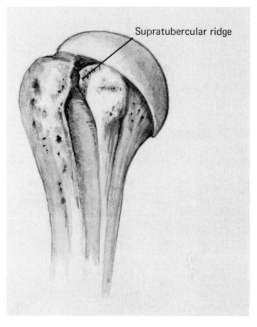

Supratubercular ridge

FIG. 4-22. Schematic drawing, showing a supratubercular ridge which may facilitate displacement of the biceps tendon out of the intertubercular sulcus.

with all three ligaments. Although rare, developmental anomalies of the biceps tendon occur. The tendon may occupy a partially intracapsular position (Fig. 4-20); it may present as a double structure; it may be absent; it may be entirely intracapsular, and occasionally a well formed mesentery exists (Fig. 4-21).

## Gliding Mechanism of the Biceps Tendon

The greater and lesser tuberosities of the humerus and the long head of the biceps tendon lying in the groove, which the tuberosities bound, form a very important gliding mechanism. The synovial lining of the glenohumeral joint continues distally in the bicipital groove and is then reflected proximally onto the biceps tendon.

The concept that the biceps tendon moves up and down the groove during motion at the glenohumeral joint must be discarded. With the bicipital tendon and groove exposed under local anesthesia, it can be

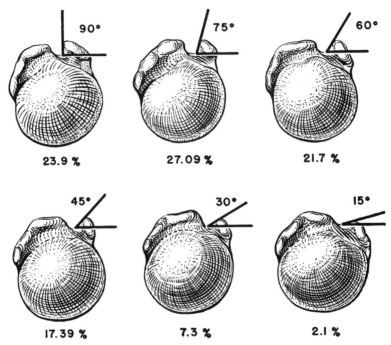

FIG. 4-23. Six variations of the angle of medial wall of the intertubercular groove, and their incidences. (Redrawn with modification from Hitchcock, H. H. and Bechtol, C. O.: J. Bone & Joint
Surg., 30-A:263, 1948)

demonstrated on living subjects that the
biceps tendon remains fixed in the groove
during motion, but the head of the humerus
glides up and down the tendon. Contraction
of the biceps muscle by supinating the forearm or flexing the elbow makes the tendon
taut but produces no motion of the tendon
in the groove. All movements at the shoulder joint, regardless of the plane in which
the arm is elevated, are accompanied by
gliding motions of the humerus on the
tendon.

Internal rotation of the arm forces the
biceps tendon to perform over the medial
wall of the groove; the lesser tubercle, from
a mechanical viewpoint, functions as a
trochlea. Such a position forces the tendon
to work at a great mechanical disadvantage.
External rotation of the arm places the tendon over the top and the center of the head
of the humerus and on the floor of the
groove. In this position the mechanical

efficiency of the tendon is greatly enhanced,
and it can act as a depressor of the head
of the humerus and participate as an abductor of the limb, a function it normally
performs in lower forms.

The bicipital groove exhibits many variations. A supratubercular ridge may be present. This is a ridge of bone continuous with
the medial wall of the groove and extending
proximally toward the articular margin of
the humeral head. Its size and configuration vary considerably (Fig. 4-22). The
author's study of this region revealed that
in 23.8 percent of the humeri studied it was
a pronounced structure; in 31.5 percent it
was moderately developed and in 43.4 percent it was absent. This bony projection
favors dislocation of the biceps tendon by
levering it out of the proximal portion of
the bicipital groove. Supratubercular ridges,
sufficiently high to displace the tendon
against the transverse humeral ligament, are

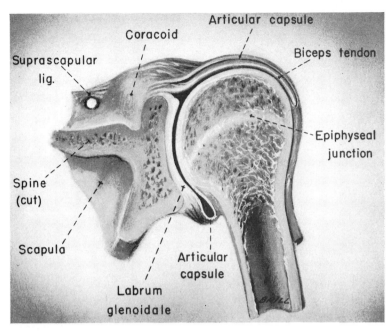

Fig. 4-24. Frontal section of the right shoulder joint, posterior view. Observe the redundancy of the capsule along the inferior aspect of the humeral neck. The fibrous capsule is lined with synovial membrane which extends downward, lining the bicipital groove as far as the surgical neck of the humerus; here it ends as a blind sac and is reflected upon the tendon. (Redrawn from W. Spalteholz: Hand Atlas of Human Anatomy. Philadelphia, J. B. Lippincott)

responsible for repeated trauma inflicted to the tendon and its sheath during joint motion.

Also there is considerable variation in the configuration of the walls of the bicipital groove. The height of the groove depends upon the obliquity of the medial wall. Of 100 humeri studied, the angle of the medial wall was 90° in 23.9 percent of the specimens, 75° in 27.09 percent, 60° in 21.7 percent, 45° in 17.3 percent, 30° in 7.3 percent and 15° in 2.1 percent. When a supratubercular ridge is present, its base also diminishes the depth of the bicipital groove. In these humeri the base of the ridge is broad and is continuous across the floor of the groove toward the lateral wall (Fig. 4-23).

The bicipital groove, especially its walls, is a frequent site for the formation of hypertrophic bony spurs which may seriously interfere with the efficiency of the gliding mechanism of the tendon. Also, the developmental variations of the groove discussed above enhance the development of these degenerative alterations. These abnormalities are discussed fully in the chapter dealing with the degenerative changes of this area.

## ARTICULAR CAPSULE OF THE GLENOHUMERAL JOINT

The fibrous capsule is a loose, redundant structure with twice the surface area of the humeral head (Fig. 4-24). Posteriorly and inferiorly, it arises from the capsular border of the labrum glenoidale and the bone immediately adjacent to it.

Synovial recesses are present when the capsule arises from the anterior neck of the scapula at varying distances from its articular surface. Thus, the presence and the size of the synovial recesses are determined by

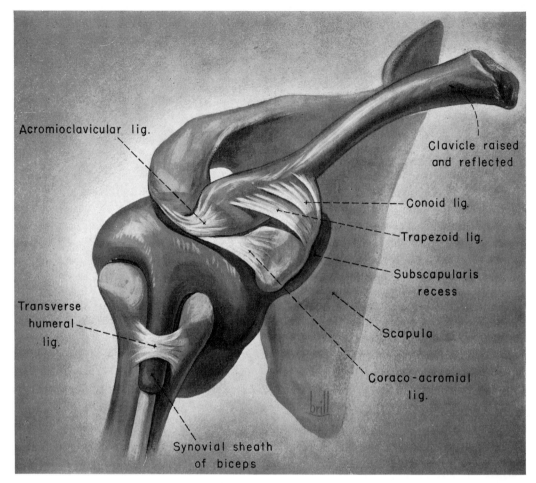

FIG. 4-25. Synovial membrane of the scapulohumeral joint. Note the extensions under the coracoid process, and downward along the walls of the bicipital groove.

how far from the articular surface of the scapula the fibrous capsule arises from the anterior neck of the scapula. In shoulder joints without synovial recesses, the fibrous capsule arises from the entire circumference of the capsular border of the labrum glenoidale, the rim of the glenoid cavity and the bone surrounding it.

Distally, the fibrous capsule inserts superiorly into the upper portion of the anatomical neck and inferiorly into the periosteum of the humeral shaft at a considerable distance from the margin of the articular cartilage of the humeral head. The fibrous capsule is lined throughout by synovial membrane that is reflected inferiorly along the anatomical neck of the

humerus toward the periphery of the articular cartilage of the humeral head, blending with the hyaline cartilage of the head. Proximally, it extends for varying distances over the labrum glenoidale and blends with its superficial fibers but fails to reach the articular cartilage of the glenoid cavity.

In the anterior region of the joint, the synovial membrane is loose and redundant; it is prolonged (in 81.8% of the shoulders) along the anterior surface of the neck of the scapula toward the root of the coracoid process, for varying distances, to form the previously mentioned synovial recesses. It is also prolonged distally to line the bicipital groove and then reflected over the

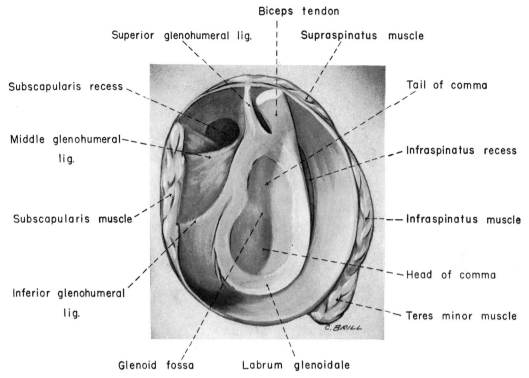

Biceps tendon

Superior glenohumeral lig.

Supraspinatus muscle

Subscapularis recess

Tail of comma

Middle glenohumeral lig.

Infraspinatus recess

Subscapularis muscle

Infraspinatus muscle

Inferior glenohumeral lig.

Head of comma

Teres minor muscle

Glenoid fossa          Labrum glenoidale

FIG. 4-26. Glenoid side of the scapulohumeral joint. This is the general arrangement of the superior, middle and inferior glenohumeral ligaments, but there are numerous variations. Note that the synovial membrane adheres closely to all the underlying structures: fibrous capsule, ligaments, labrum and biceps tendon.

biceps tendon (Fig. 4-25). The articular capsule is loose and redundant in the inferior region of the humeral neck. With the arm at the side, the capsule forms a large nictitating fold in this region. As the arm is abducted, this fold becomes smaller and disappears when full abduction is attained.

On all sides, except the inferior portion, the fibrous capsule is strengthened by the broad, flat tendons of the rotator muscles (supraspinatus, infraspinatus, teres minor and subscapularis). These tendons are approximately 2.5 cm. long. They blend with the fibrous capsule to form the musculo-tendinous cuff, also referred to as the fibro-tendinous cuff or the capsulotendinous cuff (Fig. 4-19).

## GLENOHUMERAL LIGAMENTS AND SYNOVIAL RECESSES

It was previously pointed out that the fibrous capsule is a loose, saccular, re-

dundant structure whose surface area is approximately twice that of the head of the humerus. Posteriorly and inferiorly, the capsule is continuous with the capsular border of the labrum and the bone immediately adjacent to it. Anteriorly, its relation to the labrum varies, depending upon the configurations of the glenohumeral ligaments and synovial recesses. In general, there are three glenohumeral ligaments: the superior, the middle and the inferior. Essentially they are thickened strands of the fibrous capsule which reinforce the anterior portion of the capsule and act as static checkreins to external rotation of the humeral head. From the humeral head they converge toward the anterior border of the glenoid fossa; the superior blends with the superior portion of the labrum and the biceps tendon, and the middle and inferior with the labrum at a level lower than that of the insertion of the superior. In this region are found the synovial recesses, the number, size and loca-

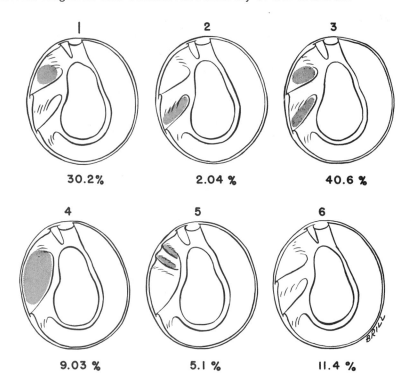

Fig. 4-27. Six types of arrangement of the synovial recesses, and their incidence: (1) Characterized by one synovial recess above the middle glenohumeral ligament. (2) One synovial recess below the glenohumeral ligament. (3) Two synovial recesses: a superior subscapular recess above the glenohumeral ligament, and an inferior subscapular recess below the glenohumeral ligament. (4) One large synovial recess above the inferior glenohumeral ligament; the middle glenohumeral ligament is absent. (5) The middle ligament exists as two small synovial folds. (6) Complete absence of synovial recesses.

tion of which depend upon the topographic variations of the ligaments (Fig. 4-26).

My study on 96 shoulders obtained from cadavers revealed that six variations, or types, are identifiable, as follows: Type 1 exhibits one synovial recess above the middle ligament; it is present in 30.2 percent of the specimens. Type 2 presents one synovial recess below the middle ligament and occurs in 2.04 percent. Type 3 discloses one recess above and one below the middle ligament; it occurs in 40.6 percent. Type 4 reveals one large recess above the inferior ligament; the middle ligament is absent; it occurs in 9.03 percent. Type 5 presents the middle ligament as two small synovial folds occurring in 5.1 percent and Type 6 has no synovial recesses; all the ligaments are well defined and this occurs in 11.4 percent (Fig. 4-27).

Study of specimens with large synovial recesses emphasizes the anatomical fact that, when these recesses are present, the fibrous capsule is not directly continuous with the anterior portion of the labrum, but rather it first extends toward the base of the coracoid process from which point it returns along the anterior aspect of the neck of the scapula as a thin fibrous sheet which finally blends with the anterior portion of the labrum. Regardless of the type in which they are found, the recesses show extreme

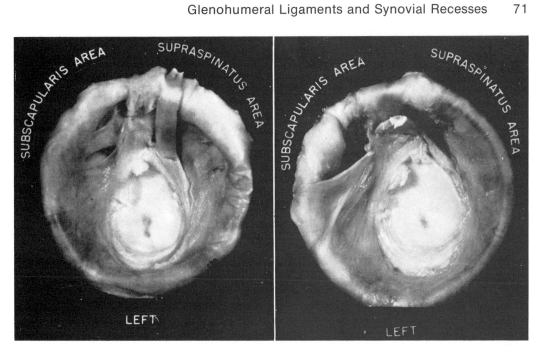

Fig. 4-28. (*Left*) Small synovial recesses above and below the middle glenohumeral ligament. (*Right*) Large synovial recess above the middle glenohumeral ligament. This recess may be interpreted erroneously as a rent in the capsule.

variability. They may be very small or very large as in the specimens shown in Figure 4-28. The ligaments themselves also exhibit many variations.

## Middle Glenohumeral Ligament

The middle ligament is a well formed, distinct structure in 68 percent of the specimens studied; it is poorly defined in 16 percent and absent in 12 percent. When present, it generally arises from the anterior portion of the labrum immediately below the superior ligament; in a few specimens it has no attachment to the labrum, and occasionally (4 to 5%) it exists as a double structure on the anterior aspect of the capsular wall, having no connection with the labrum. Also, its length, width and thickness vary considerably (Fig. 4-29).

## Superior Glenohumeral Ligament

Of the three ligaments, the superior ligament is the most constant; it is a distinct

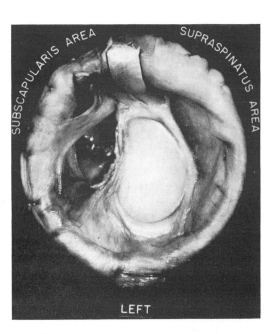

Fig. 4-29. A well formed middle glenohumeral ligament with a large synovial recess above and a still larger one below. The superior glenohumeral ligament is also a well formed structure.

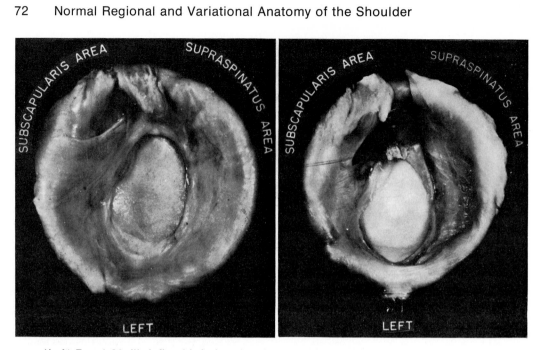

(*Left*) FIG. 4-30. Ill-defined inferior glenohumeral ligament. It exists as a diffuse thickening of the capsule between the subscapular area and the triceps area.

(*Right*) FIG. 4-31. Note the synovial tabs in the coracohumeral area. Also, in this specimen the middle glenohumeral ligament is not continuous with the labrum.

structure in 94 specimens studied and absent in 2 specimens. It arises from the upper pole of the glenoid fossa and the root of the coracoid process (Figs. 4-26 and 4-29). In 73 of the 96 specimens it is attached to the middle ligament, the biceps tendon and the labrum; in 20 to the biceps tendon and labrum; and in one, to the biceps tendon only. It inserts into the fovea capitis of the humerus adjacent to the lesser tuberosity in relation to the coracohumeral ligament. Schlemm, many years ago, considered this ligament as the deep portion of the coracohumeral ligament and in 1877 Welcher compared the ligament to the round ligament of the hip joint. During its development, it shifts from an extracapsular to an intracapsular position; accordingly, the visibility of the ligament from the synovial side of the capsule varies. Although its anatomical position is fairly constant, the superior ligament, like the middle ligament, varies considerably in size.

Ninety-four of the 96 specimens reveal the superior ligament to be attached to the labrum and biceps tendon. This observation is significant because, as will be shown later, the labrum in the region of the tail of the comma tends to pull away as early as the second decade. The frequency and the severity of the abnormality increase with each subsequent decade. These findings may indicate that the superior ligament together with the biceps tendon exerts a distracting force on the labrum, causing the structure to pull away from the tail end of the glenoid fossa.

### Inferior Glenohumeral Ligament

This is a triangular structure, with its apex at the labrum and its base blending with the capsule in the region between the subscapularis and the triceps tendon (Fig. 4-26). Often it is an indistinct structure, existing only as a diffuse thickening of the capsule (Fig. 4-30). Of the 96 specimens, it is a well defined ligament in 54, poorly defined in 18 and absent in 24.

## Synovial Membrane

In the specimens of the early decades the synovial membrane is seen in its normal state. It lines the inner aspect of the fibrous capsule and all of the intracapsular soft tissue elements: the biceps tendon, the labrum, the glenohumeral ligaments and the recesses. It is thin, smooth, glistening and closely adherent to the underlying structures (Fig. 4-26). In the bursal recesses and coracohumeral areas it is more or less a redundant structure from whose surface small tabs, fringes or villi project into the joint cavity (Fig. 4-31). The afflictions of aging produce many characteristic alterations in the synovial membrane. These will be considered later.

## Clinical Significance of the Relation of the Synovial Recesses and the Subscapularis Tendon

The relation of the subscapularis tendon to the synovial recesses and glenohumeral ligaments has great clinical significance. In shoulders with large recesses, the subscapularis tendon is not in close proximity to the anterior neck of the scapula; also the anterior capsular wall is poorly constructed or may not be present at all. Anterior stability in these joints is provided by the dynamic action of the large subscapularis muscle; the anterior capsular wall adds little or nothing to the stability of the joint. It is reasonable to assume that such joints are more likely to develop recurrent dislocations following an initial traumatic dislocation than are shoulder joints that have a strong capsular wall as when the synovial recesses are small or absent and the glenohumeral ligaments are well formed, distinct, sturdy structures. In these anatomical arrangements the subscapularis muscle hugs the anterior neck of the scapula closely and works with greater efficiency than it can if it is separated from the scapula by large synovial recesses. Also, it is reasonable to assume that less force is required

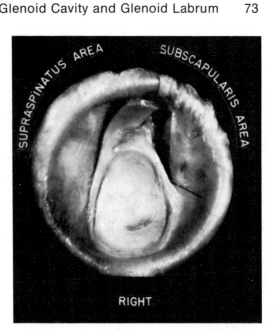

FIG. 4-32. The glenoid cavity resembles an inverted comma. Note how all three glenohumeral ligaments tend to converge toward the biceps tendon. The biceps tendon blends with the labrum which resembles a meniscus.

to dislocate shoulder joints with large synovial recesses than those with small or no synovial recesses.

## GLENOID CAVITY AND GLENOID LABRUM

This shallow fossa is shaped like an inverted comma. Its superior portion, which is designated the tail of the comma, is narrow; the inferior portion (head of the comma) is broad. It faces forward and upward and is covered by hyaline cartilage, which is thinner in the center of the head of the comma than at the outer margins of the articular cavity.

A fibrous structure, the labrum glenoidale, triangular in cross section, rims the glenoid cavity. In infant shoulders, this structure is closely attached by its base to the brim of the glenoid cavity, its glenoid edge blending with the fibrils of the hyaline cartilage, while its capsular border is continuous with

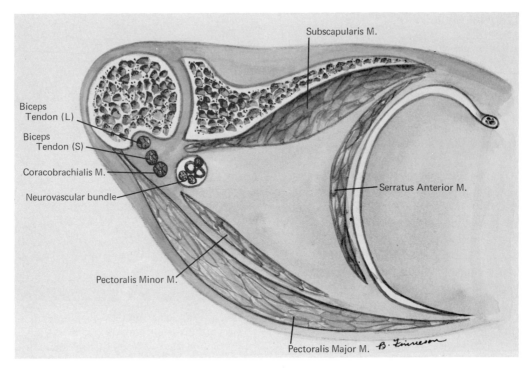

FIG. 4-33. Walls of the axilla on cross section.

the fibrous capsule. In later decades, the labrum in the region of the tail of the comma rests on the edge of the glenoid fossa like a meniscus, its glenoid border lying free (Figs. 4-26 and 4-32).

The long head of the biceps tendon inserts into the supraglenoid tubercle and is continuous with the posterior and anterior fibers of the labrum in the superior region of the comma (Fig. 4-32).

Superiorly, posteriorly and inferiorly the fibrous capsule blends with the labrum, but anteriorly this relationship changes with the presence or absence of synovial recesses and their configuration. If recesses are present, the capsule is attached to the scapula at a distance from the labrum and then reflects along the anterior neck of the scapula to reach the labrum and glenohumeral ligaments. As will be shown subsequently, the labrum in adults shows varying degrees of degenerative changes due to injury and stresses incident to function.

## BURSAE AROUND THE SHOULDER JOINT

In addition to the subacromial bursa previously described, other bursae of lesser significance may be the source of pain in the region of the shoulder. These are:

1. **The subscapularis bursa** (or bursae), which are really outpouchings of the synovial membrane of the glenohumeral joint beneath the subscapularis tendon. They do not communicate with the subacromial bursa in its normal state.

2. **Bursae beneath tendons** near their insertion into the humerus on either side of the bicipital groove, as seen under the pectoralis major, the latissimus dorsi and the teres major muscles.

3. **Supracoracoid bursa,** most likely to be found when there is an anomalous insertion of the pectoralis minor into the coracoid process.

4. **Infraserratus bursa,** located between

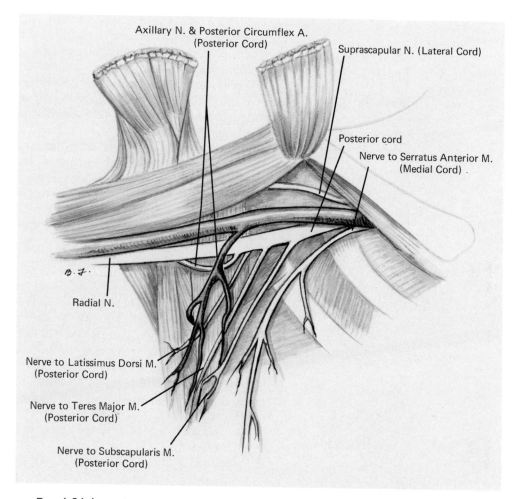

Axillary N. & Posterior Circumflex A.
(Posterior Cord)

Suprascapular N. (Lateral Cord)

Posterior cord

Nerve to Serratus Anterior M.
(Medial Cord) .

Radial N.

Nerve to Latissimus Dorsi M.
(Posterior Cord)

Nerve to Teres Major M.
(Posterior Cord)

Nerve to Subscapularis M.
(Posterior Cord)

FIG. 4-34. Important nerves in relation to the posterior and medial walls of the axilla. Note the high position of the suprascapular nerve as it runs toward the base of the coracoid process. Also note the main branches of the posterior cord: axillary nerve, and nerves to the subscapularis, latissimus dorsi and teres major.

the inferior angle of the scapula and the thoracic wall.

5. **Subscapular bursa,** situated between the upper anterior region of the scapula and the upper three ribs.

The last two bursae named have been held to be responsible for painful crepitation in the posterior region of the shoulder when the scapula is in motion, particularly during such elevation of this bone as shrugging of the shoulder.

6. **Supra-acromial bursa** (subcutanea acromialis), situated between the skin and

the dorsum of the acromion, with its base fixed to the acromion.

7. **Bursa between insertion of the trapezius** and the dorsum of the base of the spine.

## AXILLA

The neurovascular bundle streams downward under the clavicle and into a spacious compartment, the axilla. Here it begins to break up into component parts vital to the upper extremity. Many disorders of the upper extremity and the shoulder require

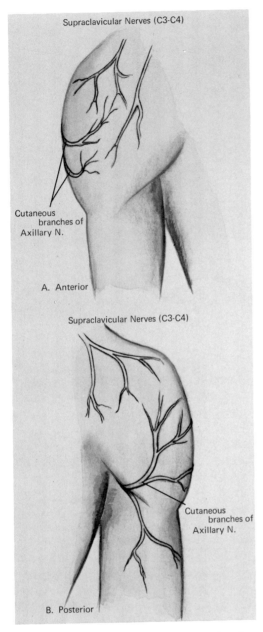

FIG. 4-35. Cutaneous nerve supply of the anterior (A) and posterior (B) aspects of the shoulder.

The axilla is cone shaped, with its apex formed by the subscapularis and the scapula, posteriorly, the serratus anterior, ribs and intercostales, medially, and the pectoralis major and minor, anteriorly (Fig. 4-33). Below the apex it rapidly expands and presents four walls: The anterior wall comprises pectoralis major, pectoralis minor and subclavius muscles; the posterior wall consists of subscapularis, latissimus dorsi and teres major; the medial wall is formed by serratus anterior and the lateral wall by the humerus in the region of the intertubercular sulcus.

### Anterior Structures of the Axilla

These elements (see Fig. 4-13) are particularly vulnerable in anterior surgical approaches to the shoulder. Immediately behind the anterior wall, under the pectoralis minor, beneath the clavipectoral fascia, lies the neurovascular bundle. A finger's breadth below the tip of the coracoid process under the pectoralis minor lies the axillary artery between the lateral and medial cords of the brachial plexus. Medial to the artery is the axillary vein.

Just below the lower edge of the pectoralis minor the lateral and medial cords give off the lateral and medial roots of the median nerve. Lateral to the lateral roots lies the musculocutaneous nerve and medial to the medial root lies the ulnar nerve.

### Posterior and Medial Walls of the Axilla (Fig. 4-34)

The posterior cord and its terminal branches the axillary and radial nerves lie immediately under the axillary artery close to the medial wall at the level of and under the pectoralis minor. In this location the cord gives off three important motor nerves, one to the latissimus dorsi, one to the subscapularis and one to the teres major. The nerve to the serratus anterior is seen coursing vertically downward, clinging to the muscle throughout its entire length.

surgical invasion of this area. Today, more and more orthopaedic surgeons are employing the axillary approach to this region. Hence it is evident that comprehension of the anatomical relationship of the structures in the axilla is essential.

The other two nerves run obliquely downward on the fleshy subscapularis muscle.

High in the axilla the suprascapular nerve is seen passing toward the root of the coracoid process on its way to the suprascapular notch. At the lower border of the subscapularis muscle, the axillary artery gives off its largest branch, the subscapular artery. The axillary nerve together with the posterior circumflex humeral artery can be seen entering the quadrangular space.

It is apparent from the above relationships that while working on the anterior aspect of the shoulder in the region of the subscapularis muscle, such as in performing a repair for recurrent dislocation of the shoulder, the musculocutaneous nerve which occupies a position high on the muscle can readily be injured. Also, just below it at the lower border of the subscapularis the axillary nerve and the posterior circumflex humeral artery as they enter the quadrangular space are vulnerable to injury.

## NERVE SUPPLY TO THE SHOULDER JOINT

Gardner has contributed much information on the nerve supply to the shoulder joint. This region, both the superficial and deep structures, is richly innervated by a network of nerve fibers derived chiefly from C-5, C-6 and C-7, although C-4 may also add a minor contribution. It is an established anatomical rule that nerves crossing a joint give off branches to the joint. Therefore, the nerves supplying the ligaments, the capsule and the synovial membrane are the axillary, suprascapular, subscapular and musculocutaneous nerves; in some instances branches from the posterior cord also reach the joint.

The size and number of fibers from these nerves to the joint is not constant. Some shoulder joints may receive a greater supply from the axillary than from the musculocutaneous nerve; in other joints the reverse is true.

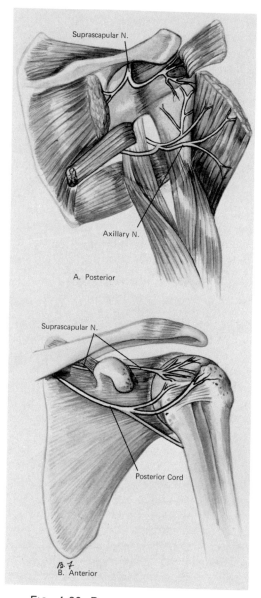

FIG. 4-36. Deep nerve supply of the posterior (A) and anterior (B) aspects of the shoulder.

### Nerve Supply to the Anterior Region of the Shoulder

The skin is supplied by the supraclavicular nerves derived from C-3 and C-4 and the terminal branches of the sensory branch of the axillary nerve, the lateral brachial cutaneous nerve. The latter nerve is a continuation of the posterior branch of the axillary which divides into an anterior and a posterior branch at its exit from the quadrangular space (Figs. 4-35 and 4-36).

The deep structures of the joint proper are innervated primarily by branches from the axillary nerve, and, to a lesser degree, by contributions from the suprascapular nerve. In some instances the musculocutaneous nerve may send some nerve twigs to the top of the joint. In addition, either the subscapular or the posterior cord may send some fibers to the anterior aspect of the joint after piercing the subscapularis muscle (Figs. 4-35 and 4-36).

## Nerve Supply to the Posterior and Superior Regions of the Shoulder

The supraclavicular nerves supply the skin of the superior and the upper posterior aspects of the shoulder. The lower posterior and lateral aspects are innervated by the lateral brachial cutaneous nerve (Figs. 4-35 and 4-36).

Superiorly the deep structures derive some of their nerve supply from the two branches of the suprascapular nerve. One branch proceeds anteriorly as far as the coracoid process and the coracoacromial ligament; the other reaches the posterior aspect of the joint. In addition, the axillary and musculocutaneous nerves and, in some instances, branches from the lateral anterior thoracic nerve contribute to the nerve supply of the superior aspect of the joint. Posteriorly the chief nerve supply is the suprascapular, supplying the upper region, and the axillary, supplying the lower region of the joint. (Figs. 4-35 and 4-36).

## BIBLIOGRAPHY

Bankart, A. S. B.: Recurrent or habitual dislocation of the shoulder joint. Brit. Med. J., 2:1-132, 1923.
_____: The pathology and treatment of recurrent dislocation of the shoulder joint. Brit. J. Surg., 26:23, 1938.

Bateman, J. E.: The shoulder and environs. St. Louis, C. V. Mosby, 1955.
Bost, F. C., and Inman, V. T.: The pathological changes in recurrent dislocation of the shoulder. J. Bone & Joint Surg., 24:595, 1942.
Broca, A., and Hartmann, H.: Contribution a l'étude des luxations de l'épaule, Bull. Soc. Anat. (Paris), (5 me. Série) 4:312, 1890.
_____: Contribution a l'étude des luxations de l'épaule (Luxations anciennes, luxations récidivantes), Bull. Soc. Anat. (Paris), (5me Série) 4:416, 1890.
Callander, C. L.: Surgical Anatomy. Philadelphia, W. B. Saunders, 1936.
Copenhaver, W. M., and Johnson, D. D. (eds.). Bailey's Textbook of Histology. Ed. 14. Baltimore, Williams & Wilkins, 1958.
Delorme, T. L.: Die Hemmungsbänder des Schultergelenks und ihre Bedeutung für die Schulterluxationen. Arch. klin. Chir., 92:79, 1910.
Fick, R.: Handbuch der Anatomie und Mechanik der Gelenke. In: v. Bardeleben: Handbuch der Anatomie des Menschen. Vol. 2, Sect. 1, Part 1. pp. 163-187. Jena, Gustav Fischer, 1910.
Finerty, J. C., and Cowdry, E. V.: A Textbook of Histology. Ed. 5. Philadelphia, Lea & Febiger, 1960.
Gardner, E.: Innervation of the shoulder joint. Anat. Rec., 102:1, 1948.
Gardner, E., and Gray, D. J.: Prenatal development of the human shoulder and acromioclavicular joints. Am. J. Anat., 92:219, 1953.
Greep, R. O.: Histology. New York, Blakiston, 1954.
Grant, J. C. Boileau: A Method of Anatomy. Baltimore, Williams & Wilkins, 1940.
_____: An Atlas of Anatomy. Baltimore, Williams & Wilkins, 1943.
Gross, C. M. (ed.): Gray's Anatomy. Ed. 28. Philadelphia, Lea & Febiger, 1966.
Haines, R. W.: The development of joints. J. Anat., 81:33, 1947.
Ham, A. W.: Histology. Ed. 6. Philadelphia, J. B. Lippincott, 1969.
Landsmeer, J. M. F., and Meyers, K. A. E.: The shoulder region exposed by anatomical dissection. Arch. Chir. Neerland., 11:274, 1959.
McGregor, A. L.: A Synopsis of Surgical Anatomy. Ed. 6. Baltimore, Williams & Wilkins, 1946.
McLaughlin, H. L.: Recurrent anterior dislocation of the shoulder. I. Morbid anatomy. Am. J. Surg., 99:628, 1960.
McLaughlin, H. L., and Cavallaro, W. U.: Primary anterior dislocation of the shoulder. Am. J. Surg., 80:615, 1950.

Moseley, H. F.: The use of a metallic glenoid rim in recurrent dislocation of the shoulder. Canad. Ass. J., 56:320, 1947.

————: Athletic injuries to the shoulder region. Am. J. Surg., 98:401, 1959.

————: Recurrent Dislocation of the Shoulder, Montreal, McGill University Press, 1961.

Moseley, H. F., and Overgaard, K.: The anterior capsular mechanism in recurrent anterior dislocation of the shoulder. J. Bone & Joint Surg., 44-B:913-926, 1962.

Olsson, O.: Degenerative changes of the shoulder joint and their connection with shoulder pain. Acta chir. scand., (Suppl.) 181, 1953.

Perkins, G.: Rest and movement. J. Bone & Joint Surg., 35-B:521, 1953.

Ranson, S. W.: The anatomy of the nervous system. Philadelphia, W. B. Saunders, 1940.

Sabotta, McMurrich: Atlas of Human Anatomy, New York, G. E. Stechert, 1932.

Schlemm, F.: Ueber die Verstärkungsbander am Schultergelenk. Arch. Anat., Physiol., wissensch. Med. p. 45, 1853.

Sutton, J. B.: On the nature of ligaments (part II). J. Anat. Physiol., 19:27, 1884.

Townley, C. O.: The capsular mechanism in recurrent dislocation of the shoulder. J. Bone & Joint Surg., 32-A:370, 1950.

Welcker, H.: Ueber das Hüftgelenk, nebst einigen Bemerkungen über Gelenke überhaupt, insbesondere über das Schultergelenk. Z. Anat. Entwicklungsgesch., 1:41, 1876.

# 5

# Biomechanics of the Shoulder

In the shoulder girdle man has evolved a delicate, intricate mechanism which permits the prehensile hand to be placed in any desired position in relation to the trunk. To achieve this, the shoulder is capable of an almost complete range of global motion. In order to gain this wide range of mobility the shoulder girdle has sacrificed much of its stability; nevertheless, it has developed active and passive mechanisms which provide optimum stability. Impairment of any one of the mechanisms is reflected in the total performance of the arm-trunk mechanism.

The multiplane action of the shoulder is a summation of movements of a complex system of joints which function synchronously to produce precise, coordinated movements. From a functional viewpoint the shoulder joint comprises four distinct articulations: (1) the scapulohumeral, (2) the sternoclavicular, (3) the acromioclavicular and (4) the scapulothoracic. Although the last-named structure is not a true joint, it must be considered as such functionally (Fig. 5-1).

Before describing the intricate mechanism of each of these components and the role they play in the overall function of the shoulder girdle, a group of simple descriptive terms must be evolved which will pinpoint the exact position of the extremity in relation to the trunk. This is a difficult task and many workers have given the problem much time and thought. The terminology proposed by Codman helped considerably to solve this enigma. Yet, it fell short of perfection because it failed to provide terms that would locate the arm

in the horizontal plane. The problem is made even more difficult by the universal adoption of certain descriptive terms such as *forward flexion, backward extension* and *abduction,* which somehow must be included in any new terminology proposed.

In 1965 the American Academy of Orthopaedic Surgeons put out a pamphlet, "Joint Motion," a product of several committees assigned to this task. The section dealing with movements of the shoulder indicates that the problem was given much thought and analyzed clearly. The committee introduced the terms *horizontal flexion* and *horizontal extension* to define the horizontal coordinates. This system adequately locates the arm in both the vertical and the horizontal planes. However, there are several terms used which I am sure will lead to confusion and will not be universally accepted. "Adduction" in the frontal plane is used to indicate "motion of the arm toward the midline of the body or beyond it in an upward plane." This gives to the term *adduction* a connotation including an element of elevation, which is contrary to the teaching of the planes of movements of all joints. Also the term *abduction* is used too loosely; it is employed to indicate elevation of the arm in the coronal plane and also elevation of the arm in varying positions of horizontal extension.

It is my opinion that by eliminating the terms *adduction* and *abduction* when the latter indicates elevation of the arm in some coordinate of horizontal extension and substituting the term *elevation* in degrees, confusion would be eliminated and the terminology would be accepted uni-

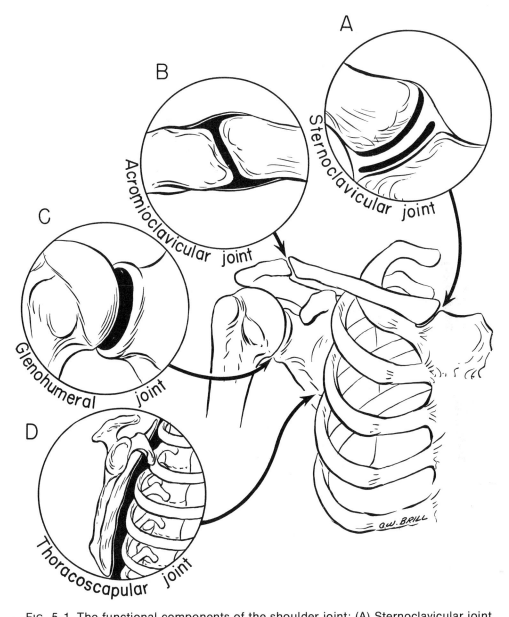

FIG. 5-1. The functional components of the shoulder joint: (A) Sternoclavicular joint. (B) Acromioclavicular joint. (C) Glenohumeral joint. (D) Thoracoscapular joint.

versally more readily. All movements of the arm are related to the planes of the body (Fig. 5-2).

## VERTICAL MOTION OF THE ARM

*Abduction:* upward motion of the arm in the coronal plane only. *This term is not to be employed for upward motion of the arm in any other plane.* The range is from 0° to 180° (Fig. 5-3).

*Forward flexion:* upward motion of the arm in the anterior sagittal plane only. The range is from 0° to 180° (Fig. 5-4).

*Backward extension:* upward motion of the arm in the posterior sagittal plane only.

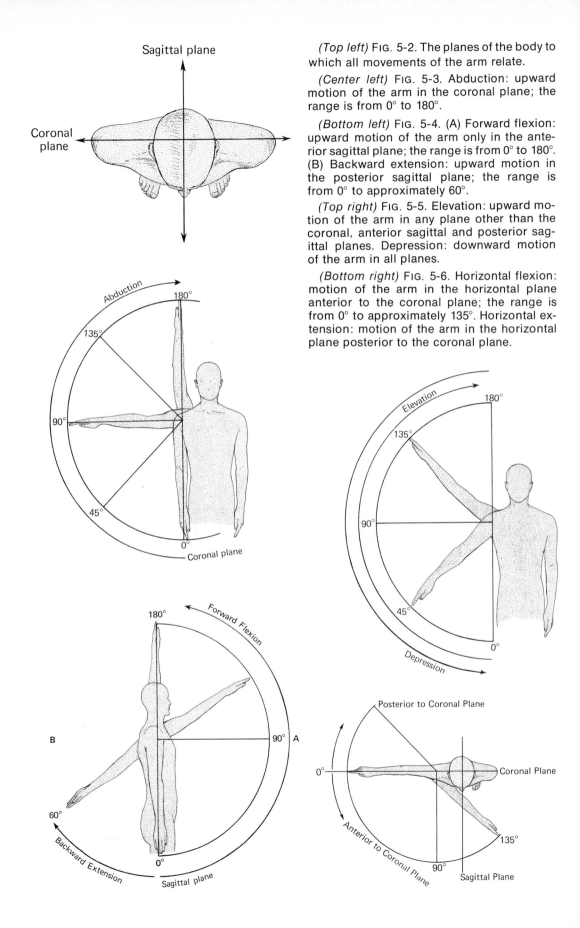

*(Top left)* FIG. 5-2. The planes of the body to which all movements of the arm relate.

*(Center left)* FIG. 5-3. Abduction: upward motion of the arm in the coronal plane; the range is from 0° to 180°.

*(Bottom left)* FIG. 5-4. (A) Forward flexion: upward motion of the arm only in the anterior sagittal plane; the range is from 0° to 180°. (B) Backward extension: upward motion in the posterior sagittal plane; the range is from 0° to approximately 60°.

*(Top right)* FIG. 5-5. Elevation: upward motion of the arm in any plane other than the coronal, anterior sagittal and posterior sagittal planes. Depression: downward motion of the arm in all planes.

*(Bottom right)* FIG. 5-6. Horizontal flexion: motion of the arm in the horizontal plane anterior to the coronal plane; the range is from 0° to approximately 135°. Horizontal extension: motion of the arm in the horizontal plane posterior to the coronal plane.

Sagittal plane

Coronal plane

Abduction
180°
135°
90°
45°
0°
Coronal plane

Forward Flexion
180°
90° A
B
60°
Backward Extension
0°
Sagittal plane

Elevation
180°
135°
90°
45°
0°
Depression

Posterior to Coronal Plane
0°
Coronal Plane
Anterior to Coronal Plane
90°
135°
Sagittal Plane

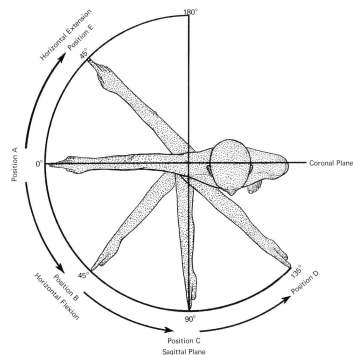

FIG. 5-7. (A–E). (A) The arm is abducted 90°; this refers to elevation only in the coronal plane. (B) Elevation of the arm in 45° of horizontal flexion. (C) The arm is elevated 90° in the anterior sagittal plane; this position is described as 90° of forward flexion. (D) The arm is elevated at 135° of horizontal flexion. (E) The arm is elevated backward at 45° of horizontal extension.

The range is from 0° to approximately 60° (Fig. 5-4).

*Elevation:* upward motion of the arm in any plane other than the coronal, anterior sagittal and posterior sagittal planes (Fig. 5-5).

*Depression:* downward motion of the arm in all planes (Fig. 5-5).

## HORIZONTAL MOTION OF THE ARM

*Horizontal flexion:* motion of the arm in the horizontal plane anterior to the coronal plane across the body. The range is from 0° to approximately 135° (Fig. 5-6).

*Horizontal extension:* motion of the arm in the horizontal plane posterior to the coronal plane (Fig. 5-6).

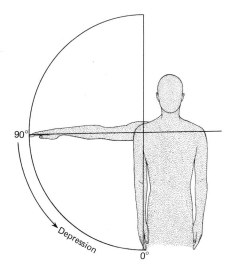

FIG. 5-8. The arm is depressed from 90° to 0° of abduction.

## APPLICATION OF PROPOSED TERMINOLOGY (Figs. 5-7, 5-8 and 5-9)

**A:** Abduction—the arm is abducted 90°; this refers to elevation in the coronal plane only.

**B:** Elevation of the arm in 45° of horizontal flexion. If the arm is elevated 90°, the arm would be located at 45° of horizontal flexion and 90° of elevation.

**C:** The arm is elevated 90° in the anterior sagittal plane; this position is described as 90° of forward flexion.

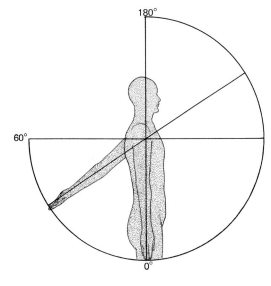

**D:** The arm is elevated at 135° horizontal flexion. If the arm is elevated 90°, the location is 90° of elevation and 135° of horizontal flexion.

**E:** The arm is elevated backward at 45° of horizontal extension. If the arm is elevated 90°, the location is 90° of elevation and 45° of horizontal extension.

### ROTATION (Fig. 5-10)

This motion can be measured, in any position, where the horizontal and vertical planes cross. As a rule, it is measured in two positions: (a) with the arm at the side, and (b) with the arm abducted 90°. The measurement is recorded in degrees of motion from the neutral starting position.

The arm can also be internally rotated behind the trunk. This motion always is accompanied by varying degrees of extension of the shoulder girdle.

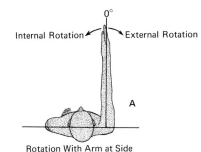

### MOTION OF THE SHOULDER GIRDLE

*Flexion and Extension* (Fig. 5-11): Forward and backward motions of the shoulder girdle are performed chiefly by the scapula and clavicle and the joints connecting them. The motions are measured in degrees, starting from the neutral position.

*Elevation and Depression* (Fig. 5-11): Upward motion of the shoulder girdle is designated elevation; and downward motion, depression of the shoulder; like flexion and extension, these motions are executed primarily by the scapula and clavicle. They are measured in degrees, starting from the neutral position.

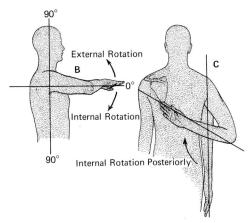

### GLENOHUMERAL MOTION (Fig. 5-12)

Elevation of the arm is a smooth, continuous, rhythmical motion from beginning to end; all the components of the shoulder joint participate, namely the glenohumeral, sternoclavicular, acromioclavicular and scapulothoracic joints. The last three articulations are concerned primarily with stabilization of the shoulder

*(Top)* FIG. 5-9. The arm is in backward extension, a term used only if the arm is elevated in the posterior sagittal plane.

*(Bottom)* FIG. 5-10. Rotation (A) with the arm at the side; (B) with the arm abducted 90°. (C) Internal rotation posteriorly.

FIG. 5-11. (A) Extension and flexion of the shoulder girdle; (B) elevation and depression of the shoulder girdle.

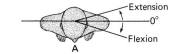

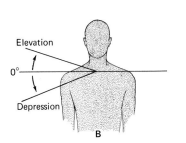

girdle and with moving the scapula upward and forward around the thoracic wall. Codman designated this complex of movements "scapulohumeral rhythm," a very appropriate term.

Under normal conditions the arm can be actively elevated from zero to 180°. One can readily determine the range of motion in the glenohumeral joint and that in the scapulothoracic joint (Fig. 5-12): With the arm at the side in the neutral position, the scapula is fixed with one hand while the other hand elevates the arm from the neutral position. With the scapula fixed, passive elevation in normal subjects is possible to approximately 90° (active elevation is possible to 120°). If the arm is raised beyond 120°, the scapula will shift up and forward under the hand; this motion of the

scapula continues until the arm reaches 180° of elevation.

## SOME PECULIARITIES OF SHOULDER MOTIONS

### Abduction

Elevation in the coronal plane is called abduction. To achieve complete elevation

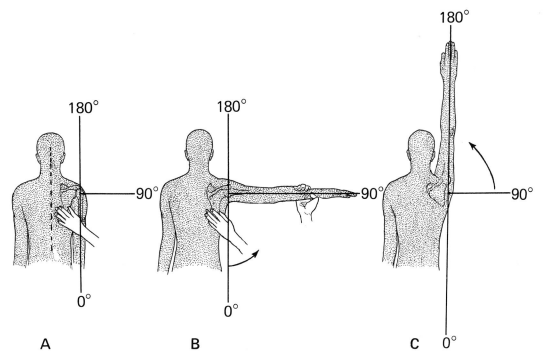

FIG. 5-12. (A and B) Motion at the glenohumeral joint. (C) Motion in the glenohumeral and the scapulothoracic joints.

in the coronal plane, the arm must be rotated externally. If the arm is fully rotated internally and then raised in the coronal plane it will lock below the horizontal position. Elevation to the vertical position can be attained only if the arm is first rotated externally 90°. Locking at the horizontal position is brought about by impingement of the tuberosities against the acromion process; by external rotation of the arm, the tuberosities are placed so that they pass beneath the acromion when the arm is elevated to 180°.

### Forward Flexion

Elevation of the extremity in the sagittal plane is termed forward flexion. This position is possible only when the arm is rotated internally. Forward flexion in man is the equivalent of extension in the quadruped. If the arm is elevated in the sagittal plane in a position of external rotation, it locks at about 45° above the horizontal and further elevation is impossible. Internal rotation of the arm (45°) permits it to be raised to complete elevation.

### Pivotal Position

Regardless of the plane in which the arm ascends to reach complete elevation, the ultimate position of the humeral head in relation to the glenoid cavity, the coracoid process and the acromion process is the same. Codman designated this the "pivotal position." In this position no rotation is possible, either internally or externally. A fracture, a dislocation or both will occur if the humerus is forced beyond the fixed position.

With the arm at the side and the elbow flexed, the condyles of the lower end of the humerus are in the transverse plane. In this position the arm can be rotated internally 90° and externally approximately 90°, a total range of roughly 180°. As the arm is elevated, regardless of the horizontal plane of ascent, the range of rotation

gradually diminishes until the arm reaches the pivotal position. Here the internal condyle of the humerus points forward, and no rotation is possible.

During elevation, the arm will lock at various levels, depending upon the degree of rotation of the humerus. If rotation in the appropriate plane is not hindered, elevation is completed in a smooth, rhythmical fashion. However, if rotation of the humerus in the correct plane is obstructed and the arm is forced beyond the locked position, dislocation or fracture of the humeral head results.

It is essential to understand these characteristics of the shoulder mechanism in order to comprehend the basic principles underlying the mechanism of dislocation and fractures of the head of the humerus.

## MOTION AT THE SHOULDER JOINT

Inman, Saunders and Abbott, in their work on the functional mechanism of the shoulder joint, carried still further the observations of Codman. They broke down the movements of the shoulder joint into successive phases and established the sequence and identified the component of the shoulder joint responsible for each phase. Moreover, they developed a fundamental principle in shoulder mechanism, the "muscle force couple."

It is fallacious that in abduction of the arm the first 90° occurs in the glenohumeral joint and the next 90° in the scapulothoracic articulation (rotation of the scapula on the chest wall). Elevation of the extremity in flexion and abduction is the result of synchronous and continuous motion of all the elements of the shoulder joint complex. Four elements or components constitute this complex: (1) the glenohumeral, (2) the sternoclavicular, (3) the acromioclavicular and (4) the scapulothoracic joint.

### Glenohumeral Joint Motion

Elevation of the arm in the coronal plane (abduction) or in the sagittal plane (forward

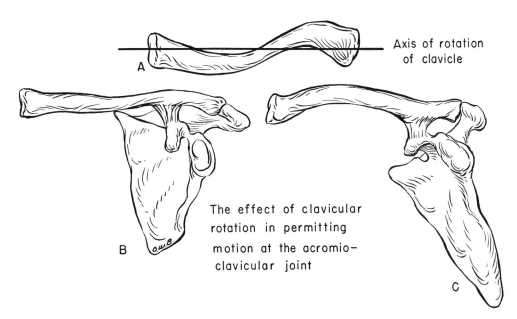

FIG. 5-13. The clavicle rotates on its long axis like a crankshaft; the configuration of the clavicle makes this possible. Its outer third is curved, producing a relative lengthening of the coracoclavicular ligaments when it rotates on its long axis. (Redrawn from Inman, V.T., Saunders, J.B., and Abbott, L.C.: J. Bone & Joint Surg., *26:2,* 1944)

flexion) is produced by simultaneous motion in the glenohumeral and the scapulothoracic articulations. During the first 30° of abduction and 60° of flexion, the scapula finds a position of stability in relation to the humerus. This is attained either by the scapula's remaining fixed (all motion occurring in the glenohumeral joint until the position of stabilization is reached) or shifting laterally or medially, or even oscillating until it is fixed by the humerus. This irregular preliminary period has been designated the "setting-stage."

From this point, the ratio of motion in the two joints is constant until full elevation is complete; the ratio is two degrees of humeral motion to one of scapular, 10° of motion occurring at the glenohumeral and 5° at the scapulothoracic articulation for every 15° of elevation of the arm. Total scapular motion is 60°; and total glenohumeral motion is 120°. Also, it was demonstrated that motion may occur independently in the above joints. By fixation of the scapula the arm can be abducted to 90°

passively and 120° actively. Loss of scapular motion, however, decreases the power of abduction by a third.

The clavicle plays a significant role in elevation of the arm. Any interference with normal motion at either end of the clavicle is reflected in the total range of elevation. Normal scapular rotation on the chest wall is dependent upon unrestricted motion at the sternoclavicular and the acromioclavicular joints.

### Sternoclavicular Joint Motion

This joint permits 40° of elevation of the clavicle during elevation of the arm, the ratio being 4° of elevation of the clavicle for every 10° of elevation of the arm. The range of clavicular elevation is expended during the first 90° of elevation of the arm.

### Acromioclavicular Joint Motion

In this joint 20° of motion occurs. Motion occurs in two separate phases of elevation; part of it takes place in the first 30° and the remainder after 135° of elevation has been attained. The clavicle is bound firmly to the coracoid process and the acromion by the coracoclavicular ligaments. Motion of this joint is made possible only by the configuration of the clavicle. Its outer third is curved, so that a relative lengthening of the coracoclavicular ligaments occurs when the clavicle is rotated on its long axis, thereby allowing a certain range of free motion at this joint.

The clavicle really acts like a crankshaft (Fig. 5-13). The amount of motion occurring in both the sternoclavicular and the acromioclavicular joints is equivalent to the amount of scapular rotation on the chest wall (60°).

### Practical Significance

It is apparent, from the preceding discussion of motion at the shoulder joint, that obliteration of motion at either end of the clavicle, surgically or by disease, results in restriction of arm elevation equal to the amount of motion lost in the affected joints. Therefore, reconstructive surgical procedures should aim to preserve or restore motion in the sternoclavicular and the acromioclavicular articulations. In these joints arthrodesing procedures or their equivalents are never justified. On the other hand, excision of the outer end of the clavicle, combined with arthrodesis of the glenohumeral joint, may be valuable to secure increase in the range of abduction.

### MECHANICAL FORCE REQUIREMENTS FOR MOTION AT THE SHOULDER JOINT

The meticulous work of Inman, Saunders and Abbott disclosed that equilibrium at the glenohumeral joint, regardless of the position of the arm, was the result of three forces: (1) the weight of the extremity, acting at its center of gravity, (2) muscular masses responsible for abduction (chiefly the deltoid), and (3) the resultant of the above two forces, which acts through a center of rotation but in a direction opposite that of the deltoid.

The third force also is the resultant of two other components, namely, (1) a passive component, the friction and the pressure of the humeral head against the glenoid cavity, and (2) the active component, the downward pull of the infraspinous muscles (infraspinatus, teres minor and subscapularis). This last force is represented by a force acting at right angles to the plane of the glenoid cavity and the other parallel to the axillary border of the scapula.

The force of elevation (pull of the deltoid), together with the active component of the third force (downward pull of the infraspinous muscles), establishes the "muscle force couple" necessary for elevation of the limb. The magnitude of the force required to bring the limb to 90° of elevation was found to be 8.2 times the weight of the extremity. Beyond 90°, the force requirements decreased progressively, reaching zero at 180°. The force requirements of the lower component of the muscle force couple (downward pull of the infraspinous muscles) attained its maximum at 60°, at which point the force requirements were 9.6 times the weight of the limb. Beyond 90° a progressive decrease of the magnitude of the force was noted, reaching zero at 135°.

The same basic principle of the muscle force couple operates in scapular rotation. Three forces are responsible for rotation of the scapula on the chest wall during elevation of the extremity: (1) a force that supports the weight of the shoulder girdle, operating in a vertical and upward direction; (2) a force acting on the acromion in a medial direction, and (3) a force acting on the inferior angle of the scapula (serratus anterior muscle).

The force operating from the region of the acromion is a resultant of a passive component, represented by the resistance of the clavicle, and an active component, the upper portion of the trapezius which, here, assumes a dual function by aiding in the support of the shoulder girdle.

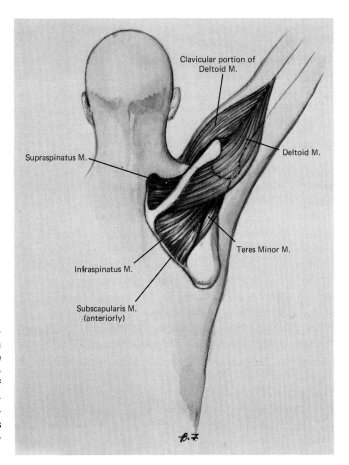

Clavicular portion of Deltoid M.

Supraspinatus M.

Deltoid M.

Teres Minor M.

Infraspinatus M.

Subscapularis M. (anteriorly)

FIG. 5-14. The upper component of the force couple in abduction and flexion of the arm is comprised of the deltoid, the clavicular portion of pectoralis major and the supraspinatus. The lower component of the unit consists of subscapularis, infraspinatus and teres minor.

The second and the third forces establish the muscle force couple essential for rotation of the scapula; they operate in opposite directions and are of equal magnitude, reaching their maximum at 90° of elevation, then dropping progressively to zero at 180°.

Some very significant characteristics are exhibited by the trapezius muscle. At rest its function is entirely supportive; during the early phase of elevation of the arm from zero to 35°, because of the shift in the angle of action of the muscle, it has two functions — supportive and rotatory. From 35° to 140° its rotatory efficiency progressively increases, reaching its maximum at 90°. Beyond 140° its supportive efficiency steadily increases, while its rotatory decreases.

By means of electromyographic studies Inman, Saunders and Abbott were able to confirm the validity of their conclusions reached in their comparative anatomical studies and analysis of the mechanical force requirements of the shoulder mechanism. As a result of these studies, muscles participating in shoulder motion were grouped into functional units. Since the publication of these observations, many electromyographers interested in the problem of shoulder movements have confirmed the classic work of Inman et al. Among these were Basmajian, Wertheimer and Ferraz; and Scheving and Pauly.

## ABDUCTORS AND FLEXORS OF THE HUMERUS

This group comprises: (1) deltoid, (2) pectoralis major and (3) supraspinatus muscles. All three act as a single functional unit in abduction and flexion of the arm. The sum of the action currents of the individual muscles of this group produces a smooth, regular curve in both flexion and abduction. The curve of flexion reaches its summit at 110°, the curve of abduction at 90°; the former is of slightly greater amplitude (Fig. 5-14).

### Deltoid

The activity of the deltoid increases progressively, reaching its peak between 90° and 180° of elevation. In abduction this muscle exhibits total potential greater than that recorded in flexion. The three parts of the deltoid are active in all movements of the arm. However, the anterior part is more active than the posterior part in flexion and medial rotation, the posterior part is more active in extension and lateral rotation, and the middle part is most active in abduction. It appears that, when one part of the deltoid functions as the prime mover, the other parts contract in order to stabilize the head in the glenoid cavity.

### Pectoralis Major

Various portions of this muscle exhibit differences in activity, depending upon the character of the motion executed. In abduction no activity is demonstrable in any portion of the pectoralis major; in flexion the clavicular portion of the muscle is most active, acting synchronously with the deltoid. Some activity, but to a lesser degree, is also discernible in the manubrial fibers of the sternocostal head. The remaining fibers of the pectoralis major disclose no activity in flexion or abduction.

### Supraspinatus

Functionally the most significant feature of the supraspinatus is that it operates synchronously and simultaneously with the deltoid in all phases of abduction and flexion. Codman was the first to observe this, but he was unable to demonstrate it experimentally. Later, Inman, Saunders

and Abbott provided such demonstration, thus dispelling the old concept that the supraspinatus muscle initiated abduction and thereafter the movement was completed by the deltoid muscle.

## DEPRESSORS OF THE HUMERUS

The infraspinous muscles including subscapularis, infraspinatus and teres minor, comprise this unit. As previously indicated, this functional unit constitutes the inferior component of the muscle force couple during flexion and abduction of the extremity. All three elements function simultaneously throughout the entire arcs of motion.

Despite the fact that teres minor, from a morphological viewpoint, originally was part of the deltoid muscle, it behaves in a fashion similar to the infraspinatus throughout its various phases of activity both in flexion and in abduction of the extremity.

## SCAPULAR ROTATORS

This important functional group comprises trapezius, serratus anterior and levator scapulae. Various portions of the trapezius and the serratus anterior perform different functions. The upper component of the muscle force couple is required for rotation of the scapula and consists of the upper portion of the trapezius, the levator scapulae and upper digitations of the serratus anterior. All three elements operate as a single unit with two functions. Besides being the upper component of the force couple necessary for scapular rotation, the unit supports the shoulder girdle passively and also elevates it (Fig. 5-15).

The inferior component of the force couple consists of the lower portions of the trapezius and the lower digitations of the serratus anterior. Both act continuously in a similar fashion, except that in abduction the lower trapezius is more active than in flexion, during which movement it relaxes in order to permit the scapula to slip forward. At this phase of flexion the serratus

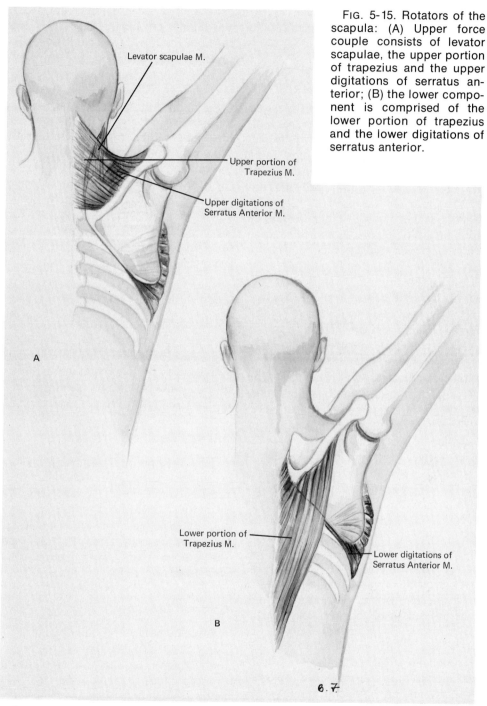

FIG. 5-15. Rotators of the scapula: (A) Upper force couple consists of levator scapulae, the upper portion of trapezius and the upper digitations of serratus anterior; (B) the lower component is comprised of the lower portion of trapezius and the lower digitations of serratus anterior.

Levator scapulae M.

Upper portion of Trapezius M.

Upper digitations of Serratus Anterior M.

A

Lower portion of Trapezius M.

Lower digitations of Serratus Anterior M.

B

anterior (lower digitations) assumes the predominant role of the lower force couple.

The middle portion of the trapezius and the rhomboids act as stabilizers of the scapula during abduction, relaxing in flex-ion to permit rotation of the scapula on the thorax.

The teres major muscle has an interesting role in the functional mechanics of the shoulder joint. It discloses no evidence of any activity during motion; activity is demonstrable only when maintenance of a static position is required.

## PRACTICAL SIGNIFICANCE OF MUSCLE FORCE COUPLE PRINCIPLE

In the light of the observations discussed in the previous section, it is clear that free, complete motion at the shoulder joint can be achieved only when efficient force couples (as described for glenohumeral motion and scapular rotation) are functioning. Therefore, all reconstructive proceddures about the shoulder aiming to restore motion in paralytic disorders of this region must re-establish the force couple mechanism which insists on "rearrangement rather than substitution" of muscles.

The belief that power in the deltoid assures abduction of the arm must be discarded. Regardless of the magnitude of deltoid activity, abduction cannot be achieved without an efficient inferior component of the force couple acting on the humeral head (depressing action of the infraspinous muscles). This essential component may be restored by transplantation of the latissimus dorsi and the teres major to the postero-inferior surface of the greater tuberosity. If these muscles are paralyzed, some stabilization of the glenohumeral joint may be attained by utilizing the biceps tendon, as in the Nicola procedure or one of its modifications.

It has been pointed out previously that only the clavicular head of the pectoralis major muscle functions as an elevator of the arm in flexion; hence, this portion alone can be utilized as an abductor, the remaining portions showing activity only in adduction and medial rotation of the limb. Any procedure designed to use the sterno-costal elements as abductors is doomed to failure. No amount of re-education will result in independent contraction of only a portion of the pectoralis major; it always performs as a whole when voluntarily contracted. Therefore, its sternocostal portion can be utilized as a lateral rotator.

The muscles supporting the scapula (leva-tor scapulae, the rhomboids and the upper and middle portions of trapezius) make it possible for the force couple essential for scapular rotation to operate. In paralysis of these supporting muscles the scapula may be stabilized by fascial transplant from the lower cervical spinous process to the base of the spine of the scapula or its upper border (Lowman), thereby re-establishing the fulcrum which is necessary for performance of the force couple.

Muscles, such as teres major, which demonstrate activity only in static positions, cannot be made to assume active roles during motion of the extremity. Therefore, teres major cannot be utilized to replace the infraspinous group.

### Adduction

Latissimus dorsi and pectoralis major produce adduction. Activity is also noted in the posterior fibers of the deltoid. This activity may be to prevent internal rotation of the arm, which would result if the action of the adductors were not resisted.

### Internal Rotation

This motion is performed primarily by latissimus dorsi and subscapularis. As mentioned previously, teres major shows no activity during any motion of the arm; activity is present only when a static position must be maintained. Pectoralis major shows activity only when internal rotation is resisted.

### External Rotation

Infraspinatus, teres minor and the posterior fibers of the deltoid are the prime external rotators of the arm. In elevation of the arm external rotation must be attained before complete elevation is achieved.

## IMPORTANT MUSCLE SYSTEMS OF THE SHOULDER GIRDLE

In order to meet the many demands of a mobile yet stable shoulder girdle some muscles have developed intricate functional systems. The muscles concerned are deltoid, trapezius, serratus anterior and pectoralis major. In general, one finds that the action of any one of these muscles differs in its individual parts. Study of the comparative anatomy of these muscles reveals that the functional changes found in man were necessary in order to free the extremity and permit it to perform in an almost complete range of global motion.

## Deltoid Muscle System (Fig. 5-16)

As previously noted, the deltoid is a massive, triangular muscle draping itself around the anterior, lateral and posterior aspects of the bony girdle of the shoulder, and its fleshy fibers converge distally, forming a stout tendon that inserts into the deltoid tubercle. The arrangement of the anterior and posterior fibers differs from that of the central fibers. The oblique central fibers arise pinnate fashion from either side of four or five tendinous bands whose proximal ends are attached to the acromion. These bands proceed distally parallel to one another and then disappear in the substance of the muscle. Three or four similar bands arise from the tendinous insertion of the muscle and pass upward into the muscle substance, alternating with those passing downward. The oblique muscle fibers arising from the descending septa insert into the ascending septa. Such an arrangement does not exist on the anterior and posterior parts of the deltoid.

Study of the comparative anatomy of this muscle discloses that its power has been increased in two ways: (1) by an increase in both absolute and relative size (it comprises 41% of the mass of the scapulohumeral group—supraspinatus, infraspinatus, teres minor, subscapularis, deltoid and teres major) and (2) by the increased leverage attained by the increase in size of the acromion and the distal migration of the deltoid insertion.

Electromyographic studies reveal that all parts of this muscle are active during

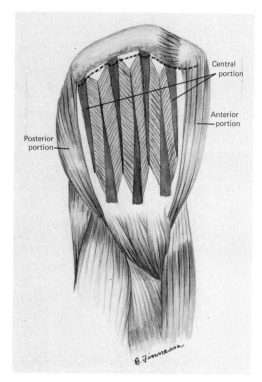

FIG. 5-16. Internal structure of central portion of the deltoid. Four septa arise from 4 bony prominences on the acromion. Three or four similar bands arise from the tendinous insertion of the muscle and pass upward into the muscle substance, alternating with those passing downward. Note how the oblique muscle fibers arising from the descending septa insert into the ascending septa.

elevation of the arm—and, also, that each part is capable of different and individual action. The anterior part is more active than the posterior in flexion of the arm and also participates in internal rotation; in extension of the arm the posterior part is more active and it participates in external rotation. In abduction the middle part is most active. As previously stated one part of the deltoid is a prime mover while the other two parts contract to fix the humeral head in the glenoid fossa. Paralysis of this muscle produces marked disturbance of function. As will be shown subsequently occasionally the supraspinatus is sufficiently powerful to achieve abduction. Also, with

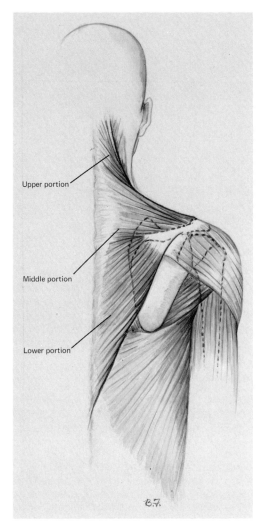

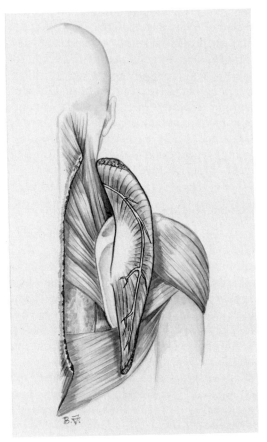

FIG. 5-18. Note the superficial course of the accessory nerve. (Trapezius has been cut and reflected downward)

FIG. 5-17. Trapezius muscle, showing its upper, middle and lower portions; the upper and lower portions are more concentrated than the middle portion.

a normal cuff mechanism abduction can be accomplished by "trick" movements employing the biceps and triceps muscles.

### Trapezius Muscle System (Fig. 5-17)

Morphologically the trapezius as found in man has changed very little from that found in the other primates. However, there has been some concentration of muscle elements along its upper and lower borders and some loss of elements in its middle

part which lies opposite the spine of the scapula. Its upper portion, through its insertion into the spine of the scapula and the acromion, functions as a suspensory mechanism for the shoulder girdle, holding it upward, backward and inward. This portion of the trapezius is also part of a functional unit acting with the levator scapulae and the upper digitations of the serratus anterior. This unit not only supports the scapula passively, but also actively elevates it (as in shrugging the shoulder), and, in addition, it is the upper component of the force couple designed to rotate the scapula. Electromyographic studies reveal activity in this unit while the arm is at rest, indicating its static postural function.

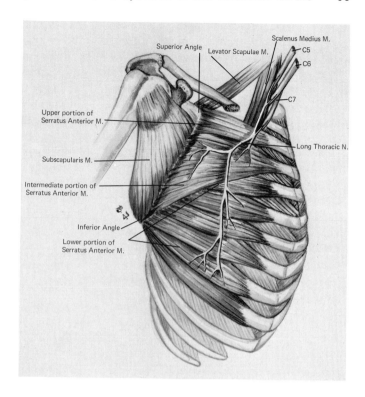

FIG. 5-19. Note concentration of the upper and lower digitations of serratus anterior; the former insert into the superior angle of the scapula and the latter into the inferior angle.

The lower portion of the trapezius works with the lower digitations of the serratus anterior, constituting the lower component of the scapular rotatory force couple. During abduction it is the more active element of the lower force couple; during flexion it has the capability to become less active and allow the scapula to slip forward. The primary function of the unit is to stabilize the scapula on the chest wall and allow only that amount of rotation of the scapula necessary for complete elevation of the arm.

The middle fibers of this system function with the rhomboid muscles, the primary role being to fix the scapula; however, they are capable of relaxing sufficiently during the early part of flexion of the arm to permit the scapula to glide forward.

Of special interest is the nerve supply to the trapezius. It is innervated by the accessory nerve, which comprises fibers from the ventral rami of C-2, C-3 and C-4. As previously noted, this nerve occupies a very superficial and vulnerable position in the posterior triangle. However, in traumatic lesions of the brachial plexus and even in paralysis following acute poliomyelitis this nerve is frequently spared, leaving the trapezius the only muscle available for reconstructive procedures (Fig. 5-18).

In the event that the muscle is paralyzed the shoulder droops downward and forward and the mechanisms producing elevation of the arm and rotation of the scapula are seriously impaired.

## Serratus Anterior Muscle System (Fig. 5-19)

Morphologically the serratus anterior has undergone considerable change. In primitive forms, levator scapulae and serratus comprise one muscle mass extending from the cervical vertebrae and the upper eight or ten ribs to the vertebral border of the scapula. In man, the muscle sheet has divided into two distinct muscles, levator scapulae and serratus anterior. The latter

exhibits even further morphological alterations; there has been a concentration of
muscle elements at the superior and inferior
angles of the scapula and a loss of elements
at its intermediate digitations. These alterations are related to the functional mechanism of the shoulder, in that the various
parts of serratus anterior differ in action.

The upper digits of serratus anterior
function as a unit with levator scapulae and
the upper part of trapezius. As previously
stated, passively, this unit supports the
scapula (and hence the shoulder girdle) and
actively, it elevates it. It is the upper component of the force couple that rotates the
scapula. The greater part of serratus anterior (its lower digits), together with the
lower part of trapezius, clamp and stabilize
the scapula to the chest wall during elevation of the arm; also it relaxes some to
permit rotation and forward and upward
displacement of the scapula. These two
muscles form the lower component of the
force couple that rotates the scapula.

Serratus anterior is supplied by the long
thoracic nerve from C-5, C-6 and C-7,
which runs superficially the entire length
of the muscle and thus is vulnerable to
trauma. Paralysis of this muscle results in
severe functional disability of the shoulder
girdle. The main stabilizer of the scapula
to the chest wall is lost and the efficiency
of the rotatory mechanism (both upper and
lower rotatory muscle force couples) is
seriously impaired.

### Pectoralis Major Muscle System

Originally the pectoral muscles were one
muscle mass. The mass separated into a
deep and a superficial stratum, giving rise
to pectoralis minor and pectoralis major.
Both show further morphological changes:
The latter shifted cephalad to gain attachment to the clavicle, and its original diffuse
insertion assumed the bilaminar configuration found in man. The insertion of the pectoralis minor became anchored to the coracoid process. Functionally the pectoralis
major has three components: the clavicular,

the manubrial and the lower sternal and
abdominal portions; these exhibit different
activity, depending upon the type of motion carried out. The clavicular portion exhibits great activity in forward flexion while
the manubrial portion shows only minimal
activity. It is apparent that in forward
flexion, the clavicular portion functions
synchronously with the anterior portion
of the deltoid. Also, as mentioned previously, the clavicular portion shows activity
only when the motion of internal rotation
is resisted.

### IMPAIRMENT OF MUSCLE FORCE COUPLE BY ISOLATED NERVE PARALYSIS AND OTHER LESIONS

Impairment of the efficiency of the muscle force couples acting upon the humerus
and the scapula by isolated muscle paralysis results in varying degrees of disability,
depending upon the muscles involved and
the importance of these components in the
performance of the force couple. Isolated
paralysis of deltoid, infraspinatus or serratus anterior causes greater disability,
whereas paralysis of supraspinatus or trapezius does not seriously impair the functional mechanism of the shoulder.

### Deltoid Paralysis

Permanent axillary nerve palsy is followed by pronounced impairment of the
upper muscle force couple necessary for
abduction and flexion of the extremity. The
deltoid mass is the most essential component of this force couple. Occasionally, a
few degrees of abduction may be achieved
by supraspinatus and the clavicular head
of pectoralis major.

In rare instances, complete abduction is
possible in spite of paralysis of the deltoid.
Abduction is accomplished by a hypertrophied supraspinatus muscle. One such case
has been studied by the author (Fig. 5-20).
The patient was able to initiate abduction
and carry the movement to completion with
normal scapulohumeral rhythm and good

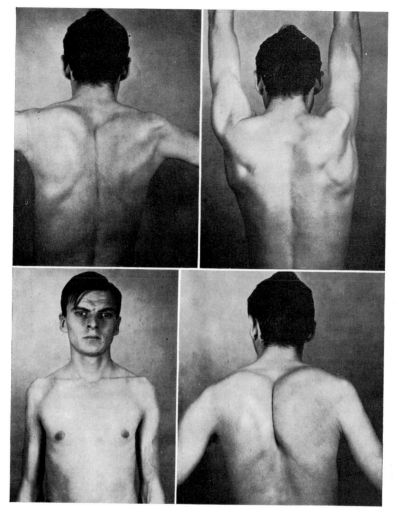

FIG. 5-20. Paralysis of the deltoid (*right*); note the complete
range of abduction of the arm produced by the supraspinatus.

power. He participated without difficulty
in athletic activities such as baseball and
golf. His only complaint was fatigue after
an unusually active day. Several such cases
have been reported in the literature. Generally, however, the supraspinatus fails to
compensate for loss of deltoid power and
the resulting impairment of function is
severe.

## Rupture of the Supraspinatus Tendon

Paralysis of the supraspinatus muscle
alone is an exceedingly rare lesion; however, rupture of the supraspinatus tendon

(a relatively common disorder) is its functional equivalent. For a long time following
the work of Codman, it was accepted that
the supraspinatus muscle played a very important part in the mechanism of elevation
of the extremity. However, clinical investigation has shown that its contribution is
relatively of minor significance.

Electromyographic studies disclose that
the supraspinatus functions simultaneously
and continuously with the deltoid muscle
and is not the initiator of abduction. This
observation is confirmed clinically in patients with rupture of the supraspinatus
tendon who possess normal scapulohumeral

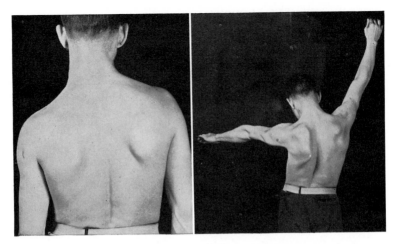

FIG. 5-21. Paralysis of left trapezius and serratus anterior. Elevation is possible to 90° only in the frontal plane. Note the pronounced flare of the inferior angle of the scapula when the arm is elevated. (Haymaker, W., and Woodhall, B.: Peripheral Nerve Injuries. Philadelphia, W. B. Saunders, 1945)

rhythm and abduction power. Further, in a series of shoulder joints obtained post mortem (see pp. 113 and 114), rupture of the supraspinatus tendon was a frequent abnormality in specimens from the later decades; yet it was known that this lesion had given rise to no demonstrable clinical dysfunction of the extremity.

It is clear that the role the supraspinatus muscle plays in regard to the efficiency of the upper muscle force couple designed for elevation and flexion of the limb is a minor one. Moreover, it is evident that the humerus can attain a fulcrum on the glenoid cavity without an intact supraspinatus tendon.

### Rupture of the Musculotendinous Cuff

It will be shown in Chapter 6 (p. 114) that the size of the tear (except in cases of complete avulsion of the cuff) is not the factor that determines the degree of functional impairment in the shoulder. The degree of loss of function depends upon the severity of muscle imbalance between the deltoid muscle and the rotator muscles that results from rupture of the cuff. Extensive tears may produce no severe impairment of func-

tion if the remaining portion of intact cuff is capable of stabilizing the head of the humerus against the glenoid cavity and balancing the power of the deltoid muscle. If a deltoid muscle is very powerful such as is found in laborers, a relatively small tear may be sufficient to disturb this muscle balance sufficiently to cause marked impairment of function.

### Paralysis of Serratus Anterior

The exposed position of the long thoracic nerve makes it vulnerable to trivial injuries, a condition frequently encountered in young athletic individuals. In one case in the author's files, paralysis resulted from direct pressure on the nerve by an osteochondroma located on the ventral surface of the scapula. Fortunately, most of the acute lesions are not complete, and recovery is the rule.

Complete lesions result in total impairment of the mechanism of scapular rotation. Both the upper and the lower force couples are affected. The trapezius muscle is unable to compensate for the loss of power of the serratus anterior muscle. Abduction is impaired severely and is accompanied by a shift of the scapula toward the vertebral column; there is marked winging of the scapula on motion, resulting from failure of the serratus anterior to fix the scapula on the chest wall (Fig. 5-21).

In incomplete lesions, weak abduction is possible, but winging of the scapula is still a prominent feature. Pushing forward against resistances causes pronounced backward displacement of the vertebral border of the scapula, accentuating the winging.

## Paralysis of Trapezius

Complete lesions of this muscle also cause serious impairment of the scapular rotatory force couple. The scapula is displaced and rotated downward and outward. Attempts at abduction, which is possible only to the horizontal or slightly lower, accentuate the deformity, whereas forward flexion diminishes it (Fig. 5-21). However, cases have been reported in which lesions of the trapezius did not disturb the normal mechanisms of the shoulder to any appreciable degree; motion in flexion and abduction was rhythmical and powerful. Apparently the serratus anterior, in certain instances, can compensate and assume the work of the trapezius in both the upper and the lower force couples.

Paralysis of both trapezius and serratus anterior results in pronounced dysfunction of the shoulder mechanism. Attempts at elevation produce a very characteristic deformity. Some abduction of the humerus occurs at the scapula, but the scapula fails to rotate outward and upward; instead, it rotates downward. Motion is accompanied by marked winging of the vertebral border and inferior angle of the scapula (Fig. 5-21).

## BIBLIOGRAPHY

Beevor, C. E.: The Crooian lectures on muscular movements and their representation in the central nervous system. Lecture II. Brit. Med. J., 1:1417-1421, 1903.

Bowen, W. P.: Applied Anatomy and Kinesiology; the Mechanism of Muscular Move-ment. ed. 4. p. 76. Philadelphia, Lea & Febiger, 1928.

Brunstrom, S.: Muscle testing around the shoulder girdle; a study of the function of shoulder blade fixators in seventeen cases of shoulder paralysis. J. Bone & Joint Surg., 23:263-272, 1941.

Cathcart, C. W.: Movements of shoulder girdle envolved in those of the arm on the trunk. J. Anat. (Paris), 18:211-218, 1884.

Codman, E. A.: The Shoulder. Boston, Thomas Todd Co., 1934.

Duchenne, G. B.: Physiologie des mouvements. Paris, Bailliere, 1867 Kaplan, E. B. (Trans.): Philadelphia, J. B. Lippincott, 1949.

Grant, J. C. B.: An Atlas of Anatomy. ed. 2. Baltimore, Williams & Wilkins, 1947.

Haymaker, W., and Woodhall, B.: Peripheral Nerve Injuries. Philadelphia, W. B. Saunders, 1945.

Inman, V. T., Saunders, J. B. deC. M., and Abbott, L. C.: Observations on the shoulder joint. J. Bone & Joint Surg., 26:1-30, 1944.

Joint Motion, Method of Measuring and Recording. Am. Acad. Orthop. Surgeons, 1965.

Lockhart, R. D.: Movements of the normal shoulder joint and a case with trapezius paralysis studied by radiogram and experiment in the living. J. Anat., 64:288-302, 1930.

Martin, C. P.: Movements of the shoulder joint, with special reference to rupture of the supraspinatus tendon. Am. J. Anat., 66:213-234, 1940.

Mayer, L.: Transplantation of the trapezius for paralysis of the abductors of the arm. J. Bone & Joint Surg., 9:412, 1927.

Milgram, J. E.: Shoulder Anatomy. Regional Orthopaedic Surgery and Fundamental Orthopaedic Problems. Ann Arbor, J. W. Edwards, 1947.

Pollack, L. J.: Accessory muscle movements in deltoid paralysis. J.A.M.A., 89:526, 1922.

Scheving, L. E., and Pauly, J. E.: An electromyographic study of some muscles acting on upper extremity of man. Anat. Rec., 135:239-246, 1959.

Staples, O. S., and Watkins, A. L.: Full active abduction in traumatic paralysis of the deltoid. J. Bone & Joint Surg., 25:85-89, 1943.

Stevens, J. H.: The action of the short rotators on the normal abduction of the arm, with a consideration of their action in some cases of subacromial bursitis and allied conditions. Am. J. Med. Sci., 138:870-884, 1909.

Wertheimer, L. G., and Ferraz, E. C. D. F.: Observacoes eletromiograficas sobre as funcoes dos musculos supra-espinhal e deltoide nos movimentos do onbro. Folia clin. biol., 28:276-289, 1958.

# 6

# Aging and the Shoulder Joint

With aging, degenerative alterations of varying degrees occur in the cartilaginous and soft tissue elements of all joints. But no joint of the human frame is more frequently involved or more severely affected than the articulations comprising the shoulder joint—i.e., the glenohumeral, the sternoclavicular and the acromioclavicular joints. This is explicable by the enormous and continuous demands made on these three articulations by the prehensile hand. In addition, the shoulder occupies a unique position in relation to the bony skeleton; it is completely exposed and is in the path of disruptive forces converging on it from all directions. There is no doubt that the many minor and major injuries inflicted on the shoulder play a role in intensifying the degenerative processes that occur naturally.

Comprehension of the nature of the degenerative processes is most essential in order to be able to distinguish which alterations are within normal limits and which

are not. In spite of advanced changes, except in the most severe disorders, the shoulder is capable of meeting the demands made upon it without producing clinical evidence of its implication. It is true also that many disorders producing dysfunction are intimately related to the degenerative process. Clearly, therefore, knowledge of the nature of the degenerative changes afflicting the shoulder joint is essential in establishing the correct diagnosis of a disabling disorder and instituting adequate and effective treatment.

In 1949 and 1950 the results of an investigation by the author into the nature and degree of the degenerative alterations occurring in successive decades in the glenohumeral joint were published. Three hundred and fifty-two joints were studied; 196 joints were obtained from cadavers ranging in age from 14 to 87 years and 12 from fetuses, 6 to 9 months old. This material provided the data on the glenoid side

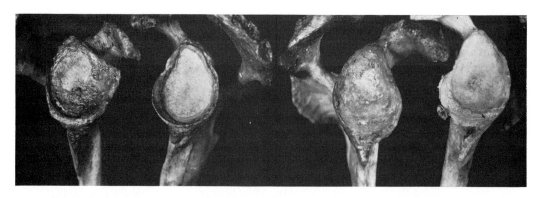

FIG. 6-1. Note advanced marginal lippings along the rim of the glenoid cavities. The new bone formation is more pronounced along the anterior and inferior borders of the glenoid fossae.

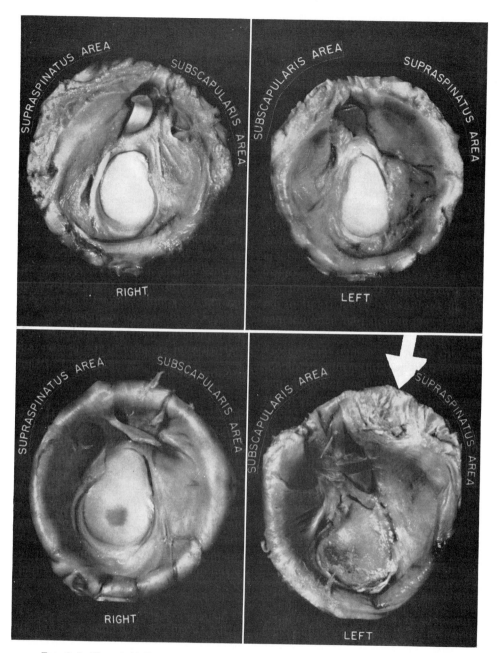

FIG. 6-2. (*Top, left*) Early detachment of the labrum from the tail of the comma in a specimen of the second decade. (*Top, right*) Further detachment in a specimen of the third decade. (*Bottom, left*) Detachment of the labrum in a specimen of the fourth decade. Note the well defined circular area in the center of the head of the comma. (*Bottom, right*) Complete detachment of the labrum from the tail of the comma and the anterior rim of the glenoid rim in a specimen of the sixth decade. This specimen also reveals thinning of the labrum along the inferior border of the glenoid fossa and the formation of numerous tabs and fringes of synovial and connective tissue. Arrow points to a large tear in the supraspinatus and the infraspinatus portion of the musculotendinous cuff.

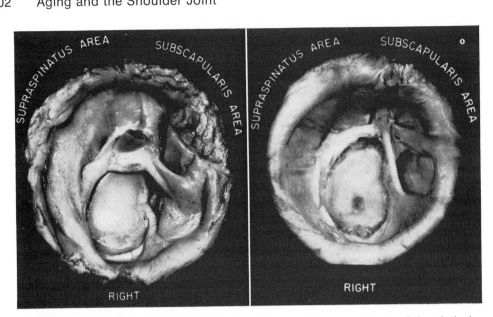

FIG. 6-3. (*Left*) Pronounced detachment of labrum in a specimen of the sixth decade. (*Right*) Detachment of the labrum in specimen of seventh decade.

of the glenohumeral joint. One hundred and forty-four joints were obtained post mortem. Of these, 96 were removed from individuals with a history of having had no serious involvement of the shoulders and, on physical examination before death, with no clinical evidence of impairment of function. The age range for this series was 18 to 74 years; there were 36 males and 14 females, 48 right and 48 left shoulders. These 96 shoulders provided the data on the humeral side of the rotator cuff. In addition, 100 scapulae devoid of all soft tissues were studied to note the physiological changes occurring with aging in the glenoid fossa.

A similar study was made by the author on the acromioclavicular and sternoclavicular joint and the observations published in 1957.

For the sake of completeness the pertinent alterations recorded in the above studies are included in this monograph.

## GLENOID SIDE OF THE GLENOHUMERAL JOINT

### Glenoid Fossa

The characteristic features of the glenoid side of the joint before the joint yields to the ravages of aging were discussed in Chapter 4 (pp. 64 to 73). It was noted that the hyaline cartilage lining the glenoid fossa was thinner in the center of the head of the comma than in the tail, leading one to assume that the thin area is the area of greater contact with the humeral head. After the second decade, the thin area is seen more readily with each successive decade. Throughout the glenoid fossa the resilient, bluish articular cartilage gives way to compact, opaque cartilage, indicating a loss of elasticity. Other alterations also occur; these comprise thinning, fibrillation and formation of small, irregularly scalloped, ulcerated areas within the substance of the cartilage. The degenerative process reaches its maximum severity in the sixth decade and is always more severe in the comma's head than in the tail. In spite of the progressive nature of the alterations, the changes are never so severe in the glenoid cavity as to involve large areas and expose subchondral bone.

Marginal proliferation of bone and cartilage is encountered along the line of attachment of the labrum to the glenoid in the later decades. The involvement is always more pronounced along the anterior mar-

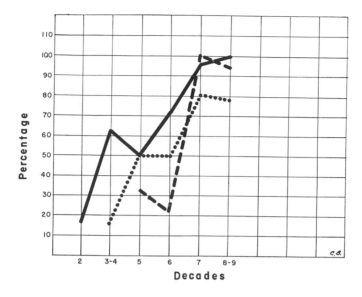

━━━ Labral detachments in each decade.
•••••• Biceps tendons in each decade showing degenerative changes.
━━━ Tears in fibrotendinous cuff in each decade.

FIG. 6-4. Rise in severity of degenerative changes in the biceps tendon and the musculotendinous cuff and the increase in the number of labral detachments in successive decades.

gin of the glenoid, especially in its lower region and along the inferior margin of the glenoid (Fig. 6-1). This response is undoubtedly the result of functional stress, cheifly traction applied by the capsule during motion. Also, the following factors may play a role in the production of the marginal osteophytes: the weight of the arm when in a dependent position, making traction on the glenoid brim through the capsule and labrum; the pull of the biceps tendon on the labrum; and the pull of the glenohumeral ligaments when the arm is externally rotated.

## Labrum

In the labrum, alterations indicative of a degenerative process at work are noted after the second decade. Whereas, prior to this period the edges of the labrum are sharply defined and its surface is smooth and glistening. After this period, small wrinkles appear on the surface which now

assumes a corrugated appearance. Also, the labrum begins to detach from the glenoid brim in the region of the insertion of the biceps tendon (comma's tail). Detachment of the labrum becomes more frequent and more pronounced with each decade; in the second decade, 16.6 percent of the specimens showed this alteration, in the third and fourth decades 63.6 percent, in the fifth decade, 50 percent, in the sixth decade, 72.2 percent and in the eighth and ninth decades, 100 percent (Figs. 6-2, 6-3, and 6-4).

From the observations on these specimens the inference is clear that detachment of the labrum from the glenoid results from traction forces acting through the capsule, biceps tendon and glenohumeral ligaments. The natural tendency for the labrum to become detached, particularly in the region of the tail of the comma, provides an explanation for the high percentage of failures following the Nicola operation for stabilization of shoulders with anterior recurrent

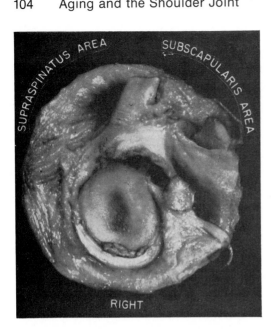

FIG. 6-5. Marked hyperplasia of detached labrum in the region of the tail of the comma and advanced hypertrophy of all the glenohumeral ligaments. Note the numerous fringes of synovial tissue in the tail of the comma between the labrum and the rim of the glenoid fossa. Also note the thinning of the labrum in the region of the comma's head.

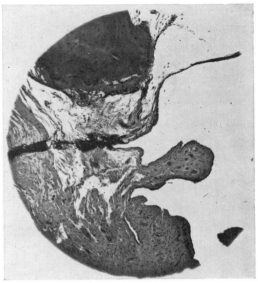

FIG. 6-6. Synovial villi and connective-tissue tabs arising from the labrum at the point of detachment from the glenoid fossa. (x 71)

dislocations. When the arm is suspended from the apex of the glenoid rim, as is done in this operation, the added pull on the labrum through the biceps tendon enhances detachment of the labrum, thereby defeating the very purpose for which the operation was performed. Remember that the goal of the Nicola operation is to stabilize the humeral head by converting the biceps tendon into an intracapsular suspensory ligament for the head.

Another phenomenon that accompanies aging is the progressive hypertrophy of the labrum, particularly in the region of the comma's tail and the anterior portion of the labrum. This alteration in later decades is associated with formation of tabs and fringes of synovial tissue, particularly along the anterior portion of the labrum. The severest alterations occur in the seventh and eighth decades (Figs. 6-5 and 6-6).

In contrast to the labral changes that occur in the region of the comma's tail, in the comma's head the characteristic findings are thinning, fraying and shredding of the labrum. These abnormalities first appear in the fifth decade and progress in intensity in the subsequent decades. They undoubtedly are the result of constant friction between the comma's head and the humeral head, again indicating that this region may be one of greater contact than elsewhere (Fig. 6-5).

### Biceps Tendon

Attritional changes in the biceps tendon are common findings after the fourth decade. They resemble those seen in the labrum: thickening, widening and shredding of the tendon fibers. The severity of the changes increases with each decade; in the fifth and sixth decade, 50 percent of the specimens exhibit the changes; in the seventh, 80 percent, and in the eighth and ninth, 78 percent. In the later decades some specimens showed total disintegration of the tendon. In these specimens the extra-

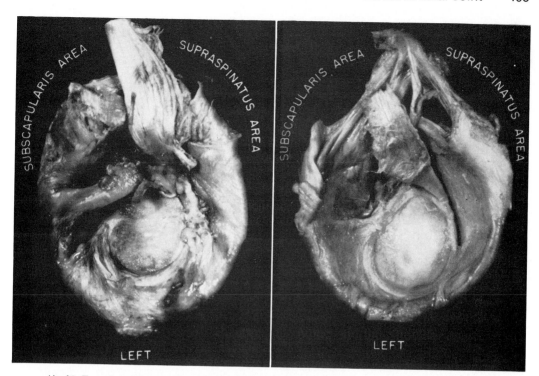

(*Left*) FIG. 6-7. Marked hypertrophy of all the intracapsular structures except the labrum in the region of the head of the comma. Also note the advanced fraying, shredding and hypertrophy of the biceps tendon and the advanced degenerative changes in the musculotendinous cuff.

(*Right*) FIG. 6-8. A specimen with complete avulsion of the cuff, advanced degenerative changes and hypertrophy and fraying of the biceps tendon.

capsular portion of the tendon attained a bony attachment on the shaft of the humerus (Figs. 6-7 and 6-8).

The severity of the changes in the biceps tendon parallel those one sees in the rotator cuff of the same specimen. This leads one to suppose that with deterioration of the rotator cuff, the biceps tendon is forced to assume a greater role in the support of the extremity and is subjected to greater attritional forces than when the rotator cuff is intact.

## Glenohumeral Ligaments, Synovial Recesses and Synovial Membrane

In the early decades (up to the third decade) the synovial membrane is a thin, glistening lining and is stretched tightly over the fibrous capsule, the glenohumeral ligaments, the labrum and the biceps tendon. Evidence of changes in the synovial membrane appear as early as the third decade; these comprise synovial tabs and fringes and synovial villi. Synovial villi appear in several forms: as fine fingerlike projections or as branching, papillary or even polypoid structures. In addition to the alterations affecting the surface of the synovial lining, gradual thickening of the synovial membrane occurs, caused by proliferations of the fibrous elements of its deeper layers.

Alteration of the synovial membrane is seen first in the subscapularis and coracohumeral regions of the joint: in the fourth and fifth decades it occurs in other areas, especially in the inferior and the anteroinferior regions which correspond to the infraspinatus and triceps area of the synovial membrane. Generally speaking, villous

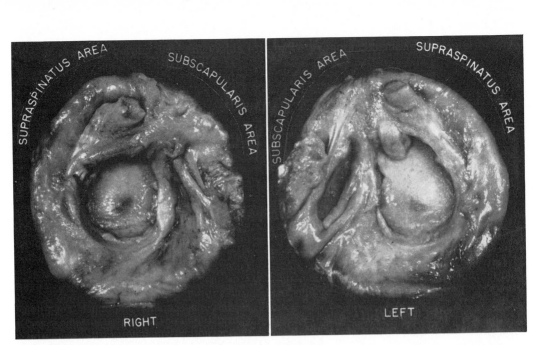

FIG. 6-9. Marked hypertrophy of the synovialis and all intracapsular elements, tending to obliterate the synovial recesses and the normal configuration of the glenohumeral ligaments.

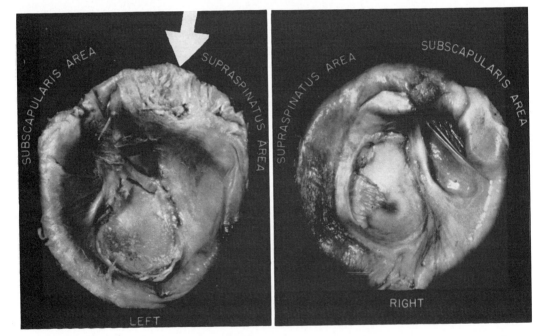

(*Left*) FIG. 6-10. The specimen reveals advanced degenerative changes in the soft tissue elements (synovial membrane, glenohumeral ligaments and labrum) and the articular cartilage of the glenoid fossa. This is the usual finding, but there are exceptions, as shown in Figure 6-11.

(*Right*) FIG. 6-11. This specimen reveals numerous tabs and fringes between the labrum and the rim of the glenoid fossa, as if an attempt were being made to reattach the labrum to the rim. Also note that the articular cartilage of the glenoid fossa is not severely involved in spite of the changes in the soft tissue elements.

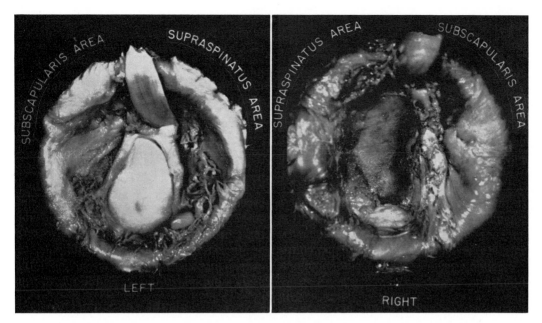

FIG. 6-12. Advanced villous proliferation and hypertrophy of the synovial membrane. These changes have obliterated the synovial recesses. The corresponding humeral heads of both these specimens exhibited evidence of severe trauma.

projections and proliferations reach their maximum in size and number in specimens of the sixth to the ninth decades.

Hypertrophy of the synovial membrane due to fibrosis of its subintimal connective tissue layer shows a progressive rise in degree after the third decade. Those structures that are subjected to constant functional stress reveal the greatest amount of thickening; thus, marked hyperplastic changes occur in the glenohumeral ligaments, the biceps tendon, the superior portion of the labrum, which is continuous with the biceps tendon and the superior glenohumeral ligament, and the anterior portion of the labrum. In some instances, the proliferative process is so thoroughgoing that any synovial recesses present are markedly reduced in size or are completely obliterated (Fig. 6-9).

In most (but not all) of the specimens exhibiting severe alterations in the synovial membrane and glenohumeral ligaments, the artcular cartilage of the glenoid fossa also disclosed advanced impairment (cf. Figs. 6-10 and 6-11). Trauma to the upper end

of the humerus, producing secondary degenerative changes in the articular surface of the humeral head, may be a factor in augmenting the severity of the synovial response. Two specimens in this study disclosed evidence of a malunited fracture of the humeral head. The articular surfaces of these humeral heads revealed advanced cartilaginous destruction and marked incongruity. The glenoid side of both of these joints revealed a profound synovial response in the form of hypertrophy of the synovial membrane and villous proliferation (Fig. 6-12).

Not infrequently, secondary changes occur in the later decades in the hyperplastic synovial membrane and villi. The most common alterations are hyaline degeneration of the connective tissue and, in some instances, formation of imperfect cartilage.

## HUMERAL SIDE OF THE GLENOHUMERAL JOINT

The observations discussed in the following sections have special clinical signifi-

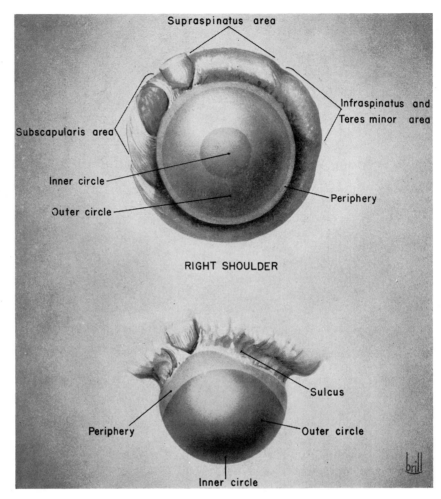

RIGHT SHOULDER

FIG. 6-13. Schematic drawing of finished mounted specimen, showing division of articular cartilage into the inner circle, the outer circle and periphery. It also shows the sulcus (produced by recession of the cuff) and the various areas of the musculotendinous cuff.

cance because they were made on shoulders from individuals who had never complained of any shoulder dysnfunction and had never sustained during life any severe trauma to the shoulders resulting in impairment of function. This material permits one to correlate the degree of abnormalities of the various elements of the shoulder compatible with good function.

As previously noted, this study was made on 96 shoulders obtained from 50 individuals, 36 males and 14 females, age range from 18 to 74 years.

In order to facilitate presentation of the findings, the articular surface was divided into three parts: the central area (or inner circle), the outer area (or outer circle), and the margin of the articular surface (the periphery). The interval between the periphery and the inner surface of the musculotendinous cuff was designated the sulcus. The musculotendinous cuff was divided into 4 areas: the supraspinatus, the infraspinatus, the teres minor and the subscapularis area (Fig. 6-13).

## Articular Cartilage of the Humeral Head

The changes in the articular cartilage of the humeral head are never extensive, even in the very late decades of life, except in

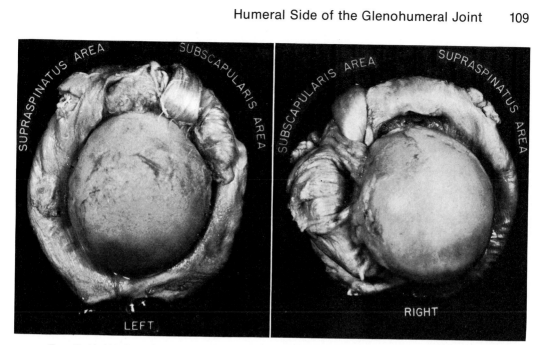

FIG. 6-14. W. S., male, age 67 years. Both humeral heads show extensive changes in the articular cartilage in the area of the outer circle; the alterations exceed by far those present in the inner circle. Also note, in the right shoulder, the formation of bony spurs and excrescences along the periphery of the articular cartilage. In addition, both shoulders exhibit extensive alterations in the musculotendinous cuffs and biceps tendons.

FIG. 6-15. R. M., female, age 55 years. Right shoulder: Changes in the articular cartilage are minimal, whereas those in the musculo-tendinous cuff are severe. Observe the changes particularly in the subscapularis and the supraspinatus regions of the cuff.

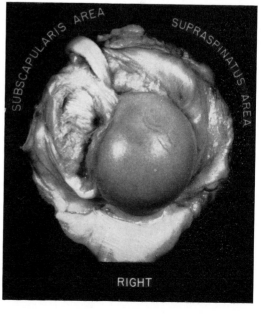

very few shoulder joints. As a rule, the cartilage within the inner circle shows the least severe alterations; the most profound lesions are encountered along the periphery of the cartilage. However, the cartilage within the outer circle invariably reveals changes of greater intensity than those in the cartilage enclosed by the inner circle. In general, the changes comprise thinning, fibrillation, pitting and erosion of the articular cartilage; along the periphery the findings consist of pitting and erosion of the cartilage and formation of bony spurs and excrescences (Fig. 6-14). Starting with the third decade, the alterations show a gradual rise in severity; however, as previously noted, they are never profound changes. Moreover, they never equal those occur-ring in the glenoid fossa of the same age period, nor do they parallel the extensive changes occurring in the musculotendinous cuffs (Fig. 6-15).

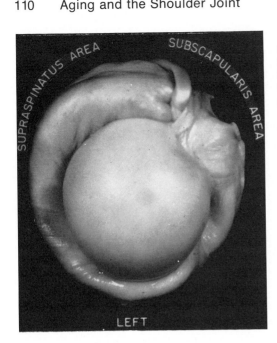

FIG. 6-16. D. A., male, age 23 years. Left shoulder: This specimen shows no macroscopic evidence of degenerative changes in the cuff or in the articular cartilage. Note that the musculotendinous cuff with its synovial lining is continuous with the articular cartilage. Nowhere is there any recession of cuff fibers.

The last-mentioned observation supports the belief that development of degenerative changes in the soft tissue components of joints is not secondary to changes in the osseous and cartilaginous tissues. Also, in the case of the shoulder joint, during motion, only a small portion of the articular surface of the humeral head is in contact with the glenoid fossa. The contact areas in the glenoid fossa are subjected to more wear and tear than are contact areas in the head of the humerus. This readily explains the discrepancies in the severity of the changes in the articular surfaces of the humeral head and glenoid fossa.

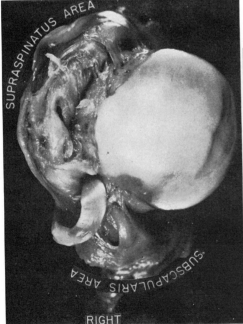

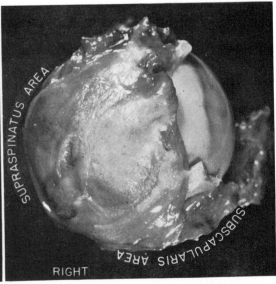

FIG. 6-17. D. F., male, age 55. Right shoulder. (*Left*) Observe the advanced degenerative lesions involving the entire cuff, particularly in the supraspinatus and infraspinatus areas. The cuff has receded a considerable distance from the margin of the articular cartilage, forming a wide sulcus. (*Right*) The cuff has been pulled over the head. Note that it is impossible to evaluate the severity of the lesions on the inner side of the cuff by the appearance of its outer surface.

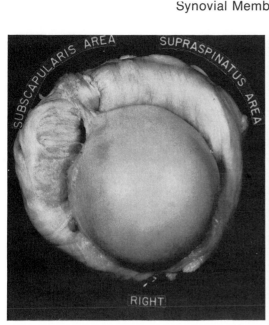

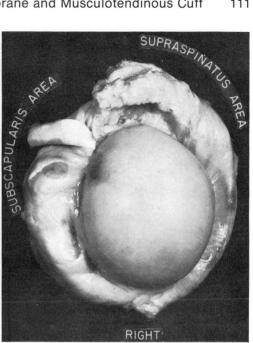

Fig. 6-18. A. G., male, age 47 years. Right shoulder: Note the large incomplete tear in the subscapularis region of the cuff. Distal to the tear, the synovial membrane is markedly thickened, forming what Codman called a falciform ligament. It is Nature's attempt to limit the extension of the tear in the cuff.

FIG. 6-19. J. S., male, age 54. Right shoulder. An unusually large incomplete tear, implicating the entire supraspinatus and a portion of the infraspinatus area of the cuff. Note the hypertrophy and thickening of the torn fibers and marked recession and thinning of the remaining intact fibers of the cuff.

## Sulcus

A sulcus is not present in shoulders of infants and of persons in the early decades of life. In these specimens the musculotendinous cuff completely fills the interval between the peripheral margin of the articular cartilage and the tuberosities (Fig. 6-16). Beginning with the third decade, the cuff, with its synovial lining, gradually pulls away from the periphery of the articular cartilage, creating the interval designated the sulcus. With each decade, the number of specimens showing this abnormality increases and the extent of the tearing away of the cuff from its attachment becomes more pronounced. The region of the supraspinatus area is involved more frequently than are other areas of the cuff. Pitting, bony spurs and excrescences are common findings in the sulcus. These alterations increase in intensity in each subsequent decade. The severity of the degenerative lesions are in direct proportion to the severity of those in the musculotendinous cuff. As more and more fibers tear away the thickness of the cuff is reduced and the sulcus becomes wider. (Fig. 6-17).

## SYNOVIAL MEMBRANE AND MUSCULOTENDINOUS CUFF

The synovial membrane is closely adherent to the inner surface of the cuff, so that any changes in the cuff produce corresponding alterations in the synovial membrane. The response in the synovial membrane comprises shredding, fraying, tabs and villous formation. A gradual progression in the severity of these changes is demonstrable in each successive decade, corresponding to the severity of the alterations in the musculotendinous cuff. The most severe changes are encountered in shoulders of the sixth decade.

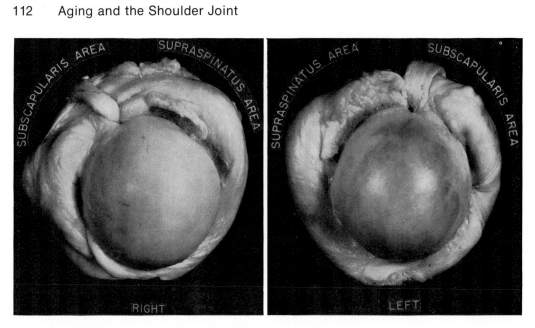

FIG. 6-20. T. C., male, age 43. (*Left*) Right shoulder. Large incomplete tear in supra-spinatus area, with recession and thickening of the torn fibers. (*Right*) Left shoulder showing an incomplete tear of both the supraspinatus and the infraspinatus areas, with thickening and recession of the torn fibers.

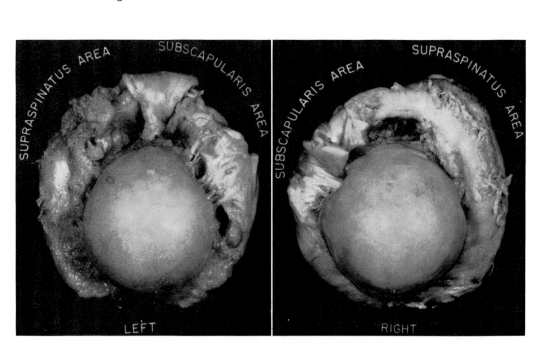

FIG. 6-21. J. S., male, age 59 years. (*Left*) Left shoulder. Except for a few fibers in the subscapularis area, the entire cuff has pulled away from the margin of the articular surface. Note the hypertrophy of the torn fibers, the deep sulcus and the widening and thickening and fraying of the biceps tendon. (*Right*) Right shoulder. In this specimen most of the cuff alterations are confined to the supraspinatus and infraspinatus areas. This is an extensive incomplete tear. In spite of the extensive changes in the cuff and the synovial membrane, the articular cartilage shows only mild alterations.

## Partial or Incomplete Tears

The innermost fibers of the cuff begin to tear away from their bony insertion into the humeral head in the fifth decade. These tears are designated partial tears of the cuff because they do not traverse the entire thickness of the cuff. A gradual increase in the size of the tears is demonstrable in each successive decade; the severest changes occur in the sixth and seventh decades. As a rule, tears in the supraspinatus region extend into the infraspinatus area for varying distances. This feature can only be appreciated by viewing the inner or synovial side of the cuff. Judgment as to the extent of the lesions cannot be made by inspecting only the outer or bursal side of the cuff (Fig. 6-17). In this series there were 35 suprainfraspinatus tears (37.3%) and 20 sub-

scapularis tears (20.8%). The extent and types of incomplete tears compatible with good function is surprising: they varied from minimal lesions to extensive areas of tearing, fraying and thinning of the cuff in all three cuff areas. Hand-in-hand with these severe alterations, pronounced hypertrophy and thickening of the torn cuff fibers and the synovial membrane proximal to the cuff lesions invariably occurs (Figs. 6-18, 6-19, 6-20 and 6-21). The shoulders depicted in Figures 6-18 through 6-21 had no impairment of function.

Since such extensive lesions of the cuff can be present without giving rise to symptoms or producing impairment of function, one is forced to look elsewhere for an explanation when pain and dysfunction do exist. I am of the opinion that although these lesions are not per se directly respon-

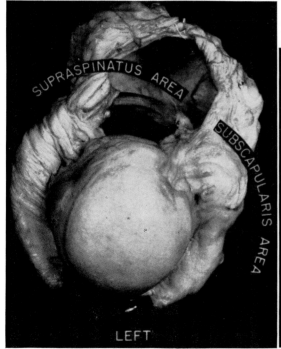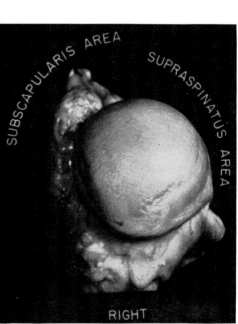

FIG. 6-22. M. A., female, age 59 years. (*Left*) Left shoulder. Note the large incomplete tear in the supraspinatus and infraspinatus areas of the cuff. The subscapularis region also shows advanced degenerative changes but the tear is incomplete. Both tuberosities are leveled off, and the walls of the enlarged subacromial bursa are irregular and thickened. (*Right*) Right shoulder. In this shoulder the complete tear includes a portion of the subscapularis and teres minor areas, yet the patient could abduct the arm freely.

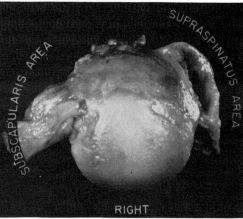

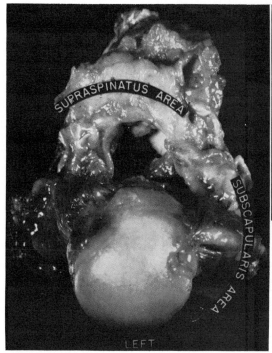

FIG. 6-23. M. W., female, age 63 years. (*Left*) Left shoulder: The complete tear included all of the supraspinatus and infraspinatus areas and part of the teres minor and subscapularis areas of the cuff. The tuberosities have disappeared and the upper end of the humerus appears like a smooth hemisphere. (*Right*) The right shoulder presents abnormalities almost the same as those observed in the left shoulder.

sible for pain and dysfunction of the shoulder, they are indirectly responsible. As the result of repeated, minor trauma to the cuff during normal or excessive function or as the result of a severe single trauma, the torn cuff fibers become markedly thickened and edematous, thereby decreasing the interval between the bursal side of the cuff and the coracoacromial arch. Now, during elevation of the arm above the horizontal, impingement of the sensitive subacromial bursa occurs when the hyperplastic portion of the torn cuff abuts against the acromion or the coracoacromial ligament, producing the painful arc syndrome. This explains why excision of the acromion or resection of a portion of the coracoacromial ligament relieves the pain.

### Complete Tears

Complete tears of the musculotendinous cuff are lesions that traverse the entire thickness of the cuff so that the joint cavity communicates with the subacromial bursa. In this series there were 9 complete tears (9.3%), ranging in size from one centimeter to massive separation of the insertion of the cuff. In the most severely affected shoulders, (of which there were 6), only a

small portion of the subscapularis tendon and a portion of the infraspinatus tendon were intact; yet, these patients were unaware of any impairment of shoulder function. Unfortunately, the power of elevation of the arm against resistance was not ascertained. I feel sure that if this test had been performed some weakness would have been elicited. Figure 6-22, depicting the cuffs of a female 59 years old, and Figure 6-23, of a female 63 years old, are examples of the profound changes that can occur in shoulder joints that can still meet the functional demands of the individual.

### Biceps Tendon

As previously stated, after the fourth decade degenerative changes in the form of thickening, widening and shredding of the biceps tendon occur. However, as this study shows, these lesions per se do not preclude good, painless function of the shoulder. Also, it was previously noted that the severity of the lesions in the biceps tendons parallels that of lesions in the cuff. Careful study of the structures adjacent to the exit of the biceps tendon from the joint cavity provides an explanation for the lack of pain and dysfunction in these affected shoulders. In each instance, the capsular and cuff fibers tear away from the anterior and posterior walls of the intertubercular sulcus, so that the tunnel which the tendon traverses is widened. Such an arrangement affords ample room for free excursion of the head of the humerus on the tendon. Figure 6-24 clearly depicts the changed relationship of the tendon to its environs.

In other instances, the intertubercular sulcus is obliterated by absorption or atrophy of the tuberosities of the humerus; now, the tendon lies in a fascial sling made by the upper border of the subscapularis tendon (Fig. 6-25).

One pair of shoulders in this series, from a male 73 years of age, are of special clinical interest. At the time of examination, this patient exhibited no pain or dysfunction in

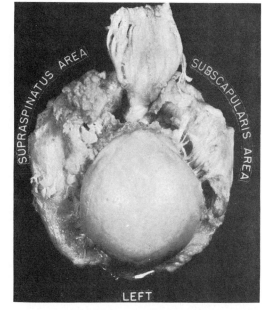

FIG. 6-24. J. F., male, age 59 years. Left shoulder. Note the advanced degenerative changes in the cuff and its synovial lining, and the extensive alterations in the biceps tendon which is shredded, thickened and widened. Note also that on either side of the exit of the biceps tendon the cuff fibers have torn away from their insertion into the anterior and posterior margins of the intertubercular sulcus, so that exit of the altered tendon is not interfered with.

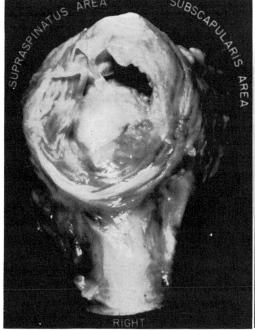

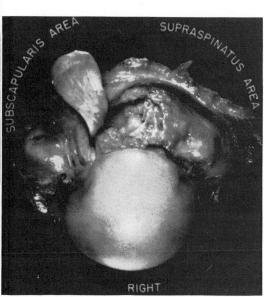

FIG. 6-25. A. R., male, age 62 years. (Left) Right shoulder. A massive complete tear of the supraspinatus and a large portion of the infraspinatus tendon. The remaining portion of the cuff shows shredding, lamination and fraying. (Right) Synovial side of the same shoulder. Observe the thickness of the biceps tendon; the tendon lies outside the intertubercular groove on a fascial sling formed by the upper border of the intact subscapularis tendon. This arrangement provides a wide exit.

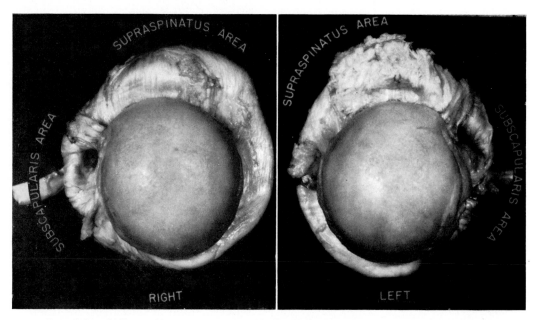

Fig. 6-26. J. F., male, age 73 years. (*Left*) Right shoulder. Note that the biceps tendon does not leave the joint cavity through its normal exit. It lies outside of the joint and is attached to the inferior aspect of the lesser tuberosity. (*Right*) Left shoulder. Again, the biceps tendon is attached to the lesser tuberosity, and its intracapsular portion is absent. This patient gave a history of having pain and dysfunction consistent with the symptoms of frozen shoulders 12 to 15 years before these specimens were obtained.

either shoulder. However, he stated that 12 to 15 years earlier he had had considerable pain and stiffness, first in the right and then in the left shoulder. After an indeterminable period, painless function slowly returned. The postmortem specimens revealed the intracapsular portion of both the right and the left tendon to be absent, while the extracapsular portion in each shoulder is attached to the upper end of the shaft of the humerus (Fig. 6-26). Both rotator cuffs show advanced degenerative changes. This may be the fate of the biceps tendon in some shoulders afflicted by the "frozen shoulder" syndrome.

**Discussion.** From a clinical point of view the assessment of the observations recorded above must be tempered with the knowledge that acute traumatic lesions of the shoulder joint differ from lesions that are the result of slowly progressing degenerative changes. In the former, disruption of tissue is sudden and violent, and the normal mechanics of the joint are immediately impaired, with no time for the shoulder to make the necessary adjustments of structures remaining intact so that function should not be seriously impaired. In the latter, as shown in this study, such compensating adjustments are possible and do take place. Also, clinical experience indicates that tears less extensive than those demonstrated in this study but produced by sudden violence may result in marked impairment of function. It is obvious, then, that (except in cases of complete avulsion of the cuff) the size of the lesion or tear is not the factor that determines the degree of dysfunction. I believe that the degree of impairment of function is directly related to the loss of muscle balance between the rotator cuff muscles, which fix and depress the humeral head in the glenoid fossa, and the deltoid muscle. For example, a complete tear implicating all of the supra-spinatus and part of the infraspinatus tendon produces loss of abduction only when the deltoid muscle is sufficiently strong and powerful to overcome the stabilizing action of the torn cuff. In such a situation, the deltoid pulls the humerus upward under the acromion when abduction is initiated. On the other hand, a more extensive tear of the cuff produces no loss of abduction if a relatively less powerful deltoid muscle is acting and the remaining intact portion of the rotator cuff is capable of stabilizing the humeral head. In other words, as long as the remaining portion of the cuff is capable of balancing the pull of the deltoid muscle no loss of abduction ensues.

It is apparent that all gradations of dysfunction may exist in different shoulders, depending on the degree of impairment of balance between these muscle groups. This provides an explanation for weak abduction or inability to maintain abduction against resistance or total loss of abduction in middle-aged persons who possess strong, powerful deltoid muscles and exhibit, at the time of operation, only small or moderate tears in the cuff. From the study discussed above it is clear that, in this group, degenerative alterations resulting from physiological wear and tear, aging and occupational traumata render the cuff weak and vulnerable. A small tear in such a cuff may be sufficient to upset the muscle balance completely. A tear of the same size produced by trauma in an elderly person with a less powerful deltoid may produce little or no impairment of function.

In view of the frequency with which complete—and, in some cases, very extensive—tears compatible with good function were found in this study, the reader may be led to conclude that, since the shoulder complex tends to restore muscle balance, it is usually only necessary to allow sufficient time to elapse to effect restoration of function. However, this may not occur if the lesion is severe, and, since fresh tears are more readily repaired than old ones, it is my opinion that repair should be effected as soon as the diagnosis of a torn cuff is made.

## Bursal Side of the Rotator Cuff

Inasmuch as many of the surgical procedures for maladies of the shoulder joint are directed to the outer or bursal aspect of the rotator cuff it is essential to have a clear concept of the changes occurring in this region with aging. For this purpose, 100 shoulders of cadavers were studied; of these, 7 were from fetuses of 6 to 9 months; the age range for the remaining specimens was 19 to 88 years.

## Subacromial Bursa

In infant shoulders and those of the second and third decades, the roof and lateral walls of the subacromial bursa consist of a filmy, transparent, delicate membrane. Occasionally, a fold is demonstrable, separating the subacromial from the subcoracoid portion of the bursa. In specimens of later decades, when degenerative alterations in the cuff are present, the bursal walls become thickened and not infrequently the bursa is divided into several compartments by thick, smooth adhesions. When the cuff exhibits a complete tear, a direct communication exists between the joint cavity and the subacromial bursa, whose capacity is markedly increased and whose walls now show marked thickening (Fig. 6-22). When the complete tear is massive, the humeral head lies directly under the roof of the bursa, this being the only barrier between the humeral head and the undersurface of the acromion. It is reasonable to assume that the increase in the size of the bursa is in response to the presence of the synovial fluid which constantly distends the bursa during elevation of the arm. A frozen shoulder is rarely seen in association with a complete tear of the cuff. I have never seen such a combination. It may be that the synovial fluid within the bursa

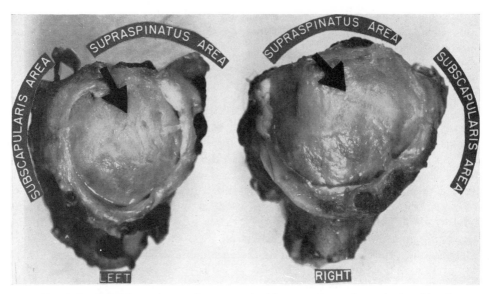

FIG. 6-27. Paired specimens from a male 48 years of age. In each shoulder the roof of the subacromial bursa has been removed and you are looking directly at the floor of the bursa overlying the cuff. The arrow points to the irregularities in the floor of each bursa; the degenerative changes are more pronounced in areas making greater contact with the acromion.

prevents formation of an adhesive type of bursitis or capsulitis, a pathological state always encountered in frozen shoulders. In this series several shoulders revealed complete obliteration of the bursa, so that sharp dissection was necessary to separate the deltoid muscle from the surface of the rotator cuff. In all these shoulders the cuff showed profound degenerative changes but no complete tear.

## Floor of the Subacromial Bursa and the Outer Surface of the Cuff

These two structures are considered together because they are intimately related. Normally, the base of the bursa is firmly adherent to the upper and outer portions of the greater tuberosity and to the rotator cuff where it inserts into the tuberosities. The base bridges the bicipital groove. In specimens of the early decades, the floor of the bursa is smooth, glistening and transparent. Palpation inside the bursa reveals the tuberosities and the edge of the acromion to be smooth and regular. Upon eleva-

tion of the arm the base of the bursa passes under the coracoacromial arch without impingement. These are not the findings noted in shoulders of later decades.

After the fifth decade the degenerative changes in the cuff increase progressively and the abnormalities in the floor of the bursa become more pronounced, paralleling those in the cuff. The lesions most prevalent in the bursal floor comprise tabs, thickening of the bursal walls and villous formations. The changes are more widespread when the cuff exhibits extensive tearing, shredding and lamination of its fibers, particularly in the supraspinatus and infraspinatus regions. Occasionally, the entire bursa is packed with numerous filmy, branching synovial villi.

The concentration of bursal changes in the region of the supraspinatus area seems to indicate that this is a region of greater stress than other regions of the cuff, and upon elevation of the arm, is more likely to impinge against the coracoacromial arch than are other regions of the cuff.

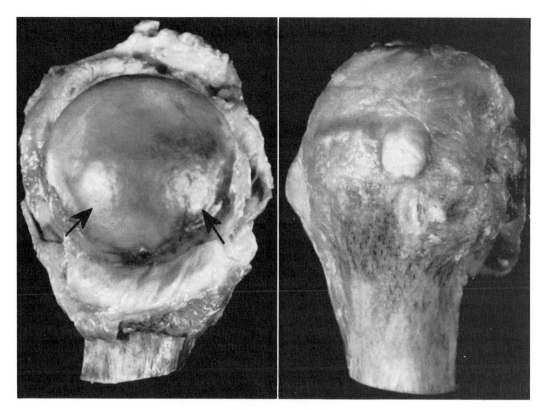

FIG. 6-28. (*Left*) Arrows point to calcareous deposits within the musculotendinous cuff. The floor of the bursa is stretched tightly over the calcareous areas. (*Right*) Large calcareous deposit in supraspinatus area of the cuff. On abduction of the arm, this mass impinges against the acromion.

Calcification within the substance of the degenerated cuff fiber is not a common finding; only two specimens reveal gross calcareous deposits in the cuff below the level of the floor of the bursa. In one of these, the deposit is sufficiently large to abut against the acromion when the arm is elevated. However, several specimens exhibit microscopic calcium deposits; these are always associated with severe cuff changes (Figs. 6-27 and 6-28).

Only three specimens disclose areas of osseous tissue within the degenerated cuff fibers; in two, the region affected is the supraspinatus area; the other specimen reveals complete ossification of the tendons of supraspinatus, infraspinatus and teres minor.

After the fourth decade, the degenerative changes in the cuff are progressively more frequent and more intense; also the supraspinatus area is involved more frequently than are other regions of the cuff. Although the appearance of the implicated cuffs varies considerably, a common pattern of involvement can be identified in most cuffs. First, thinning of the tendon occurs just proximal to this line of insertion into the tuberosity. In some instances the continuity of the cuff is maintained only by a thin ribbon of tissue. Many specimens show, just proximal to the thinned portion of the cuff, varying degrees of thickening and hypertrophy of the torn cuff fibers on the inner or synovial side of the cuff. The hyperplastic process appears to be an attempt to repair the cuff lesion. It was noted earlier that, on the inner side of the cuff, the synovial mem-

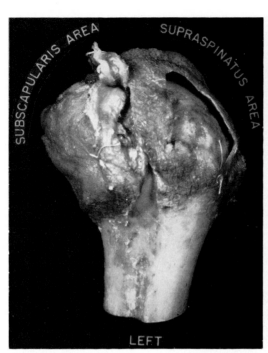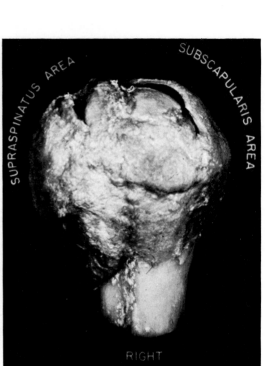

(*Left*) FIG. 6-29. This specimen shows an elongated triangular defect in the supraspinatus and infraspinatus regions of the cuff. No vestige of the distal end of the cuff remains, and the edges of the cuff defect are thin, smooth and inelastic. Note that the tuberosities are atrophic and roughened and the biceps tendon is frayed, shredded and thin.

(*Right*) FIG. 6-30. Observe the large complete tear extending across the bicipital groove and involving a portion of the subscapularis tendon. The edges of the tear are sharp, well defined, fibrotic and thin; the biceps tendon is exposed, frayed and thickened, and the tuberosities are atrophic and recessed.

brane becomes thickened, forming a falciformlike ligament just proximal to the cuff tear; this, too, is an attempt to repair the tear or limit its progress. The same pattern of involvement occurs when the cuff lesion is a complete tear. However, in the late decades, the hyperplastic process seems to come to an end and the hypertrophied torn cuff fibers now appear to wear away, leaving an atrophic or thin, scarred, inelastic cuff proximal to the insertion of the cuff if it is an incomplete lesion, or proximal to the edge of the defect in the cuff if it is a complete tear (Figs. 6-29 and 6-30).

In this series, there are 13 specimens with complete tears or 10.3 percent; the supraspinatus area is involved in 46.1 percent of the specimens with complete tears, the supraspinatus and infraspinatus areas together in 38.4 percent, the infraspinatus area alone in 0.7 percent and the entire cuff in 0.7 percent. The subscapularis region shows a complete tear in three specimens, but in each the lesion is also associated with a tear involving the supraspinatus and infraspinatus regions. The size and configuration of the tears show great variation, from small imperceptible tears to disruption of the entire cuff.

Although the small tears do not suggest the pattern of evolution of the larger lesions (except that the insertion of the cuff fibers tears just proximal to its insertion into the tuberosity), the larger, complete tears do disclose such a pattern. These reveal a tendency of the defect to develop a longitudinal extension arising from its anterior aspect and parallel to the tendon

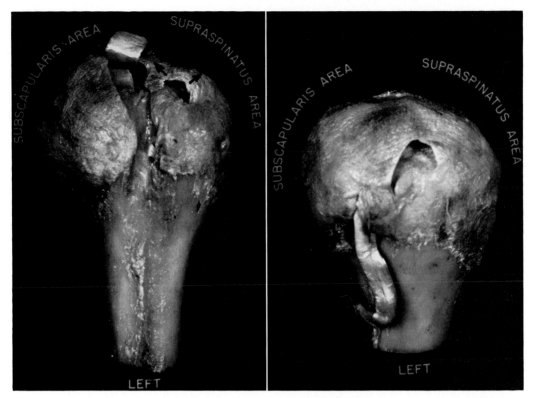

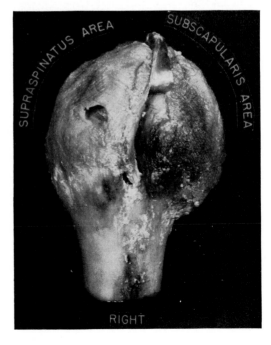

FIG. 6-31. (*Top, left*) Note the elongated cuff defect; elongation is due to pulling of the cuff fibers in the direction of the arrows. The bicipital groove has been opened for inspection; observe the well formed supratubercular ridge over which the biceps tendon lies. (*Top, right*) This specimen shows a larger complete tear in the supraspinatus region of the cuff; the edges are sharp, smooth and thin. The defect tends to elongate in the direction parallel with the muscle fibers. (*Bottom*) Small complete tear which still shows little evidence of elongation.

fibers. It appears that once the complete thickness of a portion of the cuff has pulled away from its bony insertion, opposing mechanical forces come into play splitting the cuff in a longitudinal direction. The subscapularis muscle pulls the anterior margin of the defect forward while the infraspinatus and teres minor muscles pull the posterior margin backward. At the same time, the supraspinatus muscle pulls the proximal torn fibers medially, thereby producing an equilateral triangular defect (Figs. 6-31 and 6-32).

In large defects, no vestige of the distal end of the cuff remains; in some, large

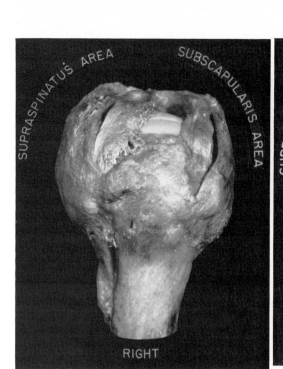

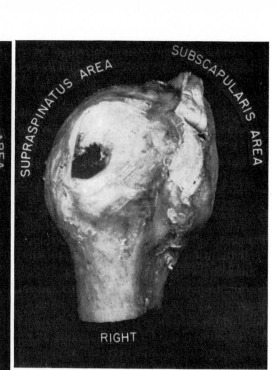

(*Left*) Fig. 6-32. Observe that the cuff has pulled away from its insertion into the humeral head and has elongated proximally, creating a triangular defect in the supraspinatus and infraspinatus regions of the cuff. The edges of the defect are thin and smooth; the tuberosities are atrophic and exhibit considerable roughening.

(*Right*) Fig. 6-33. Note the pronounced atrophy and recession of the greater tuberosity; in fact, there is a large bony defect in the head of the humerus. The bone surrounding the defect is eburnated and polished. Also note the large cuff defect in the supraspinatus and infraspinatus areas of the cuff. The edges of the defect are thin, sharp and smooth.

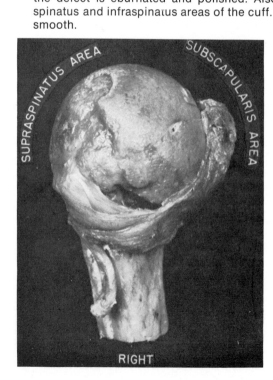

bony excrescences form on the tuberosities and appear to impinge against the acromion on abduction of the arm. Several specimens with large cuff defects show almost complete atrophy of the greater and lesser tuberosities, as if they had gradually been leveled off (Fig. 6-33). When the cuff is completely destroyed, or nearly so, the exposed head is pulled upward under the acro-

Fig. 6-34. This specimen shows a massive defect in the cuff, complete recession of the tuberosities and erosion and scalloping of the articular surface of the humeral head. Note the irregular bony excrescences at the site of the greater tuberosity; note also that only a few fibers of the subscapularis tendon remain intact. The intracapsular portion of the biceps tendon is absent and the proximal end of the extracapsular portion of the tendon is attached to the base of the lesser tuberosity.

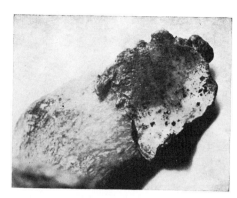

FIG. 6-35. The undersurface of the acromion of the shoulder depicted in Figure 6-34. Note the new bone formation along the margins of the acromion. Also, the undersurface of the acromion is eburnated and polished. This is the result of the constant contact of this area with the head of the humerus when there is a massive defect in the cuff.

mion by the unopposed action of the deltoid muscle. The humeral head now shows advanced degenerative changes; the cartilage is eroded away, the subchrondral bone becomes eburnated, the tuberosities wear away; even the bicipital sulcus may be obliterated. The undersurface of the acromion becomes dense, eburnated and highly polished (Figs. 6-34 and 6-35).

## Tuberosities and Bicipital Groove

Associated with degenerative alterations in the rotator cuff are changes in the regions of the tuberosities of the humerus and in and about the bicipital groove. With impairment of the cuff, the ability of the rotator muscles to depress and fix the humeral head efficiently, upon abduction of the arm,

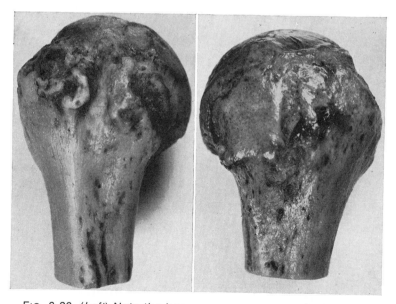

FIG. 6-36. (*Left*) Note the bony excrescences over both tuberosities. Also observe that the head of the humerus proximal to the sulcus is flattened and eburnated. The intertubercular groove is narrowed. (The biceps tendon of this shoulder showed pronounced fraying and shredding.) (*Right*) In this specimen there is complete recession and atrophy of both tuberosities, obliteration of the intertubercular sulcus, formation of bony excrescences in the bicipital groove and eburnation of the humeral head just anterior and posterior to the upper end of the bicipital groove. (The biceps tendon showed severe degeneration.)

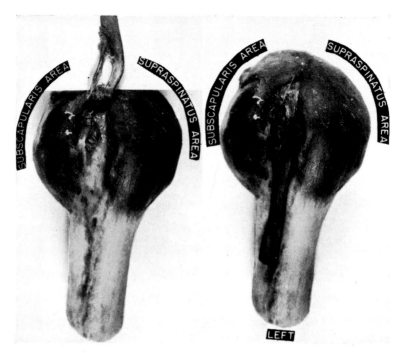

Fig. 6-37. (*Left*) Note the large bony spur in the floor of the groove and the defect in the frayed tendon. (*Right*) When the tendon is in its normal position the tendon defect fits snugly around the bony spur.

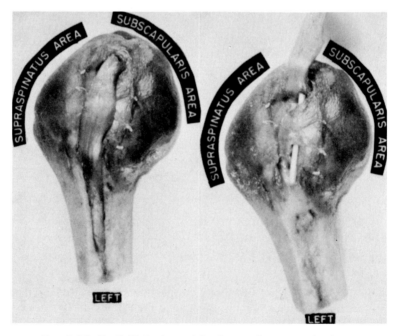

Fig. 6-38. (*Left*) Note that while the tendon occupies its normal position it lies to the inside of the lesser tuberosity. (*Right*) Observe the obliteration of the bicipital groove and that the tendon really lies on a fascial sling made by the insertion of the subscapularis tendon.

FIG. 6-39. Drawing of a sternoclavicular joint prepared for study. The disc is mobilized and the head of the clavicle is rotated upward and backward; all articular surfaces are readily visualized. (DePalma, A. F.: Degenerative changes in the Sternoclavicular and Acromioclavicular Joints in Various Decades. Springfield, Ill., Charles C Thomas, 1957)

(*Bottom*) FIG. 6-40. Drawing of an acromioclavicular joint prepared for study by sharp dissection. (DePalma, A. F.: *Op. cit.,* p. 7)

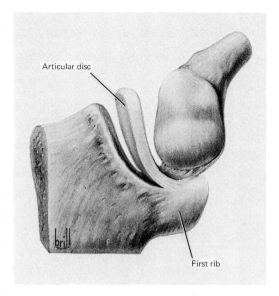

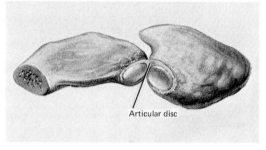

is reduced; now the deltoid muscle displaces the humeral head upward, and, on abduction of the arm, the tuberosity impinges against the acromion. Repeated trauma of this nature results in the formation of large bony excrescences over both tuberosities, such as are seen in Figure 6-36. These bony lesions may encroach upon the margins of the bicipital groove or form within the groove; in fact, the groove may be completely obliterated. Such alterations in and about the groove interfere with the normal excursion of the head of the humerus on the biceps tendon and account for severe alterations in the biceps tendon (Fig. 6-37). The tendon may be displaced from the groove and come to lie on a fascial sling made by the insertion of the subscapularis muscle (Fig. 6-38).

Continued friction between the humeral head and acromion eventually causes resorption of not only the bony excrescences but also the tuberosities themselves. In these specimens the intertubercular portion of the bicipital sulcus is completely worn away; the biceps tendon, as noted above, is always severely implicated; it may be shredded, frayed and displaced from the bicipital sulcus, or the intracapsular portion may deteriorate completely, while the extracapsular portion attains a bony attachment to the upper end of the shaft of the humerus below the lesser tuberosity. Of the adult specimens studied in two series (296 shoulders), the biceps tendon attained a bony attachment to the humerus in 10 shoulders (3.7%) (Fig. 6-26). It was previously pointed out that the supratubercular ridge

may diminish the depth of the bicipital groove; this occurs in approximately 9 percent of the shoulders. This anomaly, together with the bony changes that occur with aging in the region of the tuberosities and bicipital groove, enhances the vulnerability of the biceps tendon. This combination contributes to the development of profound degenerative changes in the tendon.

## DEGENERATIVE CHANGES OCCURRING IN THE STERNOCLAVICULAR AND ACROMIOCLAVICULAR JOINTS WITH AGING

The total performance of the hand as used by man depends not only on normal motion in the glenohumeral joint but also on normal function in the sternoclavicular and acromioclavicular joints. For example, of the 180° of elevation that the arm can

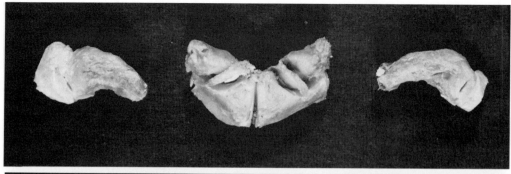

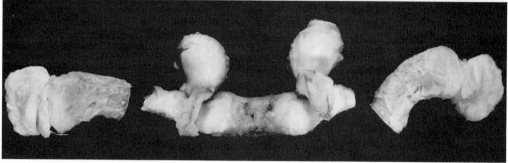

(*Top*) FIG. 6-41. Paired sternoclavicular and acromioclavicular joints of a premature infant, 7 months gestation. At this early age, in these specimens the interarticular discs of the sternoclavicular joints are well formed, dividing the joint cavity into two compartments. A flexible bar of fibrocartilage bridges the acromion and clavicle of each acromioclavicular joint. As yet a joint cavity is not grossly visible but it is discernible microscopically as a fine slit close to the acromion. (DePalma, A. F.: Op. cit., p. 18)

(*Bottom*) FIG. 6-42. Right and left sternoclavicular and acromioclavicular joints of a child, male, 3½ years of age. Observe the large synovial cavities on either side of the interarticular discs of the sternoclavicular joints and the broad areas of attachment of the discs to the clavicles. The acromioclavicular joints showed a small synovial cavity on the acromial side of the disc of the right joint, and a cavity on both sides of the disc in the left joint. (DePalma, A. F.: Op. cit., p. 21)

attain, 40° are contributed by the sternoclavicular and 20° by the acromioclavicular joint. Thus, any dysfunction in either of these two joints is reflected in the functioning of the upper extremity. The role these two joints play in shoulder motion has already been discussed. It is important to remember that the sternoclavicular joint is the only articulation between the arm and the trunk that is capable of moving about an almost infinite number of axes, and that every motion in the upper extremity is accompanied by some kind of motion in the sternoclavicular joint, in the form of impact, glide or rotation. Also, it should be kept in mind that the acromioclavicular joint is exposed and vulnerable to injuries from all directions. Although the arcs of motion in the acromioclavicular joint are smaller than those of the sternoclavicular joint, all movement in the sternoclavicular joint is accompanied by movement in the opposite direction in the acromioclavicular joint.

In view of the magnitude of the degenerative changes in the glenohumeral joint caused by aging and excessive activity, is it likely that the sternoclavicular and acromioclavicular joints respond in a like manner to these noxious agents? To answer this query, 223 sets of sternoclavicular and

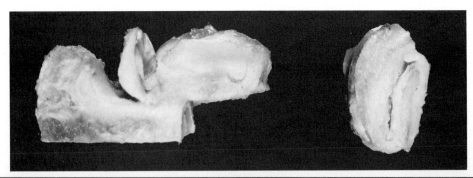

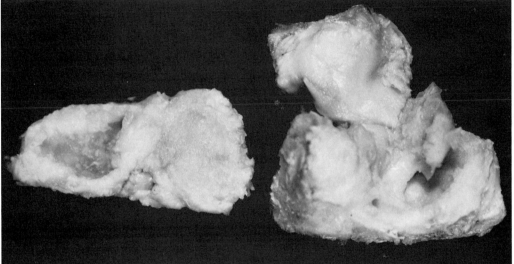

(*Top*) Fig. 6-43. Left sternoclavicular and acromioclavicular joints of female 28 years of age. The interarticular disc of the sternoclavicular joint is a complete structure and divides the joint into two separate compartments. The articular surfaces of the disc, clavicle and sternum exhibit no gross degenerative alterations. Note that the acromioclavicular joint discloses no changes in the articular surface of the clavicle and acromion but its disc exhibits far advanced degenerative changes. (DePalma, A. F.: Op. cit., p. 24)

(*Bottom*) Fig. 6-44. Right sternoclavicular and acromioclavicular joints of a male 40 years of age. The sternoclavicular disc is meniscoid in shape and permits the two compartments to communicate with one another. This is a congenital variation of the disc and not the result of degenerative changes. The acromioclavicular joint surfaces show extensive degeneration; the surfaces are granular and covered with surface and marginal excrescences. Only a small tab remains of the disc and it is markedly hypertrophied. (DePalma, A. F.: Op. cit., p. 30)

acromioclavicular joints were obtained postmortem, ranging from those of premature infants to specimens from persons 94 years of age. Only those subjects were included in this study whose hospital records showed either that routine questioning had revealed no symptoms indicative of joint involvement, or that physical examination elicited no joint abnormalities.

The observations made in this study were published in 1957\*; the reader is referred to this work if he desires to study the material in greater detail than will be presented in this monograph.

\* DePalma, A. F.: Degenerative Changes in the Sternoclavicular and Acromioclavicular Joints in Various Decades. Springfield, Ill., Charles C Thomas, 1957.

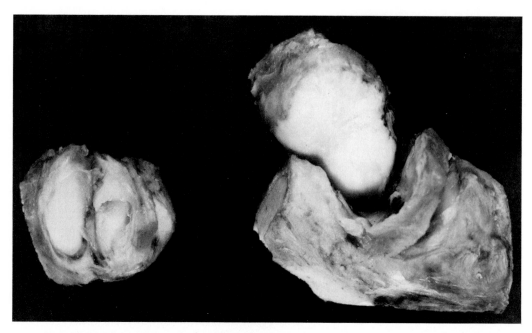

FIG. 6-45. Right sternoclavicular and acromioclavicular joints of a male 26 years of age. Observe the early changes taking place in the sternoclavicular joint. The changes are not severe. The articular surface of the clavicle shows some shredding, furrowing and fraying. The disc, a stout structure, shows some mild shredding and lamination, particularly at its center. The acromioclavicular joint shows more advanced changes than does the sternoclavicular joint. Note the severe pitting and fraying of the articular cartilage of the clavicle; the interarticular disc is meniscoid and discloses pronounced regressive changes. (DePalma, A. F.: Op. cit., p. 27)

Each sternoclavicular joint was prepared for study by removing all soft tissues down to the fibrous capsule by sharp dissection. The anterior and posterior portions of the fibrous capsule, together with the superior attachment of the disc, were severed close to the clavicle. Again, by sharp dissection, the anterior, superior and posterior portions of the capsule were cut close to the sternum. The dissection mobilized the disc completely, except at its inferior border, where it blends with the fibrocartilage of the sternum. The only connection between the clavicle and the sternum was the inferior-posterior portion of the capsule, which was used as a hinge to rotate the clavicle upward, backward and away from the midline. This brings into view the entire articular surface of the clavicle and sternum, and both surfaces of the disc (Figs. 6-39 and 6-40).

The acromioclavicular joints also were prepared for study by sharp dissection. In each instance, all the overlying soft tissues were cut away down to the fibrous capsule. Then, the superior attachment was divided close to the acromion on one side and close to the clavicle on the other. The cuts were carried directly downward so that only the inferior portion of the fibrous capsule remained; this was used as a hinge to open the joint (Figs. 6-39 and 6-40).

**Sternoclavicular Joint**

The most significant finding in specimens of the first decade is the great variation in the development of the joint. The subjects from whom the specimens were obtained ranged from premature infants to children $3^{1}/_{2}$ years of age. In one premature infant

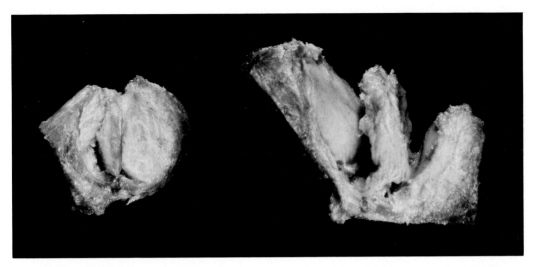

FIG. 6-46. Right sternoclavicular and acromioclavicular joints of a female 37 years of age. At this period of life the sternoclavicular joint shows little or no regressive changes; its articular surfaces show no gross alterations and the articular disc is well preserved. Observe that this is not true of the acromioclavicular joint, which shows advanced changes. (DePalma, A. F.: Op. cit., p. 30)

a well formed synovial cavity is discernible on either side of the intra-articular disc (Fig. 6-41); in contrast, the joints of a child 16 months old exhibit grossly no evidence of a synovial cavity on either side of the disc. However, after the second year all joints show well formed synovial cavities on either side of the discs which essentially divide the sternoclavicular joint into two separate compartments (Fig. 6-42). It is not until the third decade that the joints achieve the highest level of development. At that time the discs assume a convex-concave configuration, slightly thinner at the center than the periphery. They constitute stout, sturdy structures of fibro-cartilage interposed between the articular surface of the clavicle and that of the sternum. Two types of discs are discernible: the complete, and the incomplete or meniscoid. The former is found in 97 percent of the specimens of this series and the latter in 3 percent (Figs. 6-43 and 6-44). For all ages, the thickness of the superior border ranges from 4 mm. to 14 mm., that of the inferior border from 1 mm. to 1 cm.

Degenerative alterations in the articular surfaces and the discs through the first three decades are only minimal in severity. Only one disc in the third decade exhibits abnormal thinning, some shredding and lamination of its fibers, and one reveals moderate implication of the articular surfaces of the clavicle and sternum. These findings are indicative of degenerative processes at work as early as the third decade (Fig. 6-45). During the next 3 decades the degenerative changes in the discs and the articular surfaces become more marked but are never severe (Fig. 6-46). Only one specimen (from an individual 40 years of age) reveals moderate changes in the form of pitting, fraying, lamination and furrowing of the fibrocartilage of the articular surfaces and thinning and shredding of the disc. The disc in this joint is not a complete structure and has a meniscoid configuration (Fig. 6-47).

From the seventh decade onward, severe implication of the disc occurs. In addition to lamination, thinning and shredding of the disc, the frequency of perforation of the structure increases. In the fourth and fifth decades only one perforation was en-

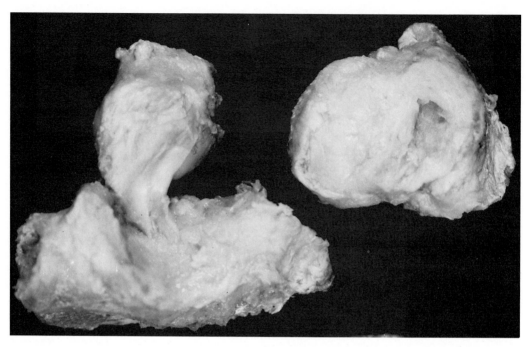

FIG. 6-47. Left sternoclavicular and acromioclavicular joints of a male 40 years of age. Note that the articular disc of the sternoclavicular joint is not a complete structure and is meniscoid in shape. Both the sternal and clavicular surfaces disclose pitting and shredding of the articular cartilage, and the disc shows some lamination. The changes in this joint were the most severe of those found in any of the specimens of the fourth, fifth and sixth decades. (DePalma, A. F.: Op. cit., p. 31)

countered, in the sixth, three, and in the seventh, eight. Thirteen of the 25 discs in the seventh decade reveal profound degenerative changes (Fig. 6-48). In the eighth decade six discs show perforations, and in the ninth and tenth, seven discs (Fig. 6-49).

Study of the articular surfaces of the clavicle and sternum of joints in various decades demonstrates clearly that the severity and extent of alterations in these areas and those of the fibrocartilaginous disc are closely parallel in gradient. As long as the disc remains a sturdy intact structure, it is capable of meeting the functional demands of the articulation and protecting adequately the articular surfaces of the joint. Up to the seventh decade, the disc is able to perform this function without difficulty; however, in most instances, at this point the degenerative processes incident to aging and function overcome the physi-

cal capacity of the disc, producing marked deterioration of the disc. It appears that, without the buffer effect of the disc, the articular surfaces alone are unable to withstand the stresses of function.

From this study one must conclude that the sternoclavicular joint is the most stable of the three true articulations of the shoulder complex. This is true in spite of its obviously unstable bony configuration. The stability of the joint is provided mainly by the tough, fibrocartilaginous disc, which functions not only as an intra-articular buffer between the articular surfaces of the clavicle and the sternum but also as a powerful intra-articular ligament, tethering the clavicle to the sternum and the first rib. It was previously noted, in the discussion on the biomechanics of the sternoclavicular joint, that the costoclavicular ligament is the most important extra-articular structure,

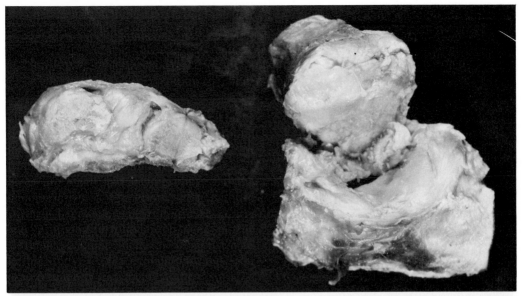

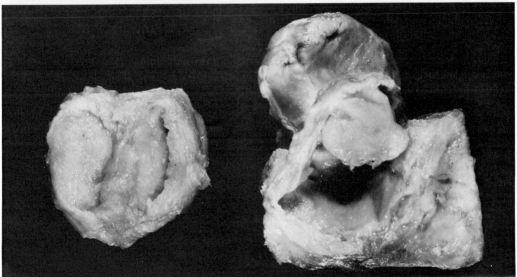

(*Top*) Fɪɢ. 6-48. Specimens of the seventh decade. Note the total disintegration of the articular disc of the sternoclavicular joint. The articular surfaces present advanced degeneration of the cartilage and surface excrescences. (DePalma, A. F.: Op cit., p. 53)

(*Bottom*) Fɪɢ. 6-49. Right joints of a female 78 years of age. Note that only a tab of disc remains which is thin and irregular. The surfaces of the sternoclavicular joint reveal severe degenerative changes. The acromioclavicular joint also shows profound degenerative alterations; the remnant of its articular disc is frayed and thickened and meniscoid in shape. (DePalma, A. F.: Op. cit., p. 67)

providing stability to the joint by firmly binding the clavicle to the sternum and the cartilage of the first rib. In the light of this knowledge one can understand why the sternoclavicular joint is so seldom a source of pain and dysfunction, compared to the frequency of disorders affecting the acromioclavicular joint.

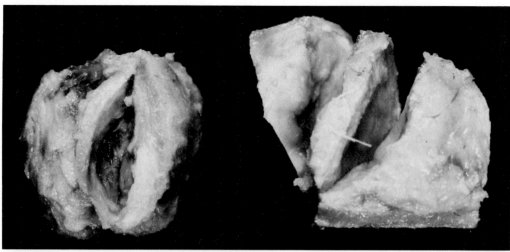

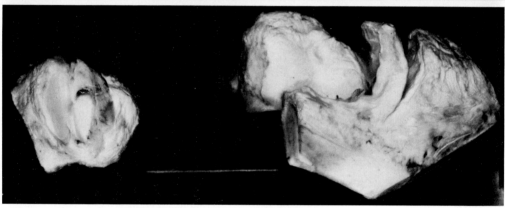

(*Top*) FIG. 6-50. Right joints from a male 94 years of age. The disc of the acromio-clavicular joint is a complete structure and divides the joint cavity into two compartments. Note that even in this late period of life, the articular disc of the sternoclavicular joint is well preserved and the degenerative changes of the articular surfaces are only moderate in degree. (DePalma, A. F.: Op. cit., p. 71)

(*Bottom*) FIG. 6-51. Right joints of a male 15 years of age. Note the complete articular disc of the sternoclavicular joint; its surfaces are smooth and glistening and exhibit no regressive changes. The same is true of the articular surface of the clavicle and the sternum. The acromioclavicular joint contains a meniscoid-type articular disc. Observe that its edges are thin, frayed and scalloped. These are the earliest degenerative changes encountered in this study. The articular surfaces of the acromioclavicular joint show no regressive alterations. (DePalma, A. F.: Op. cit., p. 21)

## Acromioclavicular Joint

As in the sternoclavicular joint, development of the intra-articular disc shows considerable variation; however, it tends to lag behind that of the sternoclavicular disc. In all the acromioclavicular joints of the premature infants a flexible band of cartilage is interposed and is continuous with the adjacent fibrocartilage of the clavicle and the acromion. In specimens from the first decade, the acromioclavicular joints of a specimen $3\frac{1}{2}$ years of age show evidence of formation of synovial cavities; in the right joint a small synovial cavity is noted only on the acromial side of the interposing fibrocartilaginous disc. The left joint exhibits a small synovial cavity on both

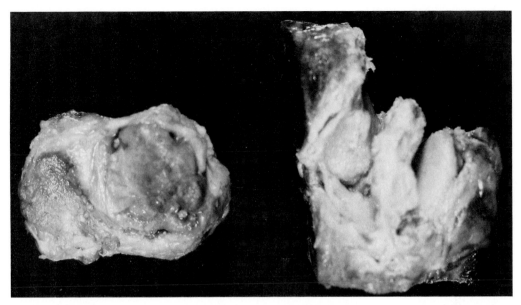

FIG. 6-52. Joints of a male 49 years of age. Note the severe implication of the articular surfaces of the acromioclavicular joint; marginal elevations and formations of bony ridges are readily discernible at the periphery and on the surfaces of the joint. The articular disc has disintegrated completely. (DePalma, A. F.: Op. cit., p. 37)

sides of the articular disc. Two types of discs were encountered: a complete disc, and a meniscoid or incomplete disc (Figs. 6-45 and 6-50). It is impossible to determine accurately the incidence of these types because of the rapid and advanced deterioration of the structures after the second decade.

All the discs of the second decade were meniscoid in form. The meniscoid variety resembles closely the meniscus of the knee joint, whereas the complete disc divides the joint cavity into two compartments. In this entire series, only 9 percent of the acromioclavicular joints contain a complete disc; in 81 percent either the structure is absent or only remnants of the disc remain; 10 percent of the specimens disclose a meniscoid type of disc. In the last-mentioned group it is impossible to determine whether the meniscoid disc is congenital in origin or the result of attritional changes.

In the second decade, whereas the intra-articular discs of the sternoclavicular joints show no regressive change, the discs of the acromioclavicular joints reveal definite evidence of degenerative alterations (Fig. 6-51). As previously noted, in 81 percent of all joints of this series the discs were either absent or in the form of irregular tabs and remnants. A high level of involvement is discernible as early as the fourth decade. In the fourth decade only one specimen presents a complete disc; the remaining discs have disintegrated completely. The response of the articular surfaces of the clavicle and sternum in the joints of this decade also reveals attritional alterations in the form of fibrillation, lamination and erosion of the articular cartilage. Although the abnormalities were only moderate in severity in the fourth decade, they increased progressively from decade to decade. Many specimens exhibit marginal osteophytes and surface excrescences, producing severe incongruity of the articular surfaces (Fig. 6-52). Whereas in the acromioclavicular joints advanced degeneration of the articular surfaces occurs in the middle decades of life, such attritional changes were not

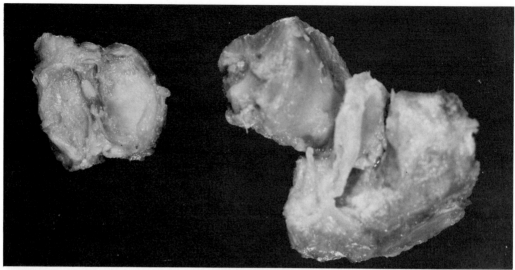

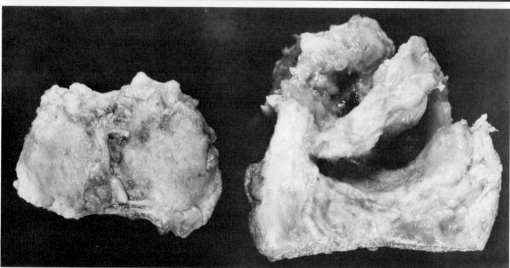

(*Top*) FIG. 6-53. Joint of a male 52 years of age. The acromioclavicular joint reveals severe, widespread involvement of its surface. Only a few tabs of tissue constitute the remnants of the articular disc. (DePalma, A. F.: Op. cit., p. 44)

(*Bottom*) FIG. 6-54. Right joints of a male 69 years of age. Observe that the surfaces of the acromioclavicular joint are devoid of cartilage; the subchondral bone is dense, pitted and nodular. The extensive marginal lipping increases the size of both the clavicular and the acromial surfaces. The articular disc has disintegrated completely. The sternoclavicular joint also shows degenerative changes, but to a lesser degree. The articular disc of this specimen showed a defect in its central and inferior portions. (DePalma, A. F.: Op. cit., p. 51)

found in the articular surfaces of the sternoclavicular joints until the seventh decade, when the intra-articular discs show extensive deterioration. This suggests that the early loss of the intra-articular discs in the acromioclavicular joints may be responsible for the early and extensive alterations in the articular cartilage of the acromion and clavicle (Figs. 6-53, 6-54 and 6-55).

It becomes apparent that the acromio-

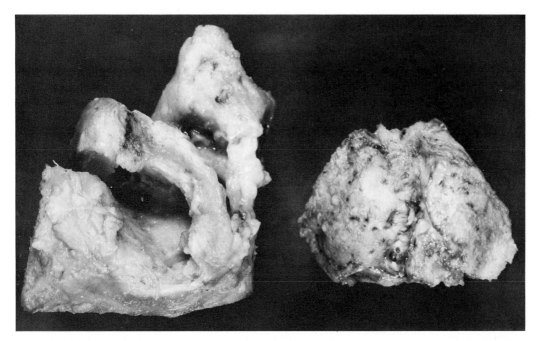

FIG. 6-55. Left joints of a male 69 years of age. Note the extensive implication of the articular surfaces of the acromioclavicular joint. The cartilage is completely destroyed, the surfaces are pitted and nodular and the articular disc has completely disintegrated. (DePalma, A. F.: Op. cit., p. 51)

clavicular joint is not very stable and lacks soft tissue elements, such as those found in the sternoclavicular joint, to protect it from early degeneration. Its articular surfaces are small and incongruous, and the manner in which it functions subjects those surfaces to constant shearing stresses. Early and profound attritional changes in the acromioclavicular joint, as demonstrated in this study, readily explain why this joint is so frequently the site of painful disorders.

## BIBLIOGRAPHY

Adams, R.: Abnormal conditions of the hip joint. *In*: Todd, R. B. (ed.): Cyclopaedia of Anatomy and Physiology. Vol. 2 pp. 780-825, London, Longmans, 1930.

Allison, N., and Ghormley, R. K.: Diagnosis in Joint Disease. New York, Wood, 1931.

Axhausen, G.: Ueber einfache, aseptische Knochen- und Knorpelnekrose, Chondritis dissecans und Arthritis deformans. Arch. klin. Chir., *99*:519, 1912.

Axhausen, G., and Pels, I.: Experimentelle Beitrage zur Genese der Arthritis deformans. Deutsch. Z. Chir., *110*:515, 1911.

Bauer, W.: Studies pertaining to the origin and nature of hypertrophic arthritis. Trans. Col. Physicians Phila. (4th Series), 7:1-20, 1939.

Bauer, W., and Bennett, G. A.: Experimental and pathological studies in the degenerative type of arthritis. J. Bone & Joint Surg., *18*:1-18, 1936.

Bauer, W., Bennett, G. A., Marble, A., and Clafflin, D.: Observations on normal synovial fluid of cattle. I. The cellular constituents and nitrogen content. J. Exp. Med., *52*:835-848, 1930.

Beitzke, H.: Ueber die sogenannte Arthritis deformans atrophica. Z. klin. Med., *74*:215, 1912.

Bennett, G. A., and Bauer, W.: A systematic study of the degeneration of articular cartilage in bovine joints. Am. J. Path., 7:399-413, 1931.

Bennett, G. A., Bauer, W., and Maddock, S. J.: A study of repair of articular cartilage and the reaction of normal joints of adult dogs to surgically created defects of articular cartilage, "joint mice," and patellar displacement, Am. J. Path., *8*:499, 1932.

Benninghoff, A.: Form und Bau der Gelenk-
knorpel in ihren Beziehungen zur Funktion. I.
Z. Anat. Entwcklungsgesch., 76:43, 1925. II.
Z. Zellforsch., 2:783, 1925.

Burckhardt, H.: Arthritis deformans. München
med. Wschr., 71:1495-1997, 1924.

Callender, G. R., and Kelser, R. A.: Degenerative arthritis: A comparison of the pathological changes in man and equines. Am. J. Path.,
14:253, 1938.

Chamberlain, E. B., and Taft, R. B.: Ancient
arthritis. Radiology, 30:761, 1938.

Charcot, J. M.: Leçons sur les maladies des
viellards et les maladies chroniques. Paris,
A. Delahaye, 1867.

Clark, H. C.: Etiologic factors in gross lesions
of the large joints, JAMA, 69:2099, 1917.

Codman, E. A.: The Shoulder. Boston, Thomas
Todd Company, 1934.

DePalma, A. F.: Surgery of the Shoulder. Ed.
Philadelphia, J. B. Lippincott, 1950.

_____: Degenerative Changes in the Sterno-
clavicular and Acromioclavicular Joints in
Various Decades, Springfield, Ill., Charles C
Thomas, 1957.

Doub, H. P., and Jones, H. C.: An evaluation
of injury and faulty mechanics in the development of hypertrophic arthritis. Am. J. Roentgenol., 34:315-324, 1936.

Elliott, H. C.: Studies on articular cartilage: I.
Growth mechanisms. Am. J. Anat., 58:127-
141, 1936.

Ely, L. W.: A study of the sternoclavicular joint.
In: Bone and Joint Studies. pp. 121-139. Stanford University Press, 1916.

Ely, L. W., and Cowan, J. F.: Experimental re-
action of the dog's knee-joint. In: Bone and
Joint Studies. pp. 5-38. Stanford University
Press, 1916.

Fisher, A. G. T.: A contribution to the pathology and etiology of osteoarthritis; with observations upon the principles underlying its
surgical treatment. Brit. J. Surg., 10:52-80,
1922.

Fletcher, E.: Herberden Lecture; Osteoarthritis; an attempt to elucidate aetiology and
pathogenesis of the condition by clinical study
and analysis. Brit. J. Rheumat., 2:62-111,
1939.

Gardner, E.: Physiological mechanisms in movable joints. Instructional Course Lectures,
10:251, 1953.

Goldhaft, A. D., Weight, L. M., and Pemberton, R.: The production of hypertrophic
arthritis by interference with the blood supply.
Am. J. Med. Sci., 180:386-397, 1930.

Harrison, M. H. M., Schajowicz, F., and Trueta,
J.: Osteoarthritis of the hip: a study of the
nature and evolution of the disease. J. Bone
& Joint Surg., 35-B:596, 1953.

Hench, P. S.: Acute and chronic arthritis. In:
Nelson's Loose-Leaf Surgery. Vol. 3. pp.
104-175. New York, Nelson, 1935.

Hippocrates: The Genuine Works of Hippocrates, translated by Francis Adams. New
York, Wood, 1886.

Jones, E. S.: Joint lubrication. Lancet, 226(1):
1426, 1934.

Kellgren, J. A., and Samuel, E. P.: The sensitivity and innervation of the articular capsule.
J. Bone & Joint Surg., 32-B:84, 1950.

Key, J. A.: The reformation of synovial membrane in the knees of rabbits after synovec-
tomy. J. Bone & Joint Surg., 7:793, 1925.

_____: Traumatic arthritis and the mechanical
factors in hypertrophic arthritis. J. Lab. Clin.
Med., 15:1145-1160, 1930.

_____: The synovial membrane of joints and
bursae. In: Cowdry, E. V. (ed.): Special
Cytology. 2nd ed. Vol. 2. p. 1053. New York,
Hoeber, 1932.

Knaggs, R. L.: A report on the Strangeways
Collection of rheumatoid joints in the Museum of the Royal College of Surgeons. Brit.
J. Surg., 20:113-129, 309-330, 1932; 425-
443, 1933.

Kuhns, J. G.: Hypertrophic arthritis of the hip:
A review of 79 patients. New Eng. J. Med.,
210:1213-1216, 1934.

Lang, F. J.: Mikrokopische Befunde bei ju-
veniler Arthritis deformans (Osteochondritis
deformans juvenilis coxae Legg-Calve-
Perthes), nebst vergleichenden Untersuchungen über die Femur kipfepiphyse mit be-
sondere Berücksichtigung der Fovea. Virchows Arch. Path. Anat. 239:76, 1922.

_____: Osteo-arthritis deformans contrasted
with osteo-arthritis deformans juvenilis. J.
Bone & Joint Surg., 14:563-573, 1932.

Langen, P.: Untersuchungen über die Altersver-
änderungen und Abnutzungserscheinungen
am Sternoclaviculargelenk. Virchows Arch.,
293:381-408, 1934.

MacConaill, M. A.: The function of intra-
articular fibrocartilages, with special refer-
ences to the knee joint and inferior radio-
ulnar joints. J. Anat., 66:210, 1932.

_____: The movement of bones and joints. The
synovial fluid and its assistants. J. Bone &
Joint Surg., 32-B:244, 1950.

Meyer, A. W.: Further evidence of attrition in
the human body. Am. J. Anat., 34:241-267,
1924. Anat. Rec., 27:211, 1924.

_____: The minuter anatomy of attrition le-
sions. J. Bone & Joint Surg., 13:341, 1931.

_____: Use-destruction in the human body.
West. Med., 47:375, 1937.

_____: Chronic functional lesions of the shoul-
der. Arch. Surg., 35:646, 1937.

Meyer, H.: Der Knorpel und seine Verknoche-rung. Arch. Anat. Physiol. wissensch. Med., pp. 292-357, 1849.

Meyer, K.: The biological significance of hy-aluronic acid and hyaluronidase. Physiol. Rev., *27*:335, 1947.

Meyer, K., and Rapaport, M. M.: The muco-polysaccharides of the ground substance of connective tissue. Science, *113*:596, 1951.

Parker, F., Jr., Keefer, C. S., Myers, W. K., and Irwin, R. L.: Histologic changes in the knee joint with advancing age. Arch. Path., *17*:516-532, 1934.

Pemberton, R.: The present status of the prob-lem of arthritis. J. Lab. Clin. Med., *15*:1055-1061, 1930.

Phemister, D. B.: Changes in bone and joints resulting from interruption of circulation. Arch. Surg., *41*:1-455, 1940.

Physics of Lubrication. A symposium. Brit. J. Appl. Physics (Suppl. I). London, the In-stitute of Physics. 1951.

Reynolds, O.: On the theory of lubrication and its application to Mr. Beauchamp Tower's experiments, including an experimental de-termination of the viscosity of olive oil. Philos. Tr. Roy. Soc. (London) A., *177*:157, 1886.

Shands, A. R.: The regeneration of hyaline car-tilage in joints. Arch. Surg., *22*:137-178, 1931.

Smith-Petersen, M. N.: Traumatic arthritis; histologic changes in hyaline cartilage. Arch. Surg., *18*:1216-1226, 1929.

Strangeways, T. S. P.: Observations on the nu-trition of articular cartilage. Brit. Med. J., *1*:661, 1920.

Trueta, J., and Harrison, M. H. M.: The normal vascular anatomy of the femoral head in adult man. J. Bone & Joint Surg., *35-B*:442, 1953.

Urist, M. R.: Complete dislocations of the acromioclavicular joint. J. Bone & Joint Surg., *28*:813, 1946.

Virchow, R.: Ueber parenchymatose Entzun-dung. Virchows Arch., *4*:261-324, 1852.

Wagoner, G., Rosenthal, O., and Bowie, M. A.: Studies of the cell in normal and arthritic bovine cartilage. Am. J. Med. Sci., *201*:489-495, 1941.

Walmsley, T.: The articular mechanisms of the diarthroses. J. Bone & Joint Surg., *10*:40, 1928.

Warren, C. F., Bennett, G. A., and Bauer, W.: The significance of the cellular variations oc-curring in normal synovial fluid. Am. J. Path., *11*:953-968, 1935.

Willis, T. A.: The age factor in hypertrophic arthritis. J. Bone & Joint Surg., *6*:316-325, 1924.

# 7

# Surgical Approaches and Procedures

Many disorders of the shoulder require surgical intervention. Among these are traumatic disruption of the articulations of the shoulder (the glenohumeral, sternoclavicular and acromioclavicular joints); certain fractures of the bony elements of the shoulder girdle; disabling disorders associated with degenerative changes involving the components of the shoulder joint (rupture of the rotator cuff, hypertrophic arthritis of the acromioclavicular joint and rupture or attritional changes of the biceps tendon); certain tumors of bone or soft tissues, treated by resection of various parts of the shoulder girdle or by amputation of the upper extremity at various levels. In addition, many forms of muscle imbalance about the shoulder joint, resulting from peripheral nerve lesions or from more widespread neurological involvement, as seen in poliomyelitis or in the various forms of birth palsies, can be treated by reconstructive procedures such as transfer of certain muscles or muscle groups, arthrodesis and arthroplasty of the glenohumeral joint. Finally, in the event of acute vascular injury jeopardizing the extremity or even the life of the patient, immediate surgical exposure of the affected vessel or vessels is mandatory.

The goal of any surgical procedure is total restoration of painless function of the implicated upper extremity. It is not always possible to attain this goal, and many compromises may have to be made. Nevertheless, a skillful and knowledgeable surgeon makes the least possible compromise and attains the best possible functional results.

To achieve the best surgical results, certain principles, which are applicable to all other areas of the body, must be adhered to: (1) The incision should be adequate to permit performance of the various operative steps with ease and without undue tension on the soft tissues. Few sights are as ridiculous — and, in a way, as sad — as a surgeon struggling in an incision too small to expose the essential anatomy adequately. The procedure becomes a tug-of-war between assistants pulling on retractors in opposite directions. (2) All tissues must be handled with gentleness. This reduces surgical trauma to tissues to a minimum and ensures healing of the wound without complication. (3) Hemostasis should be complete. If ligatures are used, only the bleeding vessels should be tied and not the vessel together with a large bite of soft tissue. Such tissue dies and must be resorbed in the wound. This is also true if a coagulating current is used to achieve hemostasis. Don't coagulate more tissue than is necessary! (4) Stretched and hypertrophic scars resulting from ill placed incisions about the shoulder may cause grave concern, especially to women. Cosmetically unacceptable scars can be avoided, provided that a few simple principles of biomechanics of the skin are not violated. Although skin exhibits great variation in tension in different parts of the body, the directional quality of skin tension in different areas is well known. The crease lines of the body correspond to the lines of maximum skin tension at that particular site. In other words, a crease line will form only if the tension at right angles to it is

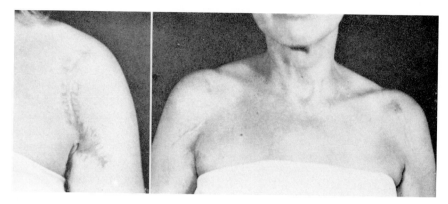

FIG. 7-1. A wide, ugly scar has formed following the use of a delto-pectoral incision. (*Right*) The scar on the left shoulder followed an anterior vertical incision; the scar on the right shoulder followed a curved incision. Although the latter is less disfiguring than the former, both scars are cosmetically unacceptable.

insignificant. Surgical experience teaches that incisions at right angles to crease lines produce ugly, stretched or hypertrophied scars; and, incisions paralleling them produce thin, fine scars, some being barely visible. Many surgeons still use the so-called Langer's lines to plan a skin incision, believing that these lines parallel skin tension lines. Nothing is further from the truth. In many parts of the body Langer's lines actually cross skin creases.

In the region of the shoulder the skin crease in the axilla is an excellent example of a line of maximum skin tension. Skin incisions in the axilla paralleling this line produce fine, almost hairline scars. On the superior and anterior aspect of the shoulder, with the arm at the side of the body, the lines of maximum skin tension parallel the axillary crease. Thus, skin incisions placed over the top of and on the anterior surface of the shoulder which parallel the lines of maximum tension are likely to heal with less stretching and hypertrophic scars than those cutting across or obliquely to them (Figs. 7-1 and 7-2). The transacromial and axillary incisions conform to the lines of maximum skin tension. They are the most widely used by surgeons who are acutely aware of how ugly an ill placed incision can be. Most surgical procedures on the superior, lateral, anterior and inferior regions of the shoulder can be performed through these approaches. I prefer these to all others.

## Position of Patient

Correct positioning of the patient facilitates surgical procedures about the shoul-

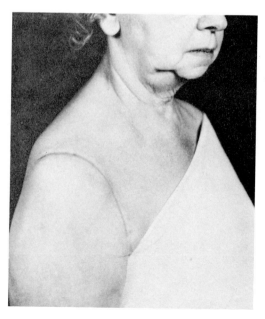

FIG. 7-2. This incision is more cosmetically acceptable by far; it is in line with the axillary crease.

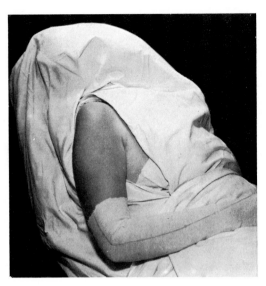

FIG. 7-3. Position of patient for surgery on the shoulder.

criteria for approaches to the superior, anterior, lateral, posterior and inferior regions of the shoulder.

The patient lies on the table with the upper part of his body elevated 45 to 60° from the horizontal. For stability, the lower part of the table is raised under the patient's knees. The arm is placed so that it rests on the edge of the table. To permit easy manipulation of the extremity it is draped separately. A sandbag is placed under the shoulder. Finally, the table is tilted slightly away from the surgeon (Fig. 7-3).

The supine position is used to approach the anterior aspect of the clavicle or the sternoclavicular joint. The patient lies on the table with a sandbag between the shoulder blades. If the arm is to be manipulated during the procedure, it should be draped separately.

For posterior approaches the patient lies in the prone position. A sandbag is placed under the chest wall of the affected side. The head of the patient is turned to the opposite side and the outstretched arm, draped separately, is placed on a table or arm board.

der. The position should be such that both surgeon and assistants can work with greatest efficiency and ease, and all the anatomical structures are readily accessible to them. The semisitting position fulfills the above

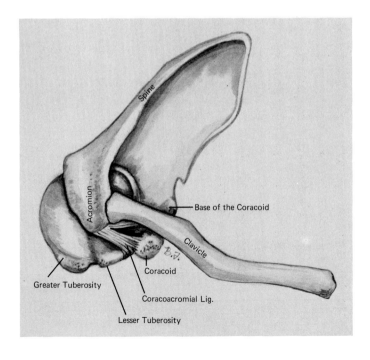

FIG. 7-4. Bony landmarks of the shoulder girdle. Note that the base of the coracoid is medial to the tip of the acromion.

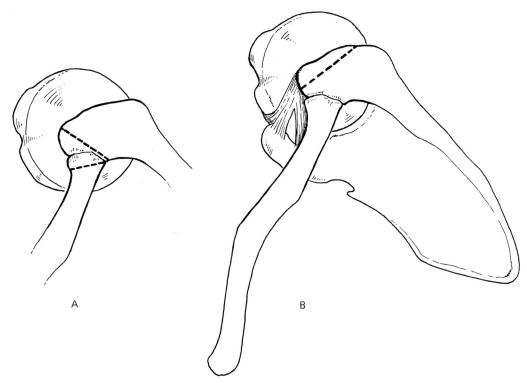

FIG. 7-5. (A) Lines of osteotomy through the acromion or clavicle adjacent to the acromioclavicular joint. (B) Line of osteotomy through the acromion; the deltoid is still attached to the distal fragment.

## Anesthesia

For extensive procedures, intratracheal anesthesia is by far the best. It eliminates the usual difficulties encountered with inhalation anesthesia. For short, simple, open procedures, such as evacuating a calcareous deposit, local anesthesia may be used.

When general anesthesia is contraindicated, brachial block anesthesia, given expertly, is excellent for both open and closed procedures.

## PERTINENT ANATOMICAL RELATIONSHIPS

### Superior and Anterior Regions of the Shoulder

Most surgical procedures on the shoulder joint are performed through superior or anterior approaches. The most common operations performed through these approaches are: (1) stabilization of anterior recurrent dislocations; (2) reduction of recent or old irreducible dislocations; (3) open reductions of fracture–dislocations of the humerus; (4) resection of the humeral head in preparation for the insertion of a prosthesis; (5) limited resections of the upper end of the humerus; (6) repair of recent or old tears of the rotator cuff; (7) arthrodesis, and (8) drainage of infected joints. Knowledge of pertinent anatomical peculiarities of the superior and anterior regions will facilitate the procedures and prevent damage to important structures—damage that may be irreversible.

### Bony Landmarks

Certain landmarks about the shoulder girdle are excellent guides to placement of the incision and also are intimately related

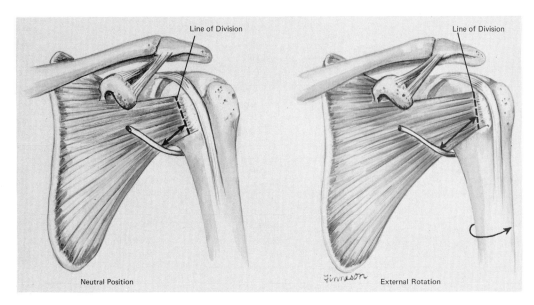

FIG. 7-6. Note that with the arm in external rotation the cut through the tendon of the subscapularis is at a greater distance from the axillary nerve than it is when the arm is in the neutral position.

to important structures encountered in developing the incision. Anteriorly, there are four prominences: the acromion, the coracoid process, the greater tuberosity and the lesser tuberosity (Fig. 7-4). The acromion overhangs the greater and lesser tuberosities and is the tip of the shoulder. The interval between the medial edge of the acromion and the coracoid is spanned by the tough, wide, triangular coracoacromial ligament. This ligament, together with its bony attachments, forms the coracoacromial arch. The edge of the arch digs into the distal end of the rotator cuff during abduction of the arm, producing attritional changes in the cuff. Frequently this overhanging structure obscures the superior and anterior aspects of the upper end of the humerus and the cuff. To obtain better exposure some surgeons remove a portion of the acromion or divide the ligament.

**Acromion.** I believe that partial or total resection of the acromion should never be done except in rare instances. In order to repair an old, severe tear of the rotator cuff adequately, partial or total excision of the acromion may be necessary. This step provides wide exposure of the region. Also, it precludes impingement of the repaired cuff against the coracoacromial arch when the arm is elevated. However, occasions for this are rare. Resection of a portion or all of the acromion produces a flat shoulder. The deltoid is weakened, by being first detached and then reattached at a more proximal site. Often the muscle pulls away from its new bony attachment, producing a sulcus. Not infrequently bony spurs form at the line of attachment; these often give rise to pain.

The deltoid muscle should never be detached from the acromion. Instead, the acromion should be divided just proximal (³/₈ to ½ inch) to the insertion of the deltoid. Reattachment of the distal end of the acromion is readily achieved by fixing it to the body of the acromion with several threaded wires. By handling the acromion in this fashion, the anatomical insertion of the deltoid is not disturbed (Fig. 7-5).

In athletes the insertion of the deltoid must never be disturbed, and, if at all possible, the end of the acromion should not be divided. Wide exposure of the superior re-

gion of the shoulder can be attained by excision of a small piece of the acromion ($3/8$
to $1/2$ inch) immediately adjacent to the
acromioclavicular joint or by excision of
approximately $3/8$ to $1/2$ inch of the distal
end of the clavicle.

Depending upon the exposure I need, I
prefer to excise $3/8$ to $1/2$ inch either of
the clavicle or of the acromion immediately adjacent to the acromioclaviclar joint
in repairing cuff tears in athletes when the
lesion is not accessible after division of
the coracoacromial ligament (Fig. 7-5A).
These procedures do not cause dysfunction of the acromioclavicular joint, and
the length of the acromion is not decreased.

**Coracoid Process and Adjacent Structures.**
The coracoid process lies in the extreme
upper portion of the deltopectoral groove.
It is readily palpable. Its base projects
straight forward but its body crooks laterally and downward towards the glenoid.
This change of direction places the tip of
the coracoid lateral to its base, which lies
directly under the clavicle. When transfixing the clavicle and coracoid with a screw,
in order to strike the base, the screw must
pierce the clavicle at a point medial to the
tip of the coracoid (Fig. 7-4).

This bony process is an important sign-
post, in respect to the nerves and vessels
that lie in close proximity to it. The relationship of these structures changes when
the arm is placed in different positions of
abduction, and internal and external rotation. Failure to appreciate this fact may result in serious injury to the neurovascular
structures. It should be recalled that the
axillary artery and vein and the cords of the
brachial plexus lie behind the pectoralis
minor. With the arm at the side these structures are relaxed and lie at a safe distance
from the coracoid process. But with the
arm abducted they are taut and lie very
close to the tip of the coracoid, rendering
them vulnerable to surgical trauma. When
detaching the coracoid or working on the
coracoclavicular ligaments, place the patient's arm down at the side of the thorax.

When the arm is adducted and the neurovascular structures are relaxed, the lateral
branch of the median nerve and the musculocutaneous nerve lie superficial to the
axillary nerve.

### Axillary Nerve

The axillary nerve lies on the subscapularis muscle; it runs downward and laterally,
paralleling the anterior rim of the glenoid
about a finger's breadth away, and then
winds around the lower edge of the subscapularis muscle. When the arm is adducted and rotated internally, the axillary
nerve approaches very closely the line of
insertion of the subscapularis tendon into
the humerus; it lies about 2 cm. away. On
the other hand, with the arm in a position of
adduction and external retation this distance is increased 5 to 6 cm. However,
there is no change in the relation of the
nerve to the lower edge of the subscapularis
(Fig. 7-6). It becomes apparent that division
of the subscapularis close to its line of insertion into the humerus with the arm adducted and rotated externally precludes injury to the axillary nerve. If the line of
division lies medial to the shaft of the humerus and close to the lower border of the
subscapularis, regardless of whether the
arm is rotated internally or externally, the
axillary nerve and the anterior and posterior
circumflex humeral vessels may be injured.

### Musculocutaneous Nerve

The muscles of the coracoid (the short
head of the biceps and the coracobrachialis)
overlie the subscapularis muscle. In order
to expose the subscapularis muscle or the
joint beneath it, the coracoid muscles must
be either retracted forcefully medially or
detached from the coracoid process. Powerful retraction may produce a traction injury
of the musculocutaneous nerve and of the
lateral branch of the median nerve. Traction on the abducted arm may produce the
same injury. To avoid this mishap and to
obtain better exposure of the region, the

coracoid process should be osteotomized and, with the coracoid muscles, it should be displaced downward and outward.

In several operative procedures the coracoid is divided close to its base and then, with the coracoid muscles still attached, is transferred elsewhere. In the Bristow operation for recurrent dislocation of the shoulder it is attached to the anterior glenoid rim. In the Bailey operation for complete separation of the acromioclavicular joint, it is anchored to the clavicle. When the process is divided close to its base, care must be taken not to injure the lateral branch of the median nerve and the musculocutaneous nerve. They are the most superficial structures below the level of the coracoid, especially when the arm is abducted.

### Suprascapular Nerve

Injury to the suprascapular nerve and vessels is not likely in these procedures. The nerve and vessels lie deep and medial to the base of the coracoid and are under the coracoclavicular ligaments. However, during reconstructive procedures or repair of the ligaments the suprascapular nerve and artery may be injured. I have seen this complication in two patients; in one the ligaments were repaired and in the other they were reconstructed.

### Bicipital Groove and Biceps Tendon

The relationship of the bicipital groove and the tendon within it changes with different positions of rotation of the arm. In internal rotation, the interval between the groove and the anterior rim of the glenoid decreases; in external rotation, it increases. When dividing the subscapularis tendon, the cut should be medial to the medial edge of the bicipital groove. If the line of division lies lateral to the medial edge of the groove, it divides the transverse ligament and capsule overlying the groove. Now, the biceps tendon dislocates from the groove. It was previously noted that, in order to prevent

injury to the axillary nerve and the anterior and posterior circumflex humeral vessels, the line of division in the subscapularis should lie close to the bone and should not be extended too close to the lower border of the muscle. Also, the arm should be adducted and rotated externally (Fig. 7-6).

## DELTOID MUSCLE AND THE AXILLARY NERVE

All approaches to the shoulder must deal with the deltoid muscle. Therefore, surgeons operating in this region should be acquainted in detail with the nerve supply of this muscle. Injury to the nerve supplying the deltoid leads to severe impairment of function of the shoulder.

The deltoid is innervated by the axillary nerve, which is composed of fibers derived from the fifth and sixth cervical nerves. It arises either as one of the terminal branches of the posterior cord of the brachial plexus or directly from the posterior divisions of the plexus. From its origin it runs downward and laterally on the subscapularis muscle to its lower border. At this point it joins the posterior humeral circumflex artery. Together they continue posteriorly around the edge of the muscle in close relation to the surgical neck of the humerus and pass through the quadrangular space. As the nerve passes through the quadrangular space it sends twigs to the capsule of the joint, and as it leaves the space it supplies the teres minor which forms the upper border of the space. On leaving the space, the axillary nerve divides; the posterior branch is the superior lateral brachial cutaneous nerve, which either passes around the posterior border of the deltoid or pierces it, to be distributed to the skin covering the deltoid. The anterior portion of the nerve, together with the posterior humeral circumflex artery, circles the humerus and enters the posterior surface of the deltoid. It then runs transversely giving off branches as it pursues an anterior course. The main trunk of the nerve lies about 5 cm. distal to the

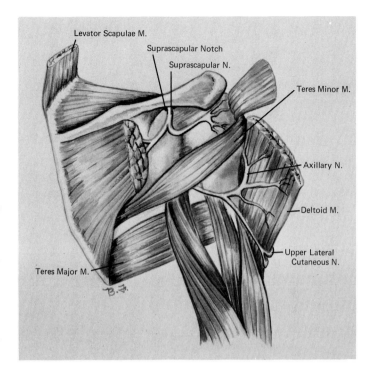

FIG. 7-7. Note that the spine of the scapula crosses the posterior surface of the scapula obliquely upward and laterally. The root or base of the spine forms the medial border of the supraglenoid notch through which pass the suprascapular nerve and vessels from the superior to the inferior fossa.

origin of the muscle; however, the small twigs it distributes to all parts of the muscle may be found close to the line of origin of the deltoid. The so-called *operable area* is a zone measuring 3 to 4 cm. from the origin of the muscle. But, as shown above, even in this zone some branches of the nerve may be severed. In all deltoid splitting incisions the path of the axillary nerve must be respected. If the main trunk of the nerve is divided, the part of the deltoid anterior to the point of severance will be denervated. The deltoid has no other nerve supply (Fig. 7-7). Also, it must be remembered that in approaches detaching the deltoid at its origin the amount of downward retraction of the muscle is limited. Forceful downward retraction of the muscle may seriously injure the axillary nerve.

## Posterior Region of the Shoulder

Not infrequently the surgeon must approach the posterior region of the shoulder. Depending upon the nature of the lesion, the surgical approaches may be limited or extensive. These approaches are employed to stabilize recurrent posterior dislocations and old posterior dislocations, to remove or reattach a fragment of bone avulsed from the posterior glenoid rim, to excise tumors of the scapula or to perform a scapulectomy for malignant lesions.

As is the case for the anterior and the superior regions of the shoulder, certain pertinent anatomical structures in the posterior region have special surgical significance. Knowledge of the relationship of these structures permits the surgeon to develop the incision with ease and precludes injury to the structures.

### Bony Landmarks

The scapula is a flat, triangular bone with three borders (the superior, the medial or vertebral and the lateral or axillary border) and three angles (the superior, the inferior and the lateral angle). Two bony prominences project from the scapula; the coracoid projects anteriorly and the spine posteriorly. The latter ends in the acromion

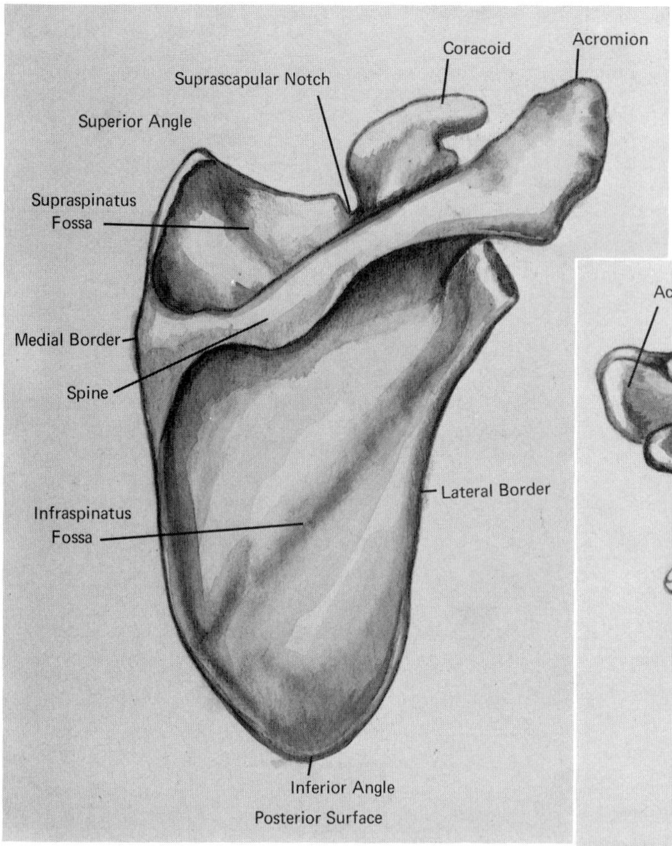

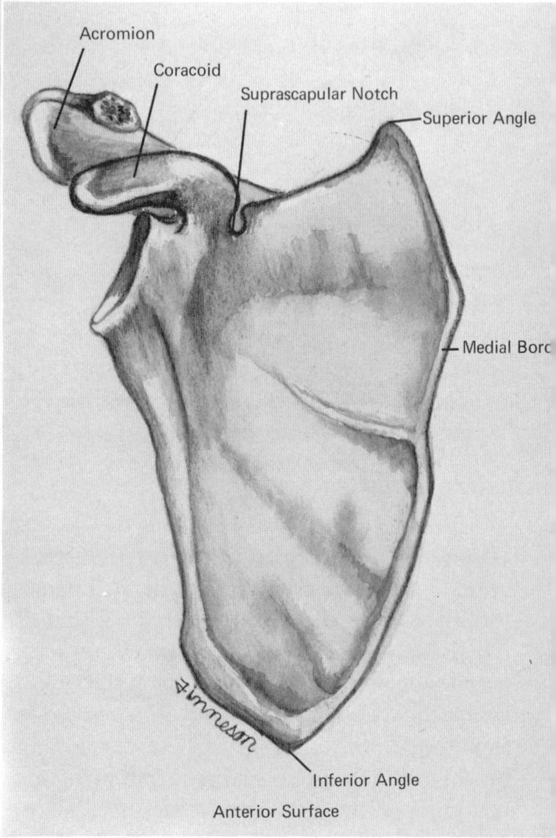

FIG. 7-8. Bony prominences and fossae of the scapula.

process. The scapula lies on the posterior aspect of the thoracic cage and covers the ribs, from the second to the seventh inclusively.

With the patient's arm at his side, one can readily palpate the spine of the scapula as far laterally as the tip of the acromion. The entire spine and the acromion (its tip, lateral border, angle and posterior border) lie directly under the skin.

Again with the arm at the side, the examiner can grasp the inferior angle of the scapula, which is thick and rounded; in fact, he can place his fingers in the interval between the chest wall and the inferior angle. This is not true when the arm is stretched in front of the thorax. In this position, serratus anterior, teres major and rhomboid major, which insert in the inferior angle, contract and hence obliterate the interval.

One can palpate the entire medial border of the scapula as it ascends from the inferior to the superior angle. The superior angle is relatively thin and acute; into it inserts the levator scapulae; one can readily feel this bony landmark. However, even with the muscles relaxed, it is difficult to palpate the lateral border.

The spine of the scapula traverses the posterior surface of the scapula obliquely upward and laterally from its medial border to a point approximately 2 cm. from the glenoid cavity. Because of its stoutness and rounded form this lateral portion of the spine is called the base or root of the spine. It forms the medial border of the spinoglenoid notch, through which the infraspinatus neurovascular structures, branches of the suprascapular nerves and vessels, run from the superior to the posterior fossa. As noted above, the spine terminates in the acromion, a stout, flat, triangular piece of bone that overhangs the glenoid cavity and the humeral head (Fig. 7-7).

The spine divides the dorsal surface of the scapula into the supraspinatus fossa above and the infraspinatus fossa below. The latter is the larger fossa (Fig. 7-8).

## Trapezius Muscle

All surgical approaches designed to expose the scapula, particularly its superior angle, must deal with the trapezius muscle. This muscle plays an important role in the total performance of the shoulder girdle. Injury to its nerve supply results in severe impairment of function. It must be remembered that the trapezius is the main suspensory muscle of the shoulder girdle, and its middle fibers help to anchor the scapula, particularly during pulling. Its lower fibers aid the upper fibers to rotate the scapula by pulling on and depressing the medial border of the scapula. The muscle is innervated by the external branch of the accessory nerve which pierces its deep surface after it crosses the superior angle of the scapula (*See* Figs. 5-17 and 5-18).

The muscle is triangular in shape. It arises from the skull and the spinous processes of all the cervical and thoracic vertebrae and the intervening supraspinous ligaments. In the cervical region it arises not from the cervical spine directly but from the ligamentum nuchae.

The fibers of the trapezius muscle are divided into three groups: the upper fibers run inferolaterally and insert into the posterior border and adjacent part of the upper surface of the flattened outer third of the clavicle. The intermediate fibers take a horizontal and lateral course and insert into the medial border and adjacent part of the upper surface of the acromion and also into the proximal edge of the crest of the spine of the scapula. The lower group, or those

arising distal to the crest of the spine, converge and proceed in a superolateral direction, forming a tough aponeurosis that inserts into the distal edge of the crest of the spine (*See* Fig. 5-17).

Any incision in the region of the trapezius must take into consideration its anatomical boundaries in order to avoid injury to its nerve supply.

## Suprascapular and Supraspinous Region

Directly under the horizontal fibers of the trapezius lie the suprascapular and supraspinous region. It includes the structures occupying and in relation to the supraspinatus fossa and the structures just proximal to the superior border of the scapula. In this area the structures of surgical importance are: the suprascapular nerve, the suprascapular artery, the accessory nerve and the fascia covering the supraspinatus and infraspinatus muscles. The region is best visualized by splitting the horizontal fibers of the trapezius at the level of the superior angle and elevating its insertion from the spine of the scapular (*See* Fig. 4-16).

**Accessory Nerve.** The accessory nerve emerges from the posterior border of the sternocleidomastoid at about its middle. Then it runs downward and backward, crossing the posterior triangle of the neck intrafascially and superficial to the levator scapulae. Finally, it dips under the anterior border of the trapezius, crossing the superior angle of the scapula, and continues downward on the deep surface of the muscle with the superficial branch of the transverse cervical artery (*See* Fig. 5-18).

**Suprascapular Nerve and Artery.** The suprascapular nerve and artery are the most important structures in the suprascapular region. The nerve arises from the upper trunk of the brachial plexus; it is its most lateral branch. The artery is a branch of the thyrocervical trunk; it passes in front of the brachial plexus. Not infrequently the artery

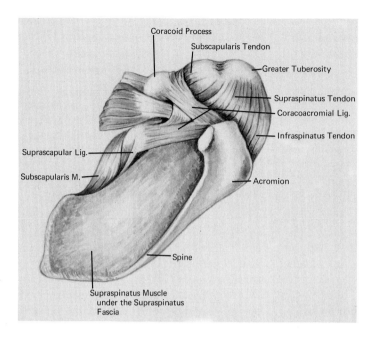

Coracoid Process

Subscapularis Tendon

Greater Tuberosity

Supraspinatus Tendon

Coracoacromial Lig.

Infraspinatus Tendon

Suprascapular Lig.

Subscapularis M.

Acromion

Spine

Supraspinatus Muscle under the Supraspinatus Fascia

Fig. 7-9. Note that the supraspinatus has a tense fascial covering extending from the upper border of the spine of the scapula to the superior scapular border. The supraspinatus tendon passes under the coracoacromial ligament.

may come off the second or third part of the subclavian, in which case it passes through or behind the plexus.

Both the suprascapular artery and nerve cross the base of the neck, passing behind the clavicle. They leave the posterior triangle, dipping under the anterior border of the trapezius. At the superior border of the scapula the artery and the nerve separate, the artery passing above the superior transverse scapular ligament (suprascapular ligament) and the nerve beneath it. The nerve continues through the scapular notch and again meets the artery; together they cross the supraspinatus fossa beneath the supraspinatus muscle and close to the bone, giving off branches to the overlying muscle. Then they pass beneath the root of the acromion and enter the infraspinatus fossa. Here the nerve terminates in the infraspinatus muscle; the artery also sends branches to the muscle and anastomoses with branches of the transverse cervical and of the scapular circumflex arteries (See Figs. 4-16 and 4-17).

**Supraspinatus Fascia.** After the intermediate portion of the trapezius is reflected upward from the spine of the scapula, the supraspinatus muscle is still not clearly visualized in its entirety. The muscle lies under cover of a dense fascia that extends from the upper border of the spine of the scapula to the superior scapular border, thereby enclosing the fossa and its contents. Also, it must be remembered that the tendon of the supraspinatus lies under cover of the tough, triangular coraco-acromial ligament which arches from the lateral border of the horizontal part of the coracoid process to the acromion (Fig. 7-9). To expose the entire supraspinatus the coracoacromial ligament and the fascia must be split.

### Infraspinatus Fascia

A similar situation exists in the infraspinatus region directly under the deltoid. A dense fascia overlies the infraspinatus fossa; it extends from the inferior border of the spine, above, to the vertebral border of the scapula. It covers both the infraspinatus and the teres minor muscles and their tendons, ending with the insertions of the tendons into the humeral head. To expose the muscles and tendons the fascia must be divided; the usual site is in the interval between infraspinatus and teres

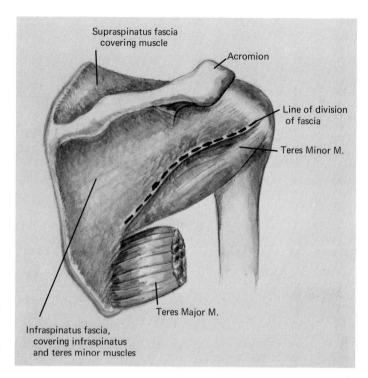

Supraspinatus fascia
covering muscle

Acromion

Line of division
of fascia

Teres Minor M.

Teres Major M.

Infraspinatus fascia,
covering infraspinatus
and teres minor muscles

FIG. 7-10. A tough, dense fascia covers the infraspinatus and teres minor muscle and tendons. The posterior aspect of the joint is readily exposed by dividing the fascia in the interval between the infraspinatus and teres minor.

minor. This is an excellent approach to the posterior region of the glenohumeral joint, especially when a limited approach is desired (Fig. 7-10).

### Posterior Subdeltoid Region

In order to expose this region one must reflect the deltoid from its insertion into the spine and from the acromion process. This route is employed in posterior approaches to the shoulder. The structures of surgical significance in this region are the contents in the quadrangular and triangular spaces. From the front, between the upper border of teres major and the lower border of subscapularis, and from behind, between the upper border of teres major and the lower border of teres minor, lies a triangular space whose apex points medially. This interval is divided by the long head of the triceps into two spaces: the triangular space on the medial side of the long head of the triceps and the quadrangular space on the lateral side (*See* Fig. 4-17).

**Quadrangular Space.** The borders of this space are teres major, below, teres minor (in back) and subscapularis (in front) above, the surgical neck of the humerus laterally and the long head of the triceps medially. Through the space pass the axillary nerve and the posterior humeral circumflex vessels which encircle the surgical neck of the humerus. As the nerve passes through the space it sends twigs to the capsule of the glenohumeral joint, and as it emerges it supplies the teres minor and then divides into two branches. One branch, the superior lateral brachial cutaneous nerve, either passes around the posterior border of the deltoid or pierces its posterior fibers to supply the skin over the muscle. The other branch encircles the humerus together with the artery and in its course sends branches into the deep surface of the deltoid. As previously mentioned, the course of the nerve is approximately 5 cm. below the insertion of the deltoid into the spine of the scapula and the acromion.

Clearly, strong downward and outward traction on the detached muscle may seri-

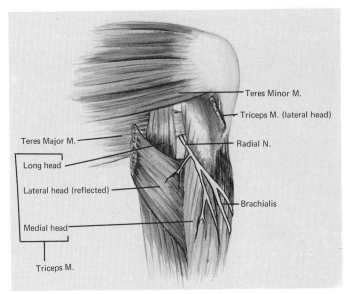

Teres Minor M.
Triceps M. (lateral head)
Teres Major M.
Radial N.
Long head
Lateral head (reflected)
Brachialis
Medial head
Triceps M.

FIG. 7-11. Course of the radial nerve.

ously injure the axillary nerve (*See* Fig. 4-17).

**Triangular Space.** Subscapularis and teres minor form the upper boundary, teres major the lower, and the long head of the triceps the lateral boundary of the triangular space. In the forepart of this space is the scapular circumflex artery, which does not traverse the space but instead winds around the lateral border of the scapula beneath teres minor and continues into the infraspinatus fossa. As the artery passes over the axillary border of the scapula, it lies in a notch (*See* Fig. 4-17).

**Humeral Triangular Space.** This interval lies on the upper and posterior aspect of the arm; essentially it is a tunnel for the radial nerve and the deep brachial artery. This area is of special surgical significance in operations on the upper end of the humerus; here the most important of the structures demanding attention is the radial nerve. In the axilla, after the radial nerve separates from the axillary nerve, it lies behind the axillary artery and successively in front of subscapularis, teres major and latissimus dorsi. As it approaches the upper part of the arm it runs behind the brachial artery and in front of the long head of the triceps. From this position it passes laterally and

posteriorly with the deep brachial artery deep to the long head of the triceps, to enter the spiral groove of the humerus. The groove is converted into a tunnel by the lateral intermuscular septum and the lateral head of the triceps. In the groove, the nerve takes almost a vertical course downward; medially it is in relation to the origin of the medial head of the triceps and laterally to origin of the lateral head of the triceps and the brachialis (Fig. 7-11).

**SUPERIOR APPROACHES**

Most of the superior approaches used today are modifications of the approaches of Kocher and Codman. None of these can be used for all lesions of the shoulder; each has its special indications. However, the approach I use and will describe first, has, in my opinion, more general use than most. In this approach the skin incision parallels the lines of greatest skin tension: hence, a more acceptable scar results. Also, the origin of the middle portion of the deltoid, which is the strongest part of the muscle and is the abductor of the arm, is not disturbed. Through this incision, ruptures of the rotator cuff, reduction and realignment of a fracture–dislocation of the humeral head and excision of the head and its replacement by a prosthesis are readily accomplished.

## Technique

With the patient's arm at the side of the trunk, first locate the exact position of the anterior part of the axillary crease. The skin incision is in line with this point and extends directly over the top of the shoulder; the incision crosses the top of the shoulder just lateral to the acromioclavicular joint.

Start the skin incision just lateral to the acromioclavicular joint and extend it downward in line with the axillary crease over the anterior portion of the deltoid for 1½ to 2 inches below the edge of the acromion. Then extend the incision backward and inferiorly over the posterior portion of the deltoid for 2 inches below the posterior edge of the deltoid (Fig. 7-12A). By sharp dissection develop a lateral skin flap by cutting the subcutaneous tissue from the top of the acromion and the tendinous line of origin of the deltoid on the lateral edge of the acromion (Fig. 7-12B). Next, divide the acromion with a sharp thin osteotome in the line of the skin incision about ⅜ to ½ inch from its outer edge. The cut extends the entire length of the acromion. Retract laterally the cut portion of the acromion with the attached deltoid; this exposes the subacromial bursa (Fig. 7-12C). In order to prevent tearing and stretching of the axillary nerve, lateral retraction must not be severe. Develop a medial skin flap by dividing the subcutaneous tissue over the proximal end of the acromion, the acromioclavicular joint and the outer third of the clavicle (Fig. 7-12D). It is essential that this medial skin flap be sufficiently mobilized, so that one has access to all the underlying structures. By sharp dissection detach the anterior longitudinal fibers of the deltoid from the outer portion of the clavicle as far medially as the deltopectoral groove. Now the entire anterior and middle portions of the deltoid

can be retracted laterally and inferiorly without danger to the axillary nerve (Fig. 7-12E).

The incision developed so far brings into view the entire anterior and superior parts of the joint, the coracoid process and the muscles attached to it, and the cephalic vein as it makes its way upward in the deltopectoral groove. By rotating the arm externally, the subscapularis muscle and its tendon inserting into the lesser tuberosity are readily identified.

Do not remove the walls of the subacromial bursa to expose the rotator cuff. The bursa provides an excellent gliding mechanism between the cuff and the overlying structures. And, if intact during the postoperative healing period, it minimizes formation of adhesions. To expose the cuff, cut the walls of the bursa in the line of the fibers of the cuff and retract the edges. To expose the joint, I prefer to make a cut along the coracohumeral ligament which lies between the upper border of subscapularis and the inferior edge of supraspinatus. In making this cut avoid injury to the intracapsular portion of the biceps tendon. It lies below and just to the outer side of the upper border of the subscapularis. If more exposure of the joint is desired, divide transversely the insertion of the musculotendinous cuff into the greater tuberosity. For even wider exposure, with the arm externally rotated, detach the insertion of the subscapularis from the lesser tuberosity.

If the need should arise, the extreme posterior portion of the joint can be exposed through this incision. To achieve this, mobilize the medial skin flap over the posterior third of the deltoid. By sharp dissection detach the tendinous origin of the deltoid from the lateral third of the crest of the spine and retract it inferiorly with the rest of the deltoid mass (Fig. 7-13).

To reattach the deltoid, anchor the cut end of the acromion to its base with two or three threaded wires. Suture the edge of the anterior portion and the edge of the posterior portion to the fascia on the clavicle

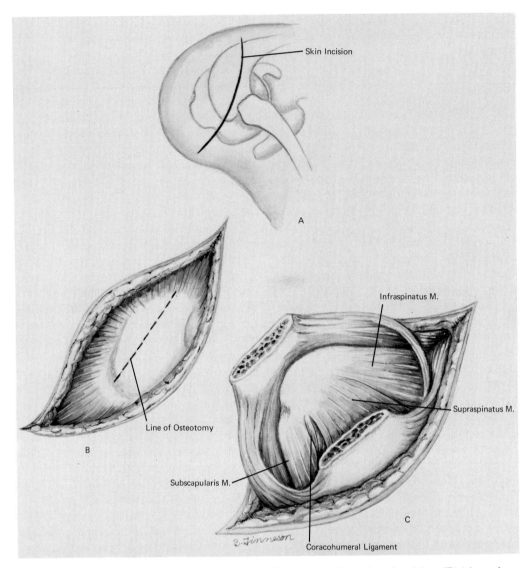

FIG. 7-12. (A) Skin incision for the superior approach to the shoulder. (B) Line of osteotomy, ⅜ to ½ inch from the outer edge of the acromion. (C) The acromion is divided and the distal end retracted laterally with the deltoid, exposing the sub-acromial bursa and the underlying structures. (D) The medial skin flap is reflected to expose the acromioclavicular joint and the distal third of the clavicle. The clavicular origin of the deltoid is detached from the clavicle (outer third) along the indicated line. (E) The clavicular portion of the deltoid is detached and reflected laterally, ex-posing the underlying structures.

and the spine of the scapula respectively.

It must be emphasized that the total incision as described above is not needed in all instances. The superior portion of the incision may suffice for the correction of some lesions; or the superior and anterior portions, or only the anterior portion, for others. In this incision the deltoid fibers are not split either anteriorly or posteriorly. It provides much mobility of the deltoid, making severe retraction in any direction unnecessary, and, hence, sparing the axillary

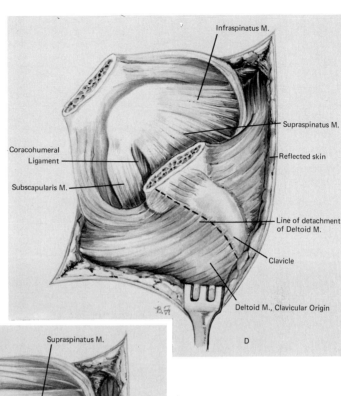

Infraspinatus M.

Supraspinatus M.

Reflected skin

Coracohumeral
Ligament

Subscapularis M.

Line of detachment
of Deltoid M.

Clavicle

FIGURE 7-12 (Cont'd)

Deltoid M., Clavicular Origin

D

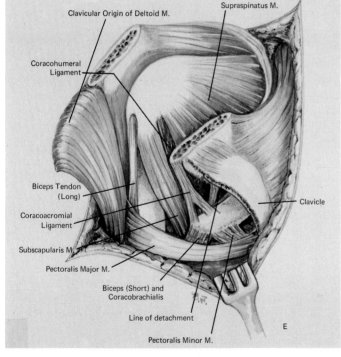

Supraspinatus M.

Clavicular Origin of Deltoid M.

Coracohumeral
Ligament

Biceps Tendon
(Long)

Coracoacromial
Ligament

Clavicle

Subscapularis M.

Pectoralis Major M.

Biceps (Short) and
Coracobrachialis

Line of detachment

E

Pectoralis Minor M.

nerve. Of course, when only parts of the incision are used the mobility of the detached deltoid is reduced. I find that the anterior and superior parts of the incision permit enough exposure of the joint to perform most operations on the shoulder joint.

## Variations of the Superior Incision

There are many variations of this incision. In my opinion some of them are useful, others are harmful. Partial or total resection of the acromion should not be done rou-

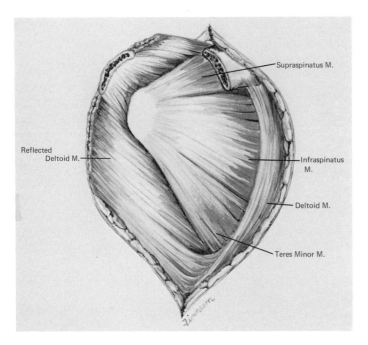

FIG. 7-13. Exposure of the posterior portion of the glenohumeral joint.

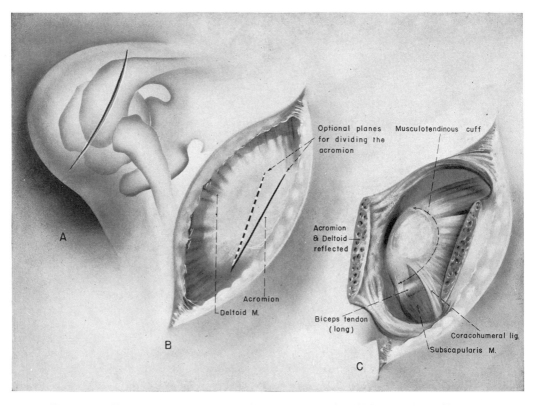

FIG. 7-14. Transacromial incision (McLaughlin). (A) Skin incision. (B) Planes through which acromion may be divided to gain access to the subacromial region. (C) Structures exposed after the deltoid is reflected downward and outward.

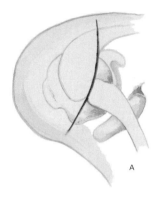

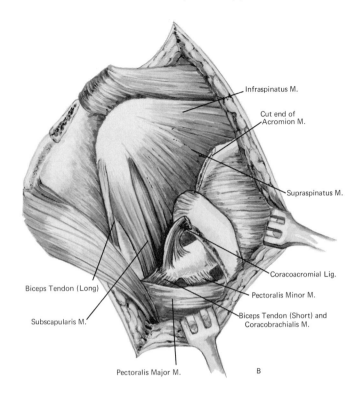

Infraspinatus M.

Cut end of
Acromion M.

Supraspinatus M.

Coracoacromial Lig.

Pectoralis Minor M.

Biceps Tendon (Short) and
Coracobrachialis M.

Biceps Tendon (Long)

Subscapularis M.

Pectoralis Major M.

B

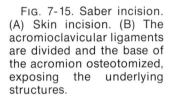

FIG. 7-15. Saber incision. (A) Skin incision. (B) The acromioclavicular ligaments are divided and the base of the acromion osteotomized, exposing the underlying structures.

tinely. On the other hand, the pathology of the cuff may be such or the mechanics of the joint may be so altered that resection of the acromion in part or totally must be done to prevent impingement of the cuff or the greater tuberosity during abduction of the arm.

**Incision of Darrach and McLaughlin (Transacromial Approach).** This incision provides ample exposure of the anterior and superior regions of the shoulder joint. My objections to it are: it detaches the deltoid from the acromion, it discards a portion of the acromion, and it splits the fibers of the anterior portion of the deltoid.

*Technique.* Begin the skin incision on the posterior aspect of the acromion just lateral to the acromioclavicular joint. Continue it over the shoulder and anteriorly, like a shoulder strap, to a point on the anterior portion of the deltoid 2 inches below the edge of the acromion. Now split the fibers of the anterior deltoid on the same line as the skin incision and detach the tendinous origin of the deltoid from the acromion.

This step brings into view the coracoacromial ligament; divide it at its acromial attachment (Fig. 7-14, A, B).

In order to obtain better exposure of the cuff (which may be necessary to facilitate its repair), osteotomize the end of the acromion. If limited exposure is desired, make the osteotomy cut in an oblique plane. This begins midway between the acromioclavicular joint and the lateral border of the acromion. It continues backward and laterally, in an oblique plane, to emerge on the lateral tip of the acromion. For wider exposure, perform the osteotomy in an anteroposterior plane, or, as recommended by Armstrong, perform a complete acromionectomy by dividing the acromion at its base on the spine after dividing the acromioclavicular ligament. When excising the acromion, the suprascapular nerve and artery may be injured as they pass through the scapular notch.

To expose the inside of the joint, make an incision in the interval between subscapularis and supraspinatus, paralleling

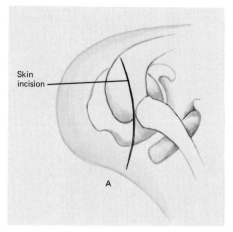

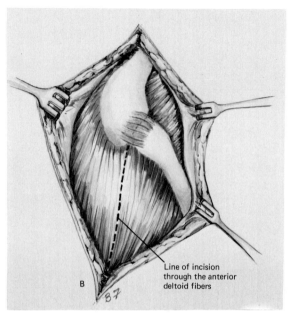

FIG. 7-16 A-D. Superoanterior incision. (A) Skin incision. (B) The skin flaps are mobilized and reflected to expose the anterior aspect of the joint. The deltoid muscle is divided in line with the acromioclavicular joint. (C) Structures exposed in the superior, anterior and medial aspects of the shoulder joint. For wider exposure a portion of the clavicle or acromion may be excised along the indicated lines. (D) A portion of the acromion has been excised to increase the exposure.

the coracohumeral ligament, or develop a line of separation between two of the tendons, or split the musculotendinous cuff in line with its fibers (Fig. 7-14C).

Later, when the deltoid is to be reattached, first bevel the remaining end of the acromion and then suture the muscle origin to the fascia on the bone. If the entire acromion is to be removed, a fascial flap must be developed from the top of the acromion and the lateral part of the spine. The edge of the deltoid is sutured to this fascial flap.

**Saber-cut Incision of Codman.** This incision, first described by Codman, provides an excellent exposure of the subacromial area. All portions of the cuff are readily visualized. And by opening the capsule, all regions of the inside of the joint can be explored. However, it is a mutilating incision; it possesses no advantages over the transacromial route and has the same unfavorable features. It splits both the anterior and the posterior portions of the deltoid. The suprascapular nerve and artery may be injured in the scapular notch when the base

of the acromion is severed; and the axillary nerve may be violated when the deltoid mass is retracted laterally and inferiorly.

*Technique.* Begin the skin incision on the anterior portion of the deltoid 1½ to 2 inches below the acromioclavicular joint. Carry the incision over the top of the shoulder in the line of the acromioclavicular joint, crossing this joint, and end it on the posterior third of the deltoid, 1½ to 2 inches below the posterior edge of the acromion. Next, by sharp dissection, develop the lateral skin flap by cutting through the subcutaneous tissue as far laterally as the tendinous fibers of origin of the deltoid on the acromion. Separate the longitudinal fibers of the anterior and posterior portions of the deltoid in the same line as the skin incision (Fig. 7-15A). Now divide the acromioclavicular ligaments, osteotomize the base of the acromion and displace the entire muscle mass laterally with the acromion still attached (Fig. 7-15B). To expose the inside of the joint, divide the superior portion of the musculotendinous cuff transversely at its line of insertion into the

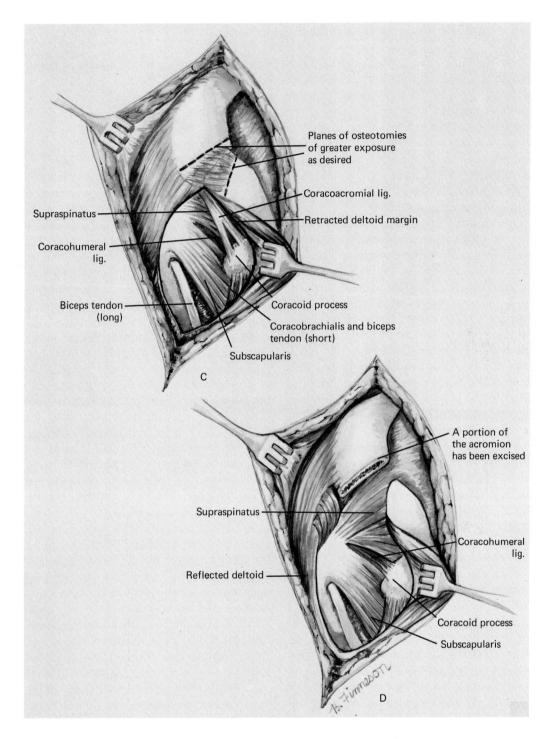

Planes of osteotomies
of greater exposure
as desired

Coracoacromial lig.

Supraspinatus

Retracted deltoid margin

Coracohumeral
lig.

Biceps tendon
(long)

Coracoid process

Coracobrachialis and biceps
tendon (short)

Subscapularis

C

A portion of
the acromion
has been excised

Supraspinatus

Coracohumeral
lig.

Reflected deltoid

Coracoid process

Subscapularis

D

greater tuberosity, or the separate tendons forming the cuff at their insertions.

Upon closure of the incision, replace the acromion in its anatomical position by sutures or several threaded wires (Codman) or excise it (Armstrong).

**Superoanterior Incision.** This is essentially the anterior limb of the superior incision. I find it very useful when I desire only limited exposure of the superior and anterior regions of the shoulder. By adding partial resection of the portion of the acromion or the clavicle forming the acromio-clavicular joint one obtains a relatively wide exposure of the superior and anterior areas of the joint. Partial resection of the clavicle or acromion is not necessary in young athletes with cuff tears and should not be done; it is an excellent procedure in older persons with extensive cuff tears.

This is the incision I prefer when operating on young people in whom the acromion must never be resected and the middle portion of the deltoid never detached from the lateral edge of the acromion. The only unfavorable feature of the incision is the splitting of the anterior deltoid for $1\frac{1}{2}$ to 2 inches. For wider exposure of the anterior aspect of the joint, the anterior portion of the deltoid may be detached from the line of origin on the clavicle. To facilitate this step the medial and lateral skin flaps of the incision must be mobilized by wide subcutaneous dissection. This modification of the incision is used only in older people and never in athletes.

*Technique.* Begin the incision over the posterior edge of the acromion just lateral to the acromioclavicular joint. Carry the incision downward over the anterior third of the deltoid in line with the axillary skin crease for 2 inches below the edge of the acromion (Fig. 7-16A). Freely mobilize the medial and lateral skin flaps by dissecting the subcutaneous layer from the underlying deltoid, the tip of the acromion and the acromioclavicular joint. Now the acromioclavicular joint is clearly seen. Develop the incision through the anterior fibers of the deltoid in line with the acromioclavicular joint for a distance not to exceed 2 inches below the edge of the acromion (Fig. 7-16B). Retraction of the muscle fibers exposes the subacromial bursa. Divide this structure in line with the muscle split; now the superior and anterior portions of the rotator cuff come into view. By rotating the arm externally, the following structures can be identified: the greater and lesser tuberosity, the biceps tendon in the bicipital groove and the tendon of the sub-scapularis inserting into the lesser tuberosity (Fig. 7-16C).

If wider exposure of the rotator cuff is desired, (e.g., when extensive tears of the cuff require repair) a portion of the acromion ($\frac{3}{8}$ inch) or of the clavicle ($\frac{3}{8}$ inch) is excised, depending upon the position of the lesion in relation to the acromioclavicular joint (Fig. 7-16D). This excision of bone from one or the other side of the acromioclavicular joint in no way affects the stability or function of the joint. The length of the acromion is not decreased. In order to expose the portion of the clavicle and acromion to be excised, the small portion of the deltoid attached to them must be peeled off; this is reattached latter.

Through this incision many operations on the anterior side of the joint can be performed, especially if the coracoid process is divided and displaced downward with the muscles attached (coracobrachialis and short head of the biceps). I prefer to divide the muscles just distal to their insertion into the coracoid process. Later the muscles are sutured to the base of the coracoid process or to a stump of tendinous tissue left behind.

This incision is suitable for any of the stabilizing operations for recurrent dislocation of the shoulder. Also, through it the biceps tendon and the tuberosities are readily accessible. To expose the inside of the joint, incise the capsule in the interval between the subscapularis and the supraspinatus paralleling the coracohumeral ligament. For wider exposure, cut the musculotendinous cuff transversely at its insertion into the greater tuberosity. To expose the anterior aspect of the inside of the joint, incise the tendon of the subscapularis at its insertion into the lesser tuberosity. When dividing the tendon, the patient's arm should be adducted and rotated externally. Take care not to carry the cut in the subscapularis tendon too far distally; otherwise the axillary nerve and the anterior and posterior humeral circumflex arteries may be injured.

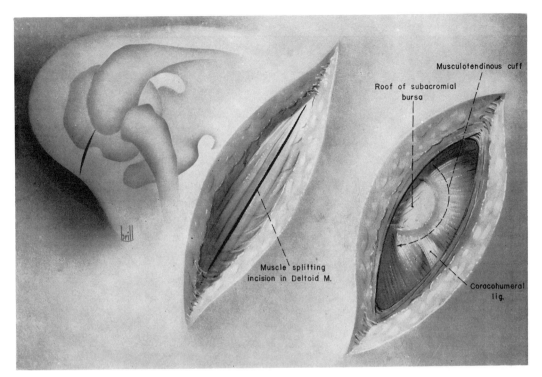

FIG. 7-17. Short deltoid splitting incision. (*Left*) Skin incision. (*Center*) Line of separation of fibers of deltoid muscle. (*Right*) Exposure of subacromial bursa and musculotendinous cuff.

**Short Deltoid Splitting Approach.** This incision provides a limited exposure and is particularly useful for procedures concerned only with the subacromial bursa or the tendons inserting into the greater tuberosity. Calcareous deposits in the tendons are readily accessible through this incision.

*Technique.* Start the incision just below the edge of the acromion and in line with the axillary crease. Carry it distally for 1½ to 2 inches. Mobilize both the lateral and medial skin flaps by dissecting the subcutaneous tissue from the anterior surface of the deltoid (Fig. 7-17, *left*). Locate, by palpation, the interval between the inner and middle thirds of the deltoid and split the muscle not more than 1½ inches from the edge of the acromion (Fig. 7-17, *center* and *right*).

Most calcareous deposits can be reached through this incision, except those in teres minor. When the deposit is in this location, place the skin incision more laterally and separate the fibers of the deltoid just beneath it.

Some recommend the use of a transverse skin incision instead of a longitudinal one, believing that it results in a more acceptable scar. I have not found this to be true and do not use it. This incision is placed on the anterior surface of the deltoid 1½ inches below the edge of the acromion.

## ANTEROMEDIAL APPROACHES

In my opinion these approaches should not be used, because of the unsightly scars they produce and also because the superior approaches provide all the exposure required for any surgical procedure, and the power of the deltoid is not jeopardized. Nevertheless, for historical reasons at least, they deserve description. There are two,

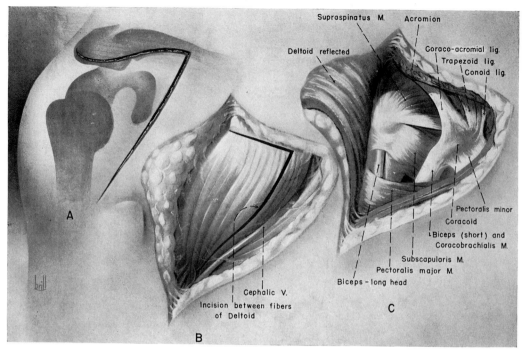

FIG. 7-18. Anterosuperomedial approach of Thompson and Henry. (A) Skin incision. If further exposure is desired the incision is continued around the acromion. (B) Line of reflection of split deltoid muscle from the clavicle. The deltoid is detached by sharp dissection. (C) Exposure of structures in the anterior, superior and medial aspects of the shoulder region.

one of which is a modification of the other.

**Approach of Thompson and Henry.** The vertical limb of the incision extends along the anterior border of the deltoid, beginning at the inferior margin of the clavicle at the juncture of its outer and middle thirds. It extends distally just proximal to the deltoid tuberosity. The horizontal limb begins over the anterior surface of the acromioclavicular joint. It proceeds medially along the anterior surface of the outer third of the clavicle and joins the vertical limb at the deltopectoral sulcus, just to the inner side of the coracoid process (Fig. 7-18A).

Next, mobilize the vertical skin flaps by dissecting the subcutaneous layer from the deltoid. This brings into view the cephalic vein traversing the deltopectoral interval. Retract the vein medially together with a few longitudinal fibers of the deltoid and the pectoralis major. Retract the deltoid mass laterally. While developing the vertical limb of the incision avoid injury to the cephalic vein and the thoracoacromial artery, which lie in the upper end of the incision (Fig. 7-18B). Now, by sharp dissection, detach the clavicular origin of the deltoid and reflect the detached deltoid downward and laterally. This step brings into view the anterior and lateral regions of the shoulder (Fig. 7-18C).

If more extensive exposure is desired, sever the coracoacromial ligament close to its insertion into the acromion. Next, osteotomize the coracoid process just proximal to the insertion of the coracoacromial ligament and displace it, with the muscles attached, downward and medially. The incision now permits ready access to the subscapularis muscle and tendon.

Henry later modified this incision. The vertical limb of the incision is the same as described above. The horizontal limb is re-

placed by an incision beginning at the upper end of the vertical incision and carried
directly over the top of the shoulder and
backward as far as the spine of the scapula.
The skin edges are mobilized by cutting
away the subcutaneous tissue from the underlying fascia so that the lateral and
posterior edges of the acromion and the adjacent spine of the scapula are exposed. By
sharp dissection, only as much of the deltoid is detached as is needed to provide the
necessary exposure.

**Approach of Cubbins, Callahan and
Scuderi.** This approach is a modification of
the Thompson and Henry incision, designed to produce an extensive exposure
of the lateral and posterior regions of the
shoulder.

The anterior limb of the incision is identi-
cal to that of the Thompson and Henry approach; it follows the anterior border of
the deltoid muscle from the clavicle to just
proximal to the deltoid tuberosity. However, the horizontal limb extends around
the acromion process and along the
lateral half of the spine of the scapula (Fig.
7-19). By sharp dissection, the tendinous
origin of the deltoid is detached from the
anterior border of the clavicle, the acromion and the spine. When the deltoid is
retracted downward, the anterior, lateral
and posterior regions of the shoulder are
clearly visualized.

To expose the joint, the tendons of the
rotator muscles are cut transversely at their
line of insertion into the greater tuberosity, or the tendons can be separated just
proximal to their insertion into the greater
tuberosity.

This extensive approach has only one
point in its favor: the deltoid fibers are not
split, thereby precluding injury to the axillary nerve.

## POSTERIOR APPROACHES

Many approaches to the posterior aspect
of the shoulder have been described. Most
are modifications of the incisions described

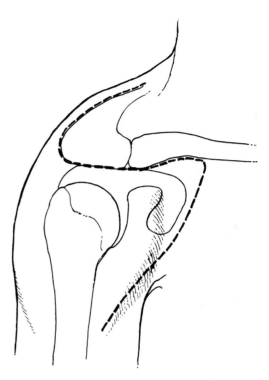

FIG. 7-19. Skin incision of Cubbins,
Callahan and Scuderi.

by Kocher, Ollier, Bennett and others. In
general, there are two groups—one for
limited exposures and the other for extensive approaches. A surgeon knowledgeable in the anatomy of the posterior region
of the shoulder can readily convert a limited
exposure to an extensive one if the need
arises. This need arises more often than is
generally appreciated, so that possession
of the skill and knowledge necessary to
shift from one incision to another can not
be overstressed. In the following description of the techniques of posterior
approaches, I shall begin with the one I
employ for limited exposure, and then indicate how it can be extended for wider and
wider exposures, including the superior,
lateral and anterior regions of the shoulder.

### Technique for Limited Exposures

This incision provides a limited but adequate exposure of the posterior rotator

cuff, the posterior glenoid rim, the posterior portion of the humeral head and the posterior region of the neck of the scapula.

With the patient's arm adducted, start the incision just below the tip of the acromion; carry it medially and posteriorly along the inferior margin of the spine to its medial angle, then curve it slightly downward, ending at the base of the spine (Fig. 7-20A). Mobilize both skin flaps freely and expose the tendinous origin of the deltoid into the spine and acromion (Fig. 7-20B). By sharp subperiosteal dissection, detach the origin of the deltoid from the spine and the acromion and displace it downward and laterally. With reflection of the deltoid the dense fascia covering infraspinatus and teres minor comes into view (Fig. 7-20C).

There are two approaches to the joint capsule. The use of one or the other depends on the extent of exposure desired.

1. Make a longitudinal incision in the fascia over the interval between infraspinatus and teres minor (Fig. 7-20C). Reflect the infraspinatus from the scapula and capsule and retract it upward. Mobilize the teres minor and displace it downward. At this point, take care that you do not injure the suprascapular nerve which lies directly under the infraspinatus muscle. It, together with the artery, comes from the supraspinous fossa through the spinoglenoid

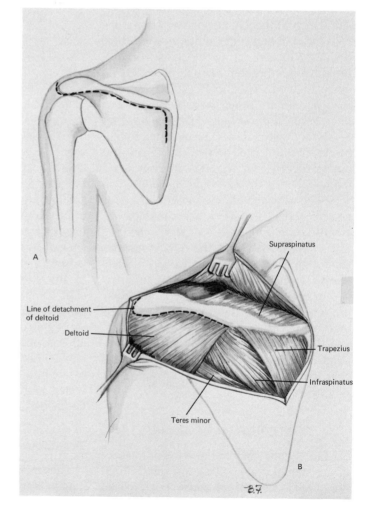

FIG. 7-20. (A) Skin incision for exposure of the posterior and superior aspects of the shoulder. (B) The skin flaps are immobilized and reflected to expose the tendinous origin of the deltoid into the spine and acromion. (C) The deltoid is reflected, exposing the dense fascia covering the infraspinatus and the teres minor. (D) The infraspinatus is retracted upward and the teres minor downward. The suprascapular nerve lies directly under the infraspinatus muscle. (E) The tendon of the infraspinatus is incised down to the capsule and retracted medially.

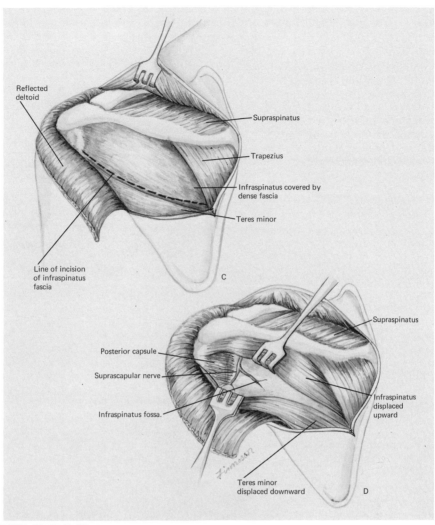

Reflected
deltoid

Supraspinatus

Trapezius

Infraspinatus covered by
dense fascia

Teres minor

Line of incision
of infraspinatus
fascia

C

Posterior capsule

Suprascapular nerve

Infraspinatus fossa.

Supraspinatus

Infraspinatus
displaced
upward

Teres minor
displaced downward

D

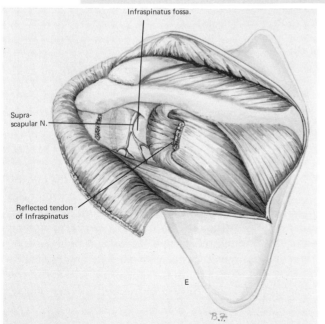

Infraspinatus fossa.

Supra-
scapular N.

Reflected tendon
of Infraspinatus

E

FIGURE 7-20 (Cont'd)

(*Right*) Fig. 7-21. The acromion is osteotomized at its base and reflected downward and laterally; this exposes the fascia lying over the supraspinatus. The tendons of the supraspinatus and infraspinatus are divided and reflected medially.

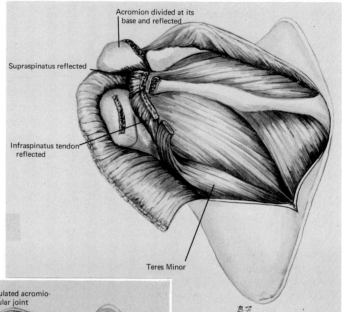

(*Left*) Fig. 7-22. Exposure can be increased by osteotomizing the base of the acromion and dividing the acromioclavicular ligaments. The acromion is retracted downward and lateralward.

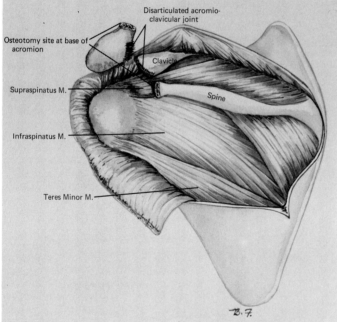

notch to the infraspinous fossa (Fig. 7-20D).

2. Incise down to the capsule the upper portion of the infraspinatus tendon near its insertion into the greater tuberosity. Dissect the detached tendon from the capsule and retract it medially (Fig. 7-20E).

In both of these approaches the capsule may be opened by an incision in the capsule paralleling the posterior glenoid brim or by a transverse or a T-shaped incision.

Although the axillary nerve is not encountered in this incision, it behooves the surgeon to keep in mind its anatomical relationship to the posterior surface of the deltoid. Severe retraction of the muscle

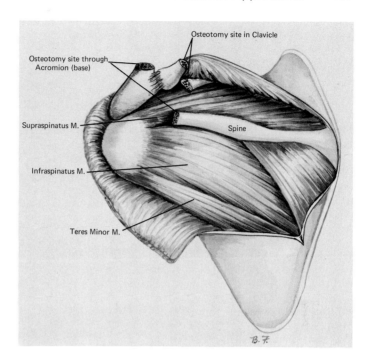

Osteotomy site in Clavicle

Osteotomy site through Acromion (base)

Supraspinatus M.

Spine

Infraspinatus M.

Teres Minor M.

B. F.

FIG. 7-23. Still wider exposure can be obtained by dividing the clavicle medial to the acromioclavicular joint.

may injure the nerve. However, safety of the nerve can be assured if the deltoid is not retracted beyond the teres minor.

## Technique for Wider Exposure of Posterior Region

If a slightly wider exposure is desired than the above incision provides, the entire width of the tendons of infraspinatus and teres minor can be cut close to their insertion into the head of the humerus and then reflected medially. This step requires great care because now you enter the quadrilateral space, through which the axillary nerve and artery pass. Open the capsule by a longitudinal or a T-shaped incision.

## Wide Exposure of Posterior and Superior Regions

If in addition to a wide posterior exposure, the superior region of the shoulder needs to be explored, several modifications of the above incision can be used.

## Osteotomy of the Acromion

As a rule, if the skin flaps of the incision described above are mobilized sufficiently, an osteotomy of the acromion can be done without further extension of the skin incision.

Divide the acromion at its base close to the spinoglenoid notch. Perform this step with care to avoid injury to the suprascapular nerve and artery as they pass through the notch. Next, divide the coracoacromial ligament at its insertion into the acromion. The supraspinatus beneath its dense fascia can be seen. To expose the tendon, incise the fascia parallel to its fibers. Now, the entire posterior and superior portions of the capsule can be exposed. Make an incision through the musculotendinous cuff perpendicular to its fibers from the anterior border of the supraspinatus tendon to the inferior margin of the teres minor tendon. Cut the cuff down to the capsule and close to its insertion into the greater tuberosity. Reflect the cuff medially, exposing the capsule. To expose

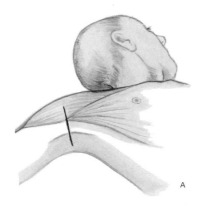

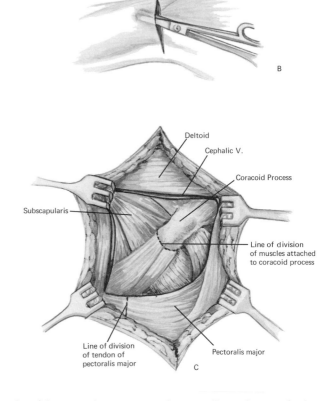

FIG. 7-24. Axillary approach. (A) Axillary incision in line with the axillary crease. (B) Undermine the skin flap over the deltoid and pectoralis major widely. (C) Develop the interval between the deltoid and the pectoralis major. Cut the tendon of the pectoralis major partially or completely.

the inside of the joint, open the capsule with a longitudinal or T-shaped incision (Fig. 7-21).

**Exposure of the Posterior, Superior and Anterior Regions**

These regions are accessible by extending the incision described on page 161. The skin incision is carried around the lateral and anterior borders of the acromion, in front of the acromioclavicular joint and along the upper border of the outer end of the clavicle. Next, divide transversely all the ligaments of the acromioclavicular joint and cut the coracoacromial ligament. Retract the disarticulated and osteotomized end of the acromion downward and laterally with the deltoid (Fig. 7-22).

Still wider exposure can be obtained by osteotomizing the clavicle medial to the acromioclavicular joint. This gives an ex-

tensive approach to all regions of the shoulder joint (Fig. 7-23). If the anterior aspect of the joint needs to be explored, detach the tendon of the subscapularis at its insertion into the lesser tuberosity.

Upon reassembling the shoulder, fix the parts of the acromion or the acromioclavicular joint or the clavicle with threaded wires. Remove the wires after bony union is attained.

**AXILLARY APPROACH**

Of the various axillary approaches described, the anterior axillary is the safest to use to gain access to the anteroinferior region of the joint. Of course, its only advantage over the other conventional anterior approaches is the nature of its scar. The greater part of the scar is hidden in the axillary crease and the visible portion is small and hairline in appearance. This

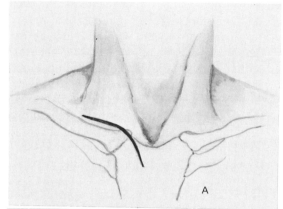

FIG. 7-25. Exposure of the sterno-clavicular joint. (A) Skin incision. (B) Exposure of insertion of the clavicular and sternal heads of the sternomastoid, the pectoralis major and the fibrous capsule. (C) The fibrous capsule is opened, exposing the interarticular disc.

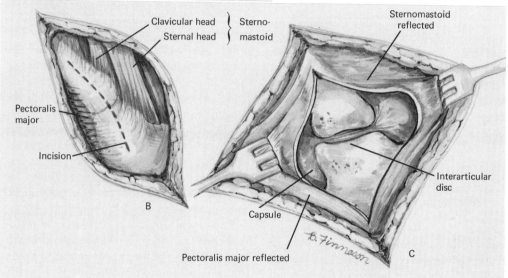

consideration is a serious one to all women and most men. My principal use of this incision is in stabilization operations for recurrent dislocations of the shoulders. Most of the accepted procedures to correct this lesion can be performed through the anterior axillary approach. This incision can be difficult or it can be easy to perform. Two steps convert a difficult procedure to a simple one. First, the anterior and lateral skin flaps must be undermined extensively in order to permit the necessary retraction of muscles; and, second, the insertion of the pectoralis major should be partially or completely severed.

## Technique

With the arm in 90° abduction and rotated externally, begin the incision at the mid point of the anterior axillary fold over the pectoralis major. Extend it posteriorly in line with the axillary crease for 2½ to 3 inches (Fig. 7-24A). Next comes the first of the two important steps mentioned above. By sharp dissection, undermine the skin over the deltoid and pectoralis major widely, so that the deltopectoral triangle and cephalic vein are reached without excessive retraction of the skin margins (Fig. 7-24B).

Develop the interval between the deltoid and pectoralis major, allowing the cephalic vein to go laterally with the deltoid. Now expose the tendon of the pectoralis major at the lower end of the deltopectoral groove and divide it partially or completely, depending on the ease with which the antero-inferior region of the shoulder can be reached. By retracting the deltoid laterally and the pectoralis major medially and inferiorly, the anterior region of the shoulder comes into view (Fig. 7-24C). In most instances, this exposure is adequate to perform the Magnuson operation. If more exposure is desired, detach the coraco-brachialis and the short head of the biceps from the coracoid process and displace them inferiorly. The other alternative is an osteotomy of the coracoid process below the insertion of the muscles. Now the exposure is adequate to perform any of the popular operations for recurrent dislocation of the shoulder.

## APPROACH TO THE STERNOCLAVICULAR JOINT

Begin the incision over the clavicular head of the sternocleidomastoid just above the upper border of the clavicle. Extend it medially to the outer border of the sternum, then curve it gently downward on the anterior surface of the sternum for $1\frac{1}{2}$ inches. Retract the skin margins, exposing the tendinous insertions of both heads of the sternocleidomastoid. By sharp periosteal dissection, reflect the sternocleidomastoid and the pectoralis major from the clavicle. This brings into view the fibrous capsule of the joint. Open the joint by a horizontal incision in the fibrous capsule (Fig. 7-25).

## APPROACH TO THE ACROMIOCLAVICULAR JOINT AND CORACOCLAVICULAR LIGAMENT

Start the incision on the posterior border of the acromioclavicular joint and carry it forward over the top of the shoulder, over the acromioclavicular joint. Extend it forward and downward $1\frac{1}{2}$ to 2 inches. By sharp dissection, reflect the skin flaps on either side, exposing the tendinous insertions of the deltoid and trapezius and the upper part of the deltopectoral groove. Develop the interval between the deltoid and the pectoralis major, exposing the coracoid process. Using subperiosteal dissection, detach the deltoid from the clavicle and the acromion and reflect it downward. In a like manner, detach the trapezius from the superior surface of the clavicle and reflect it upward. Retract the pectoralis major and the cephalic vein medially. This brings into view the coracoid process, the coracoacromial ligament, the coraco-clavicular ligament (trapezoid and conoid ligaments) and the fibrous capsule of the acromioclavicular joint (Fig. 7-26).

Adequate exposure in this incision depends on the skin flaps being mobile enough to permit wide retraction of the skin edges. I favor this incision because it follows the lines of greatest skin tension and, therefore, produces a good looking scar.

The usual approach, favored by many surgeons, provides the same exposure with less difficulty, but it results in a scar that is far less acceptable cosmetically. For this approach start the incision at the angle of the acromion and proceed medially along the lower border of the acromion, the acromioclavicular joint and the outer third of the clavicle to the deltopectoral cleft. At this point, swing it downward and outward, following the anterior border of the deltoid for 1 to 2 inches.

The rest of the technique is the same as that used in the first incision described above.

## APPROACHES TO THE HUMERUS

Many pathological conditions require exposure of the upper or middle portions of the humerus or even of the entire humerus. Some tumors of the upper end of the

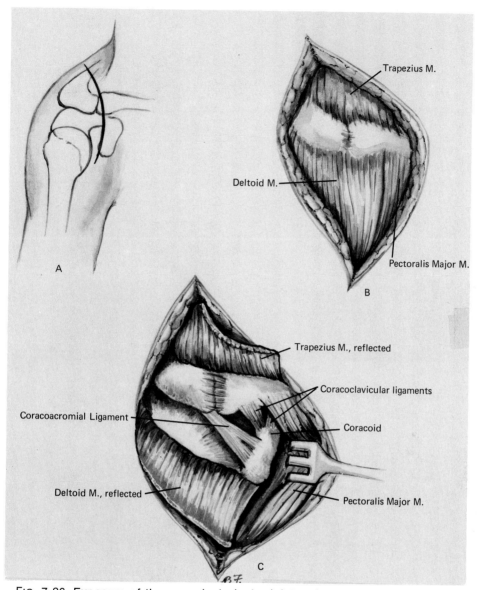

FIG. 7-26. Exposure of the acromioclavicular joint and coracoclavicular ligament. (A) Skin incision. (B) Exposure of the origins of the deltoid and trapezius. (C) The trapezius and the deltoid are reflected and the pectoralis major is retracted medially; the coracoid and coracoclavicular ligaments are in view.

humerus can be treated by local resection. Some traumatic or degenerative lesions require excision of the humeral head and replacement of the head by a prosthesis. Occasionally, as will be demonstrated, the entire diaphysis of the humerus must be removed and replaced by long tibial grafts. It is clear that one concerned with the management of these lesions must know the approaches to the different regions of the arm, and he must know in detail the regional anatomy of the part involved.

There are many approaches to the arm. However, the surgeon must choose the approach that provides adequate exposure for the work to be done and at the same time avoids injury to structures vital to function.

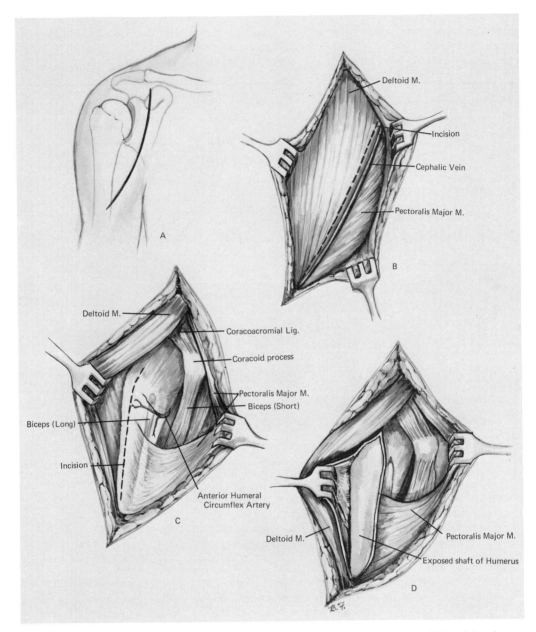

FIG. 7-27. Exposure of upper end of the humerus. (A) Skin incision. (B) Incision in the deltoid-pectoral interval. (C) Exposure of upper end of humerus, coracoid process, coracoacromial ligament and long and short heads of the biceps. (D) Exposure of the upper end of the humeral shaft.

## Approach to the Upper End of the Humerus (Anterior-Deltoid Approach)

This approach provided excellent exposure of the upper end of the humerus and to the anterior region of the joint. In addition, if the middle third of the humerus needs to be exposed, the incision can be readily carried downward along the lateral aspect of the arm in the interval between the triceps and brachialis.

*Technique.* Begin the incision at the

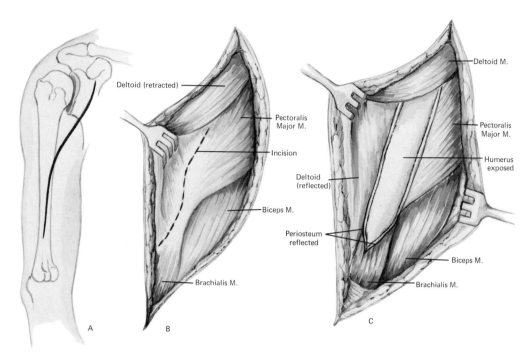

FIG. 7-28. Exposure of the proximal two thirds of the humerus. (A) Skin incision. (B) Exposure of tendinous fibers of the deltoid, pectoralis major and brachialis. (C) The periosteum over the upper two thirds of the humeral shaft is divided and reflected with the fibers of the insertion of the deltoid and the pectoralis major.

lower border of the clavicle just above the tip of the coracoid process. Extend it downward along the anterior margin of the deltoid for 5 inches (Fig. 7-27A). Divide the fascia along the line of the skin incision; this exposes the cephalic vein: retract it medially, with the pectoralis major (Fig. 7-27B). Retract the deltoid laterally, bringing into view the broad tendon of the pectoralis major as it runs to its insertion into the humerus. In the upper end of the wound, the fleshy part of the short biceps lies between the humerus and its tendon, which runs to the tip of the coracoid process (Fig. 7-27C).

On external rotation of the humerus the tendon of the long head of the biceps may be readily felt on the anterior surface of the humerus. At the lower pole of the incision the tendon dips beneath the tendon of the pectoralis major. At the upper pole, note the course of the anterior circumflex artery as it winds around the surgical neck of the

humerus. Ligate this vessel. Incise the periosteum of the humerus in a line just lateral to the tendon of the long head of the biceps above and the tendon of the pectoralis major below. By sharp periosteal dissection, expose the shaft of the humerus from the greater tuberosity above to the lower border of the tendon of the pectoralis major below (Fig. 7-27D).

A word of caution: Do not injure the axillary nerve, which lies on the anterior surface of the deltoid, by forceful retraction.

## Approach to the Proximal Two Thirds of the Humerus

Essentially this is an extension of the incision just described. Begin the incision on the anterior border of the deltoid, about 2 inches below the clavicle. Extend it distally and laterally along the anterior border

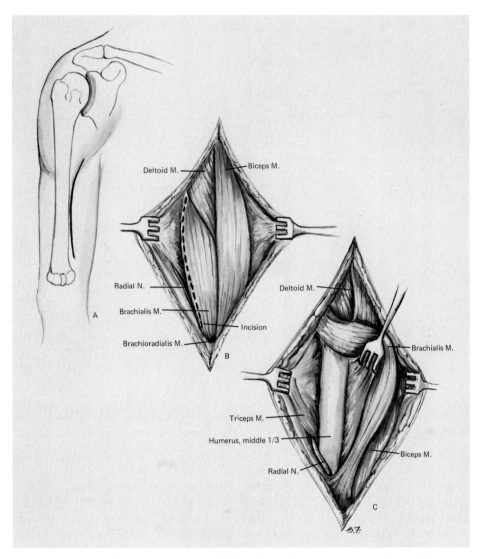

FIG. 7-29. Exposure of the middle third of the humerus. (A) Incision. (B) Exposure of the biceps and brachialis and the radial nerve lying between the brachioradialis and the brachialis. (C) Exposure of the shaft of the humerus by subperiosteal dissection. Note the position of the nerve in the lower end of the wound.

of the deltoid as far as the deltoid tubercle. Then carry it distally along the lateral border of the arm in the interval between the triceps and brachialis (Fig. 7-28A). Divide the deep fascia along the line of the skin incision and the cephalic vein in the deltopectoral groove. Retract the vein and pectoralis major medially (Fig. 7-28B). By sharp dissection down to the bone, develop the incision between the deltoid and pectoralis major. In the lower end of the incision, distal to the insertion of the deltoid,

develop the incision between the brachialis medially and the lateral head of the triceps laterally (Fig. 7-28C).

## Approach to the Middle Third of the Humerus

Begin the incision on the anterior margin of the deltoid about 2 inches above the deltoid tubercle. Curve it gently downward for 6 to 7 inches along the lateral border of the brachialis and end it over the interval between the brachialis and brachioradialis

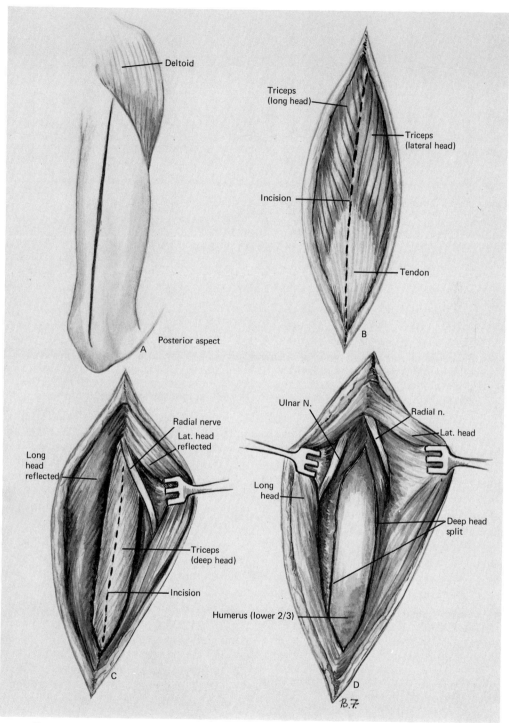

FIG. 7-30. Posterior exposure of middle and lower thirds of the humerus. (A) Incision. (B) Exposure of lateral and long heads of the triceps. (C) Lateral and long heads are reflected to expose the deep head and the radial nerve. (D) The deep head is split to expose the shaft of the humerus; the radial and ulnar nerves lie in the proximal end of the wound.

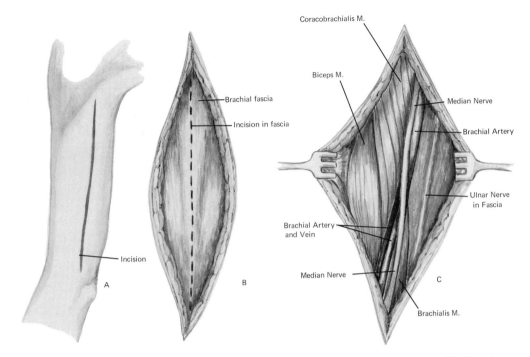

FIG. 7-31. Approach to anteromedial aspect of the arm. (A) Incision. (B) Fascia overlying the muscles and neurovascular structures. (C) Fascia is reflected. Note relation of median nerve to the brachial artery in the upper and lower portions of the incision. The ulnar nerve lies posterior to the medial intermuscular septum.

(Fig. 7-29A). By sharp dissection, divide the deep fascia and free widely the lateral and medial skin flaps; now identify the radial nerve in the lower part of the wound lying between the brachialis and brachioradialis (Fig. 7-29B). Using subperiosteal dissection, elevate the brachialis and retract it and the biceps medially. In a like manner, expose the posterior aspect of the humerus by raising the triceps and retracting it posteriorly. While elevating these muscles, always keep the radial nerve in view and protect it from the line of dissection (Fig. 7-29C).

### Posterior Approach to the Middle and Lower Thirds of the Humerus

Start the incision on the posterior surface of the arm, in the midline, at the posterior border of the deltoid and extend it to the olecranon fossa. Divide the deep fascia in the line of the incision and mobilize the skin flaps (Fig. 7-30A). Identify, by palpation, the interval between the long and the lateral heads of the triceps. By sharp dissection, separate the two heads and split the triceps tendon down to the olecranon fossa. Now the floor of the incision consists of the deep head of the triceps (Fig. 7-30B).

By careful dissection, develop the incision down to the deep head of the triceps and expose the radial nerve and the deep branch of the brachial artery in the upper end of the incision. They emerge from the medial border of the wound and run obliquely downward and laterally and dip under the lateral head of the triceps (Fig. 7-30C). To expose the humerus split the deep (medial) head of the triceps longitudinally down to the bone and by subperiosteal dissection elevate the muscle from the bone (Fig. 7-30D).

Avoid injury to the ulnar nerve which, in the upper part of the wound, lies under the long head of the triceps.

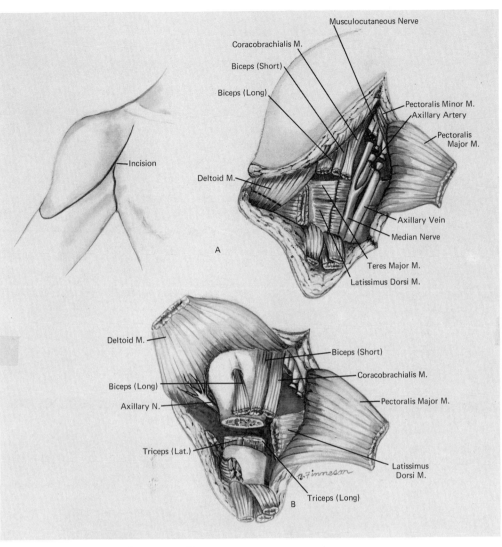

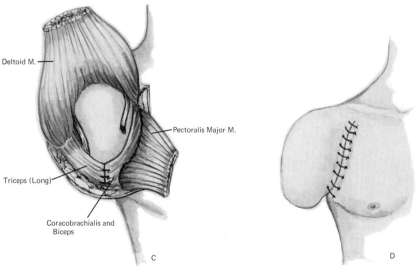

FIG. 7-32. Amputation through the upper third of the humerus. (A) Skin incision and cutting of muscles and neurovascular bundle. (B) Further division of muscles and transection of the bone. (C) Assembling the muscle around the bone. (D) Closure of the skin incision.

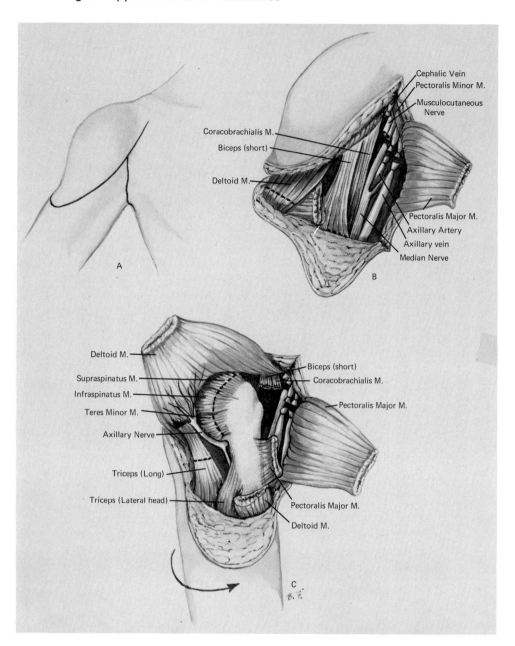

## Approach to the Anteromedial Aspect of the Arm

Begin the incision at the anterior axillary fold and extend it distally over the antero-medial border of the arm, ending just in front of the medial epicondyle of the humerus (Fig. 7-31A). Divide the deep fascia in the line of the skin incision; separate the medial skin flap from the medial border of the biceps and mobilize the lateral flap (Fig. 7-31B).

Identify the median nerve in the upper end of the wound and free it from the surrounding soft tissue. In the upper half of the wound it lies lateral to the brachial artery and veins. Then it crosses the artery and veins and runs on the medial side of the vessels. The ulnar nerve is not in the

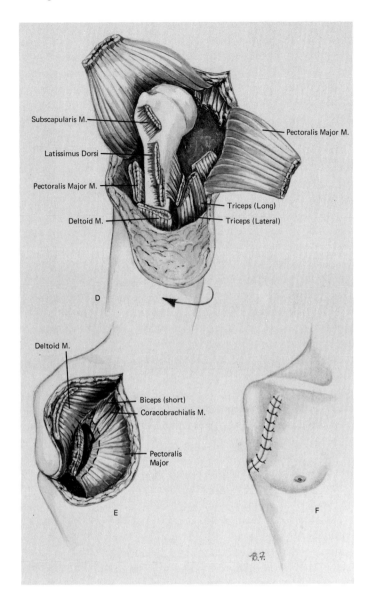

Subscapularis M.

Pectoralis Major M.

Latissimus Dorsi

Pectoralis Major M.

Triceps (Long)

Deltoid M.

Triceps (Lateral)

D

Deltoid M.

Biceps (short)

Coracobrachialis M.

Pectoralis Major

E

F

FIG. 7-33. Disarticulation of the shoulder. (A) Skin incision. (B) Exposure and division of the neurovascular bundle. (C) Division of the deltoid; the capsule and the rotator muscles (the arm is in internal rotation). (D) Division of the anterior muscles and the capsule (the arm is in external rotation) and disarticulation of the arm. (E) Assembling the muscles over the glenoid fossa. (F) Closure of skin incision.

field; it lies posteriorly to the medial intermuscular septum (Fig. 7-31C).

## SURGICAL PROCEDURES ABOUT THE SHOULDER JOINT

### Amputation Through the Upper Third of the Arm

Often, traumatic or pathological conditions arise which necessitate high amputation of the arm. The upper end of the humerus should be preserved whenever possible because it not only preserves the normal contour of the shoulder but also permits fitting of a more serviceable prosthesis. The type of incision made depends on the level of the amputation; as a rule, most amputations are performed through the surgical neck of the humerus.

*Technique.* Place the patient in the supine position with a sandbag beneath the shoulder but close to the midline, so that the patient lies at an angle of 45° with the table. Begin the skin incision at the coracoid process and extend it distally along the anterior border of the deltoid to its insertion. Then curve the incision upward and continue it along the posterior aspect of the deltoid as far as the posterior axillary fold. Connect the two ends of the incision by a horizontal incision on the medial side of the arm, about 1 inch above the level of the deltoid tubercle (Fig. 7-32A). Develop the deltopectoral interval anteriorly and isolate the insertion of the pectoralis major, now sever it and reflect it medially. Develop the interval between pectoralis minor and coracobrachialis to expose the neurovascular structures. Isolate, clamp, divide and ligate the ends of the brachial artery and vein below the pectoralis minor. Identify the median, ulnar, radial and musculocutaneous nerves, pull them down gently and inject them with procaine; then section them so that they retract above the level of the pectoralis minor (Fig. 7-32A). Now, divide the insertion of the deltoid and reflect it upward; next, section the teres major and latissimus dorsi at their site of attachment into the bicipital groove. Cut the biceps tendon, triceps and coracobrachialis three quarters of an inch below the saw line. Finally, transect the bone at the level of the neck of the humerus (Fig. 7-32B).

Pull the long head of the triceps and the coracobrachialis over the stump of the humerus and suture them to the bone; swing the tendon of the pectoralis major laterally and anchor it to the inferior pole of the bone (Fig. 7-32C). Trim the skin flap and the attached deltoid to oppose the medial flap neatly; approximate the skin flaps with interrupted sutures (Fig. 7-32D).

### Disarticulation of the Shoulder

**Technique.** The patient assumes the supine position, with a large sandbag under the shoulder close to the midline so that the patient lies at a 45° angle to the table. Begin the incision at the coracoid process and carry it downward along the border

of the deltoid to its insertion; then curve the incision upward along the posterior aspect of the deltoid to the axillary fold. Join the two ends of the incision by a horizontal incision at the level of the axillary fold (Fig. 7-33A). To expose the neurovascular structures, develop the interval between the coracobrachialis and the pectoralis minor. Isolate, clamp, divide and ligate the axillary artery and vein and allow them to retract beneath the pectoralis minor. Identify and gently pull down the median, ulnar, radial and musculocutaneous nerves. Inject them with procaine and then divide them so that they will retract upward beneath the pectoralis minor. Divide the radial nerve at the level of branching of the axillary nerve. It is essential to preserve the axillary nerve: otherwise, the deltoid will be deprived of its nerve supply (Fig. 7-33B). Divide the coracobrachialis muscles at their line of insertion into the coracoid process; sever the insertion of the deltoid from the humerus and reflect it upward to expose the capsule of the joint.

Rotate the arm internally and cut the insertions of the supraspinatus, infraspinatus and teres minor muscles, and the posterior fibrous capsule (Fig. 7-33C). Now, rotate the arm externally and divide the insertion of the subscapularis and the anterior fibrous capsule. Divide the long tendon of the biceps; then with the arm in slight external rotation, divide the long head of the triceps, and with the arm in slight internal rotation, cut the insertions of the teres major and the latissimus dorsi. Finally, sever the inferior capsule to complete the disarticulation (Fig. 7-33D).

Bring together the ends of all the cut muscles and suture them over the glenoid fossa. Suture the deltoid flap just below the inferior glenoid rim with several interrupted sutures (Fig. 7-33E). Trim the skin flap so that it neatly opposes the medial skin flap; approximate the skin edges with interrupted sutures (Fig. 7-33F). Always insert a drain into the deep regions of the wound; retain it in place for 48 to 72 hours. Apply soft, voluminous, dry dressings to obliterate all tissue spaces.

## Interscapulothoracic Amputation (Forequarter Amputation)

As a rule this is a salvage procedure, an attempt to save a life by deleting the entire shoulder girdle and arm. Unfortunately it often must be done on young people who, psychologically, react violently to this mutilating operation which, in most instances, fails to achieve its purpose. There is only one reason for doing this operation: the removal of highly malignant tumors that cannot be treated by local resection or radiation. The tumors may involve the bony elements of the shoulder or any of the muscles and other soft tissues in this region. Resection of the regional lymph nodes is a necessary part of the procedure; this includes resection of the supraclavicular nodes if they are involved. In some instances, because of the size or position of the tumor or the extent of destruction, the skin flaps must be altered to meet the situation. This may pose some difficulty at the time of closure, often necessitating skin grafting of denuded areas.

**Technique.** The patient lies on the unaffected side, with the upper end of the table elevated at an angle of 45° to the horizontal lower portion of the table. Drape the arm separately to permit easy maneuvering of the limb.

Begin the incision on the anterior surface of the clavicle close to the outer border of the sternocleidomastoid; carry it laterally on the anterior surface of the clavicle over the acromioclavicular joint. Make a second incision beginning at the lower border of the middle of the clavicle. Continue it downward in the interval between the deltoid and the pectoralis major to the lower border of the anterior axillary fold (Fig. 7-34A). Before making the posterior and axillary portions of the skin incision, direct your attention to the development of the

anterior incisions. Carry the clavicular incision down to bone, and by subperiosteal dissection detach the clavicular portion of the pectoralis major from the medial end of the clavicle and the deltoid from the lateral end. Finally, strip the clavicle of all soft tissue attachments from one end to the other. With a Gigli saw divide the clavicle close to the outer border of the sternocleidomastoid and then gently elevate it from its bed. By elevating the inner part of the clavicle, the coracoclavicular ligaments come into view; divide these. Next, section all the acromioclavicular ligaments and remove the clavicle (Fig. 7-34B). While freeing the clavicle of its soft tissue investments take the following precautions: (1) Do not injure the cephalic vein, which occasionally joins the lateral jugular vein on the anterior surface of the clavicle. (2) Remember the course of the transverse scapular vein, which runs immediately posterior to and parallel with the clavicle; laceration of this vein may cause much loss of blood. (3) The coracoclavicular ligaments are stout and strong; these ligaments must be cut to free the clavicle.

Develop the deltopectoral interval and expose the coracoid process; isolate the cephalic vein, which is the guide to the neurovascular structures. Sever the tendon of the pectoralis major close to its bony insertion and reflect the muscle medially (Fig. 7-34C). Cut the insertion of the pectoralis minor into the coracoid process. Using the cephalic vein as a guide, identify the clavicoracopectoral fascia and carefully divide it. Now, the entire neurovascular bundle is unroofed. Bear in mind that the subclavian vein is intimately related to the subclavian muscles from which the vein must be freed or the muscle cut (Fig. 7-34D).

Separate the subclavian artery and vein and divide and ligate each vessel, treating the artery first. Inject each nerve of the brachial plexus with procaine. Before cutting the nerves ligate each one with a fine silk suture; then divide the insertion of the

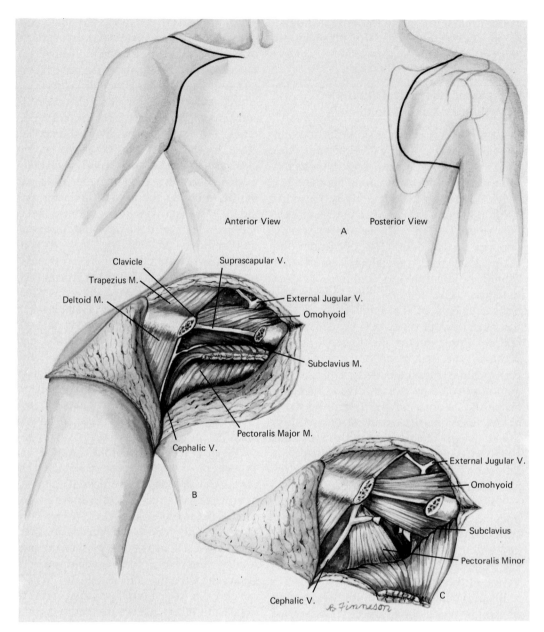

FIG. 7-34. Interscapulothoracic amputation. (A) Skin incision. (B) Resection of the clavicle and exposure of the anterior structure. (C) Exposure of the structures under the pectoralis major. (D) Division of the neurovascular structures. (E) Posterior skin incision and section of thoracoscapular muscles. (F) Closure of skin incision. (*D, E, and F on facing page*)

latissimus dorsi and allow the limb to fall away from the trunk (Fig. 7-34D).

You are now ready to complete the skin incisions. Extend the clavicular incision backward over the top of the shoulder along the vertebral border of the scapula to the inferior angle, then swing it outward to the posterior axillary fold. Now raise the arm and complete the axillary incision; continue it across the axilla to meet the

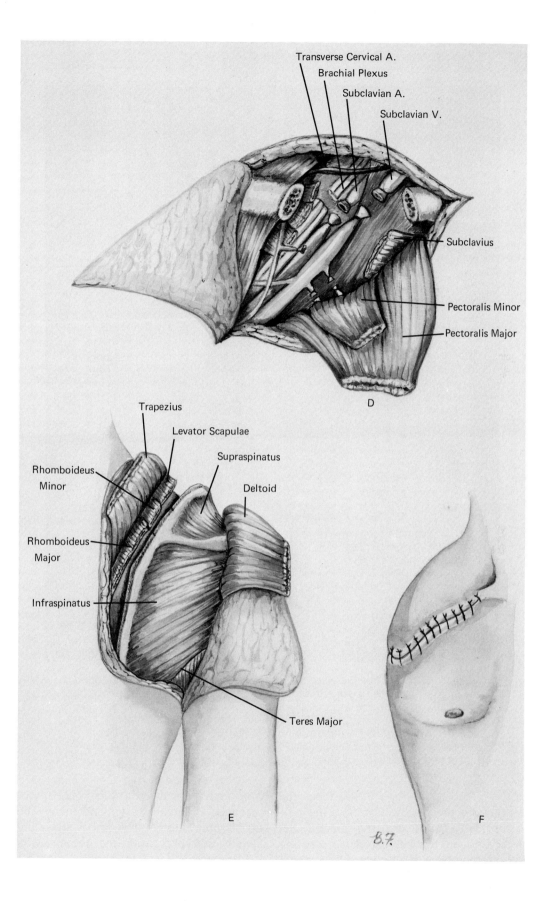

Transverse Cervical A.

Brachial Plexus

Subclavian A.

Subclavian V.

Subclavius

Pectoralis Minor

Pectoralis Major

D

Trapezius

Levator Scapulae

Supraspinatus

Deltoid

Rhomboideus
Minor

Rhomboideus
Major

Infraspinatus

Teres Major

E

F

B.7.

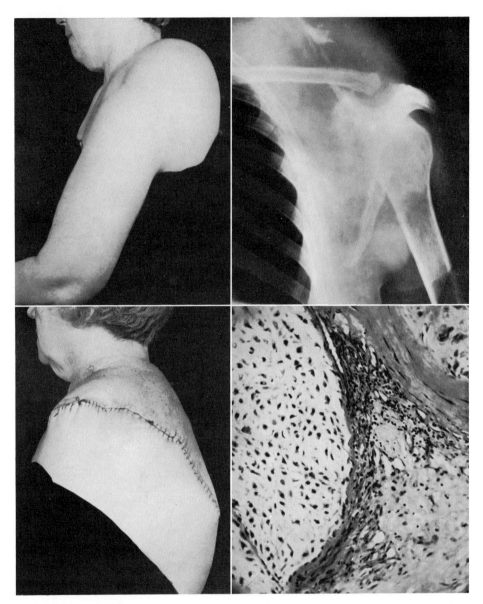

FIG. 7-35. (*Top, left*) Female, 53 years old, showing a chondrosarcoma of the scapula and the upper end of the humerus. (*Top, right*) Roentgenograph of the lesion. Note the enormous size of the lesion; most of the scapula is destroyed. (*Bottom, left*) Patient 7 days after interthoracoscapular amputation. (*Bottom, right*) Photomicrograph (× 150) of tissue obtained from the amputated extremity. Observe the pleomorphic character of the chondroblasts and the paucity of stroma.

posterior incision (Fig. 7-34A). Place the arm across the chest and reflect the posterior flap to expose the trapezius muscle; detach it from the scapula. Sever all muscles running from the thorax to the scapula from above downward: omohyoid, levator scapulae, rhomboid major and minor and the serratus anterior. The limb is now completely detached from the thorax (Fig. 7-34E).

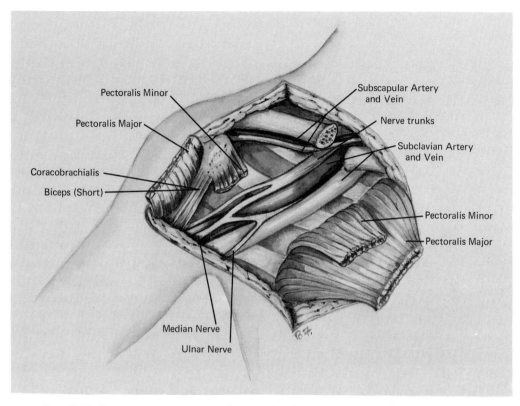

FIG. 7-36. Emergency exposure of the axilla. The clavicle is divided and the pectoralis major split to expose the underlying neurovascular structures.

Suture the pectoralis major and the trapezius and all other muscle stumps to the lateral chest wall. Ligate all bleeding vessels. Finally, tailor the skin flaps and approximate them with interrupted sutures. Place a drain deep in the wound; leave it there for 48 to 72 hours. To obliterate open tissue spaces, apply voluminous dry dressings snugly over the wound (Figs. 7-34B and 7-35).

### Emergency Approach to the Neck and Axilla

Although rare, emergencies may arise that require a speedy exposure of the large vessels and nerve trunks in the neck and axilla. This is a lifesaving procedure; therefore, the integrity of some structures lying in the path leading to the vital structures must be disregarded. For example, in the incision about to be described, the clavicle is transected and the pectoralis major is split in two from the clavicle through its tendon of insertion. Should the need arise, you can extend this incision into the neck to expose the carotid artery and the external jugular vein.

**Technique.** Place the patient in the supine position with the arm slightly away from the body, externally rotated and flexed at the elbow. In order to bring the sternocleidomastoid into relief, turn the hyperextended head and neck toward the opposite side. There are two incisions to this approach, a horizontal and a vertical limb.

Begin the horizontal limb just above the clavicle and about 1½ inches lateral to the sternoclavicular joint; continue it laterally for about 4 inches. The vertical limb starts just lateral to the beginning of the horizontal incision and runs straight down over the pectoralis major to the anterior axillary fold. Quickly reflect the skin flaps of the vertical incision, exposing the pectoralis major, and then divide the muscle in the line of the skin incision from the clavicle through its tendon of insertion. In performing this step, very likely you will encounter and sever a branch of the acromiothoracic artery. Ligate the vessel. Now you are ready to expose the depths of the supraclavicular and axillary regions. By abducting the arm, the fasciomuscular covering from the coracoid to the axilla is brought into view. Beginning below the level of pectoralis minor, penetrate this layer with the index finger; by careful, rapid, blunt dissection, work the finger upward until it reaches the clavicle. Now divide the tissues immediately above the finger, in line with the junction of the two limbs of the incision. Next, with a Gigli saw, transect the clavicle and the subclavius muscle in the same line. When the abducted and externally rotated arm drops away from the trunk, all the neurovascular structures come into view. From above downward appear the deep transverse cervical vein and artery, the suprascapular artery, vein and nerve (just behind the clavicle), and the subclavian artery, vein and the nerve trunks crossing the axillary space (Fig. 7-36).

Closure of the wound is relatively simple. Approximate the edges of pectoralis major and minor and restore alignment of the clavicle. The ends of the clavicle can be either wired together or transfixed with an intramedullary pin.

## SURGICAL MANAGEMENT OF SOME TUMORS OF THE SHOULDER

It is not my purpose in this book to delve in detail into the many tumors and tumorous lesions that can affect the shoulder region. These are no different from those occurring in other major articulations. However, I have found a number of procedures that are especially applicable to the shoulder. Some of these are lifesaving operations; others restore useful function.

## Scapulectomy

Some primary malignant tumors of the scapula can be treated by scapulectomy. Among these are chondrosarcoma, fibrosarcoma, desmoid tumors and giant cell tumors. If a patient with metastatic carcinoma of the scapula refuses a forequarter amputation, scapulectomy is the next best procedure. Scapulectomy results in severe impairment of shoulder and arm function. Nevertheless, in my experience, patients with a scapulectomy are very grateful to still have an arm and a hand. I have performed five scapulectomies (one was performed 17 years ago and another 14 years ago) and in each one I was successful in anchoring the humeral head to the clavicle. Although this appears to be a frail arrangement, in practice it has proved to be a valuable addition to the operation. Suspension of the humerus on the clavicle prevents downward migration of the arm and traction on the neurovascular bundle in the neck and axilla.

### Technique

Ollier's operation is the procedure I prefer. The scapula is removed through two incisions. Begin the first incision (horizontal limb) at the acromioclavicular joint and pass it along the spine of the scapula to the vertebral border. Start the second incision (vertical limb) on the vertebral border above the medial angle of the scapula and run it vertically downward to just below the inferior angle (Fig. 7-37A). Reflect the skin flaps of the horizontal incision and expose the acromioclavicular joint; divide the ligaments of the joint. Next, by sharp dissection, detach the insertion of the trapezius and the origin of the posterior and middle parts of the deltoid from the spine and from the acromion. Mobilize the trapezius enough to expose the medial angle when it is everted. Isolate and protect the nerve going into the trapezius; it is readily seen when the muscle is everted. Near the insertion of the levator scapulae, on the surface of the serratus anterior, the descending scapular artery appears and begins its course downward along the vertebral border of the scapula. Ligate this artery near the medial angle but spare the branch going to the trapezius. Ligate the artery before detaching any of the muscles from the vertebral border of the scapula. Retract the trapezius upward and medially and cut the muscles attached to the medial border and inferior angle of the scapula (rhomboid major and minor, levator scapulae, teres major and serratus anterior) (Fig. 7-37B).

Complete the separation of the deltoid from the acromion and also detach it from the lateral 2 inches of the clavicle. This exposes the coracoid process and the musculotendinous cuff as it inserts into the humerus. Now rotate the scapula laterally and isolate the insertions of the coracobrachialis muscles and the pectoralis minor; cut them close to the bone (Fig. 7-37C). Divide the subscapularis. Next, return the scapula to its normal position and cut the supraspinatus, infraspinatus and teres minor. Grasp and cut the tendon of the long head of the biceps which can now be seen within the joint. Hold the distal cut end of the tendon with a hemostat so that it does not retract downward beneath the transverse ligament. Complete the excision of the scapula by cutting the inferior part of the capsule and any remaining soft tissue attachments. When cutting through the rotator cuff, make the line of division about $3/4$ to 1 inch from the line of insertion into the greater tuberosity. Later this tendon flap will be used to stabilize the humeral head to the outer end of the clavicle (Fig. 7-37D).

After removal of the scapula, clamp and ligate all bleeding vessels. Do not injure the axillary nerve and artery, or the long thoracic nerve.

Anchor the humeral head to the distal end of the clavicle by suturing the tendon flap (still attached to the greater tuberosity) to the end of the clavicle. Pass the sutures through drill holes in the end of the clavicle. (Use stout nylon sutures.) Attach the distal cut end of the long head of the biceps tendon to the floor of the bicipital groove. First divide the transverse ligament spanning the groove, then scarify the floor of the groove with a curette. Place the tendon in the groove and anchor it with several interrupted sutures passing through the overlying transverse ligament and the surrounding fascial tissue (Fig. 7-37E).

Finally, bring together and suture the trapezius and deltoid. Close the skin flaps with interrupted sutures. Always place a drain in the dependent part of the wound. Leave the drain in place for 48 to 72 hours (Fig. 7-38).

### Benign Chondroblastoma

Discussion of management of this tumor is particularly appropriate in a book on the shoulder for it was first recognized and described by Codman in 1931. However, its distinct histological pattern and origin, and its clinical course and significance were first recorded by Jaffe and Lichtenstein in 1942. They named the tumor chondroblastoma and separated it from a host of other tumors containing cartilage cells.

Usually the lesion occurs in males before the age of 20, in the epiphyses. However, the literature reports several cases after age 50. The most prevalent sites are: the upper tibial epiphysis, the lower femoral epiphysis, the upper humeral epiphysis, the greater tuberosity of the humerus and the greater trochanter of the femur. It is generally believed that the lesion is benign; however, several cases of malignant transformation of the lesion are on record. Whether the tumors reported were primarily malignant and not recognized as such, or whether they actually are transformed from a benign to a malignant lesion is difficult to determine.

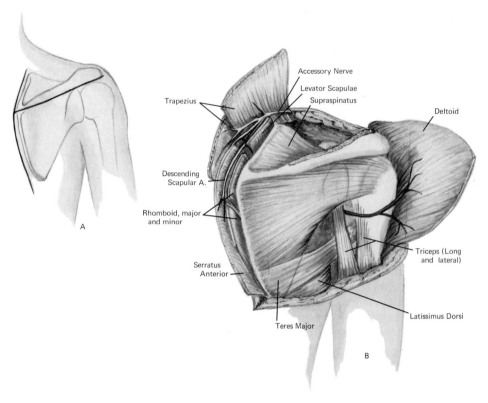

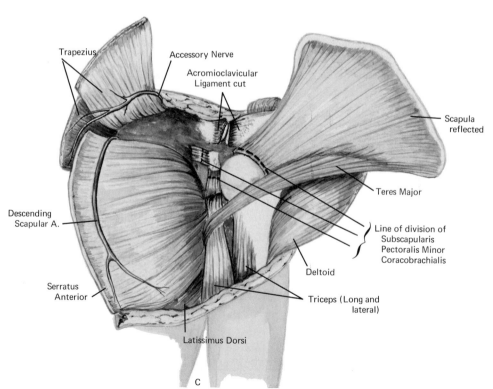

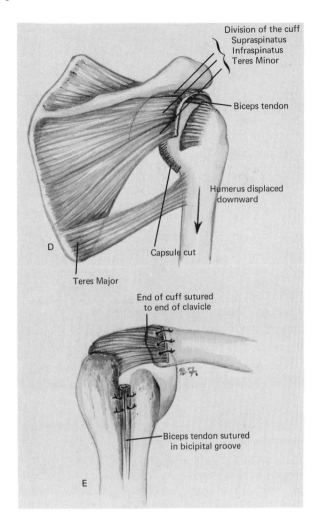

FIG. 7-37. Scapulectomy. (A) Incision. (B) The deltoid is cut at its origin on the spine of the scapula, the acromion and the outer two inches of the clavicle and is reflected outward. The trapezius is cut along its insertion on the spine of the scapula and then reflected inward. The levator scapulae, rhomboid major and minor and serratus anterior are cut from the vertebral border of the scapula. (C) The scapula is rotated outward, allowing ready access to the pectoralis minor and coracobrachialis and the tendon of the subscapularis. (D) The scapula is returned to its normal position and the remaining rotator cuff is divided ¾ of an inch from its insertion into the head of the humerus; the head of the humerus is displaced downward, exposing the biceps tendon in the joint. The remaining capsule is cut. (E) The rotator cuff on the humeral head is sutured to the end of the clavicle, and the biceps tendon is anchored in the bicipital groove.

## Clinical Features

The clinical manifestations are far from dramatic. Rarely do you see a patient with severe, excruciating pain of sudden origin; rather, the symptoms, usually a dull ache referred to the neighboring joint, appear gradually. More often than not, the pain is intermittent in nature and usually relieved by rest. The character of the disorder is such that rarely do the patients seek medical aid under two years from the time of onset of the symptoms.

## Histological Features

The histological features of the tumor are fairly characteristic. Essentially it comprises distinctive, mature chondroblasts. However, in some instances it may be difficult to distinguish the lesion from chondrosarcoma or osteosarcoma, and it may be confused with chondromyxoid fibroma or giant cell tumor (Fig. 7-39).

## Roentgenographic Features

The radiographic appearance of the lesion also is distinctive: the lesion is located in the epiphysis but occasionally it crosses the epiphyseal line; its boundaries are clearly demarcated by a thin zone of sclerotic bone; the classic finding is the presence of punctate, irregular areas of calcification, representing calcification of

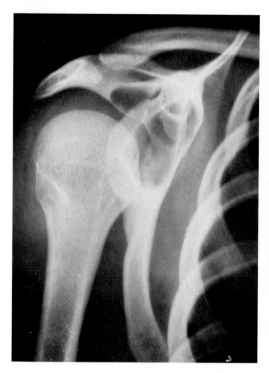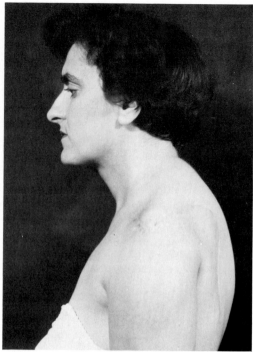

FIG. 7-38. (*Left*) Fibrosarcoma of the scapula. (*Right*) Same patient 21 years after scapulectomy. Note the cosmetic appearance following suspension of the humerus from the clavicle.

nests of cartilage cells. Occasionally, however, the radiographic picture shows some variations: the tumor may lack a delineating line of sclerotic bone and, instead, exhibit an irregular outline; some show reactive periosteal bone formation. When the variant features exist, it is difficult to make a diagnosis of a benign lesion by radiographs alone (Fig. 7-40).

### Treatment

The accepted treatment of chondroblastoma is curettement of the lesion, followed by packing with bone chips. Irradiation has no place in the treatment of chondroblastoma. When the lesion lies in the upper humeral epiphysis, the anterior limb of the superior approach usually provides adequate access to the tumor. If this approach is inadequate, the incision can be extended over the top of the shoulder; the classic superior approach is made to expose the entire upper end of the humerus.

**Technique.** Expose the upper end of the humerus by the anterior limb of the superior approach or by the total superior approach (Fig. 7-41, A and B). With the arm rotated internally, make a circular window in the center of the lateral wall of the greater tuberosity just below the insertion of the rotator cuff. Using sharp curettes, scoop out all tumor tissue down to normal bone. The curettement must be thorough because, even with the most meticulous curettage, some tumor cells remain in situ (Fig. 7-41C). Now flush out the bone cavity with normal saline in order to cleanse the area of any tissue debris. Finally, pack the defect in the humerus tightly with small bone chips obtained from the anterior iliac crest. The incision is reassembled in the usual manner.

### Giant Cell Tumor

Like benign chondroblastoma, the giant cell tumor as a distinct entity was salvaged from a heap of other and unrelated lesions. The common histological denominator in

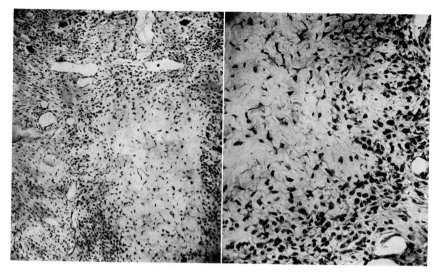

FIG. 7-39. Benign chondroblastoma. The tumor tissue comprises stellate cells, in a myxomatous stroma, fibroblastic proliferation, and numerous chondroblasts. (Photomicrographs × 125 and × 250.)

this group was the presence of numerous multinucleated giant cells. Failure to recognize the fact that giant cells are found in many unrelated lesions gave birth to the term *giant cell variants*. However, since 1940, through the efforts of Jaffe, Lichtenstein, Portis, Sutro and many others, many distinct and unrelated lesions were identified and described; among these are pigmented villonodular synovitis, nonosteogenic fibroma, chondroblastoma, chondromyxoid fibroma and aneurysmal bone cyst. Gradually the stock-pile "variant giant cell tumor" became smaller and smaller, and now such a designation applies to no tumor. Nevertheless, there still remains with us the benign and malignant giant cell tumor. Some pathologists believe that there is no such thing as a benign giant cell tumor; others think differently.

### Histological Features

Jaffe recognizes three gradations of giant cell tumors; all contain many multinucleated giant cells dispersed in a fibrous stroma. The classification is based on the nature of the stromal cells. In Grade I the stromal cells are mature, showing no atypism; in Grade II moderate atypism is present, and in Grade III atypism is pronounced and the cells appear frankly malignant. The greater number of tumors are Grade I and II; the recurrence rate of the former is estimated as high as 40 percent, of the latter 60 percent, and for both 55 percent. For Grade III tumors it is 100 percent. Of the entire group, 15 percent metastasize. Clinical experience, however, reveals that the course of Grade I and II tumors is highly unpredictable. Also, grading this tumor on its histological features is very difficult and in most cases impossible. Many factors are involved; for example, most tumors exhibit different features in different areas. The cells may be of one type in one area and of another type in a different area. Biopsy material obtained by needle aspirations and small samples of tumor tissue obtained by open biopsy are, for this reason, worthless. Also, what is even more discouraging, cases are on record in which the pulmonary metastatic lesion was Grade I.

### Clinical Features

In the region of the shoulder, as elsewhere in the body, giant cell tumors occur

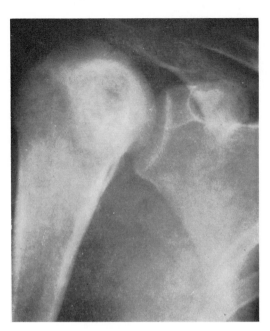

FIG. 7-40. Chondroblastoma of the humerus in a male, aged 23. Observe the mottled appearance, resulting from irregular areas of calcification within the cartilaginous tumor. Also observe the pronounced increase in cortical bone in the shaft of the humerus immediately below the tumor, a characteristic feature of this tumor.

most frequently in the third decade; they rarely occur in children and past middle life. Males and females are affected about equally. They occur in the metaphyseal area of a long bone adjacent to a closed epiphyseal plate. The common sites according to frequency are: the distal end of the femur, the proximal end of the tibia, the distal end of the radius, and the proximal end of the humerus. Not infrequently the discovery of the lesion follows trauma to the part. In general, the growth of the lesion is insidious, and the tumor, when it is detected, is considerable in size. At first, pain is not severe; it is a dull ache and is often referred to the adjacent joint. It is relieved by rest, and, in the early phases of the disease, motion of the joint is not impaired. On the other hand, the first indication of the lesion may be a fracture through the involved bone. Locally, you can palpate a swelling, usually eccentric, of the bone, and pressure causes pain. In some instances, the tumor attains a large size before it produces symptoms.

## Roentgenographic Features

Giant cell tumor has characteristic features: the lesion occurs in the metaphyseal ends of a long bone at or adjacent to an ossified epiphyseal plate. It is radiolucent and at first eccentrically located. With growth, it may involve the entire diameter of the bone. Rarely does it occur in persons under 20 years of age or when the epiphyseal plate is still open. In spite of its progressive nature, it initiates neither periosteal nor endosteal bone formation. The tumor may appear loculated, giving the impression that the lesion is traversed by trabeculae of new bone. The fact is that these fine lines are nothing more than the remains of dead bone surrounding an area of bone destruction.

The tumor is not demarcated by sharp bone margins. In fact, it may penetrate the bone cortex or (in very rare cases) even cross the articular cartilage and involve the joint. By roentgenographic study alone, it is impossible to distinguish a benign from a malignant tumor (Fig. 7-42 and 7-43).

## Surgical Management

The more giant cell tumors I encounter, the more I am convinced that the best treatment is total resection of the portion of the bone harboring it. My belief is based on the following observations: the high incidence of local recurrence following curettement or irradiation; the unpredictability of the course of tumors graded I and II; the unreliability of histological and roentgenographic examinations, and the high incidence of metastasis. The upper end of the humerus lends itself nicely to resection. And, if the resected bone is replaced by bone grafts, both length of the

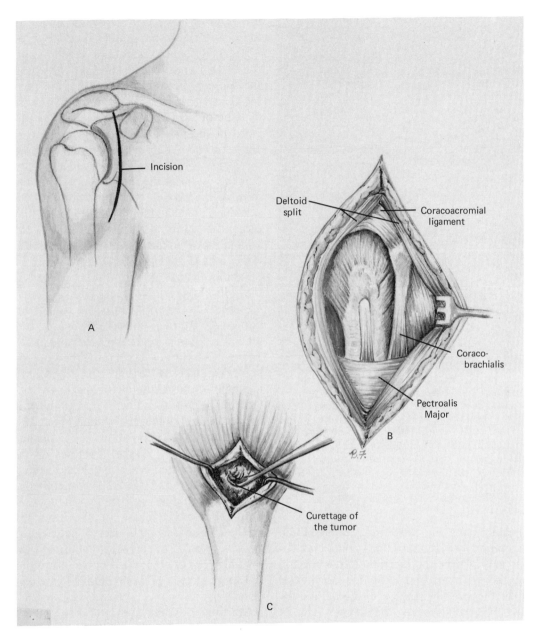

FIG. 7-41. Benign chondroblastoma. (A) Incision—anterior limb of the superior incision. (B) Exposure of the greater tuberosity and the rotator cuff. (C) Curettement of the tumor.

humerus and useful function of the arm are restored. I have employed the following technique in five cases. One of these is 17 years postoperative. All have a useful extremity. In this operation, after excision of the upper end of the humerus, the bone grafts are anchored to the anterior and posterior surfaces of the neck of the scapula. Therefore, the incision must make accessible all regions of the shoulder and upper humerus. The superior and anterior incisions combined provide this exposure.

**Technique.** RESECTION OF THE UPPER END OF THE HUMERUS. Start the incision 2

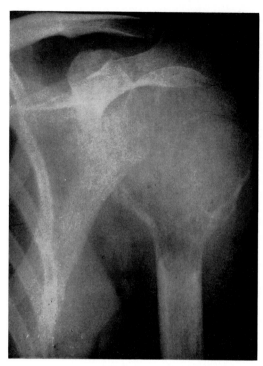

FIG. 7-42. Giant cell tumor in female, aged 26. Note the pronounced expansion of the upper end of the humerus; the remaining cortical shell is thin on the outer aspect of the humerus and absent on the inner aspect. A cartilaginous cap still remains intact; the tumor is traversed by trabeculae of varying thicknesses, giving the tumor mass a bubble-like appearance.

inches below the posterior margin of the acromion just lateral to the acromioclavicular joint. Carry the incision across the top of the shoulder and extend it downward over the anterior portion of the deltoid for 1½ to 2 inches below the anterior edge of the acromion. (Fig. 7-44A). Develop the lateral skin flap by cutting the subcutaneous tissue from the top of the acromion and the tendinous origin of the deltoid (Fig. 7-44B). With a sharp osteotome, divide the acromion in line with the skin incision about three eighths to one half of an inch from its outer edge. Now, gently retract the acromion with the attached deltoid laterally, exposing the subacromial bursa (Fig. 7-44C).

Extend the skin incision downward along the anterior margin of the deltoid as far as its insertion into the deltoid tubercle (Fig. 7-44D). By sharp dissection, develop both the medial and lateral skin flaps, exposing the interval between the deltoid and pectoralis major as far as the inferior margin of the clavicle. The cephalic vein runs upward in the interval. Develop the interval and retract the deltoid laterally and the pectoralis major and the cephalic vein medially. Cut the origin of the deltoid from the outer third of the clavicle and the margin of the acromioclavicular joint. You can now displace the entire deltoid mass downward and laterally, exposing all regions of the upper end of the humerus (Fig. 7-44E). For better exposure of the anterior aspect of the joint, divide the coracobrachialis muscles at their insertion into the tip of the coracoid. Retract them downward and medially. Do not injure the musculocutaneous nerve as it passes through the coracobrachialis muscle. Divide the transverse ligament spanning the bicipital groove, isolate and grasp the biceps tendon with a hemostat, and divide the tendon above the hemostat. If further exposure of the humerus is desired, cut the insertions of the deltoid and of pectoralis major and reflect them laterally and medially respectively. Remember that just proximal to the tendon of the pectoralis major are the branches of the thoracoacromial artery; ligate these vessels. At the upper pole of the incision the anterior circumflex artery winds around the surgical neck of the humerus; ligate this vessel.

Starting in a line just lateral to the bicipital groove above and the tendon of the pectoralis major below, by sharp dissection — preferably subperiosteally — reflect the soft tissues from the shaft of the humerus from the tuberosities above to a level well below the lesion (Fig. 7-44F). If you desire to expose the shaft below the insertion of the deltoid, develop the interval between the brachialis medially and the lateral head of the triceps laterally. Now, transect the shaft of the humerus several inches below the level of the tumor, and elevate the upper end of the humerus from its soft tissue bed. The rotator muscles still remain attached to the humerus. Cut these at their line of insertion into the tuberosities; sever the inferior fibrous capsule and remove the bone and tumor.

REPLACEMENT OF THE BONE DEFECT BY BONE GRAFTS. Two tibial grafts are used to span the bone defect. The upper ends of the grafts are fixed to the neck of the scapula, one graft end on the anterior surface of the neck and the other on the posterior surface. The distal ends of the grafts are fixed to the upper end of the remaining humerus. One graft is fixed on the anterior surface and the other on the posterior surface of the humerus.

First prepare the neck of the scapula to receive the grafts. By sharp periosteal dissection, reflect the subscapularis muscle from the anterior surface of the neck. In a like manner, expose the posterior surface of the neck. Care must be taken during this dissection to avoid injury to the suprascapular nerve—anteriorly, as it enters the suprascapular notch, and posteriorly, as it winds around the base of the spine to enter the infraspinous fossa. Next, with a sharp osteotome, shave the anterior and posterior surfaces of the upper end of the humerus. They must be flat in order to make good contact with the grafts.

Fix the lower ends of the two stout tibial grafts to the end of the humerus with 2 screws, as depicted in Figure 7-44G. Then with 2 screws anchor the upper ends of the grafts to the neck of the scapula, one graft on the anterior surface and the other on the posterior surface. Before inserting the second screw in the neck of the scapula, place the arm in the desired position of abduction and internal rotation in relation to the scapula.

When reassembling the incision, suture the coracobrachialis muscle to the tip of the coracoid process and attach the tendon of the long head of the biceps to the tendon of the short head. Reattach the lateral portion of the acromion with two or three threaded wires, cutting them below the level

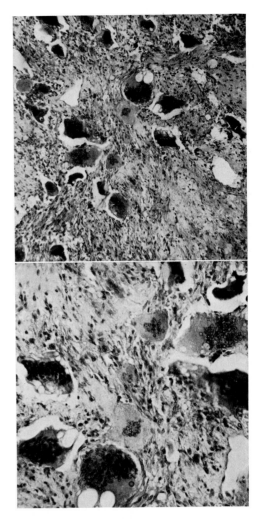

FIG. 7-43. Tissue obtained from giant cell tumor depicted in Figure 7-42. The stroma comprises mononuclear spindle and ovoid cells and small amounts of intercellular collagenous substances, consisting of fine fibers. Many multinucleated giant cells of varying sizes are distributed irregularly throughout the stroma. [Photomicrographs ($\times$ 160 and $\times$ 320)]

of the skin. After closure, apply a plaster spica, holding the arm in the desired position of abduction and foreward flexion. Remove the cast when there is roentgenographic evidence of union at both ends of the grafts and the grafts themselves show evidence of revascularization. This usually takes 4 to 5 months.

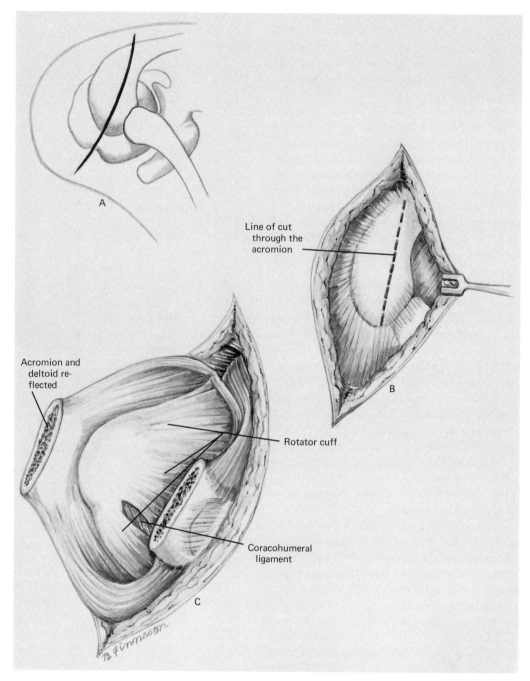

Line of cut
through the
acromion

Acromion and
deltoid re-
flected

Rotator cuff

Coracohumeral
ligament

FIG. 7-44. Excision of the upper end of the humerus and spanning the defect with tibial grafts. (A and D) Incisions. (B) Exposure of tendinous origins of the deltoid on the acromion, and line of the osteotomy through the acromion. (C) Exposure of the subacromial structures. (D) Extension of the incision. (E) Line of exposure of the upper end of the humerus. (F) Exposure of the upper end of the humerus and line of osteotomy below the level of the tumor. (G) Placement of tibial grafts.

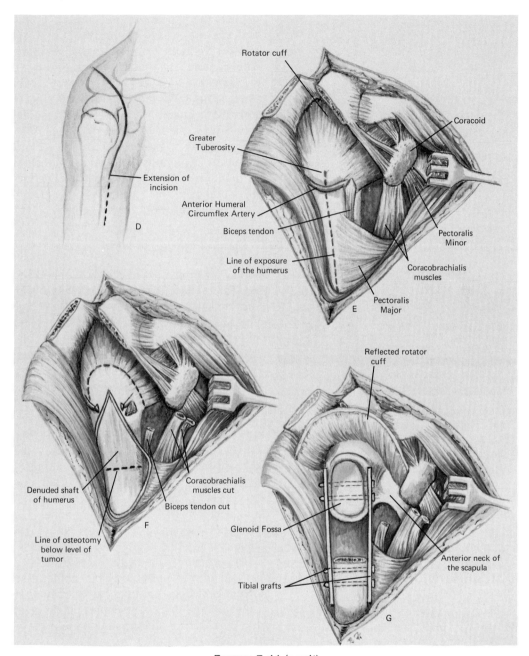

Rotator cuff

Coracoid

Greater
Tuberosity

Extension of
incision

Anterior Humeral
Circumflex Artery

Biceps tendon

Pectoralis
Minor

Line of exposure
of the humerus

Coracobrachialis
muscles

D

Pectoralis
Major

E

Reflected rotator
cuff

Coracobrachialis
muscles cut

Denuded shaft
of humerus

Biceps tendon cut

F

Glenoid Fossa

Line of osteotomy
below level of
tumor

Anterior neck of
the scapula

Tibial grafts

G

FIGURE 7-44 (con't)

## Solitary Bone Cyst

Although solitary bone cyst is not a true neoplasm, its tendency to recur, even after thorough curettement, and the ease with which fractures occur at the stie of the lesion, make it a difficult bone disease to contend with. The pathogenesis of this lesion is not known; however, it is generally accepted that the destructive nature of the lesion is the result of overactivity of many osteoclasts. Among the many theories as

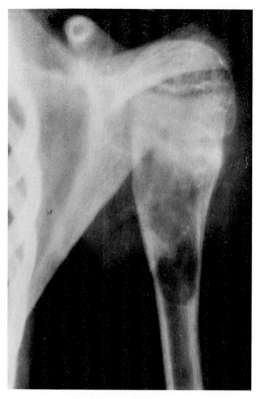

FIG. 7-45. Bone cyst in an 11-year-old girl. Note the expansile nature of the lesion, the thin cortex and the juxta-epiphyseal location. There is no roentgenographic evidence of repair.

to the cause of solitary cysts two are mentioned most frequently in the literature. (1) The cyst is the healed phase of a giant cell tumor; (2) it is the result of intramedullary hemorrhage. Two types are recognized: the active, and the latent solitary cyst.

The active cyst, as a rule, lies close to the growth plate and possesses growth potential. The latent cyst is at a distance from the plate and, with longitudinal growth of the bone migrates away from the metaphysis. After surgical excision both cysts tend to recur; however, the recurrence rate is much higher in the active than in the latent cyst. Most observers believe that there is close correlation between the activity of the cyst and the number of osteoclasts present. Grossly, the affected portion

of the bone appears expanded from within, and the cortex is very thin. In fact, it has a paper thinness and a bluish discoloration. The contents of the cyst vary. Serous or sanguineous fluid may fill the cyst cavity or there may be very little fluid, if any. In the latter cases, some reddish granular tissue lines the cyst. The cyst wall comprises fibrous tissue harboring varying amounts of hemosiderin and aggregates of giant cells. The general histological appearance resembles giant cell tumor and local tissue reaction to hemorrhage.

**Clinical Features**

The lesion occurs in early childhood and in adolescence; however, cases have been reported in persons over 50 years of age and in an infant 2 months old. It is more prevalent in the male than the female, the ratio being 2 to 1. Most cysts cause no pain; occasionally swelling of the bone may direct attention to the lesion. In many instances the first manifestation of the cyst is a fracture of the involved bone. Solitary cysts usually occur at the ends of the long bones; the upper end of the humerus and the upper end of the femur are the most common sites; here 75 percent of all solitary cysts occur. Solitary cysts occasionally occur in the shafts of long bones and have been reported in the ribs, ilium, calcaneus and talus.

Bone repair and healing progress at a normal rate after fracture, but obliteration of the cyst does not take place. Only after repeated fractures does some filling-in of the cyst occur, but the new bone appears defective.

**Roentgenographic Features**

The lesion is very radiolucent and is oval in shape, and its long axis parallels the long axis of the bone. It lies close to the epiphyseal plate and is sharply demarcated by a fine line of sclerotic bone. Thin, irregular septa may cross the cyst. These are not

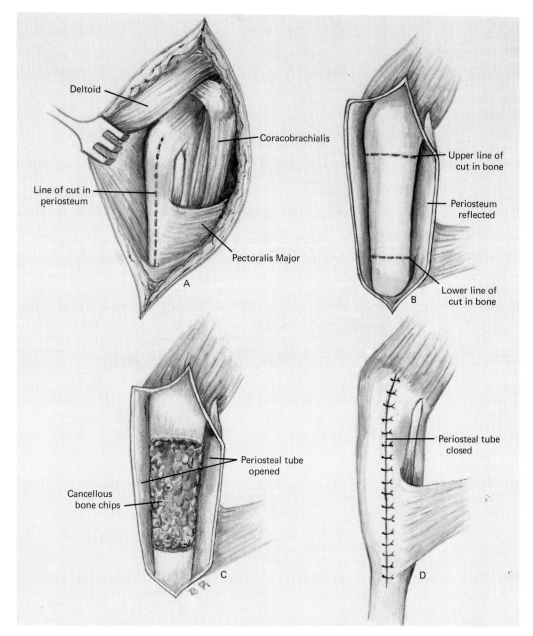

FIG. 7-46. (A) Exposure of the upper end of the humerus through an anterior incision. (B) Reflection of periosteum from around the entire circumference of the shaft of the humerus. (C) Resection of the defective bone and filling of the defect with cancellous bone. (D) Closure of the periosteal tube.

bony trabeculae dividing the cyst into many chambers; rather they are linear areas of erosion of the underlying cortex. Calcification rarely occurs in this lesion.

Penetration of the cortex and extension into the soft tissues never occurs. The cortex appears thin and expanded from within. When fracture does occur, the periosteum remains intact; therefore, displacement of the fragments is never severe.

The size of the cysts varies considerably. As a rule, when first seen, the cyst is 2 to 4 cm. in length; on the other hand, it may occupy the greater part of the length of the bone. Following fracture the healing process may produce a loculated appearance of the lesion.

In the differential diagnosis the following lesions must be considered: enchondroma, fibrous dysplasia, eosinophilic granuloma, giant cell tumor and aneurysmal bone cyst (Fig. 7-45).

### Surgical Management

The conventional method of treatment of this lesion is curettement of the cyst walls, followed by packing of the cyst cavity with bone chips. However, this method of treatment does not preclude recurrences. In 1965 Agerholm and Goodfellow described a method of treatment that reduced the incidence of recurrences drastically. Essentially it comprises resection of the affected diaphysis subperiosteally and filling of the periosteal tube with bone chips. In my opinion, this method of treatment is far superior to simple curettement of the lesion. In 6 cases treated by this method I have had no recurrences and no fractures through the affected bones. Although total resection of several inches of the humerus appears to be a radical approach to the problem, in no case treated by me has nonunion occurred. Also, normal growth of the humerus has never been interfered with, no matter how close the lesion was to the epiphyseal plate.

**Technique.** If the upper end of the diaphysis is to be resected, employ the anterolateral approach described on page 170. If more of the diaphysis must be exposed, extend the incision downward in the interval between the triceps and the brachialis.

Deepen the incision down to the bone and incise the periosteum on its anterior surface (Fig. 7-46A). By sharp subperiosteal dissection reflect the periosteum from the entire circumference of the diaphysis to be resected (Fig. 7-46B). The lines of transection through the diaphysis should be 2 to 3 cm. above and below the limits of the cyst. If the proximal limit of the cyst cavity is next to the epiphyseal plate, the diaphysis is removed at the distal end of the plate and the cyst lining curetted from the plate. Exposure of the growth plate does not interfere with normal growth of the humerus.

After the diseased bone is removed, pack the empty periosteal sheath with cancellous bone chips removed from the side of the ilium (Fig. 7-46C). Now close the sheath with a continuous suture, converting it into a tube (Fig. 7-46D). It appears that the function of the bone chips is mainly to maintain the periosteal tube patent. Restoration of the diaphysis is achieved by rapid and abundant subperiosteal new bone.

At the end of the operation apply a light hanging cast and place the arm in light overhead traction for 5 to 7 days. Then allow the patient to be up with the arm in a sling. The plaster cast, together with gravity, is sufficient to maintain bone length in the upright position during consolidation of the new bone. Remove the plaster cast at the end of 7 weeks; at this time union is usually complete.

### Fibrous Dysplasia

In 1937 Albright described a disease entity which he designated *osteitis fibrosa disseminata* and described it as a distinct disease in no way related to hyperparathyroidism. Later it became known as Albright's Syndrome. Three features are characteristic of this syndrome: (1) bone lesions that tend to be unilateral (i.e., affecting one side of the skeletal system), (2) the presence of isolated areas of pigmentation of the skin (café-au-lait spots) having an irregular outline often compared to the coast of Maine, and (3) endocrine disturbances which in females may cause precocious puberty. The essential pathological lesion is replacement of portions of the medullary cavity of one or more bones with fibrous tissue.

Lichtenstein in 1938 described the same bone lesions without the presence of café-au-lait spots or any evidence of endocrine disturbance. He named the new entity *polyostotic fibrous dysplasia*. Further clarification came in 1946 when Schlunbeger noted the same pathological process in single bones. Although he believed that no relation existed between the monostotic and polyostotic processes, most workers are of the opinion that there is some relationship between the two.

The cause of the disease is not known. Apparently, it is the result of some developmental abnormality of the bone-forming mesenchyme, resulting in replacement of the spongiosa and filling the medullary cavity with fibrous tissue. Also, scattered throughout the tissue, defective bony trabeculae form by osseous metaplasia. The process is neither neoplastic nor inflammatory.

## Clinical Features

As noted previously, two forms of fibrous dysplasia are recognized: monostotic and polyostotic. In both types, males and females are equally affected. The lesion begins early in life, often in infancy, but, because it is often asymptomatic, its recognition may be late in life. The symptoms vary greatly from a mild ache to a severe limp. In females, vaginal bleeding may occur early in life, even in infants. Fracture of the affected bone may be the first indication of the disease, and in the polyostotic form it occurs in 40 percent of the patients at some time during life. On the other hand, a bone may exhibit extensive involvement and yet never suffer a fracture. When the lower extremity is involved, difference in leg lengths is a common finding; it is caused by deformity of the upper end of the femur (the "shepherd's crook"). Malig-

nant transformation is indeed rare, as is death due to the disease. Death may come a few months or many years after the disease is recognized. In most patients the process becomes quiescent at puberty, but in a few the active stage extends beyond this period, and a quiescent lesion may be reactive during pregnancy.

Patients afflicted with the monostotic form of fibrous dysplasia may be completely asymptomatic. When the disease manifests itself, some local swelling usually becomes noticeable in the subperiosteal bones. Not infrequently pain is referred to the adjacent joint, mimicking an arthritic process. Fracture through the site of the lesion may be the initial presenting complaint. The prognosis is good; the monostotic form does not go on to involvement of other bones. Moreover, no café-au-lait spots appear, and no changes in the blood chemistry and no dysfunction of the endocrine system occur.

In marked contrast to the monostotic, in the polyostotic variety of fibrous dysplasia 35 percent of patients reveal areas of pigmentation. Usually the spots are on the affected side of the skeleton, but occasionally they appear on the other side. Twenty percent of these patients show evidence of sexual precocity. In addition, at the end of skeletal maturity, males are shorter than average because of premature closure of the epiphyseal plates. The mechanism producing this disturbance is not clear but it is supposed that the onset of puberty is triggered by the release of gonadotrophic hormones from the anterior pituitary as a result of stimuli traveling through the hypothalamic pituitary nervous humeral pathway. It is of interest that sexual precocity rarely occurs in males and, when it does, presents in a mild form. Hyperthyroidism may occur in both sexes, before or after the bone lesions appear.

Like monostotic fibrous dysplasia, the polyostotic form may exhibit minimal or extensive involvement of the bones on one side of the body. Also, in the polyostotic

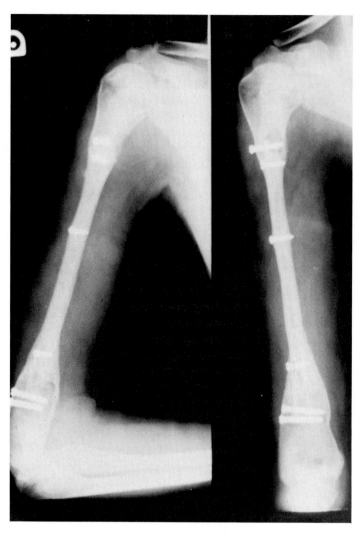

FIG. 7-47. Fibrous dysplasia of all bones of the right upper extremity in a female 21 years old. The characteristic roentgenographic features of this lesion are distinctly seen in the lower end of the humerus and the proximal ends of the radius and ulna. Note the homogeneous "ground glass" appearance of the medullary canals and the expansion of the affected bones. The normal delineation between cortex and medullary cavity has disappeared. Because of severe pain in the arm the diaphysis of the humerus was resected and the defect spanned by two tibial grafts. The operation was performed 4 years prior to the taking of this roentgenogram. Since the operation, the patient has had a painless extremity and has regained full function.

variety no skin pigmentation or endocrine disturbances may occur. When the skull is involved the features are characteristic: the outer table of the calvaria expands and the foramina become distorted, often producing neurological manifestations.

### Pathological Features

Grossly, the medullary cavity of the affected bone is replaced by a whitish-gray tissue, rubbery in consistency and permeated with spicules of bone. Microscopically, the tissue occupying the medullary canal comprises fibrous tissue, throughout which are scattered nests of osteoid tissue. These areas may contain cartilage cells and even some giant cells. The total pattern is variable; it may resemble Paget's disease, metastatic carcinoma and ostitis fibrosa cystica, depending upon the ratio of fibrous to osseous elements.

### Roentgenographic Features

Although marked variations exist, the roentgenographic appearance of fibrous dysplasia presents some fairly characteristic features. The medullary cavity shows evidence of replacement by a tissue whose density may vary from complete radiolucency to a homogeneous "ground glass"

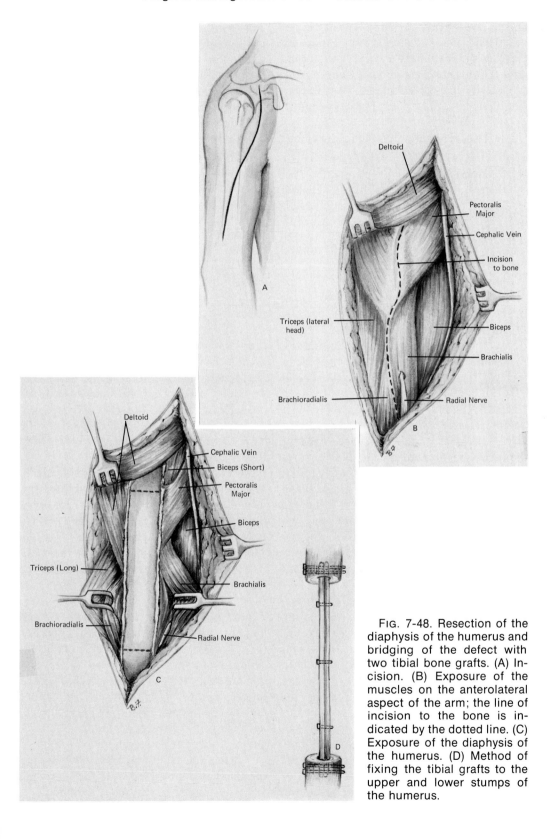

FIG. 7-48. Resection of the diaphysis of the humerus and bridging of the defect with two tibial bone grafts. (A) Incision. (B) Exposure of the muscles on the anterolateral aspect of the arm; the line of incision to the bone is indicated by the dotted line. (C) Exposure of the diaphysis of the humerus. (D) Method of fixing the tibial grafts to the upper and lower stumps of the humerus.

appearance. This variation is dependent upon the amount of fibrous tissue occupying the medullary cavity. The normal delineation between the cortex and medullary cavity may disappear, so that the entire diameter of the bone appears homogeneous in texture.

On the other hand, radiolucent areas may be present in which the cortex is markedly thinned on its medial border. If a fracture has occurred, the cortex may be thicker than normal. The deossified area not infrequently exhibits well delineated sclerotic borders, of which the inner surface is dense and the outer surface blends into normal bone.

Substitution of the elements of the medullary cavity tends to expand the diameter of the bone. This is true especially in the ribs and the skull and, to a lesser degree, in the long bones. In the long bones, expansion generally occurs in the metaphyseal regions rather than in the diaphysis, but the shaft also may be involved. In the lower extremity, the femur is most commonly affected, usually the neck and the metaphysis; however, implication of the ilium and tibia on the same side is not unusual. In the long bones, bowing is a common finding, resulting, as a rule, from fracture. In the upper end of the femur the resulting deformity is known as the shepherd's crook. Usually, healing at the site of fracture occurs as in normal bones; occasionally, however, pseudarthrosis occurs.

At times the only evidence of fibrous dysplasia is the presence of small, spotting lesions of increased density on the opposite side of extensive involvement. Evidence of malignant transformation in fibrous dysplasia is exceedingly rare.

## Surgical Management

Occasionally, fibrous dysplasia may produce intense pain in the affected bone. If the lesion is confined to a limited area of a long bone, the best surgical treatment is extraperiosteal resection of the involved portion of the bone and spanning of the remaining defect with a bone graft. That the resection is performed extraperiosteally is most important, for I have seen recurrence of the lesion in the graft following subperiosteal resection of the affected bone. On the other hand, when the entire long bone is implicated, the entire diaphysis can be resected and replaced by bone grafts. Again, extraperiosteal resection reduces the chances of recurrences. It is true that implication of a long bone usually means involvement of the metaphyseal regions; but, in my experience, after resection of the diaphysis and implantation of the bone grafts into the proximal and distal metaphyses, the healing process overcomes the pathological activity and the grafts are incorporated into the metaphyses without further reactivation of the basic pathological lesion. I have performed this operation in the femur, the tibia, the radius and the humerus. In the case of the femur, 17 years have passed without evidence of recurrence; in the tibia, 7 years; in the radius, 8 years and in the humerus, 4 years (Fig. 7-47).

**Technique.** To expose the entire diaphysis of the humerus, employ the anterolateral approach (p. 170) and extend it downward in the interval between the triceps and the brachialis (Fig. 7-48A). Deepen the incision down to the periosteum on the anterior surface of the humerus (Fig. 7-48B). Then, by sharp dissection reflect the soft tissues from the periosteum for the entire length of the diaphysis and from its entire circumference (Fig. 7-48C). In the lower end of the incision avoid injury to the radial nerve in the interval between the brachialis and brachioradialis. Now transect the upper end of the humerus through its surgical neck and the lower end about 1½ to 2 inches above the humeral epicondyles.

A large defect now remains between the proximal and distal ends of the humerus. With a curette excavate the medullary cavity of each bone end for a distance of 1½ to 2 inches. Take two tibial grafts and insert them into the bone ends. The grafts are so placed that their medullary surfaces are in apposition and their ends are deeply seated into the medullary cavities of the upper and lower stumps of the humerus. The lengths of the grafts is enough to restore the normal length of the humerus. To obtain even better fixation, transfix the graft ends by two screws passing through the entire thickness of the humeral stumps and passing at the same time through the ends of the tibial grafts (Fig. 7-48D).

After closure, apply a shoulder plaster spica, holding the arm in about 30° of abduction. After consolidation remove the plaster shoulder spica and allow motion at the shoulder and elbow within the tolerance of pain. In the case mentioned above, revascularization of the tibial grafts and incorporation of the graft ends by the host bone were accomplished in 4 months. The patient returned to full activity at the end of six months.

## PROSTHETIC REPLACEMENT OF THE ARTICULAR SURFACE OF THE HUMERAL HEAD

Replacement of the articular surface of the humeral head was first described by Neer in 1955. It has proved to be a valuable procedure when the only alternatives are resection of the head or arthrodesis of the glenohumeral joint. It is indicated in severe traumatic lesions of the joint when the articular surface is severely comminuted or the blood supply of the humeral head has been disrupted. Also, it can restore painless motion in a joint extensively affected by degenerative changes, as in osteoarthritis, post-traumatic arthritis, irradiation necrosis, sickle cell infraction or gout. It is contraindicated in neurotrophic arthropathy, osteomyelitis and active rheumatoid arthritis and in shoulders with paralysis of the deltoid or with large complete tears of the rotator cuff.

The Vitallium prosthesis is available in four stem sizes, with perforations in the upper part of the stem to permit ingrowth of bone. The difference in stem sizes is necessary because of the great variation of the diameter of the medullary cavity in different persons. In order to prevent rotation and to ensure fixation of the device, the upper end of the stem has three flanges that fit in slits in the cancellous bone when the prosthesis is seated in its final position. It is best to determine the proper stem size before the operation. Tape the prosthesis to the lateral surface of the arm in the plane it is to occupy and take anteroposterior roentgenograms. Now, by comparing the size of the medullary canal with that of the stem, determine the stem size to be used. To prevent subluxation or dislocation of the device, it must be placed in slight retroversion, usually about 20°.

## Technique:

The supero-anterior approach (p. 157) provides adequate exposure to insert the prosthesis. However, when a fresh fracture–dislocation is being explored, the superior incision (p. 149) gives even better exposure of the upper end of the humerus. I routinely use this incision in all cases of fracture–dislocations. It should be remembered that the supero-anterior incision is the anterior limb of the full superior incision.

Begin the incision on the posterior edge of the acromion just lateral to the acromioclavicular joint. Carry the incision over the top of the shoulder and then downward over the anterior portion of the deltoid in line with the axillary crease. Terminate the skin incision 2 inches below the edge of the acromion (Fig. 7-49A). Now, freely mobilize the medial and lateral skin flaps by dissecting the subcutaneous layer from the deltoid, the top of the acromion and the acromioclavicular joint. Develop the incision through the anterior fibers of the deltoid in line with the acromioclavicular

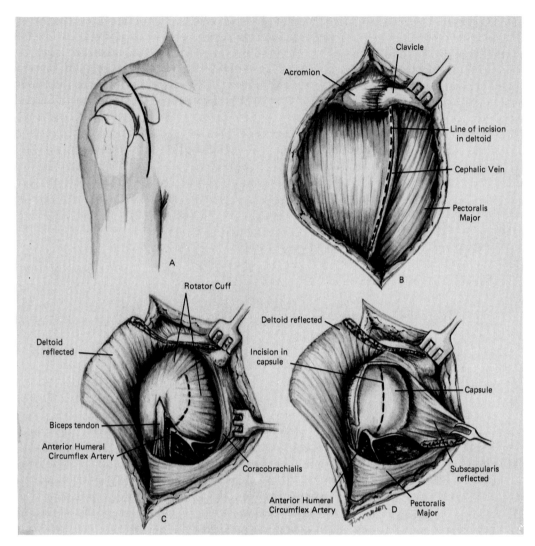

FIG. 7-49. Insertion of humeral head prosthesis. (A) Incision. (B) Line of incision through the deltoid. (C) Exposure of the subdeltoid region. (D) Exposure, division and reflection of the subscapularis tendon. (E) Humeral head is delivered into the wound by rotating the arm externally; the articular surface is removed with a broad osteotome. (F) The medullary canal of the neck of the humerus is cleared of cancellous bone, the three slots to receive the flanges of the prosthesis are made in the base of the neck, and the biceps tendon is divided at its insertion into the superior glenoid rim. (G) The prosthesis is seated on the humeral neck. (H) The biceps tendon is anchored in the bicipital groove.

joint for 2 inches (Fig. 7-49B). By sharp dissection detach the anterior insertion of the deltoid from the clavicle and the acromioclavicular joint and displace it laterally. Now the entire upper end of the humerus comes into view (Fig. 7-49C).

With the arm in external rotation iden-tify the insertion of the subscapularis ten-don into the lesser tuberosity. Divide the tendon along its line of insertion and re-flect it medially; now divide the anterior capsule transversely (Fig. 7-49D). The humeral head can now be dislocated into the wound by further external rotation of

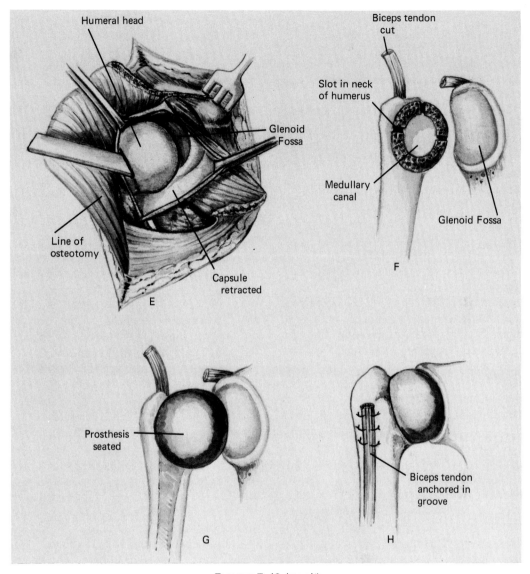

FIGURE 7-49 (con't)

the arm and by prying it with a blunt elevator. Remove the articular surface of the humeral head with a broad, sharp osteotome (Fig. 7-49E). Next locate the biceps tendon in the joint, cut its insertion into the superior rim of the glenoid fossa and displace it from the bicipital groove. With a small curette pierce the cancellous bone of the neck until the medullary canal is located. Now, with large curettes, enlarge the opening in the neck until it will accept the stem of the prosthesis (Fig. 7-49F). Place the stem in the medullary canal so that its flanges rest on the neck, but make sure that the articular surface is retroverted about 20°. This is best determined by turning the prosthesis posteriorly about 20° to a plane passing through both epicondyles of the humerus. Mark off on the neck the exact sites of the flanges; then make slits in the cancellous bone with a fine osteotome. Seat the flanges in their respective slits and drive the prosthesis to its final position (Fig. 7-49G).

In reassembling the incision, the subscapularis must be firmly reattached to its original site, the biceps tendon is anchored in the bicipital groove and the anterior fibers of the deltoid are reattached to the clavicle (Fig. 7-49H).

After closure of the wound, place the arm in a sling and swathe. Start pendulum exercises after the third day but prohibit external rotation movements for $3\frac{1}{2}$ to 4 weeks. Discard external fixation after 4 weeks and permit full use of the arm, but insist on a progressive exercise program.

## ARTHRODESIS OF THE SHOULDER

Arthrodesis of the glenohumeral joint is a valuable procedure in properly selected cases. In the western world the decrease in the number of patients afflicted with tuberculosis and anterior poliomyelitis has reduced the number of patients requiring arthrodesis of the shoulder. However, elsewhere in the world this is not true. The indications for this procedure are: tuberculosis of the glenohumeral joint, flail joint caused by anterior poliomyelitis, flail joint following injury to the brachial plexus and degenerative lesions of the joint caused by either osteoarthritis or trauma. The few cases of tuberculosis of the joint that I have seen in recent years have responded to chemotherapy and rest. Also, today, most cases of osteoarthritis or traumatic disruption of the joint can be salvaged by replacing the articular surface of the humeral head with a Vitallium prosthesis provided the power of the rotator muscles is not impaired.

Before an arthrodesis is effected certain criteria must be met. The patient must demonstrate unrestricted motion of the scapula on the thoracic cage, and the axioscapular muscles must have adequate power. This means that the trapezius and serratus anterior must be strong enough to elevate and rotate the scapula against resistance. (At least 75% of normal strength must be present.)

Once a decision to perform an arthrodesis is made, the position of the humerus in relation to the scapula must be given much thought. Many factors govern this decision: the sex and occupation of the patient, and the strength of the trapezius and serratus anterior muscles. A joint fused so that the arm when at rest is in slight abduction (away from the trunk) provides more elevation of the extremity but produces more winging of the scapula than if the arm is close to the trunk. This winging of the scapula is not acceptable to most women. The controversy in regard to the best functional position of the humerus in relation to the scapula in a fused shoulder is still with us. In 1942 a research committee of the American Orthopaedic Association, after intensive study, found that the most serviceable position of the arm in relation to the scapula to be 50° of abduction, 20° of forward flexion and 25° of internal rotation; further, that this fixed position makes possible 90 to 95° of active abduction, 80° of flexion and 90° of internal rotation. However, I have found that this position is not applicable to all patients. The needs of the different patients vary and a given position may produce excellent function in one person and poor function in another. In 1964, Charnley and Houston aimed for a fusion with the arm at 45° of abduction, 45° of flexion and 45° of medial rotation. Their patients had difficulty in doing their hair and coping with back fastenings of their garments.

In general, women desire a position of the fused shoulder which permits reaching the hair and face and the back of the head. However, these requisites demand more abduction which, in turn, means winging of the scapula, a feature women dislike. Men desire a position providing more power; this means less abduction of the fused joint. Patients with extensive paralysis and weak axioscapular muscles tolerate poorly a position of marked abduction (over 45°) and external rotation. This position places a strain on the scapulothoracic muscles beyond their tolerance. The result is pain and fatigue. Deformities of the thorax, such as occur in scoliosis, interfere with the normal movements of the scapula and hence restrict abduction and external rotation of the limb after shoulder fusion. The operation may be performed in all age groups. The techniques in current use can be performed on children as young as 6 years without fear of interfering with bone growth. There is sufficient evidence to indicate that a screw or nail across the epiphyseal plate causes no growth disturbances.

Function of the elbow in patients with paralysis may be improved by shoulder fusion. With the arm at the side a patient may not be able to flex the elbow against gravity. However, if the same arm is elevated and is fixed in that position, active flexion of the elbow may return.

Because it is so difficult to determine the correct position of fusion for any one person, especially for patients with extensive paralysis of the upper extremity, it is helpful to determine the most functional position before the operation. This can be done as follows: Under local anesthesia, fix the humerus to the glenoid cavity by two short Steinman or Knowles pins and have the patient put the arm through the different arcs of movements. The procedure may have to be done several times before the best position for the patient can be determined. Before removing the pins apply a plaster shoulder spica which holds the arm in the desired position. After removal of the pins, perform the arthrodesis through an opening in the cast. In general, unless there is weakness of the scapulothoracic muscles, I prefer the following position of fusion in men: 60° of abduction, 20° of forward flexion and 45° of internal rotation. In addition, in males, I resect the distal end of the clavicle just beyond the coracoclavicular ligament. This is done several months after a solid bony fusion has occurred. By so doing, both abduction of the arm toward the chest and flexion increase; also, an in-

crease of a few degrees of internal rotation and extension occurs. Excision of the outer end of the clavicle forces the scapula to shift around the thorax and, hence, causes some winging of its vertical border. Women do not like this deformity. In women I place the arm in 45° of abduction, 20° of forward flexion and 45° of internal rotation.

## Methods of Arthrodesis

Over the years many techniques have evolved to achieve arthrodesis of the glenohumeral joint. Some are extra-articular fusions, some are intra-articular and others are a combination of both. Fusion by extra-articular methods alone is difficult to attain; the combined procedures give the best results. If to the combined methods internal fixation is added, the results are even better. I prefer a combined intra-articular and extra-articular fusion in which two Knowles pins are employed across the joint for internal fixation. Instead of internal fixation appliances, Charnley uses an apparatus to produce compression at the sites of contact between the denuded humeral head and the glenoid fossa, and the head and the undersurface of the acromion. According to Charnley, by this method the incidence of failure of arthrodesis is drastically reduced and, on the average, bony fusion is demonstrable and all external fixation can be discarded in only 10 weeks. Twenty-two of his 23 cases showed clinical union when the compression clamps and pins were removed after an average of 4.8 weeks. These data differ from those of the Research Committee of the American Orthopaedic Association. They found an overall incidence of non-union in 22 percent, and, if fixation was discarded at 10 weeks or less, the incidence rose to 42 percent. They recommended a minimum of 3 months in plaster and, if union was doubtful, 5 months.

## Technique

Essentially, the shoulder fusion I perform is a modification of the Watson-Jones

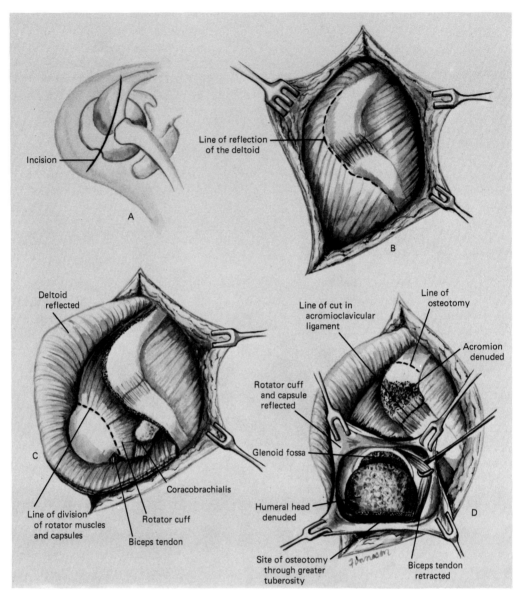

FIGURE 7-50, A–F (*Caption on facing page*)

operation. Also, I use two short Knowles pins to transfix the joint. A day or two before operation apply a plaster cast to the trunk which includes the normal shoulder but leaves the shoulder to be fused, and the arm, free. Be sure that the entire posterior aspect of the scapula is accessible in order to determine the final position of the arm at the time of operation. Place the patient on the table just short of a full sitting position, with the body tilted slightly away from the surgeon. This position makes all regions of the shoulder accessible to the surgeon.

Use the superior approach (p. 149). Make the skin incision directly over the top of the shoulder just lateral to the acromioclavicular joint and in line with the axillary crease. Extend it downward on the anterior surface of the deltoid for at least 2 inches below the edge of the acromion. Posteriorly, extend the incision backward and downward over the posterior portion of

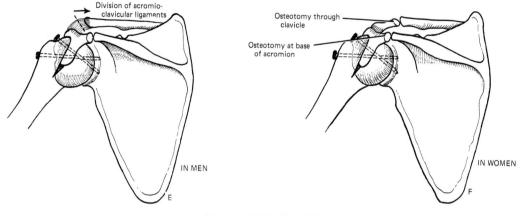

FIGURE 7-50 (Cont'd)

FIG. 7-50. Arthrodesis of the glenohumeral joint. (A) Incision. (B) Skin is reflected to expose the origin of the deltoid. (C) Reflection of the deltoid, exposing the subacromial region. (D) Division and reflection of the cuff and capsule. The articular surface of the humeral head is denuded of cartilage, as is the glenoid fossa; the top of the acromion is scarified to raw bone. An osteotomy at the base of the acromion is made and the acromioclavicular ligaments are cut. (E) In men, the end of the acromion is wedged under the greater tuberosity and the humeral head is fixed to the glenoid with two Knowles pins. (F) In women, the outer end of the clavicle is also osteotomized and tilted downward with the acromion.

the deltoid for two inches (Fig. 7-50A). By sharp dissection develop the lateral and medial skin flaps to expose the tip of the acromion, the scapular spine, the acromioclavicular joint and the outer third of the clavicle (Fig. 7-50B). By sharp subperiosteal dissection detach the deltoid from the outer third of the clavicle, the acromioclavicular joint, the acromion and the spine of the scapula. Now reflect the deltoid downward, exposing the subacromial region (Fig. 7-50C). To expose the humeral head and glenoid fossa, resect the tendons of the rotator cuff, along with the joint capsule. Locate the long head of the biceps tendon. Sever it at its insertion into the superior glenoid rim and remove it from the bicipital groove. With a curette scarify the bottom of the groove. Now place the biceps tendon into the groove and anchor it there with several interrupted sutures passing through the transverse ligament and adjacent soft tissues. Denude the humeral head and the glenoid fossa of all

cartilage, exposing bleeding bone (Fig. 7-50D). The following steps of the operation depend upon whether or not resection of the outer end of the clavicle is anticipated. As a rule, in men the outer end of the clavicle is resected at a second operation, whereas in women this is not done.

**In Men.** Disarticulate the clavicle from the acromion by dividing transversely all the ligaments and the capsule of the acromioclavicular joint. Next, denude the superior and the inferior surface of the acromion to raw bone, and, with a fine sharp osteotome, partially divide the acromion at its base. Angulate the acromion downward, creating a greenstick fracture at its base. The next step is elevation of the greater tuberosity, in the manner of a trap door, and insertion of the acromion under it (Fig. 7-50E). In order to obtain a snug fit, the angles of the cut through the greater tuberosity must be made accurately. To achieve this, place the humerus in relation to the glenoid fossa in the desired position

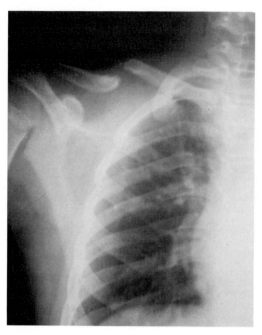

FIG. 7-51. Congenital pseudarthrosis of the clavicle in a boy 5 years of age.

After closure of the wound, while the arm is held in the desired position, apply a plaster cast to the arm and join it to the trunk cast. At the end of two weeks, replace the spica by another spica extending from just behind the metacarpal heads to well below the iliac crests and including both shoulders. Solid bony fusion is usually attained 10 to 12 weeks after the operation. At this time remove the cast and institute exercises to restore motion at the wrist, elbow and thoracoscapular joints.

In men, after solid fusion is demonstrable, wait another 3 months, during which the patient exercises the extremity to regain muscle strength and motion in the joints; then remove the Knowles pins and excise the clavicle distal to the coracoclavicular ligament. In women, merely remove the Knowles pins, in order to prevent formation of a painful bursa over the pin heads.

of fusion and mark off the angle of the cut in the greater tuberosity. Beginning just distal to the articular margin of the head, with a sharp, broad osteotome, cut and raise the greater tuberosity as a bone flap, 1 inch wide and 2 inches long and attached at its base. Wedge the acromion under the bone flap and place the arm in the desired position of arthrodesis. Now, fix the head to the glenoid cavity with two small Knowles pins passing from the lateral surface of the head to the neck of the scapula. Leave the heads of the pins under the skin so that they are accessible when they are to be removed (Fig. 7-50E).

In Women. Denude the superior and inferior surfaces of the acromion and the clavicle. Partially divide the base of the acromion and also the clavicle at the juncture of its middle and outer thirds. Now angulate them downward enough to wedge the acromion under the bone flap made from the greater tuberosity. The rest of the operation is the same as described above (Fig. 7-50F).

## PARTIAL RESECTION OF THE SCAPULA

Because of the presence of benign tumors, tuberculosis or osteomyelitis, it may be necessary to resect a part of the body of the scapula. The function of the shoulder girdle is not seriously impaired after such procedures, because the muscular attachments to the coracoid process and the acromion are not disturbed; the relationship of the rotator muscles to the humeral head is still intact and the humerus remains in its normal relation to the glenoid fossa. The first steps of the operative procedure are similar to those described for scapulectomy (p. 184).

### Technique

Begin the skin incision on the posterior edge of the acromion and extend it along the spine of the scapula to its medial border, then curve the incision downward, paralleling the vertebral border of the scapula, and terminate it at the inferior angle of the scapula. Dissect the skin flaps away from the underlying muscles. By sharp subperiosteal dissection detach the trapezius from the spine of the scapula and retract it upward and inward. Develop the interval on the posterior aspect of the vertebral border of the scapula between the infraspinatus and the rhomboid major down to the periosteum. Then divide the periosteum and reflect it from the infraspinatus fossa, thereby elevating the infraspinatus from its fossa. In a similar manner detach the rhomboids, serratus anterior, teres major, teres minor and latissimus dorsi. Next detach, subperiosteally, the subscapularis. On the ventral surface of the scapula you may extend the subperiosteal dissection as far as the neck of the scapula. The entire body of the scapula is exposed and any portion of it can be removed below the level of the spine.

When all of the scapula below the level of the spine is removed, function can be preserved if the muscles are reassembled in the following manner. Bring together the lateral border of the subscapularis and the teres major and the medial border of the subscapularis and the serratus anterior. Suture the axillary border of the infraspinatus to the teres minor, and its medial border to the serratus anterior; then suture the above combined attachments to the rhomboids. Finally, cover the rhomboids with the trapezius and reattach it to the spine of the scapula.

## REPAIR OF CONGENITAL PSEUDARTHROSIS OF THE CLAVICLE

In the chapter concerned with congenital abnormalities of the shoulder, congenital abnormalities of the clavicle were discussed. It was pointed out that pseudarthrosis tends to implicate the middle third of the clavicle, and the sternal portion usually lies in front and above the acromial portion. Up to 1969, 20 cases of this lesion

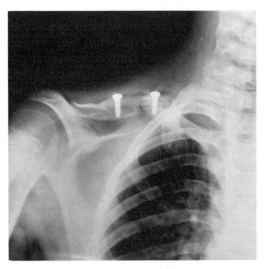

Fig. 7-52. The defect in the clavicle is spanned with an onlay bone graft.

have been reported in the literature. I have seen and treated one case, making the total 21. The right clavicle only was affected in all patients except one, in whom both clavicles were involved. Essentially the lesion is the result of failure of ossification during the 19 mm. stage of the precartilaginous bridge spanning the sternal and acromial segments of the clavicle. The cause is not known. Gruenberg believed that the lesion is not due to any aberrant systemic genes; yet, in one family reported, several children were affected. It is not clear whether the lesion is related to craniocleidodysostosis. On the other hand, patients with simple pseudarthrosis of the clavicle do not show the stigmata so commonly associated with craniocleidodysostosis.

Some patients exhibit no impairment of function and have no pain; others do complain of dysfunction and increasing pain in the affected shoulder girdle. The patient I treated was a male, 5 years of age, who complained of pain over the right clavicle. The pain was aggravated by those activities little boys engage in. It is the general belief that the continuity of the clavicle should be restored. The most common method of repair is spanning of the defect

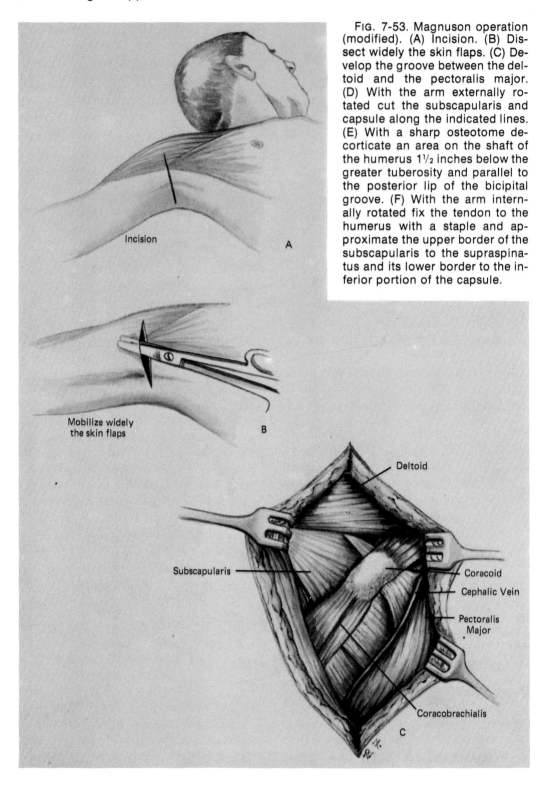

Fig. 7-53. Magnuson operation (modified). (A) Incision. (B) Dissect widely the skin flaps. (C) Develop the groove between the deltoid and the pectoralis major. (D) With the arm externally rotated cut the subscapularis and capsule along the indicated lines. (E) With a sharp osteotome decorticate an area on the shaft of the humerus 1½ inches below the greater tuberosity and parallel to the posterior lip of the bicipital groove. (F) With the arm internally rotated fix the tendon to the humerus with a staple and approximate the upper border of the subscapularis to the supraspinatus and its lower border to the inferior portion of the capsule.

Incision

A

Mobilize widely
the skin flaps

B

Deltoid

Subscapularis

Coracoid

Cephalic Vein

Pectoralis
Major

Coracobrachialis

C

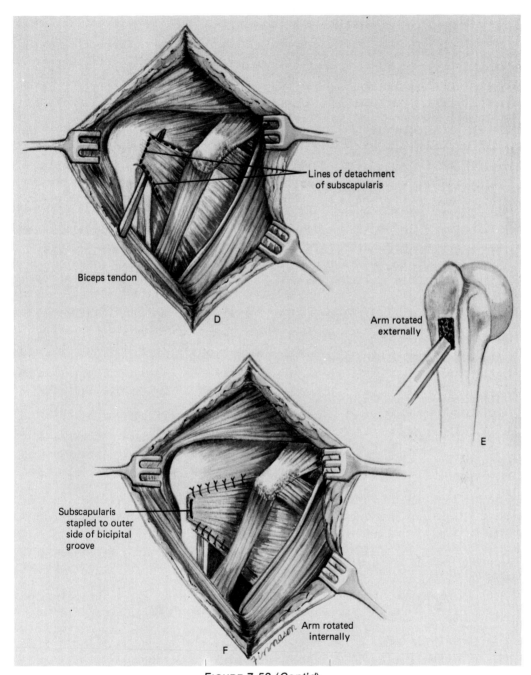

Lines of detachment of subscapularis

Biceps tendon

D

Arm rotated externally

E

Subscapularis stapled to outer side of bicipital groove

Arm rotated internally

F

FIGURE 7-53 (Cont'd)

with a bone graft; this was the procedure I used with my patient (Fig. 7-51).

## Technique

Make a skin incision along the inferior border of the middle third of the clavicle. Reflect the skin flaps upward and down- ward, exposing the clavicular defect. By subperiosteal dissection, expose the bones, which are usually covered with dense fibrous tissue and imperfect cartilage. Between the bone ends a space may exist, containing synovial fluid. The ends of the bones are usually sclerotic.

Resect the ends of the bones back to normal bone and also resect any scar tissue and cartilaginous tissue found between the two segments of the clavicle. Span the defect with an onlay graft obtained from the iliac crest. Now fix the graft with one or two screws in the acromial end and one or two screws in the sternal end. Fill the gap between the bones with cancellous bone chips (Fig. 7-52).

After the wound is closed apply a plaster posterior figure-of-eight to the shoulders.

Union, in my patient, was complete at the end of 8 weeks.

An alternate method may be used. Fix the bone ends with an intramedullary rod, then place cortical and cancellous bone chips across the defect.

## OPERATIONS TO STABILIZE THE UNSTABLE SHOULDER

The indications and merits of each of the following operations are discussed in Chapter 10, "The Unstable Shoulder."

### Magnuson-Stack Operation (Modified)

The axillary incision provides ample exposure to perform this operation and it precludes cosmetically poor scars on the anterior aspect of the shoulder. I now use it routinely for all patients. The anterior portion of the superior incision is an excellent alternate incision. It should be made in line with the axillary crease. It begins just medial to the acromioclavicular joint and extends downward on the anterior aspect of the shoulder for 3 to 3½ inches.

**Axillary Incision.** With the arm in abduction and external rotation, make an incision in the center of the axillary crease (Fig. 7-53A), beginning at the upper border of the pectoralis major. Now, undermine the skin all around the incision widely, by cutting the subcutaneous tissue (Fig. 7-53B). This is an important step because it permits wide retraction of the incision without tension on the skin. Next, develop the interval between the deltoid and the pectoralis major. Take care not to injure the cephalic vein which lies in the deltopectoral groove; retract the vein medially with the pectoralis major. At this point the coracoid process comes into view (Fig. 7-53C).

Externally rotate the arm and identify the tendon of the subscapularis. Insert a blunt dissector under the tendon and capsule of the joint. Now make a ¾ inch incision in the interval between the subscapularis and the supraspinatus and a second incision of the same length along the lower border of the tendon. Incise the tendon and capsule between the two incisions along the anterior lip of the bicipital groove. Do not cut the biceps tendon (Fig. 7-53D).

Rotate the arm internally and, with a sharp osteotome, remove the top layer of cortical bone from an area 1½ inches below the greater tuberosity and parallel with the posterior lip of the bicipital groove (Fig. 7-53E).

With the arm rotated internally pull the subscapularis tendon downward and outward and determine the site on the shaft of the humerus to which the tendon is to be anchored. The site should be such that the subscapularis forms a cup around the inferior border of the humeral head. Next, approximate the freed subscapularis tendon to the predetermined site on the humeral shaft and fix it there with a staple. Finally, with interrupted sutures approximate the upper border of the subscapularis to supraspinatus and the lower border to the inferior portion of the capsule (Fig. 7-53).

**Postoperative Immobilization.** Place a cotton pad in the axilla and encircle the arm and trunk with a 6-inch elastic bandage. Support the arm in a triangular sling. Sometimes I use a Nicola sling to immobilize the arm. I think it is more comfortable than the sling and swathe.

**Postoperative Management.** The arm should be fixed to the side in internal rotation for 4 weeks. During this period encourage motion at the elbow, wrist and fingers. At the end of 4 weeks discard the sling and swathe and start the patient on pendulum exercises in ever increasing arcs on a regulated regimen (5 to 10 minutes every hour).

Do not permit external rotation of the arm until the end of the fifth week; and then it should be performed always within the patient's tolerance of pain. Do not forcefully rotate the arm externally at any time. At this point add wall crawling and wheel exercises to the rehabilitation program. Full restoration of function should be achieved in 8 to 10 weeks.

## Bankart Operation

To perform this operation adequate exposure of the anterior aspect of the joint is essential. The anterior limb of the superior incision provides the necessary exposure. The axillary incision does not provide the wide exposure the anterior incision does. Yet, in females, the axillary incision should be used.

**Anterior Incision.** Begin the incision just lateral to the acromioclavicular joint and extend it downward in line with the axillary crease for 3 to 3½ inches (Fig. 7-54A). Next, develop the interval between the deltoid and the pectoralis major and retract the cephalic vein with the pectoralis major medially and identify the coracoid process. If more exposure is needed, free the origin of the deltoid from the clavicle and retract the muscle laterally (Fig. 7-54B). Next, drill a hole in the longitudinal axis of the coracoid process 1 inch deep and one eighth of an inch in diameter. This facilitates reattachment of the tip of the coracoid to the base. Now, with a sharp osteotome, divide the coracoid process just proximal to the insertions of the short head of the biceps and the coracobrachialis and retract it inferiorly (Fig. 7-54B). The last step is important because it reduces the amount of traction necessary to expose the anterior

aspect of the joint and hence precludes possible injury to the musculocutaneous nerve.

Rotate the arm externally and locate the subscapularis tendon. Next, beginning along the inferior edge of the tendon, with a blunt dissector, develop the interval between the tendon and the capsule. At the inferior edge of the tendon lies a plexus of veins; ligate these vessels before beginning the dissection. After the entire width of the tendon is separated from the capsule place two sutures in the medial portion of the tendon and then divide it vertically close to the lesser tuberosity (Fig. 7-54C). Retract the tendon medially in order to expose the underlying capsule.

Through the capsule identify the anterior rim of the glenoid; now divide the capsule vertically for approximately 2 inches, about ½ inch from the glenoid rim. This brings into view the interior of the joint. Inspect the joint carefully, identify the pathology and remove loose bodies if present (Fig. 7-54C).

Now roughen the rim of the glenoid with an osteotome or a sharp curette and then make three or four holes in the rim with a sharp spike or dental drill (Fig. 7-54D). With the arm in about 45° of abduction and slight external rotation, anchor the lateral edge of the capsule to the glenoid rim with interrupted sutures passing through the drill holes in the glenoid rim (Fig. 7-54E). Next, lap the medial edge of the capsule over the lateral portion and fix it there with interrupted sutures (Fig. 7-54F). Finally, suture the tendon of the subscapularis to its normal position and with one screw fix the coracoid process to its base (Fig. 7-54G).

Postoperative immobilization and rehabilitation are the same as those described for the Magnuson-Stack operation.

The Johannesburg Stapling Operation is a modification of the Bankart operation. In it the torn capsule or detached labrum is reattached by being stapled to the glenoid rim. The staples may be inserted extra- or intracapsularly, depending on the nature of the pathology.

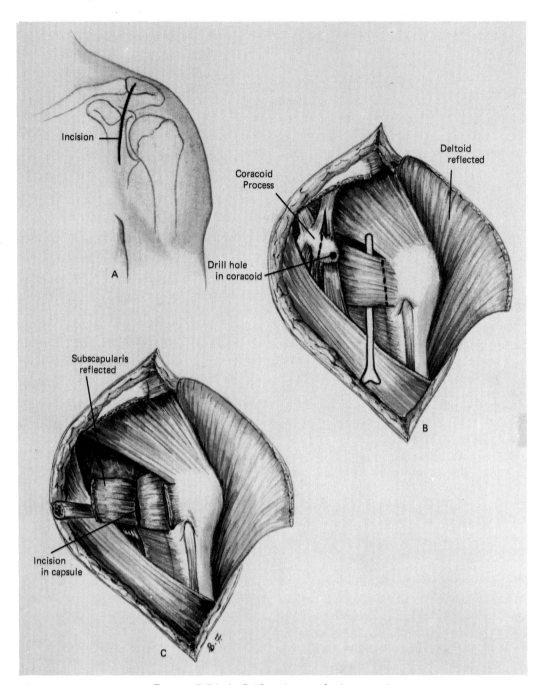

FIGURE 7-54, A–C (*Caption on facing page*)

## Putti-Platt Operation

This operation can be performed through either an anterior incision or an axillary incision.

**Anterior Incision.** Begin the incision on the inferior edge of the clavicle just lateral to the acromioclavicular joint. Extend it downward in line with the axillary crease for 3 to 3½ inches (Fig. 7-55A). Develop the interval between the deltoid and the pectoralis major and retract the cephalic vein and the pectoralis major medially. Now identify the coracoid process. Next,

FIGURE 7-54, D–G

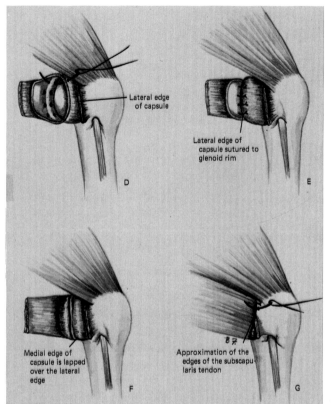

Lateral edge
of capsule

Lateral edge of
capsule sutured to
glenoid rim

D

E

Medial edge of
capsule is lapped
over the lateral
edge

Approximation of the
edges of the subscapu-
laris tendon

F

G

FIG. 7-54. Bankart operation. (A) Incision. (B) Exposure of the anterior structures of the shoulder. (C) The coracoid process is divided and reflected downward with the conjoined tendon; the subscapularis is divided close to the lesser tuberosity and reflected medially; the anterior capsule is divided 2½ inches from the glenoid rim. (D) Three or four holes are made through the glenoid rim. (E) Suture the lateral edge of the capsule to the glenoid rim. (F) Overlap the medial edge of the capsule over the lateral edge and fix it with interrupted sutures. (G) Approximate the edges of the subscapularis tendon.

drill a hole in the longitudinal axis of the coracoid process, 1 inch long and one eighth of an inch in diameter. With a sharp osteotome divide the coracoid process just proximal to the insertions of the short head of the biceps and the coracobrachialis and retract it inferiorly (Fig. 7-55B).

Rotate the arm externally; this brings into view the subscapularis tendon. Isolate the upper and lower margins of the tendon, then divide it and the capsule 1 inch medial to its insertion. The joint is now exposed; identify the pathology present (Fig. 7-55C).

When the labrum and capsule are intact, suture the free edge of the lateral part of the subscapularis tendon to the soft tissues and labrum along the anterior glenoid rim. If the labrum and capsule are detached or torn away from the glenoid rim, first roughen the anterior surface of the neck of the scapula, then suture the free edge of the lateral portion of the subscapularis tendon to the undersurface of the capsule and sub-

scapularis muscle (Fig. 7-55D). In either case, place the arm in internal rotation before the sutures are tied, then tie the sutures. Next, lap the medial portion of the capsule over the lateral part of the subscapularis tendon and suture it in place (Fig. 7-55E). Lastly, pull the medial part of the subscapularis laterally and suture it to the cuff at the greater tuberosity or at the bicipital groove (Fig. 7-55E).

Reattach the tip of the coracoid to its base with a screw and some interrupted sutures.

Postoperative immobilization and rehabilitation are the same as those described for the Magnuson-Stack operation.

## Eden-Hybbinetti Operation

This operation can be performed through either an anterior or an axillary incision, as has been described for the Bankart and

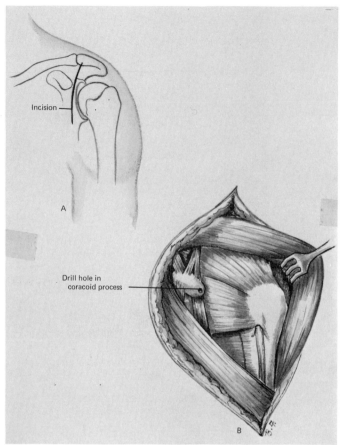

FIG. 7-55. Putti-Platt operation. (A) Incision. (B) Exposure of subdeltoid region of the shoulder. (C) The coracoid process is divided proximal to the insertion of the conjoined tendon; the subscapularis tendon and capsule are divided 1 inch medial to their bony insertion. (D) The lateral edge of the tendon is sutured to the undersurface of the capsule and subscapularis tendon. (E) The medial edge of the tendon is lapped over the lateral edge and sutured to the cuff in the region of the greater tuberosity or at the bicipital groove.

the Putti-Platt operation. I always combine this operation with the Magnuson-Stack operation.

**Anterior Incision.** Begin the incision on the inferior edge of the clavicle just lateral to the acromioclavicular joint and in line with the axillary crease. Extend it downward for 3 to 3½ inches (Fig. 7-56A). Develop the interval between the deltoid and the pectoralis major, exposing the coracoid process. Now detach the tip of the coracoid process just proximal to the insertions of the coracobrachialis and the short head of the biceps. Retract the detached bone and muscles inferiorly (Fig. 7-56B).

Externally rotate the arm and bring into view the subscapularis tendon. Make an incision three quarters of an inch long in the interval between the subscapularis and the supraspinatus and isolate the lower border

of the subscapularis tendon. Now divide the tendon and the underlying capsule ¼ inch medial to the insertion of the tendon (Fig. 7-56B). This brings into view the inside of the joint. Explore the joint and note the existing pathology.

Displace the head of the humerus downward and outward with a Bankart retractor; this gives excellent exposure of the joint. With a fine, sharp osteotome make a subperiosteal pocket along the inferior aspect of the anterior glenoid rim. If the labrum is intact, place the pocket between the labrum and the rim (Fig. 7-56C).

Remove from the outer table of the iliac crest a graft 1½ inches long and three quarters of an inch wide. Shape the graft and fit it into the subperiosteal pocket so that it lies against the rim and projects beyond it one quarter of an inch. The graft

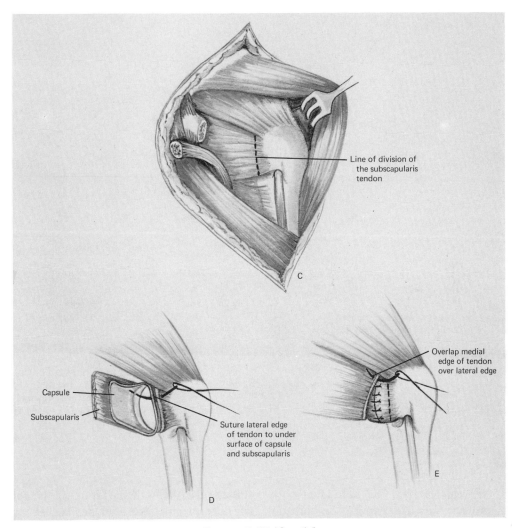

Line of division of
the subscapularis
tendon

Capsule

Subscapularis

Suture lateral edge
of tendon to under
surface of capsule
and subscapularis

Overlap medial
edge of tendon
over lateral edge

FIGURE 7-55 *(Cont'd)*

forms an excellent buttress on the anterior-inferior part of the rim. It usually fits so snugly in the pocket that it needs no additional fixation (Fig. 7-56D).

Next, rotate the arm internally and with a sharp osteotome remove the top layer of bone from an area 1¹/₂ inches long below the greater tuberosity and parallel to the posterior lip of the bicipital groove (Fig. 7-56E). With the arm still internally rotated approximate the cut edge of the subscapularis tendon to the raw surface and fix it in place with a staple. Now with interrupted sutures approximate the upper border of the subscapularis to the lower margin of the

supraspinatus, and the lower margin to the inferior capsular tissues (Fig. 7-56E). Reattach the tip of the coracoid to its base with one screw and interrupted sutures.

Postoperative immobilization and rehabilitation are the same as those described for the Magnuson-Stack operation.

**Bristow Operation**

**Anterior Incision.** Start the incision along the inferior edge of the clavicle just lateral to the acromioclavicular joint. Extend it downward in line with the axillary crease for 3 to 3¹/₂ inches (Fig. 7-57A). Develop

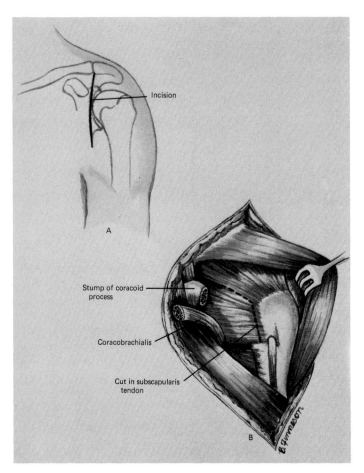

Stump of coracoid process

Coracobrachialis

Cut in subscapularis tendon

FIG. 7-56. Eden-Hybbinetti operation. (A) Incision. (B) Exposure of subscapularis tendon. (C) A subperiosteal pocket is developed on the antero-inferior aspect of the neck of the scapula; the osteotome is under the labrum. (D) The iliac graft is shaped and inserted into the subperiosteal pocket. (E) The subscapularis tendon is stapled to raw bone, below the greater tuberosity and parallel to the posterior lip of the bicipital groove.

the interval between the deltoid and the pectoralis major and expose the coracoid process. With a sharp osteotome divide the coracoid process just proximal to the insertion of the tendons of the short head of the biceps and the coracobrachialis. Retract the bone and muscles downward; do not injure the musculocutaneous nerve (Fig. 7-57B).

Bring the subscapularis tendon into view by rotating the arm externally. Make a vertical slit 1 to 1¼ inches long in the middle ⅔ of the musculotendinous junction of the muscle and through the capsule (the capsule is adherent to the undersurface of the tendon at this site) (Fig. 7-57B). Explore the joint cavity identify the type of pathology and remove loose bodies, if present. Next, dissect the capsule free from the

subscapularis muscle as far as the glenoid rim; the capsular flap includes the labrum. This brings into view the neck of the scapula and glenoid rim (Fig. 7-57C). If the labrum is detached from the glenoid, the neck of the scapula is covered with thick periosteal tissue which must be elevated so that an area of raw bone three quarters of an inch in diameter is exposed. Now close the capsule and with a sharp gouge or osteotome roughen the exposed area of bone on the neck of the scapula (Fig. 7-57D).

Pass the coracoid process through the slit in the subscapularis and press it firmly against the raw surface on the neck of the scapula (Fig. 7-57E). Maintain this contact by incorporating the conjoined tendon in the interrupted sutures which approximate

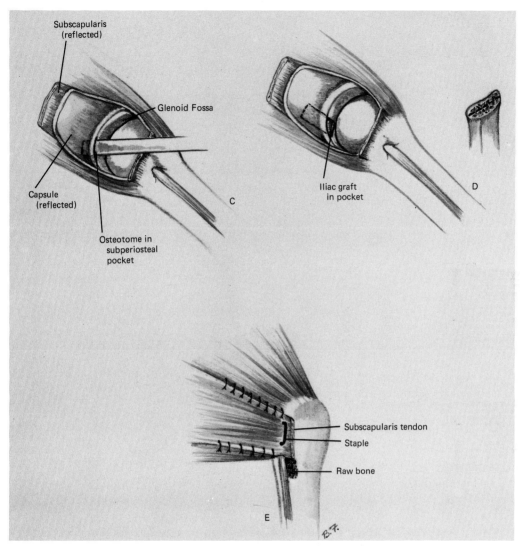

Figure 7-56 (*Cont'd*)

the edges of the cut in the subscapularis (Fig. 7-57F).

Postoperative immobilization and rehabilitation are the same as those described for the Magnuson-Stack operation.

## Bone Block Operation for Posterior Recurrent Dislocations

**Posterior Incision.** Make an incision 4 to 5 inches long, over the top of the acromion and extend it posteriorly over the spine of the scapula; then gently curve it toward the axilla (Fig. 7-58A). Split the posterior fibers of the deltoid for 2½ inches and expose the conjoined tendon of the infraspinatus and teres minor (Fig. 7-58B). Next, divide the conjoined tendon vertically ½ inch from its insertion (do not injure the axillary nerve in the quadrilateral space) and deepen the incision through the capsule. Retract the muscles and capsule medially to expose the posterior aspect of the neck of the scapula and the posterior

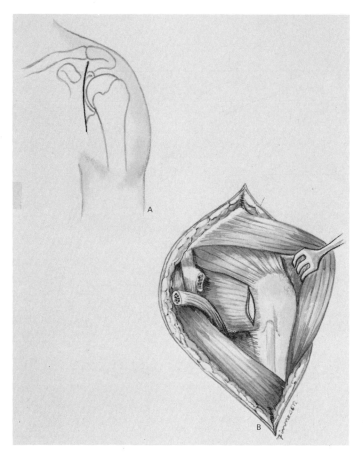

A

B

FIG. 7-57. Bristow's operation. (A) Incision. (B) The subscapularis tendon is exposed, the coracoid process is osteotomized proximal to the insertion of the conjoined tendon and a vertical slit is made in the tendon of the subscapularis. (C) The capsule is peeled off the subscapularis beyond the attachment to the labrum, exposing the anterior surface of the neck of the scapula. (D) Expose an area of raw bone ³/₄ of an inch in diameter on the neck of the scapula. (E) The coracoid is passed through the slot and pressed against the raw area of bone. (F) It is anchored in this position by incorporating the conjoined tendon in sutures which approximate the edges of the cut in the subscapularis.

rim of the glenoid. To gain a good view of the joint, retract the head of the humerus laterally. With a sharp, fine osteotome make a subperiosteal pocket at the inferior part of the posterior rim of the glenoid. If the labrum is intact, make the pocket between the labrum and the posterior glenoid rim (Fig. 7-58C).

Insert into the pocket an iliac bone graft approximately 1½ inches long and three quarters of an inch wide. Place the graft so that it lies against the posterior rim and projects beyond it one quarter of an inch. No sutures or screws are needed to hold the graft in place (Fig. 7-58D). Finally, advance and lap the severed conjoined tendon and capsule over the posterior aspect of the greater tuberosity and fix them in place with interrupted sutures (Fig. 7-58E).

**Postoperative Immobilization and Management.** Immobilize the arm with a sling and swathe. Keep the arm at the side for 3 or 4 weeks; but during this period allow free motion at the elbow, wrist and fingers. Discard the sling at the end of 4 weeks and start pendulum exercises in ever increasing arcs on a regulated regimen—5 to 10 minutes every hour. During the first 5 weeks prohibit forceful internal rotation of the arm; the arm should always be exercised within the patient's tolerance. Now add wall crawling, pulley and wheel exercises.

### Anterior and Posterior Bone Block Operation

For habitual dislocations in which the humeral head displaces both anteriorly and posteriorly, the anterior and posterior bone block operations described above can be

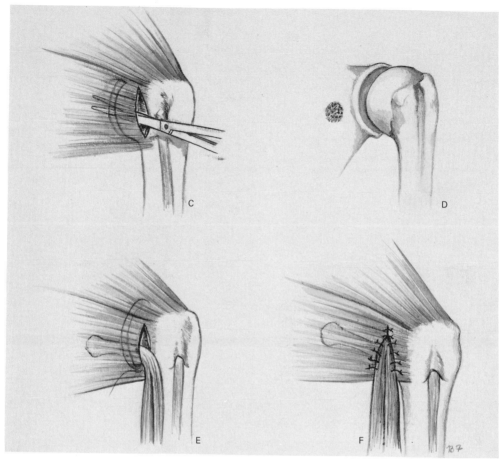

FIGURE 7-57 (*Cont'd*)

performed in one operation. Use the superior incision with an anterior and a posterior extension. First the deltoid muscle is split anteriorly and the anterior bone block operation is performed. Then the deltoid is split posteriorly and the posterior bone block is inserted. In front the subscapularis tendon is advanced as in the Magnuson-Stack operation, and posteriorly the conjoined tendon of the infraspinatus and teres minor is advanced.

## REPAIR OF TEARS OF THE ROTATOR CUFF

The majority of surgical procedures on the rotator cuff can be performed through the supero-anterior approach. In this incision the attachment of the central portion of the deltoid muscle is not disturbed. In young people the incision is adequate to perform any procedure on the cuff; in older people more exposure may be necessary to repair a massive tear. In these instances, resection of a portion of the clavicle or the acromion forming the acromioclavicular joint provides the necessary exposure of the superior and anterior areas of the joint.

### Incomplete Tears

### Repair of Incomplete Tears on Inner Side of the Cuff

It should be remembered that in many instances the appearance of the outer surface of the cuff may give no indication of an incomplete tear, even a massive one,

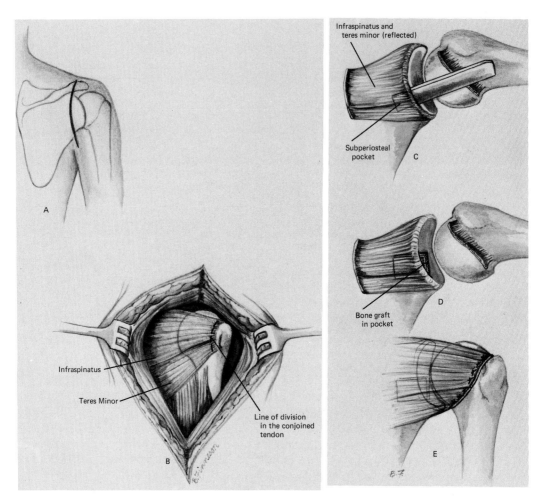

FIG. 7-58. Posterior bone block for recurrent dislocation. (A) Incision. (B) The deltoid is split to expose the conjoined tendon of the infraspinatus and teres minor. (C) The infraspinatus and teres minor are reflected medially and a subperiosteal pocket is made at the inferior aspect of the glenoid rim. (D) An iliac graft measuring 1½ by ¾ inch is inserted in the pocket. (E) The conjoined tendon is lapped over the posterior aspect of the greater tuberosity and fixed with interrupted sutures.

on the the synovial side of the cuff. In fact, the floor of the subacromial bursa and the musculotendinous cuff may appear normal. The following tests may identify and localize incomplete tears.

1. Normally, upon abduction of the arm in various planes of rotation, the musculotendinous cuff passes under the coracoacromial arch without a wrinkle on its superficial surface. However, if a tear or rim rent is present and the arm is abducted, a wrinkle or blister forms at the site of the

lesion as the lesion approaches the falciform edge of the coracoacromial ligament.

2. Simple palpation of the subacromial bursal floor may reveal thinning of the cuff, irregularity of the inner side of the cuff, a sulcus and, at times, both sulcus and eminence at the site of insertion of the cuff into the humeral head.

3. If a flat instrument is passed laterally toward the tuberosities over the surface of the cuff, a blister appears over the site of the tear.

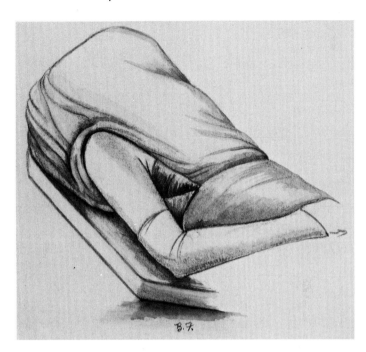

FIG. 7-59. Position of patient.

4. When grasped with a forceps a defective portion of the cuff moves freely on the humerus, whereas the normal cuff on either side of the defect fails to show this mobility.

5. Make a small longitudinal incision through the entire thickness of the cuff and insert a probe into the joint. The probe may identify the irregularities on the deep surface of the cuff produced by incomplete tears. Also through this slit the inner side of the cuff can be inspected.

6. Arthrography will clearly show most incomplete tears of the cuff.

**Position of Patient.** I have found the position of the patient to be most important in order to have free access to the rotator cuff. For the reader's convenience, the description of the most useful position is repeated here.

Place the patient in the sitting position with the trunk inclined 45 to 60 degrees from the horizontal. In order to prevent the patient from slipping on the table elevate the lower part of the table under the knees (Fig. 7-59). Place the patient on the table so that the arm rests on the edge of the table; the arm is draped separately. Turn the head of the patient to the opposite side and tilt the table slightly away from the side of the surgeon.

**Supero-Anterior Incision.** Begin the incision over the posterior edge of the acromion just lateral to the acromioclavicular joint. Carry the incision downward over the anterior third of the deltoid in line with the axillary skin crease for 2 inches below the edge of the acromion. Freely mobilize the medial and lateral skin flaps by dissecting the subcutaneous layer from the deltoid, the tip of the acromion and the acromioclavicular joint. Now, the acromioclavicular joint is clearly seen (Fig. 7-60A).

Develop the incision through the anterior fibers of the deltoid in line with the acromioclavicular joint for a distance not to exceed 2 inches below the edge of the acromion. Retract the muscle margins medially and laterally so that the subacromial bursa comes into view. Divide the superior bursal wall in line with the muscle split. Now, by rotating the arm internally and externally, the superior and anterior portions of the cuff come into view. Also, the biceps tendon in its groove and the subscapularis

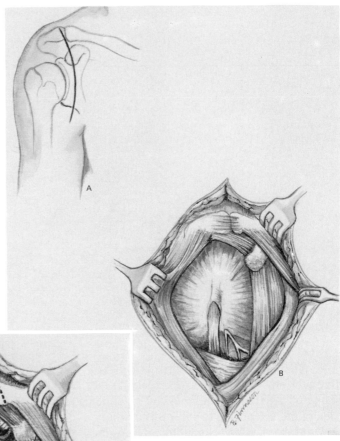

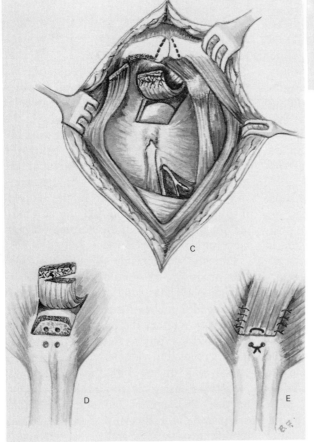

FIG. 7-60. Repair of incomplete tears on the inner side of the cuff. (A) Incision. (B) Exposure of the subacromial region. (C) Lines of excision of the acromion or clavicle from either side of the acromioclavicular joint, and mobilization of the portion of the cuff with the incomplete tear. (D) Excision of the defective portion of the cuff and preparation of the trough in which the flap will be sutured. (E) Reattachment of the cuff flap to the bone and to the adjacent sides of the cuff.

tendon as it inserts into the lesser tuberosity can readily be seen (Fig. 7-60B).

Wider exposure can be attained by excising a portion of the acromion or of the clavicle forming the acromioclavicular joint. If a wider exposure of the cuff is desired, determine on which side of the acromioclavicular joint the exposure should be increased. Then, in order to expose the portion of the clavicle or acromion to be excised, detach by sharp subperiosteal dissection of the portion of the deltoid attached to them. Next, with a sharp osteotome excise three eighths of an inch of the acromion or the clavicle (Fig. 7-60C).

Whether a portion of the acromion is resected or not, I always divide the coracoacromial ligament close to its insertion into the medial edge of the acromion, and, in many instances, I excise a portion of the ligament. This step increases the interval between the acromion and the tuberosities. Also it permits the arm to abduct freely without the cuff's impinging against the acromion or the falciform edge of the coracoacromial ligament.

At this point try to localize the lesion by performing the tests mentioned previously. Next, make a longitudinal incision through the fibers of the coracohumeral ligament (it lies between the subscapularis and the supraspinatus) and visualize the tear. Then make a transverse incision through the whole thickness of the cuff, extending posteriorly for a distance equal to the length of the incomplete tear and, as a rule, terminating just beyond the juncture of the supraspinatus and infraspinatus tendons. Make a second longitudinal incision, beginning at the posterior edge of the transverse incision and paralleling the first longitudinal incision. (Fig. 7-60C). This step mobilizes the affected portion of the cuff. Excise transversely the degenerated portion of the mobile flap; the stump of the flap should consist of healthy tendon fibers throughout its entire thickness (Fig. 7-60D).

You are now ready to reattach the stump of the cuff to the humerus. Make a trough in the anatomical neck of the humerus; then drill holes through the lateral surface of the greater tuberosity, emerging at the base of the trough (Fig. 7-60D). Anchor the stump of the cuff into its new bed by mattress sutures passing through the drill holes and tied on the outer surface of the greater tuberosity. Finally, attach the lateral margins of the flap to the adjacent subscapularis and infraspinatus tendons by interrupted side-to-side sutures (Fig. 7-60E).

### Repair of Incomplete Tears on the Bursal Side of the Cuff

Once the subacromial area is exposed, incomplete tears on the bursal side of the cuff are easily detected and identified as to type and size. Treat the incomplete transverse tears in the same manner that you treated incomplete tears on the synovial side of the cuff.

However, some tears are within the substance of the cuff or are superficial tears running parallel with the cuff fibers. Excise these lesions by elliptical incisions paralleling the tendon fibers. Then close the remaining gap with interrupted side-to-side sutures.

In all the repairs described above, the sutures should never be under tension. The arm should come to the side without straining the suture line.

Also, unless the subacromial bursa is severely diseased, its walls should not be removed. Preservation of the bursa prevents formation of postoperative adhesions and permits early painless movements of the shoulder.

**Postoperative Management.** No rigid external immobilization is necessary; a simple sling provides adequate support of the arm. Pendulum exercises are started as soon as the postoperative pain and muscle spasm subsides, usually within 36 to 48 hours. They should always be performed within the tolerance of the patient. After 3 weeks institute a program of active exercises on a regulated regimen.

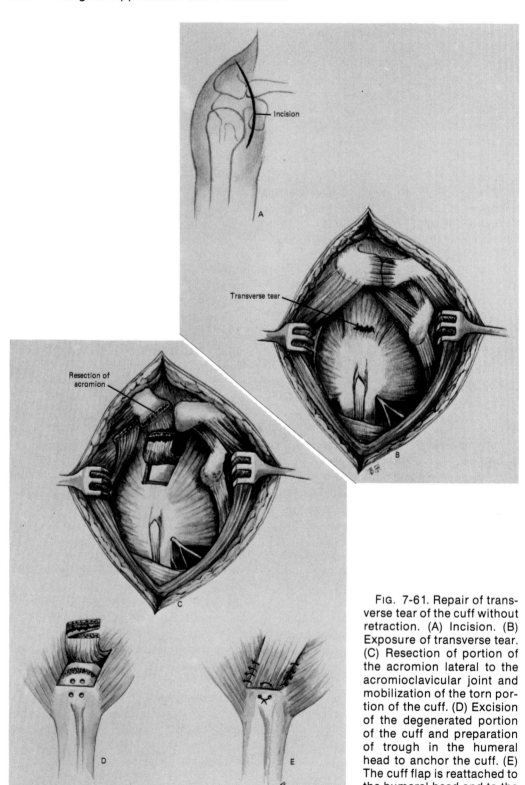

FIG. 7-61. Repair of transverse tear of the cuff without retraction. (A) Incision. (B) Exposure of transverse tear. (C) Resection of portion of the acromion lateral to the acromioclavicular joint and mobilization of the torn portion of the cuff. (D) Excision of the degenerated portion of the cuff and preparation of trough in the humeral head to anchor the cuff. (E) The cuff flap is reattached to the humeral head and to the adjacent sides of the cuff.

## Repair of Complete Tears of the Rotator Cuff

### Transverse Tears of the Cuff

Expose the rotator cuff by the supero-anterior incision (Fig. 7-61). Identify the tear in the cuff and determine whether or not more exposure is necessary to do an adequate repair. Also determine on which side of the acromioclavicular joint more exposure is desired and, accordingly, remove approximately three eighths of an inch of the clavicle or acromion as described on page 157 (Fig. 7-61B).

Next, extend the transverse tear anteriorly and posteriorly until healthy cuff tissue is encountered. Then mobilize the portion of the affected cuff by an anterior and a posterior incision parallel with the cuff fibers (Fig. 7-61C). Excise transversely the degenerated tissue on the lateral end of the flap (Fig. 7-61D).

With a fine, sharp osteotome make a trough in the humerus at the level of the anatomical neck. Next, drill holes through the lateral surface of the greater tuberosity; these should emerge at the base of the trough (Fig. 7-61D). Anchor the stump of the cuff into the trough by mattress sutures passing through the drill holes and tied on the outer surface of the greater tuberosity (Fig. 7-61E). Finally, attach the anterior and posterior margins of the flap to the adjacent cuff fibers by interrupted side-to-side sutures.

The repair described above must be made with the arm at the side and in such a way that there is no tension at the line of suture where the flap is attached to the bone. As a rule, the mobilized flap stretches sufficiently and without undue tension to meet the raw bony surface in the trough.

**Postoperative Management.** A sling to support the arm is adequate external immobilization. Just as soon as the patient can tolerate pendulum exercises, they should be started on a regulated regimen. But they should never exceed the patient's tolerance of pain. After 2 to 3 weeks institute active exercises. Within 6 to 8 weeks the patient should have a free, painless range of abduction.

### Complete Tears with Retraction

Expose the rotator cuff by a supero-anterior incision as described on page 157. Repair of these lesions usually requires a wide exposure of the cuff; therefore, routinely excise three eighths of an inch of the clavicle or of the acromion, depending on which side of the acromioclavicular joint the exposure needs to be increased (Fig. 7-62A). Next, identify the limits of the tear; then gently manipulate the shoulder through its full range of motion in order to break up any adhesions that might fix the cuff to the surrounding tissues.

Now, cut away all degenerated tissue from the margins of the cuff. The new margins should consist of healthy cuff fibers. The resulting defect in the cuff is triangular (Fig. 7-62B). Beginning at the apex of the defect, approximate the edges of the cuff with strong nylon interrupted sutures up to the point of tension. Now, a small triangular hiatus remains in the cuff (Fig. 7-62C).

With the arm at the side, determine just where the cuff reaches the head of the humerus; then, immediately below the cuff defect remove the articular cartilage from the head of the humerus and drill holes through the lateral surfaces of the tuberosity, emerging through the raw bone in the humeral head. Anchor the edges of the cuff to the raw bone by mattress sutures passing through the drill holes and tied on its lateral surface (Fig. 7-62D). When the remaining defect is large, additional mattress sutures may be necessary to bring the edges of the cuff tightly against the raw bone.

### Massive Avulsions of the Cuff

The repair of this lesion is the same as that for transverse tears with retraction described above. However, in these instances,

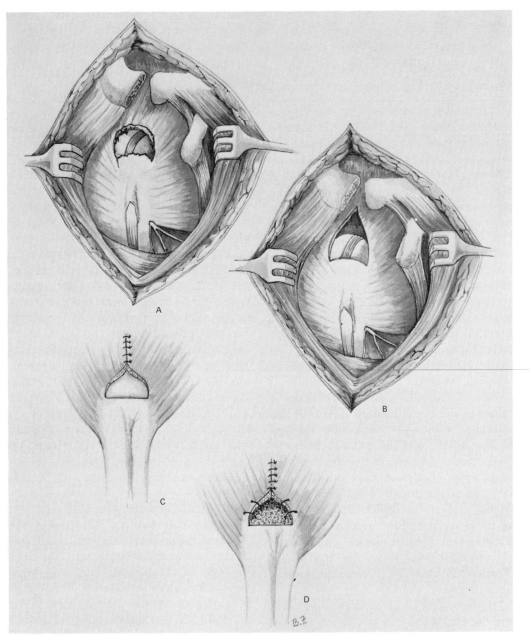

FIG. 7-62. Repair of complete tear of the cuff with retraction. (A) A portion of the acromion lateral to the acromioclavicular joint is removed to increase the exposure; the cuff tear is now clearly visible. (B) The degenerated edges of the cuff are cut away to healthy tissue. (C) The edges of the tear are approximated with interrupted sutures up to the point of tension. (D) The articular cartilage is removed immediately below the triangular defect and the edges of the defect are attached to the raw bone by mattress sutures passing through drill holes.

it may be necessary to remove cartilage from an area of the humeral head much more proximal than the area denuded in transverse tears; also, as a rule, the raw area is larger (Fig. 7-63A). The most important point to remember is that the cuff must be attached to that area on the head that allows anchoring of the edges of the

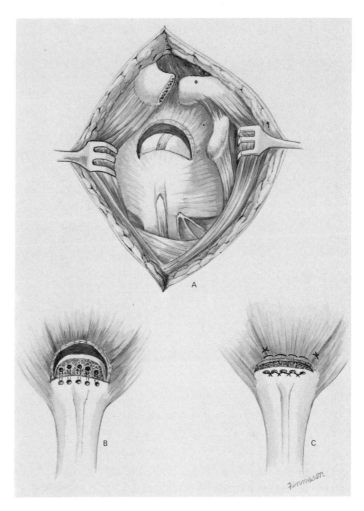

FIG. 7-63. Repair of massive avulsions of the cuff. (A) Exposure of the massive avulsion of the cuff. (B) preparation of the trough in the humeral head to receive the edges of the cuff. (C) The cuff is reattached by mattress sutures to the humeral head, passing through drill holes.

cuff defect without tension while the arm is at the side (Fig. 7-63, B and C).

When it is obvious that the cuff edges cannot be approximated to the humeral head without tension, considerable length may be gained by elevating the supraspinatus from its bed in the supraspinous fossa. This is readily achieved by extending the posterior limb of the skin incision along the spine of the scapula as far as the medial vertebral angle. Divide the fibers of insertion of the trapezius, and by sharp subperiosteal dissection elevate the trapezius from the spine of the scapula. Now, the dense fascia overlying the supraspinatus comes into view; divide this fascia in a line parallel to the spine. By blunt dissection, preferably digital dissection, raise the supraspinatus from its bed. This step

must be done with great care so that the suprascapular nerve is not injured as it passes under the suprascapular ligament to enter the supraspinous fossa.

I have found this step most useful for mobilizing the cuff and gaining length. However, in some instances, it is impossible to reattach the cuff without tension; there is entirely too much degeneration and shortening of the cuff. In these instances, arthrodesis of the shoulder is justified.

**Postoperative Management.** Immediately after operation I prefer to immobilize the arm in a brace that holds the arm in 30° to 45° of abduction, 30° of external rotation and 30° of forward flexion. The brace is made for the patient before the operation and is applied at the end of the operation. Within 36 to 48 hours after surgery the

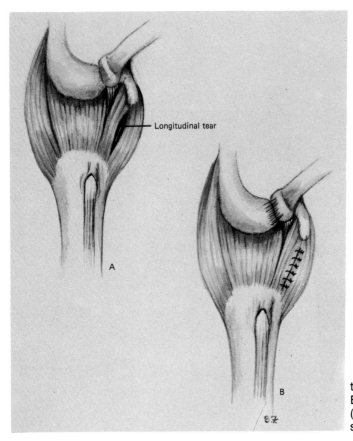

FIG. 7-64. Repair of longitudinal tears of the cuff. (A) Exposure of longitudinal tear. (B) Tear is repaired by side-to-side sutures.

straps holding the arm to the brace are released and the patient is encouraged to shrug the shoulder and to flex and extend the elbow. This is done several times each day. Do not allow active abduction of the arm for 4 to 6 weeks.

At the end of this period the patient attempts to abduct the arm in the brace. When he can abduct the arm freely and with good strength, remove the brace and institute a program of pendulum exercises and, later, wall crawling and pulley exercises. The exercise program should be carried out regularly for 4 or 5 minutes of each hour. Keep the exercises within the patient's tolerance.

### Longitudinal Rents (Complete Tears)

These lesions usually occur in young people. As a rule, they occur through the interval between the supraspinatus and the subscapularis, splitting the fibers of the coracohumeral ligament. Great exposure of the cuff is not needed to do a repair of the cuff.

Expose the anterior region of the cuff by the supero-anterior incision. Visualize the longitudinal rent and repair it with side-to-side sutures (Fig. 7-64, A and B).

In the event that the tear extends into the bicipital groove, the repair may compromise the gliding mechanism of the biceps tendon. This may cause bicipital tenosynovitis. In these instances, the intra-articular portion of the biceps tendon must be excised and the tendon anchored into the bicipital groove. This can be done either by interrupted sutures passing through drill holes in the humerus or by stapling the tendon into the groove.

**Postoperative Management.** The postop-

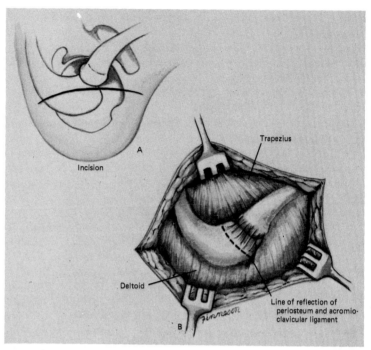

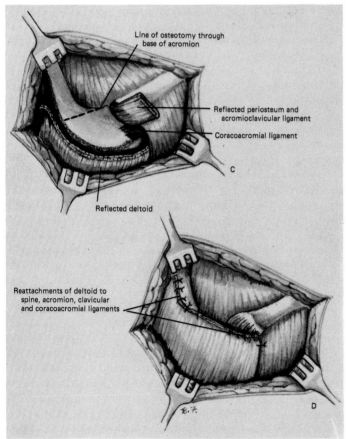

FIG. 7-65. Acromionectomy. (A) Incision. (B) Exposure of acromioclavicular ligament and origin of the deltoid muscle. (C) Reflection of the periosteum and acromioclavicular ligament; reflection of deltoid from acromion and osteotomy of the acromion at its base. (D) Reattachment of the deltoid to the spine of the scapula, the periosteum and the acromioclavicular ligaments.

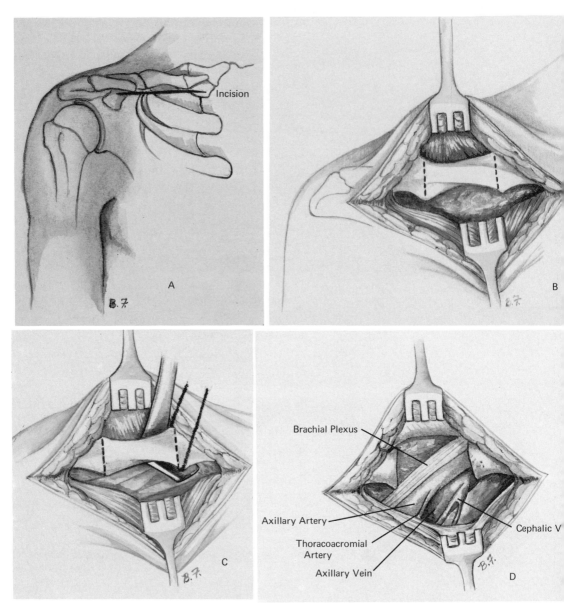

FIG. 7-66 (A–D). Technique of excision of the middle portion of the clavicle for massive callus formation.

erative management is the same as that described for the repair of incomplete lesions of the cuff.

## ACROMIONECTOMY AND ACROMIOPLASTY

I consider acromionectomy a radical and mutilating procedure; yet, in certain instances, it is the most satisfactory operation for elimination of friction between the cuff and the acromion. If any portion of the acromion is to be removed, I prefer acromionectomy to acromioplasty. It is my opinion that if an acromioplasty will relieve pain due to pathology in the subacromial region so will simple resection of the lateral portion of the coracoacromial ligament. If this procedure is not adequate, then acromionectomy is indicated.

Many surgeons are of the opinion that

acromioplasty is not harmful and does not impair the power of the deltoid. This is not my experience. After acromioplasty many patients have considerable pain over the stump of the acromion. The edge of the remaining acromion may show considerable spurring and most patients with acromioplasties have some reduction in the power of the deltoid, regardless of the method of reattachment of the muscle to the bone.

When a shoulder with a supraspinatus syndrome is explored and the cause of the pain and disability is found to be marked degeneration of the cuff and a secondarily inflamed bursa, and if the subacromial tissues cannot be relieved of undue compression and friction by excision of the outer portion of the coracoacromial ligament, then I prefer to do an acromionectomy instead of a resection of the outer end of the acromion. In my hands, this has been the more gratifying procedure.

Moreover, I do not believe an acromioplasty or an acromionectomy should be performed when the primary lesion is a calcific deposit in the cuff. Simple excision of the degenerated cuff containing the calcific deposit, together with resection of a portion of the coracoacromial ligament, effects a cure in most instances. If, in addition to the calcific deposit in the cuff, the cuff is severely degenerated and the walls of the overlying bursa are inflamed, edematous and hypertrophied, acromionectomy is justified. This procedure eliminates all friction against the subacromial tissues when the arm is abducted; however, some strength in the power of abduction of the deltoid is lost.

## Acromionectomy

Make a superior skin incision centered over the acromioclavicular joint and in line with the axillary crease (Fig. 7-65A). One half inch lateral to the joint incise the periosteum and by sharp dissection reflect it medially (Fig. 7-65B). With a fine, sharp osteotome divide the acromion in the line extending directly posteriorly from the acromioclavicular joint. Take care not to injure the structures immediately below the acromion. By sharp dissection free the acromion from its attachment to the deltoid and the subacromial bursa and divide the acromioclavicular and coracoacromial ligaments. Do not excise the walls of the bursa unless they are seriously inflamed, thickened and hypertrophied; if they are healthy, close the bursa with a fine suture (Fig. 7-65C).

Now, reassemble the attachment of the deltoid. Using strong nylon interrupted sutures, reattach the deltoid to the acromioclavicular ligament and to the reflected periosteum. Be sure that the central tendon of the deltoid is firmly anchored in the suture line. If the suture line does not provide a strong reattachment of the deltoid, reinforce it by sutures passing through drill holes in the spine of the scapula (Fig. 7-65D).

At the end of the operation support the arm in a sling. Institute pendulum exercises just as soon as the operative pain subsides, but do not allow active abduction of the arm for 3 to 4 weeks. Then institute a graduated program of active exercises, always within the tolerance of the patient.

## Acromioplasty

Make a superior incision centered just lateral to the acromioclavicular joint and in line with the axillary crease. Incise the periosteum and by sharp dissection reflect it medially. Also by sharp dissection free the deltoid from its acromial origin and divide the coracoacromial ligament just lateral to the acromioclavicular joint. With a sharp osteotome, divide the acromion on a line beginning anteriorly midway between the acromioclavicular joint and the lateral margin of the acromion and extending directly posteriorly. Now, bevel and make smooth the medial fragment of the acromion. With strong interrupted nylon sutures reattach the deltoid to the acromion; take care that the central tendon of the deltoid is firmly anchored. If necessary, anchor the central tendon by sutures passing through

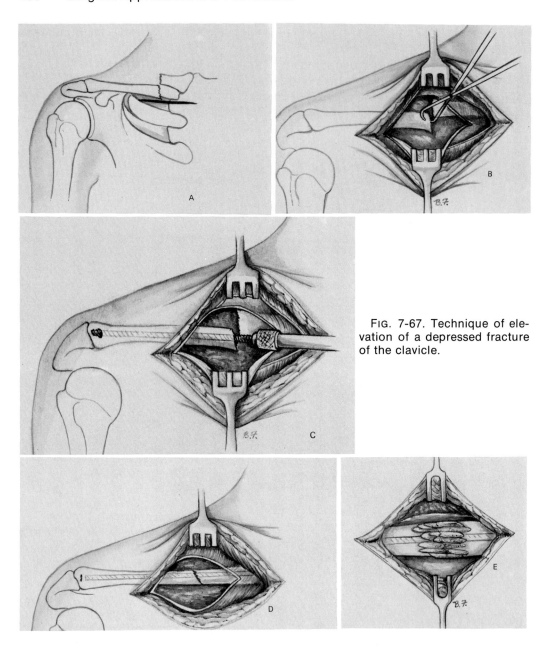

FIG. 7-67. Technique of elevation of a depressed fracture of the clavicle.

drill holes in the medial portion of the acromion.

The postoperative management is the same as that described for acromionectomy.

## EXCISION OF THE MIDDLE PORTION OF THE CLAVICLE

Certain conditions that cause pressure on the neurovascular structures in the thoracic outlet may require excision of the middle portion of the clavicle. Some of the lesions are: displaced fragments of bone, excessive callus formation, and tumors.

## Technique (For Massive Callus Formation)

Expose the clavicle by a 4-inch incision along its inferior border (Fig. 7-66A). By

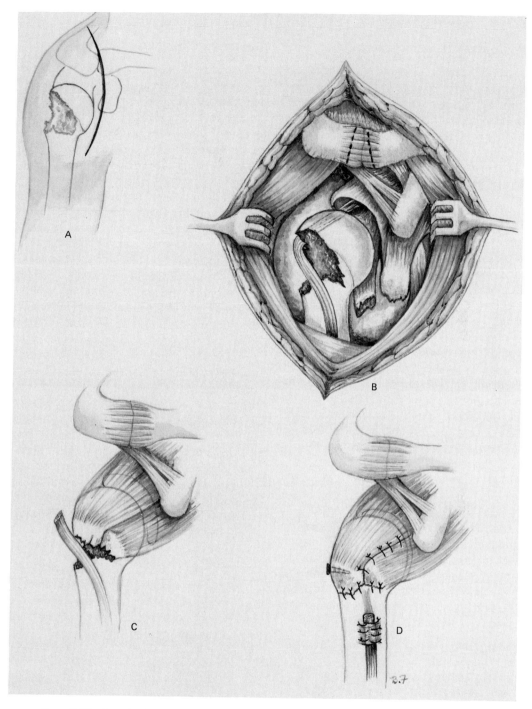

FIG. 7-68. Surgical management of anterior dislocation complicated by a Type II fracture of the greater tuberosity.

extraperiosteal dissection carefully free the clavicle from all surrounding soft tissues and mark off the segment of the clavicle to be excised (Fig. 7-66B). Place a retractor between the clavicle and the underlying soft tissues at the site of severance of the clavicle; with a Gigli saw divide the bone at both sites (Fig. 7-66C). The middle third of the clavicle has been excised; the underlying structures are free (Fig. 7-66D).

## Postoperative Management

Apply a figure-of-eight plaster cast and maintain this fixation for 10 to 14 days, until soft tissue healing is complete. During this period, institute a program of exercises for the arm, the hand and the fingers.

## ELEVATION OF A DEPRESSED FRACTURE OF THE CLAVICLE

Make an incision 4 inches long along the inferior border of the clavicle (Fig. 7-67A). Expose carefully both fragments by sharp subperiosteal dissection; grasp the lateral fragment with a medium size towel clip, elevate it and deliver it into the wound (Fig. 7-67B). Insert a threaded Kirschner wire ($^7/_{64}$ inch) in the medullary canal of the lateral fragment and advance the wire until it appears medial to the acromioclavicular joint (Fig. 7.67C). Reduce the fracture, then insert the wire into the medullary canal of the medial fragment and advance it $1^1/_2$ inches (Fig. 7-67D). Place slabs of cancellous bone around the fracture site; cut the wire just below the skin (Fig. 7-67E).

## Postoperative Management

Apply a figure-of-eight plaster cast and maintain this fixation until there is roentgenographic evidence of healing—at least 8 to 10 weeks. Remove the wire only after bony union is complete. During this period, the arm, hand and fingers should be exercised on a regulated regimen.

## SURGICAL MANAGEMENT OF ANTERIOR DISLOCATION COMPLICATED BY A TYPE II FRACTURE OF THE GREATER TUBEROSITY

In this complication the biceps tendon falls behind the humeral head, and the tuberosities, with the cuff attached, drop in front of the glenoid fossa.

## Operative Procedure

The supero-anterior approach provides adequate exposure of this lesion. Make an incision on the top of the shoulder just lateral to the acromioclavicular joint and extend it downward on the anterior aspect of the shoulder for 2 to $2^1/_2$ inches (Fig. 7-68A). Split the fibers of the deltoid vertically for 2 inches below the edge of the acromion and open the subacromial bursa in the same line as the muscle split. If more exposure is needed, resect three eighths of an inch of either the clavicle or the acromion adjacent to the acromioclavicular joint. Now explore the subacromial region and identify the pathology (Fig. 7-68B). Disengage the biceps tendon from behind the humeral head and sever its attachment to the superior glenoid rim. Remove the cuff from between the glenoid fossa and the humeral head and reduce the dislocation (Fig. 7-68C). Reattach the cuff and tuberosities to the surrounding soft tissue by interrupted sutures. It may be necessary to fix the greater tuberosity to the shaft by a transfixation screw. Cut away the intracapsular portion of the biceps tendon and anchor the proximal end of the remaining tendon in the intertubercular groove by interrupted sutures passing through the overlying transverse ligament (Fig. 7-78D).

## Postoperative Immobilization

Apply an abduction brace (made before the operation) which holds the arm in 45° of abduction, 30° of external rotation and 30° of forward flexion.

## Postoperative Management

The brace is worn until the patient can actively abduct the arm out of the brace (6 to 8 weeks). Attempts at active abduction should begin at the end of the fourth week. During this period, motion is allowed daily at the elbow, wrist and fingers. After removal of the brace institute an intensive program of gravity-free pendulum exercises

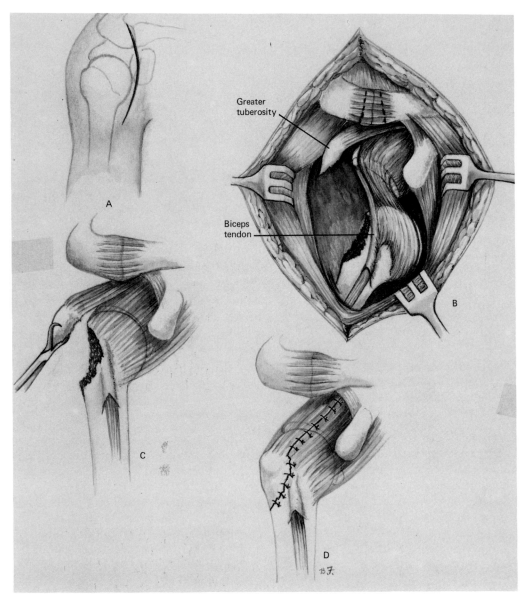

FIG. 7-69. Surgical management of an anterior dislocation complicated by a Type III fracture of the greater tuberosity.

(5 minutes every hour). Later, wall crawling and pulley exercises are added.

## ANTERIOR DISLOCATION COMPLICATED BY A TYPE III FRACTURE OF THE GREATER TUBEROSITY

In this lesion the greater tuberosity is pulled under the acromion; the lesion is comparable to a massive rupture of the cuff.

### Operative Procedure

Employ a supero-anterior incision to expose the subacromial region. The incision begins on the top of the shoulder just lateral to the acromioclavicular joint and extends downward on the anterior aspect of the shoulder for 2 to 2½ inches (Fig. 7-69A). Next, split the fibers of the deltoid for 2 inches below the level of the acromion; open the subacromial bursa in the same plane. The entire subacromial region now can be visualized and the pathology identified (Fig. 7-69B). Grasp the retracted tuberosity and cuff with a towel clip and pull the tuberosity down to its anatomical position (Fig. 7-69C). Anchor the tuberosity with interrupted sutures to the adjacent soft tissues (or fix it with a screw). Repair any rent in the cuff (Fig. 7-69D).

The postoperative immobilization and management are the same as those described for repair of complications associated with Type II fractures of the greater tuberosity.

## SURGICAL MANAGEMENT OF FRACTURES OF THE HEAD AND NECK OF THE HUMERUS WITH DISLOCATION

Expose the subacromial region through a supero-anterior incision, and develop the anterior portion of the incision by splitting the anterior fibers of the deltoid 1 cm. from its medial border. Retract the deltoid mass downward and laterally, exposing the entire subacromial region. Next, identify the pathology and the position of the humeral head (Fig. 7-70A).

Now make gentle traction on the arm in the axis of the body (Fig. 7-70B), and lever the head into the glenoid fossa. Assemble the fragments of the tuberosities and suture them to one another and the adjacent tissues with interrupted sutures, or with sutures passing through drill holes in the bone. Finally, repair all tears in the cuff. Occasionally, the proximal assembled fragment is still very unstable. In such instances, the proximal fragment and the distal shaft fragment can be aligned and stabilized by passing a Rush nail through the head into the medullary canal. The nail is removed after 4 to 6 weeks (Fig. 7-70C).

## Immobilization

Following the operation place a cotton pad in the axilla, fix the arm to the chest wall with a 6-inch elastic bandage that encircles the arm and chest and support the arm with a triangular sling.

## Postoperative Management

Immobilize the arm to the side for 10 to 14 days; during this period exercise the elbow, wrist and fingers 5 to 10 minutes every hour. After 10 to 14 days, start gentle pendulum exercises and, at the end of the fourth week, discard the sling and add to the exercise program wall-crawling exercises. If a Rush nail is used, remove the nail after 4 to 6 weeks.

## FRACTURE OF THE ANTERIOR PORTION OF THE GLENOID

### Operative Procedure

Make an anterior incision, beginning in line with the acromioclavicular joint, and extend it downward in line with the axillary crease for 2½ inches (Fig. 7-71A).

Split the anterior fibers of the deltoid and expose the subacromial bursa; open the bursa in the line of the muscle-splitting incision. Retract the edges of the deltoid and bursal sac, exposing the subacromial region (Fig. 7-71B).

Isolate and divide the coracoid process proximal to the insertion of the conjoined tendon (short head of the biceps and the coracobrachialis) (Fig. 7-71C). Retract the detached portion of the coracoid process, with its muscular attachments, medially. One half inch from the lesser tuberosity divide the subscapularis tendon down to the capsule and by sharp dissection reflect it from the capsule beyond the anterior rim of the glenoid. Isolate the site of fracture; the displaced fragment will be found still attached to the capsule (Fig. 7-71D). Restore the fragment to its anatomical posi-

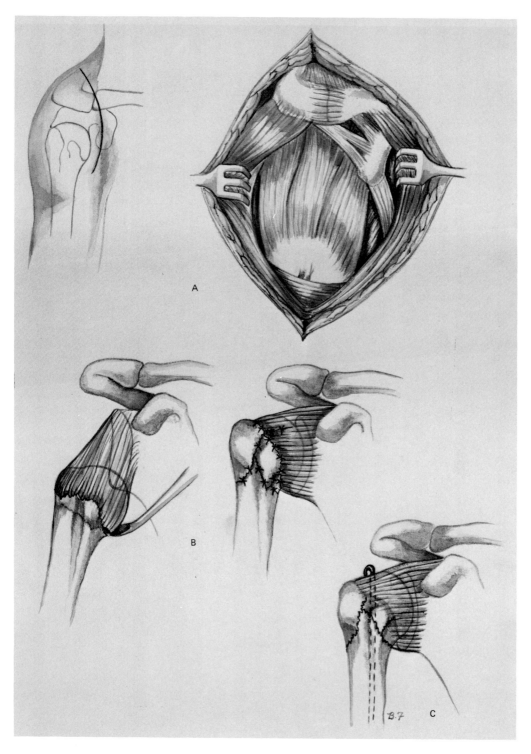

FIG. 7-70. Surgical management of fractures of the head and neck of the humerus with dislocation.

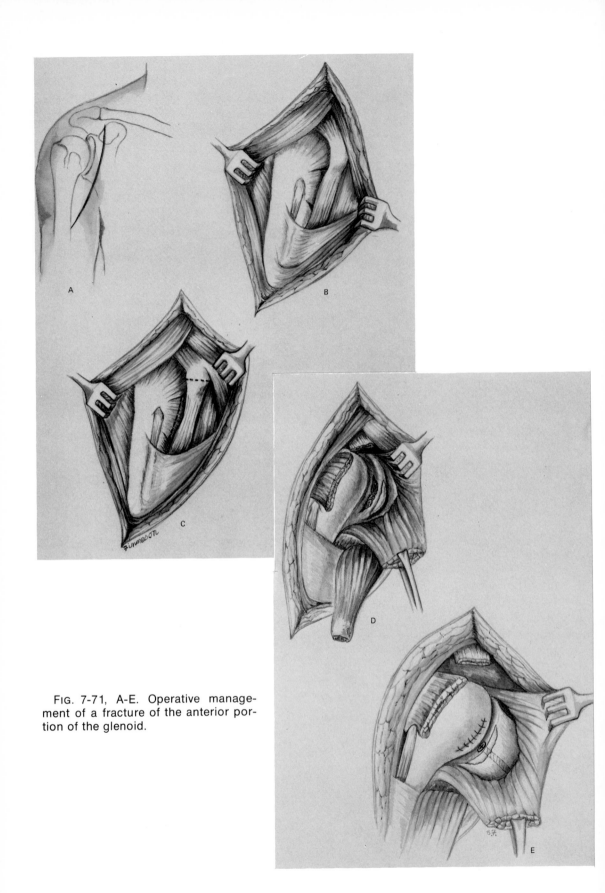

FIG. 7-71, A-E. Operative management of a fracture of the anterior portion of the glenoid.

tion and fix it with a screw (Fig. 7-71E). Repair any existing rent in the capsule.

### Postoperative Immobilization

Place a pad of cotton in the axilla, encircle the arm and trunk with a 6-inch elastic bandage and apply a triangular sling; or apply a Nicola sling.

### Postoperative Management

The arm must be fixed to the side in a position of internal rotation for at least 4 weeks. During this time allow motion at the elbow, the wrist and the fingers. After 4 weeks discard all external immobiliation and begin pendulum exercises in ever increasing arcs on a regulated regimen (5 to 10 minutes every hour).

After 5 weeks encourage active external rotation of the arm within the patient's tolerance. Also, at this time, add crawling up the wall, pulley and wheel exercises. The exercises should be increased progressively in range and frequency until all movements are restored to normalcy.

## FRACTURES OF THE POSTERIOR PORTION OF THE GLENOID

### Operative Procedure

Place the patient in the prone position with a sandbag under the affected shoulder. Drape the arm separately and place it on an arm board in the abducted position. Begin the skin incision at the acromioclavicular joint and continue it posteriorly over the top of the acromion to the spine of the scapula, then curve it downward and outward to a point 4 cm. above the posterior fold of the axilla (Fig. 7-72A).

Mobilize the skin flaps sufficiently to expose the entire posterior and central portion of the deltoid. By blunt dissection, develop the interval between the deeper muscles and the deltoid. Detach the central portion of the deltoid by an osteotomy through the acromion $3/8$ inch to $1/2$ inch

from its tip; then cut the posterior portion of the deltoid $1/2$ inch from its bony attachment. Retract the muscle mass laterally and downward (Fig. 7-72B).

Divide the conjoined tendon, including the infraspinatus and the teres minor and a portion of the supraspinatus (*caution:* do not sever the axillary nerve in the quadrilateral space), $1/2$ inch from its insertion and reflect the muscles medially as far as the posterior aspect of the glenoid. Isolate the posterior detached fragment of the glenoid (Fig. 7-72C). Restore the fragment to its anatomical position and fix it with a screw and repair any rents in the capsule by interrupted sutures (Fig. 7-72D).

Reattach the conjoined tendon with interrupted sutures and the central position of the deltoid by passing two or three threaded wires through the rim of the acromion that is still attached to the muscle and the acromion.

The postoperative immobilization and management are the same as those described for fractures of the anterior portion of the glenoid.

## SURGICAL TECHNIQUE OF OPEN REDUCTION OF OLD ANTERIOR DISLOCATION OF THE SHOULDER

Expose the subacromial region through a supero-anterior incision and split the anterior deltoid fiber vertically downward for 2 inches. If necessary, for more exposure divide the proximal half of the tendon of the pectoralis major (Fig. 7-73A). Next, expose the tendon of the subscapularis and divide it $1/2$ inch from its insertion into the lesser tuberosity; retract the muscle medially (Fig. 7-73, B-1). At this point, take care not to injure the axillary nerve. Remove all fibrous tissue from the glenoid fossa (Fig. 7-73, B-2); at this point, it may be necessary to cut part or all of the pectoralis major tendon in order to mobilize the head of the humerus (Fig. 7-73, B-3).

If the tendon of the long head of the biceps muscle is displaced posteriorly and is

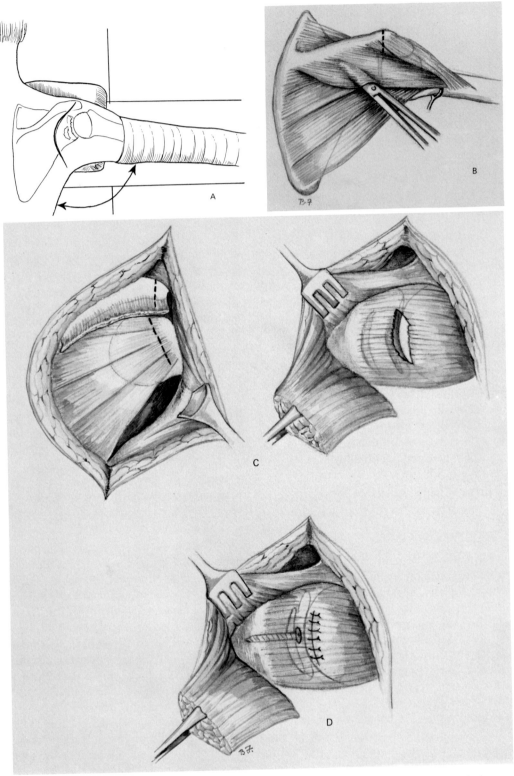

FIG. 7-72. Operative management of fractures of the posterior portion of the glenoid.

preventing reduction, divide it at its superior attachment to the glenoid rim and resect the intracapsular portion of the tendon. After the humeral head is mobilized, effect a reduction of the dislocation by using the Kocher maneuvers as described on page 375. After the reduction is achieved, anchor the proximal end of the remaining biceps tendon in the bicipital groove either by a staple or by interrupted sutures passing through the transverse ligament covering the bicipital groove.

Following reduction the joint may in some cases tend to redislocate. As a rule, if the arm is kept in extreme internal rotation, redislocation does not occur. On the other hand, particularly in old dislocations, the configuration of the glenoid fossa and the humeral head may be severely altered so that redislocation can be prevented only by some form of internal fixation, such as transfixion of the humeral head and acromion with two cruciate threaded wires, ($\frac{5}{64}$ inch in diameter) (Fig. 7-73, C-1), or by a Steinman pin traversing the humeral head and glenoid (Fig. 7-74).

Finally, suture the divided tendons of the subscapularis and the pectoralis major and, repair any defect found in the cuff (Fig. 7-73, C-2). The wires and the pin are cut below the level of the skin.

### Postoperative Immobilization

Postoperatively, a cotton pad in the axilla and a 6-inch elastic bandage encircling the arm and chest (holding the arm internally rotated) and a triangular sling to support the forearm afford adequate external immobilization.

The postoperative management must permit active exercises of the elbow, wrist and fingers. If wires or pins were used for internal fixation, remove them at the end of 3 weeks. At this time or within another week discard the external apparatus and sling and increase the intensity of the exercise program. Allow free use of the arm within the painless arcs of motion and in-stitute antigravity exercises (in the stooped position) which must be performed every hour for 5 to 10 minutes. Later, add wall-crawling and pulley exercises. Daily use of radiant head and gentle massage gives the patient much comfort. Do not permit strenuous activity or sports for a minimum of 3 months.

### SURGICAL TECHNIQUE OF OPEN REDUCTION OF OLD POSTERIOR DISLOCATION

Expose the subacromial region through a supero-anterior incision and split the anterior deltoid fibers vertically downward for 2 to 2½ inches. If more exposure is necessary, divide the proximal half of the tendon of the pectoralis major (Fig. 7-75A).

Next, divide the subscapularis tendon close to its insertion and retract the muscle medially; do not injure the axillary nerve in performing this step of the operation (Fig. 7-75B), and note the position of the humeral head in relation to the glenoid. Place a small bone skid between the humeral head and the glenoid and disengage the posterior glenoid rim from the defect in the humeral head; then, rotate the arm externally to complete the reduction (Fig. 7-75C).

Visualize the defect in the head and with a sharp curette scarify its surface; now anchor the tendon of the subscapularis in the base of the defect by mattress sutures passing through drill holes in the bone (Fig. 7-75D). Finally, if the tendon of the pectoralis major was divided, restore its continuity by mattress sutures.

The postoperative immobilization and management are the same as those described for old anterior dislocation treated by surgical reduction.

### SURGICAL TREATMENT OF CONGENITAL ELEVATION OF THE SCAPULA

Many surgical procedures have been designed to decrease the deformity and dis-

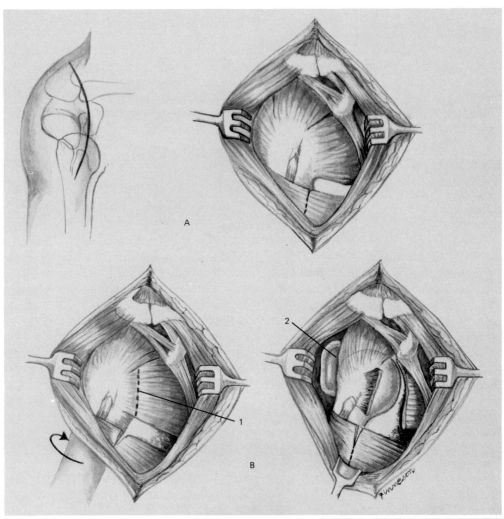

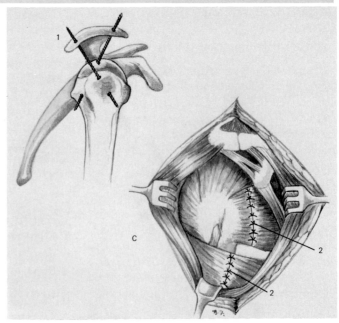

FIG. 7-73. Operative management of old anterior dislocation. (A) Incision and exposure of subacromial region. (B) Division of the subscapularis tendon (1); exposure of the humeral head and excision of all fibrous tissue in the glenoid fossa (2). (C) Internal fixation of the relocated humeral head by transfixion of the head of the acromion with two threaded wires (1); and resuturing of the subscapularis and pectoralis major tendons (2).

ability of the congenitally elevated scapula. One of the first was performed by Schrock (1926). Essentially the operation consists of freeing the scapula subperiosteally of all muscle and soft tissue attachments, excising the omovertebral bone, if present, and resecting the prominent parts of the scapula, especially the supraspinatus area. The entire scapula is then pulled downward and its inferior angle is anchored to the lowest rib possible.

The end results of the operation are far from satisfactory. In many instances, much of the cosmetic improvement is lost because of regeneration of bone at the site of resection. Also, many patients still have winging of the inferior angle or of the medial border of the scapula, or of both. Finally, scarring is unsightly in most patients and some may develop a prominence of the sternoclavicular joint. Because of these results, Schrock recommended that in children over 6 years of age no surgery other than extraperiosteal excision of the supraspinatus area and of the omovertebral bone should be performed.

A popular operation in Europe is Koenig's operation, later modified by Wittek. In this procedure, the scapula is divided ½ inch lateral and parallel to its vertebral border. All muscles attached to the medial border are left intact. The lateral segment of the scapula is pulled inferiorly and its inferior tip is anchored in a slit made in the superior belly of the latissimus dorsi. The medial and lateral segments of the scapula are sutured to the infraspinatus and subscapularis respectively. Finally, the projecting superior end of the medial segment of the scapula is resected (Fig. 7-76).

The operation devised by Woodward (1961), produces satisfactory results in most patients; however, I have had two patients with a transient brachial palsy following this operation. Woodward reported one such case in his series. The following are the essential features of the operation. The origins of all the muscles attached to the vertebral border of the scapula and of the trapezius are freed by sharp dissection

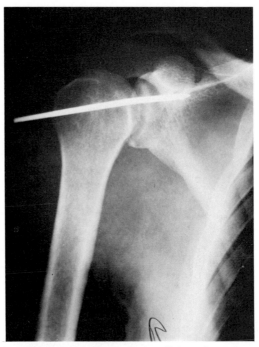

FIG. 7-74. Old anterior dislocation of the shoulder: Following open reduction the head was fixed to the glenoid with a Steinman pin.

from the spinous processes. If present, the omovertebral bone is excised and the prominent supraspinous area is resected extraperiosteally. Then the scapula is pulled inferiorly and the muscles released from the spinous processes are reattached at a lower level.

In my hands, Green's operation (1957) has given the most consistently satisfactory results. However, this is a difficult operation to perform. In this operation the muscles on the vertebral and superior margins of the scapula are freed extraperiosteally; the supraspinous portion of the scapula is exposed extraperiosteally and resected and the omovertebral bone is excised. Then the scapula is displaced inferiorly and the muscles are reattached.

## Surgical Technique of the Woodward Operation

Place the patient in the prone position and drape the shoulder and arm separately

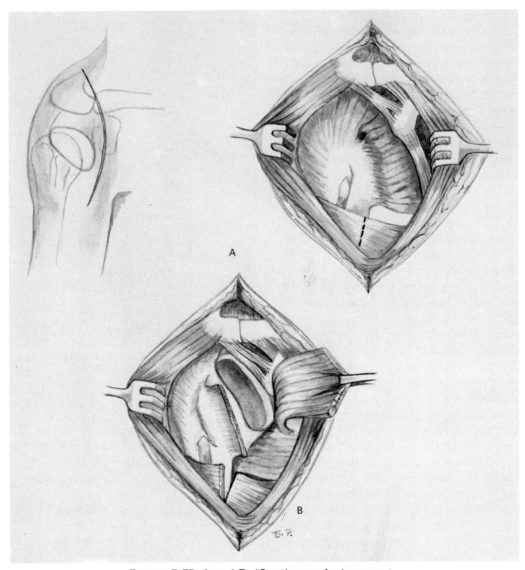

FIGURE 7-75, A and B. (*Caption on facing page*)

so that the extremity can be manipulated during the operation. Make a midline skin incision extending from the spinous process of the first cervical vertebra to the spinous process of the ninth thoracic. By sharp dissection reflect the skin and subcutaneous tissue from the underlying fascia laterally to the vertebral border of the scapula. Next, identify the medial border of the trapezius in the lower end of the incision and free it from the underlying latissimus dorsi. Cut the fascial sheath of origin of the trapezius from the spinous processes and reflect the muscle laterally, exposing the origins of the rhomboid major and minor (Fig. 7-77A). Free the origins of the rhomboids from the spinous processes and reflect the rhomboids and the superior part of the trapezius from the muscles of the chest wall (Fig. 7-77B).

Retract the entire sheet of muscles laterally; if the omovertebral bone is present, attached to the superior angle of the scapula, it will now lie exposed. Excise this bone extraperiosteally; also excise any fibrous bands attached to the angle of the scapula

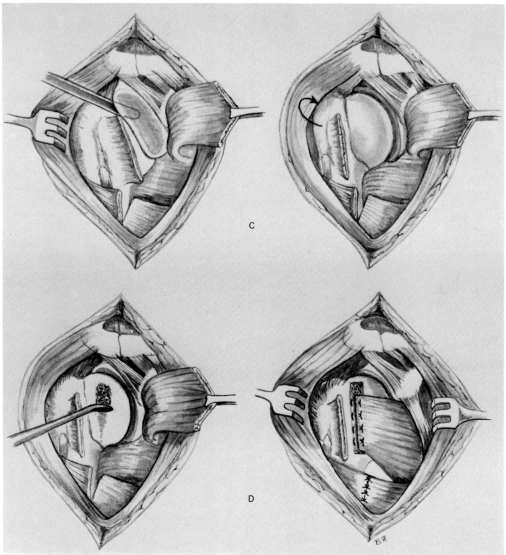

C

D

FIGURE 7-75 (*Continued above*)

FIG. 7-75. Operative management of old posterior dislocation. (A) Incision and exposure of the subacromial region. (B) Division of the subscapularis tendon to expose the humeral head. (C) Mobilization and relocation of the humeral head. (D) Transfer of the tendon of the subscapularis into the defect in the humeral head.

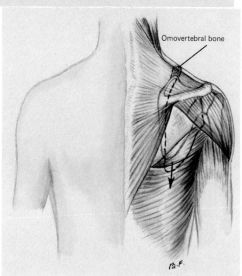

Omovertebral bone

(*Right*) FIG. 7-76. Koenig's operation modified by Wittek for congenital elevation of the scapula.

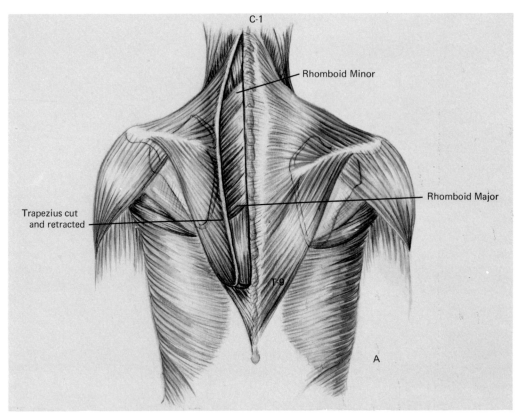

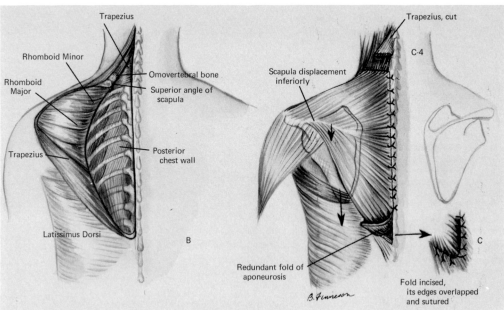

FIG. 7-77. Woodward operation for congenital elevation of the scapula. (A) The fascial sheath of origin of the trapezius is divided at the spinous processes and reflected laterally, exposing the rhomboid major and minor muscles. (B) The rhomboids and the trapezius are reflected from the posterior chest wall. (C) The trapezius is divided at the level of the fourth cervical vertebra and the scapula with the attached muscles is pulled distally until it lies at the same level as the opposite scapula. Finally, the trapezius and rhomboids are reattached to the spinous processes at a lower level.

or contracted levator scapulae muscle. In performing this step, take care to protect the spinal accessory nerve and the nerves to the rhomboids from injury. Inspect the supraspinous part of the scapula and, if it is deformed, resect it extraperiosteally. This step freely mobilizes the scapula. Now divide the attachment of the trapezius transversely at the level of the fourth cervical vertebra (Fig. 7-77C).

Pull the scapula with the attached muscles distally until it lies at the same level as the opposite scapula. While holding the scapula in this position, suture the fascial origins of the trapezius and rhomboids to the spinous processes at a lower level. The distal origin of the trapezius now presents a fold of aponeurosis; either excise the excess tissue or incise it, overlap the edges and suture the free edges in place (Fig. 7-77C).

**Postoperative Management.** After the operation, apply a Velpeau bandage; remove the bandage after 2 weeks and institute a program of mild active exercises to improve motion in the shoulder girdle.

## Surgical Technique of the Green Operation

Begin the skin incision one finger's breadth above the middle of the spine of the scapula; extend it medially paralleling the spine to the vertebral border of the spine; curve it around the border and continue it distally one finger's breadth medial to and parallel with the vertebral border; terminate the incision 2 inches below the inferior angle of the scapula (Fig. 7-78A). By sharp dissection, reflect the deep fascia, exposing the insertion of the trapezius on the spine of the scapula, and free the insertion extraperiosteally. Next, reflect the trapezius medially, exposing the supraspinatus, the rhomboid major and the rhomboid minor (Fig. 7-78B). Elevate the supraspinatus from its fossa extraperiosteally, as far laterally as the scapular notch, and displace it laterally. Identify the suprascapular nerve and transverse scapular artery passing through the notch and protect them

from injury. Next, free the origins of the levator scapulae and the rhomboids extraperiosteally from the superior and medial borders of the scapula and the part of the subscapularis lying above the level of the spine on the anterior surface of the scapula (Fig. 7-78C).

Tilt the upper part of the scapula backward to expose its anterior surface above the level of the spine, and with a fine, sharp osteotome divide the scapula along the base of the spine as far laterally as the scapular notch (Fig. 7-78C). Do not injure the neurovascular structures traversing the notch. Remove the supraspinous portion of the scapula extraperiosteally and if the omovertebral bone is present, excise it and any fibrous bands anchoring the scapula to the vertebrae. Now, in the lower end of the incision, identify the origin of the latissimus dorsi and divide it from the spinous processes distally to a point just beyond the most inferior fibers of origin of the trapezius. Next, by extraperiosteal dissection, free the origin of the serratus anterior from the medial border and the inferior angle of the scapula. Cut any dense fibrous bands binding the inferior angle to the chest wall.

Now, just beyond its middle, make a drill hole in the base of the spine and pass through the drill hole a stout wire 3 feet long. Direct both ends of the wire distally, posterior to the infraspinatus and beneath the latissimus dorsi. Pull the wire through the skin about 3 inches distal to the anticipated level of the inferior angle of the scapula and pointing toward the middle of the buttock on the opposite side (Fig. 7-78D).

With its inferior angle beneath the latissimus dorsi, pull the scapula inferiorly to its new position and reattach the muscles in the following order (Fig. 7-78E): Suture the supraspinatus to the scapular spine. Reattach the origin of the serratus anterior in the natural pull of its fibers to a more superior position on the medial border of the scapula. Likewise, reattach the levator scapulae and the rhomboids (the levator scapulae may need lengthening). Reattach

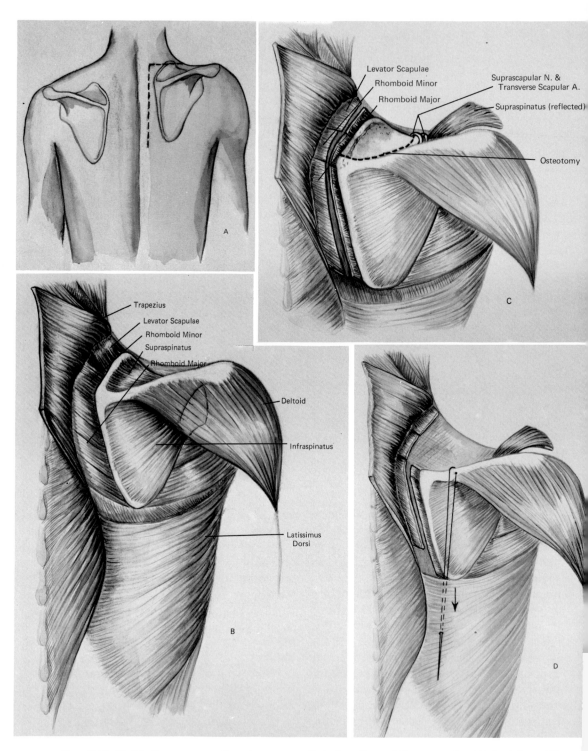

Fig. 7-78 (A-E). Green operation for congenital elevation of the scapula. (A) Incision. (B) The trapezius is reflected medially, exposing the supraspinatus and rhomboids. (C) The supraspinatus is elevated from its fossa and reflected laterally and the levator scapulae and rhomboids are detached from the superior and the medial border of the scapula. The supraspinatus portion of the scapula is resected and the serratus anterior is freed from the medial border and the inferior angle of the scapula. (Continued on facing page.)

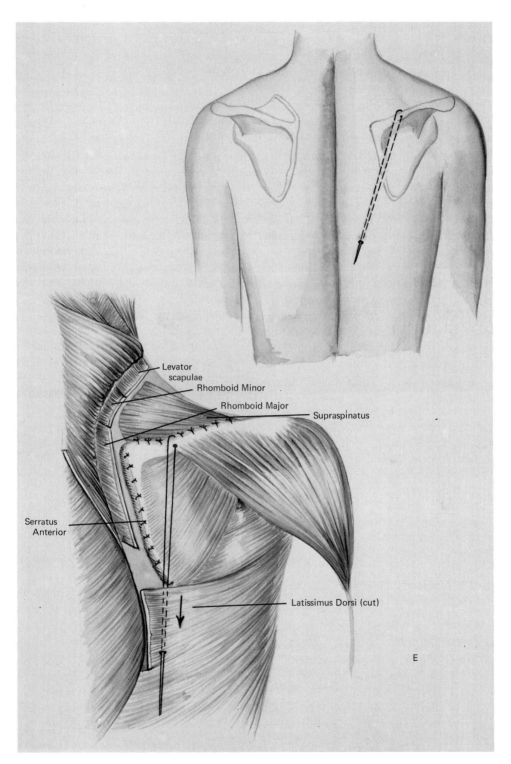

Levator
scapulae

Rhomboid Minor

Rhomboid Major

Supraspinatus

Serratus
Anterior

Latissimus Dorsi (cut)

E

(FIG. 7-78, Cont'd.). (D) A drill hole is made in the base of the spine, through which is passed a stout wire; the wire passes beneath the latissimus dorsi and pierces the skin about 3 inches distal to the anticipated level of the inferior angle of the scapula; it points toward the middle of the opposite buttock. (E) After the scapula is pulled to its new position the muscles are re-attached to the scapula.

the trapezius to the spine so that its new insertion is displaced about 1 inch more medially than its natural insertion and its inferior fibers more laterally and superiorly than before. Lap the divided portion of the latissimus dorsi over the inferior portion of the trapezius and suture it to the spinous processes in its natural position; it should completely cover the inferior angle of the scapula; if it does not, advance its reattachment more superiorly. Finally, suture the upper portion of the latissimus dorsi to the inferior outer edge of the trapezius.

After the operation, place the patient in a bivalved plaster spica (prepared beforehand) that includes the leg on the opposite side. Fix the ends of the wire attached to the scapula to a spring scale and attach the other end of the scale by means of a strap to a ring in the spica. Adjust the strap so that approximately 3 pounds of pull is made on the scapula.

**Postoperative Management.** After 4 or 5 days begin active exercises of the arm to maintain and improve motion in the shoulder girdle. At the end of 3 weeks remove the spica and the wire and place the arm in a sling for several weeks. During this period, continue and increase the active exercises. After 3 months, institute a program of strenuous overhead and abduction exercises.

## MUSCLE TRANSFERS FOR PARALYSIS ABOUT THE SHOULDER

It must be conceded that the results of muscle transfers for paralytic disorders about the shoulder have been disappointing. However, in selected instances and if properly performed, some transfers do improve function and reduce the disability of the shoulder. Steindler pointed out that a trapezius transfer is beneficial only because it produces a tenodesis effect. The type of transfer selected depends upon the extent of involvement of the muscles about the shoulder and, like arthrodesis of the shoulder, depends, above all, upon the usefulness of the forearm, elbow and hand. Mus-

cle transfers about the shoulder are useless operations if there is a flail elbow and hand. Muscle and tendon transfers to improve the function of a paralyzed or weak deltoid are successful only when the upper trapezius, serratus anterior, pectoralis major and the short external rotators of the shoulder have fair or better power. And in the trapezius transfer designed by Mayer, the other supporting muscles of the girdle, the levator scapulae and the rhomboids, must have good motor power. In the event that the external rotators are weak, they can be reinforced by transfer of the latissimus dorsi or the teres major to the outer aspect of the humerus.

Some paralytic disorders are complicated by an anterior or posterior subluxation or dislocation of the shoulder. To stabilize the humeral head, some surgeons transfer the long head of the biceps as in the Nicola procedure for recurrent dislocations of the shoulder. The value of this procedure is indeed questionable. The best results follow when the posterior deltoid is transferred anteriorly to the acromion and outer third of the clavicle to substitute for a paralyzed anterior third.

### Deltoid Paralysis

Of the operations designed for complete paralysis of the deltoid, transfer of the trapezius is the most effective. Mayer successfully transferred the trapezius to the region of the deltoid tubercle by using a fascial graft to increase its length. More recently, Bateman modified this operation by transferring the acromion and part of the spine of the scapula, with the trapezius attached, to the lateral aspect of the humerus.

The Ober operation, which is a modification of the operation designed by Slomann, transfers the short head of the biceps and the long head of the triceps to the acromion. Later, first Ober and then Harmon transferred the posterior portion of the deltoid to substitute for a paralyzed anterior portion.

## Transfer of the Trapezius (Mayer)

The success of this procedure depends upon good power in the pectoralis major, the trapezius and the scapular muscles—the levator scapulae and the rhomboids. Subluxation of the humeral head is not corrected by this operation; its existence is a contraindication.

**Surgical Technique.** Make a U-shaped incision around the shoulder girdle, extending along the anterior surface of the clavicle, around the acromion and along the spine of the scapula. Make a second vertical incision on the lateral surface of the shoulder, beginning at the acromion and ending at the deltoid tubercle (Fig. 7-79A). Reflect the skin on the top of the shoulder to expose the trapezius (Fig. 7-79B). Divide the trapezius from its insertion into the clavicle, the acromion and 3 to 4 inches of the spine. Reflect the detached muscle upward until the nerves and vessels that penetrate it are exposed. Anteriorly, develop the plane between the trapezius and the outer border of the sternocleidomastoid and, posteriorly, the plane between the trapezius and the supraspinatus. Dissect the anterior and posterior flaps of the vertical incision from the top of the deltoid, until the entire muscle is exposed. Make a vertical slit 1½ to 2 inches long down to the bone in the insertion of the deltoid (Fig. 7-79C). Through this slit elevate a bone flap from the lateral aspect of the humerus (Fig. 7-79D).

Remove from the lateral aspect of the thigh a graft of fascia lata measuring 3½ to 4 inches in width and 9 inches in length. Cut the graft into a long and a short piece as shown in Figure 7-79E. Place the rough side of the longer graft on the under side of the trapezius and fix it to the muscle with fine interrupted sutures (Fig. 7-79F). Now place the outer surface of the smaller graft on the top of the trapezius and suture it to both the muscle and the longer graft. The muscle is now enveloped in two layers of fascia lata (Fig. 7-79G).

With the arm abducted 135° and flexed forward 20°, suture the edges of the long graft to the anterior and posterior borders of the deltoid (Fig. 7-79H). Finally, with strong mattress sutures, anchor the end of the long graft in the muscle slit and beneath the bone flap on the lateral side of the humerus near the deltoid tubercle. The fascia should be taut when the arm is abducted (Fig. 7-79I).

**Postoperative Management.** Apply a shoulder spica plaster cast holding the arm in 135° of abduction and 20° of forward flexion. After 4 weeks remove the cast and apply a brace holding the arm in the same position and begin graduated active abduction of the arm. Protect the arm in the abducted position for 4 months. During this period the intensity of the exercises should be progressively increased and the arm gradually lowered to the side.

## Transfer of the Trapezius (Bateman)

**Surgical Technique.** Make a T-shaped incision. Extend the upper limb of the incision around the shoulder, starting anteriorly over the outer third of the clavicle and continuing around the acromion and over the spine of the scapula. Place the vertical limb on the lateral aspect of the shoulder extending distally from the acromion for 2½ inches (Fig. 7-80A). Free all the flaps from the underlying muscles and split the deltoid in the line of the skin incision. Dissect away all soft tissues from the undersurfaces of the acromion and the spine of the scapula. Next, starting at the base of the spine of the scapula, perform an oblique osteotomy of the spine, directed distally and laterally (Fig. 7-80B). This step mobilizes a large portion of the trapezius.

Next, excise the distal three quarters of an inch of the clavicle (stay lateral to the coracoclavicular ligament) and scarify the undersurface of the acromion and spine. With the arm abducted 90°, choose the site of the new insertion of the transfer on the lateral aspect of the humerus; thoroughly roughen this area (Fig. 7-80C). Finally, with

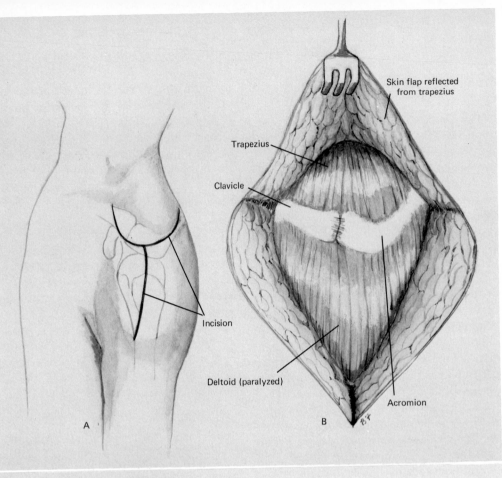

A

Incision

B

Skin flap reflected
from trapezius

Trapezius

Clavicle

Deltoid (paralyzed)

Acromion

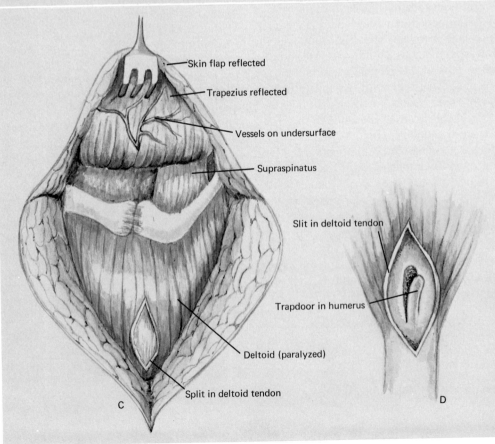

C

Skin flap reflected

Trapezius reflected

Vessels on undersurface

Supraspinatus

Deltoid (paralyzed)

Split in deltoid tendon

D

Slit in deltoid tendon

Trapdoor in humerus

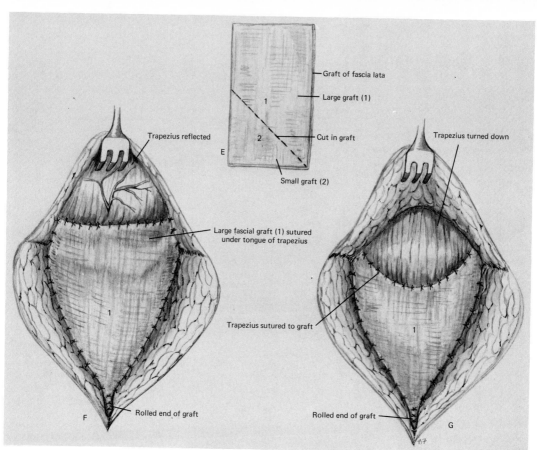

- Graft of fascia lata
- Large graft (1)
- Cut in graft
- Small graft (2)

E

Trapezius reflected

Large fascial graft (1) sutured under tongue of trapezius

1

Trapezius turned down

Trapezius sutured to graft

1

F · Rolled end of graft

Rolled end of graft

G

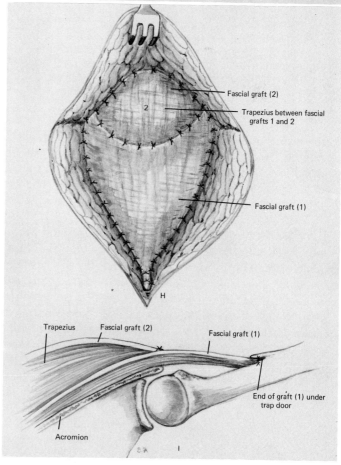

FIG. 7-79. Transfer of the trapezius (Mayer). (A) Incision. (B) Reflection of skin to expose the trapezius. (C) The insertion of the trapezius into the clavicle, acromion and spine of the scapula is divided and the muscle is reflected. (D) A bone flap is elevated from the lateral side of the humerus at the insertion of the deltoid. (E) Fascia graft removed from the lateral aspect of the thigh and cut into a long and a short graft. (F) The large fascia graft is sutured to the under surface of the trapezius. (G) The small graft is sutured to the top of the trapezius. (H) The edges of the long graft are sutured to the anterior and posterior borders of the deltoid. (I) The end of the long graft is anchored under the bone flap in the humerus, while the arm is abducted 135° and flexed forward 20°. (Redrawn from Mayer, L.: *In:* Lewis Practice of Surgery, W. F. Prior, Hagerstown, Md., 1947).

Fascial graft (2)

Trapezius between fascial grafts 1 and 2

2

Fascial graft (1)

H

Trapezius   Fascial graft (2)

Fascial graft (1)

End of graft (1) under trap door

Acromion

I

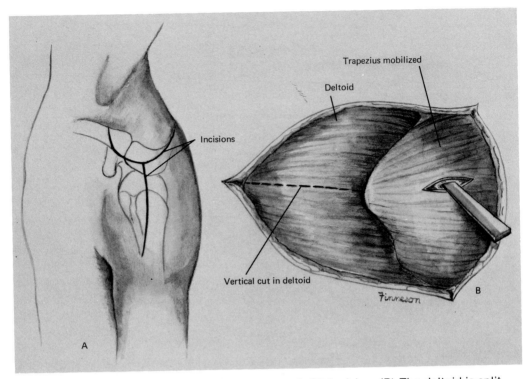

FIG. 7-80. Transfer of the trapezius (Bateman). (A) Incision. (B) The deltoid is split and the trapezius mobilized together with the acromion and a portion of the spine of the scapula. (C) The undersurface of the acromion is roughened, as is the corresponding area on the lateral aspect of the humerus. (D) With the arm abducted the acromion is fixed to the lateral aspect of the humerus with two or three screws. (Redrawn from Bateman, J. E.: The Shoulder and Environs. St. Louis, C. V. Mosby, 1954.)

the arm abducted make strong lateral traction on the cuff of the trapezius and pull it distally over the head of the humerus; anchor the acromion to the lateral aspect of the humerus as far distally as possible with two or three screws (Fig. 7-80D).

**Postoperative Management.** Apply a shoulder spica cast holding the arm in 90° of abduction. After 4 to 6 weeks bivalve the shoulder and arm part of the spica and allow active movements of the arm and shoulder. At the end of 8 weeks, at which time the acromion should be well anchored to the humerus, remove the cast and apply an abduction brace. During this period institute a program of progressive active exercises and allow the arm gradually to come to the side.

## Transfer of the Biceps and the Triceps to the Acromion (Ober)

The success of this procedure, as in the transfer of the trapezius, depends upon good power in the triceps and biceps and in the pectoralis major and scapular muscles. The best results follow when the deltoid has some power.

**Surgical Technique.** Make a superior skin incision over the top of the shoulder directly over the acromion. Extend the anterior limb downward 3 inches over the anterior aspect of the shoulder. Carry the posterior limb downward and slightly inward for 3 inches over the posterior aspect of the shoulder. Deepen the anterior portion of the incision through the fibers of the

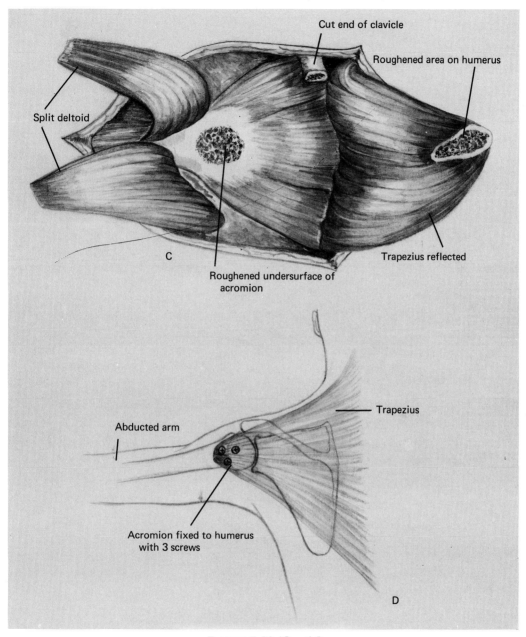

Cut end of clavicle

Roughened area on humerus

Split deltoid

C

Trapezius reflected

Roughened undersurface of
acromion

Trapezius

Abducted arm

Acromion fixed to humerus
with 3 screws

D

FIGURE 7-80 (Cont'd)

deltoid to expose the coracoid process and its muscular attachments. Dissect free the tendon of the short head of the biceps from the tendons of the coracobrachialis and the pectoralis minor; then detach it from the coracoid with a small portion of its bony insertion. Now, carefully separate the bi-

ceps from the surrounding structures as far as the tendon of the pectoralis major.

In the event that the short head of the biceps is too short to reach the top of the acromion, use the upper half of the tendon of the pectoralis major to lengthen it. Now, direct your attention to the posterior por-

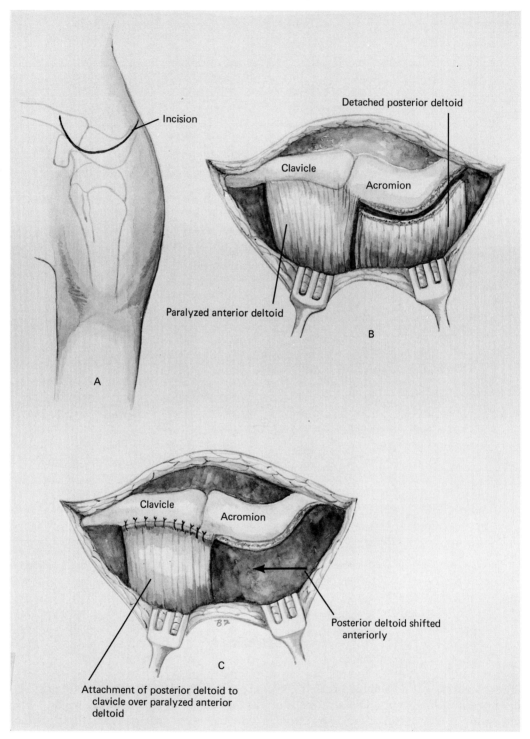

FIG. 7-81. Transfer of posterior portion of deltoid (Harmon). (A) Incision. (B) The posterior deltoid is detached from the acromion and spine of the scapula and mobilized. (C) The posterior deltoid is shifted anteriorly and sutured to the clavicle over the paralyzed anterior deltoid.

tion of the incision and develop the posterior limb to expose the long head of the triceps muscle at its origin on the scapula. Isolate the tendon and detach it from the scapula, with a small piece of bone attached. Dissect the triceps tendon and muscle free from the surrounding tissues on the upper end of the humerus.

With a sharp, fine osteotome make two cuts in the acromion—an anterior one for the biceps tendon and a posterior one for the triceps tendon. Make the cuts parallel to the flat surfaces of the acromion and spread their edges to receive the tendons. But first, the tendons must be passed through the fibers of the deltoid to emerge near the top of the acromion opposite their respective bone cuts. With the arm in abduction, anchor the tendons to the acromion with stout interrupted sutures.

The postoperative management is the same as that described for the transfer of the trapezius muscle.

### Transfer of the Posterior Portion of the Deltoid (Harmon)

Abduction power can be improved in instances of paralysis of the anterior portion of the deltoid by transferring the posterior portion to a postion of better mechanical advantage. This procedure may be used in obstetric palsy when the anterior deltoid is paralyzed.

**Surgical Technique.** Make a semicircular incision around the shoulder just below the acromion. Extend the incision along the lower border of the middle third of the clavicle, and around the acromion to the middle of the spine of the scapula (Fig. 7-81A). Reflect the skin flaps up and down to expose the entire origin of the deltoid. By subperiosteal dissection, free the scapular portion of the deltoid origin and mobilize the upper half of this portion from the surrounding tissues. Do not injure the axillary nerve and posterior circumflex artery as they emerge from the quadrilateral space (Fig. 7-81B).

By sharp subperiosteal dissection, prepare the new site of the insertion on the anterior surface of the outer third of the clavicle. Shift the posterior deltoid anteriorly and anchor its origin by interrupted sutures to the periosteum on the superior surface of the clavicle (Fig. 7-81C).

After the operation immobilize the extremity in a plaster shoulder spica holding the arm in 105° of elevation.

### FASCIAL TRANSPLANTS IN PARALYTIC DISORDERS ABOUT THE SHOULDER GIRDLE

Muscle imbalance resulting from infantile paralysis in the cervical region and the scapular muscles may be responsible for extensive deformities of the cervicothoracic and the upper thoracic regions of the trunk and the shoulder girdle. Such deformities are difficult to control and more difficult to correct.

### Paralysis of the Spinal and the Elevator Muscles of the Scapula

Paralysis or weakness of the spinal and the elevator scapular muscles may lead to severe high cervicothoracic scoliosis and dropping of the shoulder on the affected side. In these cases the goal is to elevate the depressed shoulder and to stabilize the deformity, which is progressive in nature, by creating a fixator action against the pull of the unaffected muscles on the convexity of the cervical curve. Moreover, the function of the entire upper extremity improves and fatigue and neck pain are lessened.

**Operative Technique (Dickson).** Two long strips of fascia lata rolled into tubes, with the gliding surfaces out, are employed in this operation. A skin incision of from 3 to 4 inches is made over the outer extension of the spine of the scapula close to the acromial end; the spine is exposed subperiosteally, and a slot is made through it. A second incision is made from the spine to the apex of the cervical curve on the concave side, exposing the underlying cervical fascia. The end of one of the fascial tubes is now laced to the cervical muscles at the apex of the curve on its concave side. The dropped scapula is elevated as high as possible, and, while this position is being maintained, the other end of the fascial tube is passed through the slot in the spine and sutured to itself with interrupted silk sutures.

A third incision is made over the spinous process of the first thoracic vertebra; the spine is exposed and a hole is drilled through its base. One end of the second fascial tube is drawn through a slot made in the vertebral end of the spine and anchored to itself. The other end traverses a subcutaneous tunnel, emerging at the spinous process of the first thoracic vertebra; it is passed through the hole and is sutured to itself under tension.

**Postoperative Management.** The arm is immobilized in a plaster spica in from 40° to 50° of abduction; alternatively, the arm may be tied to the head of the bed. Active exercises are begun after 3 weeks. All support is discontinued after 5 to 6 weeks.

## Paralysis of the Serratus Anterior Muscle

Weakness or paralysis of the upper spinal and scapular muscles is responsible for pronounced hypermobility of the scapula and promotes high thoracic and cervico thoracic curves. The serratus anterior functions primarily as a stabilizer of the scapula. In pushing movements it draws the scapula toward the thoracic cage; in elevating movements it rotates the inferior angle upward and forward. If the serratus anterior is implicated, the scapula shifts toward the vertebral column and rotates downward and inward. Marked winging of the scapula occurs during arm elevation. The deformity is particularly striking in the movements of pushing. In the operation about to be described, an attempt is made to stabilize the scapula; this, in turn, improves shoulder function and also acts as a check to further progression of the spinal curvatures.

**Operative Technique (Dickson).** First, the scapula is displaced forward to the position desired in relation to the thoracic wall. While it is held in this position, an incision is made above the lower axillary border of the scapula, and a drill hole is passed through the inferior angle. Through this hole, the end of a tube made of fascia lata is passed and sutured to itself.

A second incision is made on the lateral aspect of the thorax over the origin of the pectoralis major muscle; the two skin incisions are connected by a subcutaneous tunnel, through which the distal end of the fascial tube is passed. The end of the tube is split in half; one half is laced into the lowermost fibers of the pectoralis major, the other into the anterior border of the latissimus dorsi. Then the ends of the fascial tube are anchored under considerable tension while the scapula is held in the desired position. Added stability of the scapula may be attained by running a second fascial tube from the cervical muscles to the spine of the scapula.

## Paralysis of the Rhomboidei and the Levator Scapulae Muscles With Good Power in the Serratus Anterior Muscle

With paralysis or weakness of the levator scapulae and the rhomboidei muscles, the scapula shifts laterally toward the axilla. During arm elevation, its upper vertebral border is pulled downward and inward by the unopposed serratus anterior, in addition to a lateral shift of the scapula. High thoracic scoliosis may be a concomitant finding; the deformity tends to be progressive.

**Operative Technique (Dickson).** Two fascial transplants in the form of tubes are used in this procedure. One extends from the lower vertebral border of the scapula to the spinal muscles, the other from the inferior angle of the scapula to the latissimus dorsi. A small incision is made over the lower vertebral border of the scapula, and a hole is drilled through the bone; another

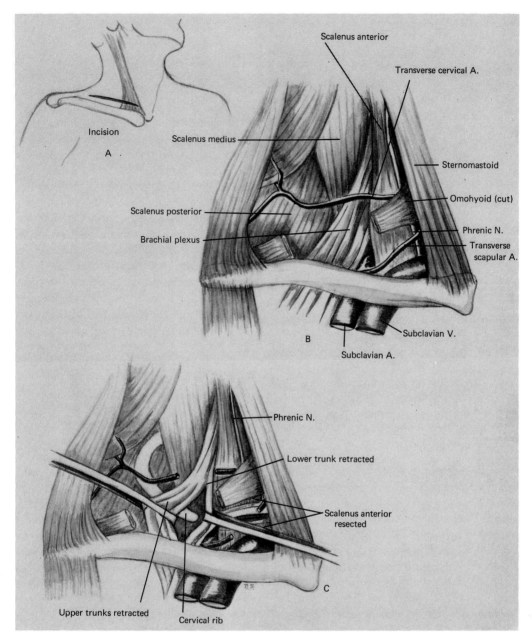

FIG. 7-82. Operation for neurovascular compression. (A) Incision in the supra-clavicular area. (B) Normal anatomy in the supraclavicular region. (C) The upper and lower nerve trunks are retracted in opposite directions to expose the underlying cervical rib. The anterior scalenus has been divided and the cervical rib isolated and is now ready for partial or total resection.

small incision is made over the spinal mus-cles, opposite and slightly inferior to the first incision. The two incisions are con-nected by a subcutaneous tunnel. One end of a fascial tube is laced into the spinal muscles, the other end traverses the sub-cutaneous channel, proceeds through the hole in the vertebral border of the scapula and is sutured to itself under tension.

A third incision is made over the inferior angle of the scapula. The bone is exposed and a hole is drilled through its substance. Another small vertical incision is made 3 inches medial and inferior to the inferior angle of the scapula, exposing the fibers of the latissimus dorsi. Both incisions are also connected by a subcutaneous tunnel. One end of the second fascial tube is laced into the fibers of the latissimus dorsi. The other passes through a tunnel hole in the inferior angle of the scapula and is sutured to itself under tension.

The aforementioned procedures are useful in improving the overall function of the extremity. They stabilize the scapula and may arrest partially the development of spinal deformities. More study of the usefulness and the indications of fascial transplants is necessary before definite conclusions can be drawn as to the merit of the procedures.

## SURGICAL MANAGEMENT OF COMPRESSION OF THE NEUROVASCULAR ELEMENTS IN THE ROOT OF THE NECK

In my experience most of the compression syndromes in the neck requiring surgical intervention can be managed adequately through the supraclavicular approach. However, in patients exhibiting evidence of pronounced vascular compression and objective evidence of secondary changes in the hands, decompression of the neurovascular structures is best achieved by excision of the first rib through the transaxillary approach. The transclavicular approach is indicated in those instances in which the clavicle is the primary site of the pathology responsible for the compression of the neurovascular structures, or in which the pathology in the root of the neck is such that a wide exposure is mandatory for an adequate exploration of the area, or when a portion of the subclavian artery or axillary artery is so involved as to require resection and replacement with a graft.

### Supraclavicular Approach

Make a 6- to 8-cm. transverse incision in the supraclavicular fossa, beginning just above and lateral to the sternoclavicular joint and extending slightly upward and backward (Fig. 7-82A). Divide the platysma in the line of the skin incision and identify the clavicular insertion of the sternocleidomastoid muscle; retract this muscle medially or divide it. Identify the external jugular vein and the transverse scapular and transverse cervical arteries lying anterior to the anterior scalene; divide and ligate these vessels. Isolate the omohyoid as it courses obliquely across the anterior scalene and retract it out of the field or divide it. Now the phrenic nerve comes into view as it courses downward and obliquely across the anterior scalene; free it and retract it medially. Isolate the anterior and posterior borders of the anterior scalene and divide the muscle close to its attachment. Avoid injuring the subclavian vein, which lies anterior to the muscle and inferior to the site of division of the muscle (Fig. 7-82B). Directly posterior to the anterior scalene lies the subclavian artery and the brachial plexus; note if division of the anterior scalene relieves pressure on these structures. Carefully identify and explore the neurovascular elements lying medial to the medial scalene; note if there are any fibrotendinous bands compressing these elements; look for anomalies of the scalene muscles, the presence of cervical ribs or a large transverse process of the seventh cervical vertebra (Fig. 7-82C).

The commonest type of cervical rib arises from the seventh cervical vertebra; its length and termination vary considerably. From its origin it extends laterally, then curves inferiorly and anteriorly and traverses the interval between the medial scalene and anterior scalene. The lowest root of the brachial plexus and the subclavian artery arch over the rib. The end of the rib may be free or it may join the first thoracic rib. Often a short anomalous rib may exhibit a fibrotendinous band, ex-

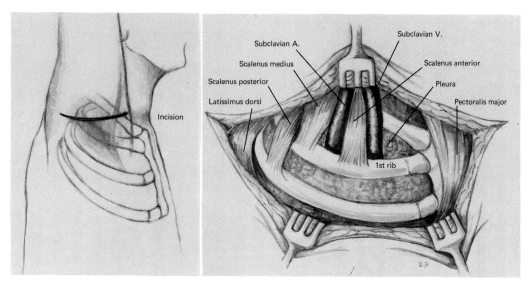

FIG. 7-83. (*Left*) Incision for the transaxillary approach. (*Right*) Cardinal structures in the axilla visualized by the transaxillary approach.

tending from its tip to the first thoracic rib or to the sternum.

The goal of the operation is to free the plexus and the vascular structures of any existing compression. If a cervical rib is present, carefully isolate it and remove part or all of it. Resect all fibrous bands. Inspect the medial scalene; if it is constricting the plexus, excise enough of the muscle to relieve the pressure. Before dividing any structure be sure to identify the components of the plexus and subclavian artery. Remember that, in some instances, elements of the plexus penetrate the scalene; blind sectioning of these muscles may injure the plexus.

### Transaxillary Approach (Roos)

Place a small sandbag under the patient's shoulder and drape the arm separately so that it can be manipulated easily during the operation. Make a transverse incision across the axilla, following the skin crease; begin the incision well over the anterior border of the pectoralis major and extend it slightly downward across the posterior border of the axilla (Fig. 7-83A). Freely mobilize the skin flaps by sharp dissection; this step facilitates retraction of the edges of the incision. Develop the incision toward the costal cage and expose the second and third ribs and the scalenus anterior (Fig. 7-83B).

Develop the plane between the axillary fascia and the costal cage in an upward direction until the first rib comes into view. Now raise the arm completely and open the axillary tunnel; carefully isolate the first rib from all surrounding soft tissue. Identify the structures in the operative field; the brachial plexus lies posteriorly, the subclavian vein lies anteriorly, and the subclavian artery and the scalenus anterior lie in the middle of the field.

Isolate and divide the tendons of insertion of the scalenus anterior and the scalenus medius from the first rib and divide the subclavius muscle; do not injure the internal jugular vein while isolating the scalenus anterior. Carefully expose the first rib by sharp subperiosteal dissection; avoid injury to the pleura, which is in close proximity to the posterior surface of the rib. Now cut the rib close to the costochondral junction and disarticulate its posterior end from the transverse process.

Should the pleura accidentally be opened, place a small catheter in the opening and close the pleura around the catheter. Attach the other end of the catheter to a water-seal drainage system until the lung expands; this usually occurs within 2 or 3 hours.

**Transclavicular Approach (See p. 183)**

## BIBLIOGRAPHY

Agerholm, J. C., and Goodfellow, J. W.: Simple cysts of the humerus treated by radial resection. J. Bone & Joint Surg. (Brit.), *47-B*:714, 1965.

Brittain, H. A.: Architectural principles in arthrodesis. ed. 3. Edinburg, E. & L. Livingstone, 1952.

Charnley, J., and Houston, J. K.: Compression arthrodesis of the shoulder. J. Bone & Joint Surg. (Brit.), *46-B*:614-620, 1964.

Codman, E. A.: Epiphyseal chondromatous giant cell tumors of the upper end of the humerus. Surg., Gynec., Obstet., *52*:543, 1931.

Davis, J. B., and Cottrell, G. W.: A technique for shoulder arthrodesis. J. Bone & Joint Surg., *44-A*:657-661, 1962.

Déjerine-Klumpke, A.: Des polynévrites en général et des paralysies et atrophies saturnines en particulier. Étude clinique et anatomopathologique. Paris. Baillière, 1889.

Duchenne, G. B.: De l'électrisation localisée, et de son application à la pathologie et à la thérapeutique, 1855.

Duchenne, G. B. (Kaplan, E. B., trans. and ed.): Physiology of motion demonstrated by means of electrical stimulation and clinical observation and applied to the study of paralysis and deformities. Philadelphia, J. B. Lippincott, 1949.

Edeiken, J., and Hodes, P. J.: Roentgen Diagnosis of Diseases of Bone. p. 6.588. Baltimore, Williams & Wilkins, 1967.

Fairbank, H. A. T.: Birth palsy: subluxation of the shoulder joint in infants and young children. Lancet, *1*:1217, 1913.

Gill, A. B.: A new operation for arthrodesis of the shoulder. J. Bone & Joint Surg., *13*:287-295, 1931.

Gruenberg, H.: The genesis of skeletal abnormalities. Second International Conference on Congenital Malformations. New York, International Medical Congress, 219, 1963.

Harmon, P. H.: Anterior transplantation of the posterior deltoid for shoulder palsy and dislocation in poliomyelitis. Surg., Gynec. Obstet., *84*:117, 1947.

_____: Muscle transplantation for triceps palsy. The technique of utilizing the latissimus dorsi. J. Bone & Joint Surg., *31-A*:409, 1949.

_____: Surgical reconstruction of the paralytic shoulder by multiple muscle transplantations. J. Bone & Joint Surg., *32-A*:583, 1950.

Jaffe, H. L.: Tumors and tumorous conditions of the bones and joints. Philadelphia, Lea & Febiger, 1958.

Jaffe, H. L., and Lichtenstein, L.: Benign chondroblastoma of bone. Am. J. Path., *18*:969, 1942.

_____: Solitary unicameral bone cyst, with emphasis on the roentgen picture, the pathologic appearance and the pathogenesis. Arch. Surg., *44*:1004, 1942.

Jaffe, H. L., Lichtenstein, L., and Portis, R. B.: Giant cell tumor of bone: its pathological appearance, grading, supposed variants and treatment. Arch. Path., *30*:993, 1940.

Jaffe, H. L., Lichtenstein, L., and Sutro, C. J.: Pigmented villonodular synovitis, bursitis, tenosynovitis. Arch. Path., *31*:731, 1941.

Kendrick, J. I.: Changes in the upper humeral epiphysis following operations for obstetrical paralysis. J. Bone & Joint Surg., *19*:473, 1937.

Kleinberg, S.: Reattachment of the capsule and external rotators of the shoulder for obstetric paralysis. JAMA, *98*:294, 1932.

Klumpke, A. Contribution à l'étude des paralysies radiculaires du plexus brachial. Paralysies radiculaires totales, paralysies radiculaires inférieures. De la participation des filets sympathiques oculo-pupillaires dans ces paralysies. Étude clinique et expérimentale, Rev. Méd., 1885. pp. 591, 736.

L'Episcopo, J. B.: Restoration of muscle balance in the treatment of obstetrical paralysis. N. Y. J. Med., *39*:357, 1939.

Lombard, P.: La paralysie dite obstetricale du membre superieur (The so-called obstetrical paralysis of the upper extremity). Rev. orthop., *33*:235, 1947.

Mayer, L.: Tendons, ganglia, muscles, fascia. *In*: Lewis' Practice of Surgery. vol. 3. Hagerstown, Md., W. F. Prior, 1942.

_____: The significance of the iliocostal fascial graft in the treatment of paralytic deformities of the trunk. J. Bone & Joint Surg., *26*:257, 1944.

Monckeberg: Ueber Cystenbildung bei Ostitis fibrosa, Verh. Deut. Ges. Path., *7*:232, 1904.

Moore, B. H.: A new operative procedure for brachial birth palsy — Erb's paralysis. Surg., Gynec. Obstet., *61*:832, 1935.

Moore, B. H.: Brachial birth palsy. Am. J. Surg., *43*:338, 1939.

Moore, J. R.: Bone block to prevent posterior dislocation of the shoulder. (Personal communication)

Neer, C. S.: Articular replacement for the humeral head. J. Bone & Joint Surg., *37-A*:215-288, 1955.

Ober, F. R.: An operation to relieve paralysis of the deltoid muscle. JAMA, *99*:2182, 1932.

———: Transplantation to improve the function of the shoulder joint and extensor function of the elbow joint. American Academy of Orthopaedic Surgeons Instructional Course Lectures, vol. II. Ann Arbor, J. W. Edwards, 1944.

Phelps, W. M.: A method of resection of the infraspinous portion of the scapula without impairment of shoulder muscle function. Yale J. Biol. Med., *2*:39, 1929.

Platt, H.: Opening remarks on birth paralysis. J. Orthop. Surg., *2*:272, 1920.

Pommer. G.: Zur Kenntnis der progessiven Hamarton- und Phlegmasieveränderungen der Rohrenknochen, Arch. Orthop. Unfall chir., *17*:17, 1920.

Putti, V: Arthrodesis for tuberculosis of the knee and of the shoulder. Chir. organi mov., *18*:217, 1933.

Report of the Research Committee of the American Orthopaedic Association: The survey of end results on stabilization of the paralytic shoulder. J. Bone & Joint Surg., *24*:699-707, 1942.

Rogers, M. H.: An operation for the correction of the deformity due to "obstetrical paralysis." Boston M. & S. J., *174*:163, 1916.

Scaglietti, O.: Ricupero funzionale di un arto poliomielitico, Boll. e mem. Soc. Emiliano-Romagnola di chir. vol. I, 4-5, 1935.

———: Lesioni ostetriche della spalla. Chir. organi mov., *22*:183, 1936.

———: The obstetrical shoulder trauma. Surg., Gynec. Obstet., *66*:878, 1938.

Schottstaedt, E. R., Larsen, L. J., and Bost, F. C.: Complete muscle transposition, J. Bone & Joint Surg., *37-A*:897, 1955.

———: The surgical reconstruction of the upper extremity paralyzed by poliomyelitis. J. Bone & Joint Surg., *40-A*:633, 1958.

Sever, J. W.: Obstetric paralysis. Am. J. Dis. Child., *12*:541, 1916.

———: The results of a new operation for obstetrical paralysis. Am. J. Orthop. Surg., *16*:248, 1918.

———: Obstetric paralysis. JAMA, *85*:1862, 1925.

Slomann, H. C.: Kobenhavns med. selskabs forhandl., 1916-17, p. 95. Quoted by Toft, G.: On obstetrical paralysis of the upper extremities. Acta orthop. scandinav., *13*:218, 1942.

Steindler, A.: The reconstruction of upper extremity in spinal and cerebral paralysis. American Academy of Orthopaedic Surgeons Instructional Course Lectures. vol. 4. Ann Arbor, J. W. Edwards, 1949.

———: Reconstruction of the poliomyelitic upper extremity. Bull. Hosp. Joint Dis., *15*:21, 1954.

———: Reconstructive surgery of the upper extremity. New York, Appleton, 1923.

———: Operations on the upper extremity; problems in kinetics; end results. J. Bone & Joint Surg., *9*:404, 1927.

Taylor, A. S.: Results from surgical treatment of brachial birth palsy. JAMA, *48*:96, 1907.

———: Brachial birth palsy and injuries of similar type in adults. Surg., Gynec. Obstet., *30*:494, 1920.

Thomas, T. T.: Laceration of the axillary portion of the capsule of the shoulder joint as a factor in the etiology of traumatic combined paralysis of the upper extremity. Ann. Surg., *53*:77, 1911.

———: Obstetrical or brachial birth palsy. Am. J. Obstet., *73*:577, 1916.

———: Traumatic brachial paralysis with flail shoulder joint. Ann. Surg., *66*:532, 1917.

———: Brachial birth palsy: a pseudo-paralysis of shoulder joint origin. Am. J. Med. Sci., *159*:207, 1920.

Toft, G.: On obstetrical paralysis of the upper extremities. Acta orthop. scand., *13*:218, 1942.

Watson-Jones, R.: Extra-articular arthrodesis of the osteoarthritic shoulder. J. Bone & Joint Surg., *15*:862-871, 1933.

Wickstrom, J. Haslam, E. D., and Hutchinson, R. H.: The surgical management of residual deformities of the shoulder following birth injuries of the brachial plexus. J. Bone & Joint Surg., *37-A*:27, 1955.

Zachary, R. B.: Transplantation of teres major and latissimus dorsi for loss of external rotation at shoulder. Lancet, *2*:757, 1947.

# 8
# Injuries of the Shoulder in Sports

Next to the knee, the shoulder sustains the greatest number of soft tissue injuries. This is true for all age groups, and there are reasons for this. The shoulder is a complex system of joints, all working harmoniously to meet the demands of the hand. In fact, it is the base from which the arm and hand function; without the shoulder the hand would be a useless organ. Obviously the shoulder plays an important role in all human activities, be they related to work or play. The competitive sports so popular with the American public make great demands on the shoulder joint. And, because the public has become so conscious of physical fitness, strenuous athletic competition has become a way of life. A large segment of all age groups in one way or another participates in some kind of athletic endeavor. For children of school age, organized athletics is a must. In 1965 Wheatley reported that of 17 million children in the United States under 15 years of age, 6 million are injured sufficiently, at least once a year, to seek medical treatment.

Shoulder action occurs virtually in all sports, in baseball, football, basketball, softball and bowling it plays a major role. It also contributes significantly in sports that propel heavy objects, such as discus throwing, javelin and hammer throwing and shot putting. In all these sports the act of throwing is involved. The various soft tissue elements of the shoulder may be injured during execution of the act. The resulting disorders are produced by indirect forces expended at the site of the lesion. However, in contact and collision sports serious lesions may occur when great forces are applied directly to the shoulder.

In general, two forms of trauma produce the various lesions of the shoulders: direct trauma and indirect trauma. In direct trauma the force is applied directly at some area of the shoulder and the resulting lesion is at the point of contact. In indirect trauma the disruptive force generates at a distance from the shoulder—for example, the elbow or the hand. Then it courses up the arm to the shoulder, where it expends itself. In general, indirect mechanisms produce the following soft tissue lesions: strains of the musculotendinous units, sprains of varying degrees of the ligaments and capsules of joints which may be associated with subluxations and dislocations of the glenohumeral, acromioclavicular or sternoclavicular joints, and stretching or contusion of nerves in the region of the shoulder. Direct mechanisms cause contusions of soft tissues (muscles and nerves) and subluxation or dislocation of the acromioclavicular joint. (Direct mechanisms causing subluxation and dislocation of the glenohumeral and sternoclavicular joints are rare, but occasionally they do occur.) Both types of forces may produce fractures of any of the bony elements of the shoulder. The fracture may be an isolated lesion, such as fracture of the clavicle or of the upper end or shaft of the humerus. On the other hand, it may be associated with disruption of the ligamentous and capsular apparatus of one of the joints, as in fracture-dislocations.

Many variables influence the nature and severity of the injuries. These relate to the individual and to his environment. Age is very significant. Certain anatomical features render the adolescent prone to athletic injuries. The insertion of tendons into traction epiphyses is a weak point and a frequent site of injury. The muscle-tendon unit is far stronger than the junction of the pressure epiphysis and its metaphysis. This is the basis for epiphyseal separation such as occurs in the proximal end of the humerus. The epiphyses are relatively plastic and their blood supply is critical. Severe single trauma or repeated subclinical traumata may injure the epiphysis per se or its blood supply, causing its disintegration. Congenital anomalies previously unrecognized or considered insignificant (short leg, mild scoliosis, etc.) may mar the performance of the young athlete.

The adolescent athlete is mentally and physically immature. He lacks the professional's respect for body conditioning; therefore, he overextends his efforts, well beyond his physical tolerance which leads to fatigue, overstretching, and incoordination. All these factors make him more vulnerable to injury than his older counterpart.

Body type and body conditioning are very significant factors in the effectiveness of the athlete's performance. The tight athlete, whose joints lack complete mobility because of muscle contractures, is more prone to injury than the athlete with no muscle contractures and with freely movable joints. Fatigue definitely impairs athletic performance. Agility and good coordination of movements reduce the incidence of injury. And existing injuries, masked or unknown, render the athlete vulnerable to trauma.

Certain circumstances influencing the nature of an injury to the shoulder are beyond the individual's control. The position of the arm and forearm in relation to the shoulder at the moment of injury determines the type of the lesion. Also, in this regard, the momentum and direction of the body are significant considerations. Finally, the type and effectiveness of the protective gear that the athlete wears may determine the nature of the injury.

## THE THROWING ARM

Many disorders of the shoulder, especially in the athlete, are produced by the "throwing act." In order to identify these disorders understanding of the biomechanics of the throwing act and the various structures involved is essential.

The goal of the act is the propulsion of an object away from the body. It is achieved by transference of momentum generated by certain body elements to the object to be propelled. In sports such as baseball and football, the act must also impart direction to and control the trajectory of the object. The heavier the object to be propelled the greater the number of body elements that come into play. Also, more parts of the body are involved when speed and distance are desired.

The act from start to finish is the product of smooth rhythm and delicate coordination of all the body structures concerned. All body parts work synchronously or sequentially and with perfect timing. It reaches its highest level of perfection in competitive sports; baseball is an excellent example.

In the throwing act—the pitching of a baseball, for example—the shoulder is the principal performer; all other body elements play secondary roles. As pointed out by Slocum and Bateman, the shoulder provides (1) a base for the arm, which works as a lever, and (2) a fulcrum on which the whole arm can swing. The fulcrum action is most important, because it provides a specific region at the base of the lever for the institution of direction and control. The stage is now set for delivery of the ball. The wrist and the fingers execute the finer direction and control of the ball. The entire act brings into play movements of feet, legs and hips, rotation of the trunk, shifts of the body weight and even motion of the opposite arm. In this manner momentum is generated progressively and finally expended as the ball leaves the fingers.

## THE THROWING ACT: BASEBALL

The actual mechanism of the act comprises four stages: (1) the initial stance, (2) the wind-up and leg-kick (preparatory phase), (3) the initial forward action of the body and arm prior to release (downswing to release), and (4) the follow through.

In the initial stance, the trunk twists forward with the shoulder rotated internally. In the wind-up–leg-kick phase, the trunk twists backward, the arm is extended and then abducted and rotated externally, raising the extended wrist, forearm and elbow above the head. The weight shifts to the contralateral leg. The stage is now set for the powerful forward action of the body and arm comprising the last two steps of the act. In the downswing to release stage, the body initiates powerful, forward motion of the arm by first moving forward, then pivoting and finally rotating on the trunk. In the follow-through stage the humerus is whipped into extreme internal rotation and it flails the forearm and hand forward. The momentum generated by this act reaches its peak when the elbow is forcefully whipped into extension by the humerus. Throughout the throwing act the shoulder functions like the handle of a whip; it lashes the forearm and hand forward. This is truly a dynamic action produced by tremendous muscle effort.

None of the components of the shoulder possesses a stable, bony configuration. Stability of all elements depends upon the ligamentous and capsular structures and on the muscle masses that are the motors of the shoulder girdle. The platform of the arm is the scapula, which is held firmly against the thorax by the trapezius and the serratus anterior. During the preparatory phase of throwing, the arm is extended, abducted and externally rotated by the middle and posterior deltoid, the latissimus dorsi and the infraspinatus muscles. Synchronously, the anterior deltoid and the pectoralis major are stretched in readiness for their extreme effort to move the arm forward, and the posterior scapular muscles (levator scapulae and the rhomboids) pull the scapula backward.

Forward movement and internal rotation of the arm in the last two phases of the act are executed primarily by the anterior deltoid, the pectoralis major and the internal rotators of the rotator cuff. The great momentum generated during the throwing act puts tremendous strain on all the muscle-tendon units and capsular systems of the shoulder girdle and arm. Further, for the pitch to be effective, all muscle-tendon units must work smoothly, sequentially and without impediment. There is considerable variation in the throwing act in the different sports, depending upon the path the object is to travel and the distance it is to be thrown and, also, upon its weight, size and configuration. Thus the muscle-tendon units and ligaments subjected to great stress vary from sport to sport.

## PHYSIOLOGICAL PRINCIPLES OF MUSCLE-TENDON UNITS

Comprehension of the basic physiological principles governing the function of muscle-tendon units is essential to decipher the mechanism of injury. The dynamic structure of the muscle-tendon unit is the muscle, which converts chemical energy into mechanical energy. Synchronous movements are made possible by the reciprocal contraction-relaxation of antagonistic muscles, the rhythmic innervation of muscles supplying motor power to one or more joints and the intrinsic proprioceptive senses inherent in all joints.

The muscle-tendon unit consists of contractile and elastic elements, and the total tension curve of muscle is the sum of the contractile tension plus the elastic tension within the muscle. The connective tissues in the muscle determine the elastic tension, which is maximal at the unit's greatest length. The elastic components also provide the resistance of the muscle-tendon unit, in which the contractile elements play

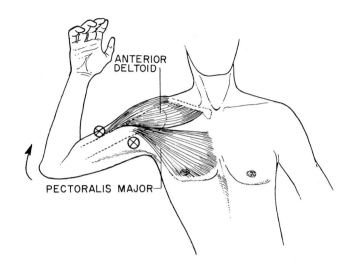

FIG. 8-1. During the preparatory phase of the throwing act when the arm has reached the extremes of abduction, extension and external rotation, the anterior deltoid and the pectoralis major are at their maximal length. With forward movement of the body more tension is applied to the muscle-tendon units and injury may result at their insertions.

an insignificant role. Extrinsic overload of a unit means uncontrolled overstretching of the unit when it is already stretched to a point near or at its greatest length. The tissues affected are the elastic tissues of the muscle, and tears may occur at the musculotendinous junction in the elastic tissue within the muscle or the tendon of origin or insertion may tear away from the bone. Essentially the mechanism is stretching of the tissues beyond their elastic limits by an external force. Besides external forces, other factors play a role in this mechanism of injury, and these factors render the person more vulnerable to injury. Some of the more common ones are: loss of normal joint motion, regardless of the cause: contracture of a muscle-tendon unit: fatigue, which not only reduces the alertness and agility of an athlete but also produces shortened muscles owing to incomplete relaxation: and degenerative alterations in muscles and tendons, owing either to aging or to repetitive trauma.

If a muscle is released at its extended length it will contract to a point known as the "rest-length"; this corresponds to the mid point of the contractile curve of the muscle. The contractile elements produce muscle tension and are the elements injured when the muscle is overloaded.

Intrinsic overloading means an injury to the contractile elements of muscle. If a muscle, at the mid point of the contraction or the contractile curve, is suddenly subjected to over-vigorous muscle effort, tearing of the contractile units of the muscle may occur. The injury occurs during the dynamic effort of muscle. An example of this is the sudden pain a pitcher experiences in the elbow joint (common flexors of the elbow) when he throws an overpowering pitch. Repetitive acts, as in throwing, produce fatigue of the muscle which results in the inability of the muscle to return to its normal rest-length. In the young pitcher this state produces some soreness and inability to extend the elbow completely for 24 to 48 hours. In the seasoned pitcher fibrosis occurs within the muscle, producing a chronic myostatic contracture. Subsequently, the elbow develops a permanent contracture; this limitation is accepted as normal and may be painless.

## INJURIES TO THE ANTERIOR MUSCLE-TENDON UNITS

Essentially these units comprise the anterior deltoid, the pectoralis major and the biceps. In the throwing arm, injuries rarely occur during the early stage of the preparatory phase of throwing. However, at the very end of this phase, when the arm reaches the extremes of abduction, extension and external rotation, the anterior units are at their maximal lengths. At this point, forward movement of the arm is started by a powerful forward and twisting movement of the body. This act puts even more tension on the muscle units, and injury may occur. The resulting injury may be caused by: (1) overpowering of the muscle-tendon units by a powerful force when the units are already at their maximal lengths, and (2) repeated forceful stretching of shortened muscles caused by myostatic contractures within the muscle (Fig. 8-1).

Other factors, both extrinsic and intrinsic, may render the units vulnerable to injury. In the presence of hidden or unknown disabilities, such as poor posture, loss of flexibility of the limb caused by myostatic contractures, scoliosis, or a short leg, the athlete may exert unusual power in an effort to compensate for the disability. Also, poor conditioning, fatigue and poor coordination may be responsible for exerting overpowering stress on the units and hence may reduce the effectiveness of the pitch and expose the units to injury.

As a result of overloading of the pectoralis major and anterior deltoid, tears may occur in the elastic components of the unit; they usually occur at or near the insertion of the tendon into the humerus. When the pectoralis major is involved, the athlete feels varying degrees of soreness in the upper and inner aspects of the humerus, and pressure over the posterior aspect of the bicipital groove elicits marked tenderness. Although an acute episode may cause only temporary impairment, repeated episodes may produce a subacute or chronic tendinitis which may result in prolonged or even permanent dysfunction. This condition is frequently encountered in javelin throwers as well as in baseball pitchers.

When the arm is in the extremes of extension, abduction and external rotation, great stress falls on the biceps muscle. Also, in this position the long head of the biceps presses firmly against the outer surface of the lesser tuberosity. Overloading of the muscle-tendon unit when the arm is in this position may result in tears of the tendon fibers, producing, clinically, bicipital tenosynovitis. Tenderness can be readily elicited along the course of the tendon in the intertubercular groove and along the anterior border of the deltoid. This lesion is commoner than is generally appreciated. When it occurs, it is usually during the conditioning period of the season, but it may occur at any time. In some instances it may be persistent, and even render the performance of the athlete totally ineffective (e.g., a javelin thrower, tennis player, or a baseball pitcher). Because strains of the long head of the biceps tendon are invariably associated with an inflammatory response of the synovial membrane lining the bicipital groove and of the synovial sheath of the tendon itself (tenosynovitis), all motions of the arm produce pain. Also, forceful flexion of the biceps and supination of the forearm against resistance accentuate the pain.

As a rule, displacement of the tendon from the intertubercular groove or rupture of the tendon does not occur in young athletes. However, when certain variations of the intertubercular sulcus are present, slipping and even complete displacement of the tendon out of the sulcus may occur. If the bicipital groove is very shallow, overloading the bicipital muscle-tendon unit when the arm is in extreme abduction and external rotation may force the tendon out of the groove. Although a shallow groove favors displacement of the biceps tendon, it may occur when the groove is anatomically adequate. The intertubercular fibers (transverse ligament) may be either attenuated or ruptured. The episode is usually associated with sudden stabbing pain in the anterior region of the shoulder and acute tenderness along the course of the tendon. All shoulder motions are painful. Later, some crepitus in the front of the shoulder can be palpated when the arm is abducted

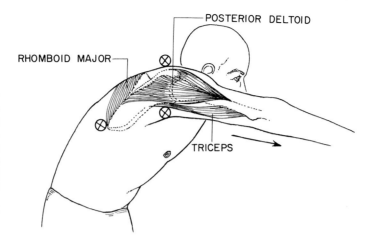

FIG. 8-2. During the follow-through phase the posterior muscle-tendon units reach their maximum tension and elongation; these are the posterior deltoid, the triceps and the rhomboid major. A powerful pitch may overpower the muscle units, causing an injury to their insertions.

and externally rotated. Occasionally, upon internal and external rotation of the arm, the tendon can be felt slipping in and out of the groove.

Underhand throwing, such as in softball and bowling, is a common cause of injury to the biceps muscle-tendon unit. In this act forceful supination and flexion of the forearm are the principal movements; but powerful internal rotation of the arm may also occur. The biceps is a powerful supinator as well as the most powerful flexor of the elbow. Overloading this muscle, as may occur in underhand throwing sports, may cause strains at either the proximal or the distal end of the muscle unit. In all such instances, an associated tenosynovitis exists. When the proximal portion is involved, the clinical manifestations are typical of the lesion and are readily identified. Repeated forceful internal rotation of the arm may strain or even tear some of the fibers of the tendon of the long head of the biceps as it is stretched against the greater tuberosity.

## INJURIES TO THE CONTRACTILE ELEMENTS OF THE DELTOID

Acute strains of the contractile elements of the anterior, middle and posterior portions of the deltoid muscle also may occur,

following sudden, over-vigorous muscle effort. These are dynamic strains. Acute strains of the anterior deltoid are by far the commonest and occur when the muscle is called to exert an extreme abduction effort against resistance in the frontal plane. The lesion is relatively common in football players. Not infrequently the unit is injured when a tackler with one laterally outstretched arm attempts to stop or impede the forward progress of a charging ball carrier. Pain and dysfunction may not be immediate. But, within 6 to 8 hours, the anterior portion of the deltoid becomes very painful, abduction in the frontal plane, especially against resistance, is weak, and demonstrable swelling of the anterior deltoid appears. The middle deltoid muscle sustains a similar injury when it contracts over-vigorously against resistance in the lateral plane. The injury may occur in any sport. As a rule, the immediate clinical manifestations are insignificant. Later, within 6 to 8 hours, soreness of the middle deltoid appears. The middle muscle mass is tender and abduction in the lateral plane is weak and painful.

Acute strains of the posterior deltoid muscle occur when it contracts over-vigorously, carrying the arm in a posterior direction; the butterfly stroke in swimming is a typical example. The clinical pattern is similar to that seen in strains of the anterior and middle deltoid except that the pain and tenderness are localized to the posterior portion of the deltoid.

## INJURIES TO THE POSTERIOR MUSCLE-TENDON UNITS

During the follow-through phase in the throwing act, the posterior units reach their maximum tension and elongation. The units primarily concerned at this point are: (1) the posterior deltoid, (2) the triceps, and (3) the rhomboid major. Injury to the posterior deltoid occurs at its site of insertion into the spine of the scapula. It is usually the result of throwing an overhand pitch and occurs at the end of the forward motion of the arm, at which point the muscle is at its maximum length. Not infrequently the injury occurs when, for some reason, the shoulder lacks a complete, free range of motion and timing and coordination are off (Fig. 8-2).

Injury to the triceps is usually associated with curve ball pitching. Again, tearing of the unit occurs at the extremes of forward motion when the muscle is fully elongated and an extra strain is placed on it when the elbow is forcefully flexed. The site of the tearing is at the scapular attachment of the long head of the triceps. The pitcher experiences a sudden, sharp, ripping pain in the region of the posterior axillary fold just under the glenohumeral joint. The area becomes painful and tender. Repeated episodes of this injury are often associated with periosteal bone formation and bony spurs at the scapular insertion of the triceps.

Again during the follow-through phase, the rhomboid major may sustain tears at or near its insertion into the lower portion of the vertebral border of the scapula. This type of injury, as a rule, occurs in discus throwers, who employ underhand throwing. Pain and tenderness is delineated to the scapular insertion of the muscle.

## INJURIES OF THE ROTATOR MUSCLES IN THE THROWING ARM

The internal group of muscles that produce the finer movements of the throwing act also may sustain tears in the act of throwing.

### Subscapularis

The subscapularis is a large, fan-shaped muscle lying directly in front of the shoulder joint and inserting into the lesser tuberosity by means of a flat, broad tendon. Together with the teres major and the latissimus dorsi it rotates the humerus inward. At the extreme of the preparatory phase of throwing when the arm is at the height of abduction and external rotation, the muscle-tendon unit is at its maximum length. With the initiation of the dynamic phase of throwing, the subscapularis contracts suddenly and powerfully, creating a tremendous load, and, hence, minute tears may occur at or near its bony insertion, giving rise clinically to a localized tendinitis. Repeated episodes create a subacute or chronic tendinitis which produces varying degrees of soreness or an aching discomfort on the anterior aspect of the shoulder and tenderness over the lesser tuberosity of the humerus.

### Supraspinatus, Infraspinatus and Teres Minor

These muscles, together with the subscapularis, are powerful fixers of the humeral head when abduction is initiated. In addition, supraspinatus is an abductor, and infraspinatus and teres minor are external rotators. In this group, minute tears within the muscles or at their insertions rarely occur during the preparatory phase of throwing. However, in the follow-through phase the pitcher actually "throws his arm at the batter." This maneuver creates a tremendous distraction force acting on all the structures attached to the posterior aspect of the shoulder joint, particularly the capsule, and causes severe stretching of the rotator muscles. Repetition of this maneuver is capable of producing not only minute tears and even avulsion of some fibers at the insertions of the tendons but also local attritional changes in the musculotendinous cuff. Again, clinically, a chronic form of tendonitis is established. Attrition need not be the result of recurrent acute episodes but may be subclinical in nature, caused by repeated strains which had given rise to no disability. However, in such circumstances, an acute superimposed episode may result in chronic disability. Healing is then slow and inadequate and the lesion may be refractory to all forms of treatment.

Fortunately, throwing does not produce massive cuff lesions very often. However, incomplete or partial tears, especially in the region of the supraspinatus, are not uncommon. Over-vigorous throwing before the muscles are fully flexible or unwise hard pitching in the preconditioning period are usually the responsible causes.

Occasionally, a terrific, powerful delivery may actually produce a complete tear of the cuff. This lesion differs from that seen in cuff avulsions of older persons. It usually is a linear defect in the cuff or a small complete avulsion of a small portion of the cuff from its bony insertion. The athlete is capable of full abduction of the arm, but, after a few innings, the arm becomes weak and, if tested against resistance, a decrease of abduction power is evident.

## CAPSULITIS OF THE POSTERIOR ASPECT OF THE SHOULDER

The tremendous follow-through effort stretches the posterior attachments of the capsule severely, producing minute tears at its site of insertion into the glenoid brim. The lesions are more prevalent in the postero-inferior region of the capsule.

Generally, there is always an associated involvement of the scapular insertion of the triceps. Repeated stretching produces osteophyte formation which is more prominent in the region of the triceps insertion. If some of the spurs become detached, loose bodies may be found in the joint.

Associated with attritional changes in the rotator cuff are alterations occurring in the humeral head. At the extremes of the preparatory phase, the arm is in extreme abduction and external rotation. A strenuous wind-up may jam the humeral head against the posterior lip of the glenoid fossa, causing furrowing or indentation of its articular surface. Repeated activation of this mechanism is capable of producing extensive secondary degenerative changes in the articular cartilage of the humeral head.

### Acute Deltoid Bursitis

Any of the strains I discussed in the previous section may be associated with implication of the subacromial bursa; careful examination usually discloses a strain of one of the muscle-tendon units either of the large external or of the short internal muscle groups.

Another cause of subdeltoid bursitis is excessive friction between the rotator cuff and the acromion. The bursal walls become irritated and thickened, thereby increasing the pressure between the cuff and the acromion. The thickened, pulled-up synovium may produce a painful arc syndrome or may even restrict the range of abduction by impinging against the acromion. Generally, the clinical manifestations are not severe; they are rather diffuse in nature and in some instances the pattern is subclinical. In the athlete, acute subacromial bursitis differs obviously from that form seen in clinical practice. The characteristic findings are: a deep seated ache in the shoulder, diffuse tenderness over the entire anterior aspect of the shoulder and, not infrequently, some palpable distention of the bursal sac. Rotation of the humerus forces the walls of the bursa into close contact; therefore, rotation of the arm—internal rotation especially— is particularly painful.

## SHOULDER INJURIES IN OTHER THROWING SPORTS

The previous sections have dealt primarily with lesions of the muscle-tendon units occurring in the baseball pitcher's shoulder. Injuries of the shoulder occur in the other throwing sports, such as football, javelin, discus and hammer throwing, bowling and softball. In each of these the mechanism of throwing differs as does the size, shape and weight of the object to be propelled. In each sport different muscle-tendon units are called upon to perform under maximum stress; hence, the injuries resulting from the throwing act differ in each sport.

### Football

#### Muscle Strains and Capsular Tears

Essentially the mechanism of throwing a football is similar to that of pitching a baseball, but there are considerable differences in each phase of the act in the two sports. In football, the windup is far less extreme than in baseball and the forward action of the body prior to the downward swing of the arm is less powerful. Also the arm in the follow-through phase travels a shorter distance; a football passer does not throw his arm at the receiver as does a pitcher at a batter. Nevertheless, extrinsic overloading of both the anterior and the posterior muscle units of the shoulder may occur, resulting in muscle strains and stretching and tearing of the capsule of the glenohumeral joint. The lesions are never as severe as they are in baseball and rarely produce chronic disability. This is understandable when the difference in the frequency of the throwing act in the two sports is taken into account.

## Subluxation and Dislocation of the Glenohumeral Joint

Subluxation and dislocation of the glenohumeral joint are relatively frequent in football players, more so than in baseball players. Undoubtedly, the nature of the preparatory phase of throwing in football, which brings the arm into a position of wide abduction and external rotation, plus the weight of the football are contributing causative factors.

Subluxation occurs when the arm is suddenly and forcefully abducted and externally rotated. The passer experiences a slipping sensation on the anterior aspect of the shoulder. By internally rotating and lowering the arm he is able to reduce the subluxation, usually with an audible click. As a rule, each episode is associated with varying degrees of soreness about the shoulder and weakness of the arm which subsides after a period of rest of 10 to 14 days. If properly treated, an initial episode of subluxation may be cured, but this is rare. Generally, it becomes recurrent in nature and, if not treated surgically, will go on to recurrent dislocation.

Recurrent dislocation of the glenohumeral joint is produced by the same mechanism that produces recurrent subluxation. The initial lesion is rarely produced by the mechanism of throwing alone; usually some external force is applied to the abducted and externally rotated arm. Once an initial dislocation has occurred the chances of it becoming a recurrent lesion are extremely high in young athletes. If the player desires to continue playing the sport, the shoulder should be stabilized surgically. The problems related to subluxation and dislocation of the glenohumeral joint are discussed in detail in Chapter 10.

### Hammer, Javelin, and Discus Throwing and Shot Putting

In these sports the objects to be thrown are relatively bulky and heavy. And, although the act of throwing is basically the same as in pitching a baseball, the tremendous strain of propelling the objects falls on the posterior muscle-tendon units of the shoulder, especially those anchoring the scapula to the trunk. The injuries occur when the momentum of the follow-through phase reaches its peak; at this point the units are stretched tremendously. Repeated acute episodes of muscle strains occur frequently in these sports.

The common sites of injury are the interscapular and scapulocostal regions. In the former, the origin of the trapezius into the spinous processes of the cervical and dorsal vertebrae may suffer tears varying from minute tears to gross avulsion of its fibers. In the latter, the same lesions may occur at the insertion of the levator scapulae, rhomboid minor and rhomboid major into the vertebral border of the scapula and at the insertion of the serratus anterior into the inferior angle of the scapula. The patient has localized tenderness at the site of the lesion along the vertebral border of the scapula or over the spinous processes of the cervical and dorsal vertebrae. There may be local swelling at these points and the entire shoulder aches and is weak. Repeated episodes may result in a chronic tendonitis which may seriously impair the effectiveness of the throwing act.

Rotator cuff lesions may also occur in these sports, but they are rare. This is also true of capsular strains. When they do occur in the capsule, it is chiefly the posterior insertion of the capsule into the glenoid brim that is affected.

### Bowling, Curling and Softball

In these sports the objects to be propelled are heavy and the delivery is accomplished by a flexion mechanism. This puts tremendous strain on the anterior muscle-tendon units of the shoulder and the anterior portion of the capsule of the glenohumeral joint. The biceps tendon is frequently involved because the forearm action is a dominant factor in the act which places tremendous stress on the biceps. Uncontrolled deliveries, especially those associated with extreme internal rotation and flexion of the arm, may severely stretch the biceps tendon in its groove. Repetition of the act may result in a chronic form of bicipital tenosynovitis; or the tendon may undergo degenerative changes and even rupture. Many participants of these sports are middle aged or older. In these, physiological degenerative alterations in the tendon are common findings. Such circumstances increase the vulnerability of the tendon.

When the act is associated with powerful flexion and supination of the forearm, the biceps tendon tends to slip out of the groove. This mechanism places considerable strain on the transverse ligament which spans the groove and fixes the tendon in place. Repetition of the act may stretch and even tear the fibers of the transverse ligament, allowing the tendon to slip out of the groove. This is especially true if the groove is congenitally shallow.

### INJURIES OF THE SHOULDER IN CONTACT SPORTS

These injuries are sustained by the application of a powerful force to some region of the shoulder girdle. They occur infrequently in baseball except when a runner trips and falls, landing on the point of his shoulder. However, in football, soccer and hockey they are relatively common lesions. Little damage occurs if the force is applied to the anterior or posterior aspects of the shoulder. When the force is applied to the lateral aspect, great damage may ensue. The direction of the force (it may be applied from above directly to the lateral portion of the shoulder or obliquely from behind) and the intensity of the force govern the type of the resulting lesion. Violent contact with the lateral aspect of the shoulder results in injuries of the acromioclavicular joint or the coracoclavicular ligament or fracture of the clavicle. If the force is applied from above, the acromioclavicular joint may be sprained in varying degree and the injury may be associated with a fracture of the outer end of the clavicle. Forces applied obliquely from behind may dissipate at the sternoclavicular joint; the resulting injury varies with the severity of the acting force.

Such are the injuries sustained when a forward rushing ball carrier tries to knife through the line and instead meets the padded shoulder of a burly tackle or guard. The same lesions result when a player falls and his shoulder is the part of his body to first make contact with the ground. The momentum of the player and his weight, together with the angle of contact the shoulder makes with the ground, determine the type of injury to the shoulder girdle. The diagnosis and management of lesions of the acromioclavicular and sternoclavicular joints are discussed in detail in Chapter 9.

### Strains of the Trapezius

The trapezius, because of its size and exposed position, is frequently injured in contact sports. This muscle and the levator scapulae are the only structures that suspend the shoulder and keep the scapula in normal relationship with the thoracic cage. The muscle has two anatomical components, the proximal portion and the distal portion. The former extends from the occipital protuberance and ligamentum nuchae to the posterior border of the outer end of the clavicle, the acromion and the spine of the scapula. The latter lies below the spine of the scapula. Forceful depression of the shoulder can be restrained or prevented only by the action of the proximal portion of the trapezius and the levator scapulae. It is evident that injuries to this suspensory apparatus must occur frequently in collision sports such as football and hockey.

A powerful blow depressing the shoulder while the head is forced to the opposite side may result in severe stretching of the proximal portion of the trapezius. The same mechanism is at work when the head is suddenly twisted to one side while the arm is pulled in the opposite direction. Occasionally the violence is so overwhelming that the shoulder is displaced far downward and forward, causing avulsion of the fibers of insertion of the muscle into the clavicle. This lesion may be complicated by a contusion or stretching of the brachial plexus.

The clinical manifestations vary from simple soreness on the side of the affected muscle, with little or no spasm, to muscle spasm so severe that the neck and head are fixed, the shoulder droops and effective use of the girdle and arm is impaired.

### Muscle Contusions

Certain muscles of the shoulder girdle are especially vulnerable to contusion injuries in collision sports such as football, hockey and lacrosse. The trapezius is such a muscle. The portion of the muscle most likely to be contused is the proximal portion. The contusions are usually the result of direct impacts from above. In most violent injuries, the pain is excruciating and localized swelling and tenderness are usually readily demonstrable. In addition, the pain may be of such intensity that abduction of the arm is weak and painful. This lesion frequently is erroneously diagnosed as a sprain of the acromioclavicular joint.

Direct, violent blows from above contuse not only the trapezius but also the posterior portion of the deltoid just lateral to the trapezius. The lesion is frequently referred to as the "shoulder pointer" and may be difficult to distinguish from a minor sprain of the acromioclavicular joint with no clinical evidence of laxity. Careful examination reveals acute tenderness and swelling localized to the muscle fibers affected, whereas tenderness over the acromioclavicular joint is minimal or absent. The joint exhibits no clinical evidence of laxity and no tenderness over the region of the coracoclavicular ligament.

## DIAGNOSIS AND MANAGEMENT

In this section I shall discuss only the diagnosis and management of strains and contusions of the muscle-tendon units about the shoulder joint. The diagnosis and management of sprains of the articulations comprising the shoulder girdle are dealt with in Chapter 9.

In order to make an accurate diagnosis of any injury and to institute adequate management, a clear understanding of the actual pathology of the lesion and of the nature of the healing process is essential. This is especially important in athletic injuries, because time is such a precious commodity, and earliest possible return to full participation the goal.

### Pathology of Injury

The basic pathological lesion of injury is dissolution or disruption of normal tissue in varying degrees. In athletic injuries this may result from intrinsic or extrinsic overloading of the muscle-tendon units or crushing of a local area of tissue by direct violence such as occurs in a contusion. As previously noted, dissolution of a small area of the contractile unit of a muscle as a result of intrinsic overloading is associated with pain on stretching the muscle and severe muscle spasm; this comprises the "charley-horse."

Likewise, injuries designated as sprains of various degrees are dissolutions or disruptions of the ligamentous fibers and of capsular structures. The lesions may be of microscopic or of gross dimensions. In certain locations, complete disruption of the ligamentous and capsular structures indicates a dislocation or subluxation of a joint. It is important to appreciate and be able to evaluate the great variability of tissue disruption in soft tissue injuries, because closely correlated with the severity of the lesion are the amount of tenderness and swelling, the intensity of the pain, the degree of dysfunction, the response to treatment, the time required for complete healing and the prognosis.

### The Healing Process In Injury

The healing process comprises many stages which follow consecutively until final repair of the tissue is achieved. If not interfered with, the process is completed in a relatively short period of time. In every injury vascular channels are disrupted; these may be veins, arteries and capillaries. Before healing can begin bleeding must cease. This is achieved by formation of intravascular clots or thrombi. With cessation of bleeding organization of the thrombi begins, the area is permeated by capillaries and vascular granulation tissue appears. Numerous macrophages and inflammatory cells invade the traumatized tissue and remove the remnants of dead tissue cells and the products of extravasated blood. The entire area is now invaded by young fibroblasts dispersed in a fine network of fibrin which restores continuity between the disrupted elements. Also, depending on the type of tissue involved, regeneration of traumatized elements occurs. The end result is a mass of closely knit fibrous tissue occupying the entire interval between the disrupted elements; this varies with the size of the lesion. With maturation of the fibrous tissue, the granulation tissue and the inflammatory elements disappear, reduction in the number of vascular channels occurs rapidly and the entire mass of scar tissue contracts precipitously.

In general, the stages of repair occur sequence, but there is considerable overlap in different areas of the same lesion and considerable variation in time in different tissues. Good, firm fibrous union occurs within 10 to 12 days.

As the healing process progresses from stage to stage, the clinical appearance and the feel of the area also change. This is of utmost importance: the changing characteristics of the lesion provide the physician with a yardstick with which to measure the extent of healing from day to day. Since most injuries in athletes are superficial, they can readily be inspected and palpated; this should be done daily in order to determine the state of healing, knowledge of which is essential to further treatment.

Often the physician is tempted to stimulate the progress of healing. Remember, however, that athletic injuries occur in youths in prime physical condition, whose healing powers are at the highest possible level. The wise doctor allows nature to take its course, for no further stimulation is necessary. All the various modalities, such as whirlpool, deep radiant heat, and ultrasonics, do nothing to increase the rate of healing and may overtax the natural processes. Also, the local administration of steroids is definitely contraindicated because they tend to suppress the inflammatory process that is so essential in the healing process of acute injuries.

If the injured area is carefully inspected and gently palpated every day—and this should be done routinely for all athletic injuries—an accurate appraisal of the state of healing is readily made. At the initial stage, when bleeding has stopped, there is local swelling but no increase in tenderness. In the next stage, evidence of an inflammatory reaction appears; the area is red, the skin temperature rises and the entire area becomes more tender. In the final stage, recession of the inflammatory process may be observed: the skin loses its redness, the area is thickened, brawny and rubbery in consistency, and pain decreases steadily. There is considerable variation in these clinical manifestations, depending on the severity of the lesion and the tissue affected.

## Diagnosis of Injuries to the Shoulder

In order to make an examination of the shoulder that will produce meaningful results, the physician needs to be thoroughly familiar with the detailed anatomy of the region. Lack of this knowledge can only lead to a vague, slip-shod diagnosis without full appreciation of the structures involved or the extent of the injury. In addition, he should have a clear understanding of the components of the act of throwing and the muscle-tendon units vulnerable to injury in each component.

A detailed history of the mechanism of the injury is mandatory; it should include the position of the extremity at the time of injury, the manner in which the injury occurred and, if there was an impact, the angle of the impact. If an injury occurred during throwing, the exact point in the act at which maximum pain occurred gives a clue to the structures involved. Sudden pain on the anterior aspect of the shoulder during the entire stage of forward movement of the body indicates either a tearing of the fibers of insertion of the anterior deltoid or the pectoralis major or both, or an injury to the biceps tendon, which tends to subluxate when the arm is in the position of abduction and full external rotation. On the other hand, pain in the posterior aspect of the arm during the follow-through phase of throwing implicates the insertion of the posterior deltoid into the spine of the scapula or the tendon of insertion of the long head of the triceps into the scapula just beneath the glenohumeral joint or the insertion of the rhomboid major into the vertebral border of the scapula. Also, some fibers of the posterior capsule may stretch and tear.

Careful inspection of the shoulder girdle will often reveal swelling at the site of impact, or deformity of one of the articulations. In the absence of any visible evidence of injury, meticulous and gentle palpation of the elements of the girdle, particularly along the sites of insertions of the muscle-tendon units, is the most important part of the examination. First palpate the clavicle over its entire length, beginning over the sternoclavicular joint, then proceeding to the acromioclavicular joint and the region of the coracoclavicular ligament. Palpate all margins of the acromion process, beginning anteriorly, passing around to the lateral and posterior borders and continuing posteriorly along the entire spine of the scapula. Now, palpate along the entire vertebral border of the scapula. Next, inspect the region of the biceps tendon; palpate over the course of the tendon itself and the areas just anterior and posterior to the bicipital groove. A tenderness just posterior to the groove indicates an injury to the pectoralis major, whereas tenderness directly over the lesser tuberosity implicates the insertion of the subscapularis muscle. Finally, palpate all regions of the glenohumeral joint, with the arm in different degrees of rotation. Localization of tenderness in this small area must be precise to be meaningful. Is the tenderness directly over the insertion of the infraspinatus, or slightly more posterior, over the insertions of the infraspinatus and teres minor: or is it still more posterior and inferior, over the scapular insertion of the triceps?

The next step is appraisal of the movements of the arm, first without resistance and then with resistance. Test the power of the arm in all planes: abduction, forward flexion, backward extension, horizontal flexion and extension and, finally, rotation. While the patient executes the movements, note if there is any limitation of motion in any of the planes of movement. Also note if there is pain in only a small arc of the total range of a specific movement (painful arc syndrome) such as occurs in partial tears of the rotator cuff.

Finally, note if there is any winging of the scapula, indicating a lesion of the serratus anterior. Have the patient "wall walk" both hands. This test reveals even minor degrees of winging of the scapula.

Roentgenograms should be made of all injured shoulders. Besides the conventional anteroposterior views, supero-inferior views and views with the humerus in varying degrees of rotation should be taken. Also, roentgenograms of the acromioclavicular joint should be a part of the routine examination.

Arthrograms of the glenohumeral or acromioclavicular joint are done only if implication of these joints is suspected. An arthrogram is a useful tool for making a diagnosis of a partial or complete tear of the rotator cuff.

From the history and the examination, establish whether there has been an acute injury or an exacerbation of a chronic lesion. Also, determine the severity of the injury to the muscle-tendon unit. Does the dissolution of fibers of the unit involve a small area or a large area, or is there complete dissolution of the tendon at some point? Correct evaluation of the nature and extent of the injury is mandatory in order to institute a logical, effective regimen of therapy.

### Management of Acute Strains

**Partial Dissolution of the Muscle-Tendon Units.** In this category the injuries may vary from dissolution of only a few fibers to a great many fibers of the unit; however, complete rupture of the tendon has not occurred. The intensity of the symptoms and the resulting dysfunction of the shoulder depend upon the severity of the lesion. Regardless of the extent of these injuries, specific principles of treatment that have proved to be effective in practice should be followed. Because acute rupture of fibers within a unit is accompanied by hemorrhage and swelling, the first step in the management of all acute injuries is to control bleeding and reduce swelling. By so doing the first stage of healing is enhanced. (Remember that the healing process begins with cessation of bleeding.) This is achieved by the application of cold, by applying either ice bags or cold packs. Cold causes local vasoconstriction and favors the formation of thrombi necessary to stop bleeding. It should be continued as long as necessary —at least 24 to 48 hours, and as much as, 72 hours if necessary. Some form of pressure over the swelling should be used if it can possibly be applied. This, too, helps to stop further extravasation of blood and reduce swelling. It is difficult to apply localized pressure to the shoulder girdle; here the use of sponge rubber pads held in place by adhesive tape is effective.

The next important step in therapy at this stage of the injury is rest to the part. This cannot be overemphasized. Rest prevents further bleeding and controls forces that cause further tissue disruption. In the shoulder, the use of a sling places the extremity and shoulder girdle at rest. At this point, it should be remembered that prolonged immobilization of the shoulder, regardless of the injury, is harmful and must be avoided. The exception to this is disruption of the articulations of the shoulder, such as dislocation of the glenohumeral, acromioclavicular or sternoclavicular joints. Such lesions require significant time for the disrupted ligaments and capsular tissues to heal; hence, long periods of immobilization are unavoidable.

For the injuries under discussion, graduated motion should be started as soon as there is clinical evidence that bleeding has stopped and swelling is subsiding. This entails constant, daily surveillance of the injury by the physician. If local swelling and tenderness do not increase, the activity will enhance the healing process and prevent loss of muscle tone and power not only of the affected muscle unit but of the other units of the shoulder girdle as well. It should be remembered that the athlete expends much time and effort in attaining the level of body conditioning necessary for him to perform effectively. A setback in his physical conditioning means loss of time and denial of participation in the sport.

For most athletes, this is hard to take. On the other hand, increased tenderness and local swelling following activity indicates that the muscle unit is being overtaxed; this is a signal to enforce rest and reduce the activity.

Just as soon as the injured tissues become brawny, thickened and less tender, as revealed by careful clinical examination, the controlled rehabilitation program can be intensified. By adhering to these principles the healing process is greatly accelerated, healing occurs with minimal fibrous tissue, all muscles of the shoulder girdle remain in top conditioning and the athlete loses very little time.

Finally, full participation in athletics is not resumed until the area affected is no longer tender, the muscle-tendon unit is not painful on effort and muscle strength returns to normal. The participation should be gradual, working up to the anticipated demands on the arm. In baseball pitchers, the gradual rehabilitation program must be carefully supervised and controlled. Too often the entire healing process is completely disrupted by one hard pitched ball.

A word should be said about the various modalities and drugs, chiefly steroids, so frequently employed to accelerate healing and relieve pain. In acute injuries, I believe that the many highly advertised modalities—ultrasonics, diathermy, infrared, hydrocollators and the like—in no way enhance the healing process; if anything, they deter it. They should be avoided assiduously. Likewise, steroids in acute injuries retard healing because of their anti-inflammatory action. The injection of anesthetic agents into an acute injury for the purpose of relieving pain and returning the player to the game is deplorable treatment. Pain and tenderness are signals indicating tissue disruption and the degree of progress of healing. If they are nullified by anesthetic agents, there is no index of the extent of the injury or the progress of the healing process.

## Management of Specific Minor Injuries of the Muscle-Tendon Units

The mechanism of injury and the pertinent clinical manifestations of most of the units of the shoulder girdle have been discussed previously. The management of the lesions to be considered here is remarkably similar, following the principles of treatment noted above.

**Acute Strains of the Deltoid Muscle.** Acute strains may occur in the anterior, lateral or posterior portion of the deltoid, depending upon vigorous muscle effort in differing planes. These are relatively common injuries in baseball and football. Disabling symptoms, as a rule, are not immediate: however, within 6 to 10 hours they may become severe. During this time, a palpable and visible swelling may appear in the portion of the muscle involved and the player has weak elevation of the arm in the appropriate plane. Pain is intensified when the arm is raised against resistance.

The immediate treatment consists of the application of cold to the affected part either by ice bags or cold packs, shoulder-cap strapping to make compression and a sling to rest and support the arm. Within 24 to 48 hours allow active motion of the arm under a hot shower and full activity after the third or fourth day. This does not mean that a pitcher returns to hard ball-throwing at this time; rather, the rehabilitation must be gradual in nature. Throwing is discontinued until all soreness disappears; then gentle tossing of the ball is permissible. This is followed by progressively harder throwing until the pitcher reaches his maximal level of performance. During the rehabilitation period the doctor keeps the athlete under close surveillance, making sure that the arm shows no evidence of reinjury and does show evidence of increasing strength and tolerance and that both the athlete and the coach do not push the program too fast. It may require two to three weeks, and more at times, to return a player to full participation.

Local administration of steroids in a true acute injury is of doubtful value; I do not believe it should be done. Nor should anti-inflammatory drugs be prescribed. As previously noted, physical therapy modalities in these injuries are worthless and may do harm.

Deltoid strains occurring in athletes other than baseball players respond, strikingly and rapidly, to the above program of treatment. Many players can return to full activity within four to seven days, depending upon the severity of the initial acute injury and the position they play on the team.

**Acute Subdeltoid Bursitis.** This lesion is never primary; it is invariably secondary to a deltoid strain or a strain of one of the rotator muscles of the shoulder or of the biceps tendon. The initial lesion of the muscle-tendon units is never severe, so that in many instances the player is able to continue full activity with only minor discomfort.

Clinically, the pain or discomfort is deep seated, vague and diffuse. However, aggravation of the symptoms occurs when certain movements are made, especially against resistance. Often a diffuse swelling of the entire subdeltoid region is palpable.

The treatment is similar to that described for deltoid strains: ice bags, sling and complete rest for 24 to 48 hours; then a program of graduated, increasing activity under close supervision. Generally, the player returns to full participation in four to seven days.

**Acute Strains and Contusions of the Trapezius Muscle.** As previously stated, the proximal portion of the trapezius (that portion between the occiput and the spine of the scapula) together with the levator scapulae comprise the true suspensory apparatus of the shoulder girdle. Also, these are the muscles that resist depression of the girdle. Both muscle units are frequently injured in collision sports, and, because they are exposed, they are frequently the recipients of powerful blows from above, as often occurs in hockey. Direct blows from above may contuse not only the trapezius but also the posterior portion of the deltoid. Not infrequently these lesions are erroneously diagnosed as sprains of the acromioclavicualr joint.

The clinical manifestations are variable. They may range from simple soreness on the affected side, with little if any dysfunction, to severe pain, muscle spasm, weak abduction and drooping of the shoulder.

The management is similar to that of deltoid strains. It consists of ice bags to the area and the wearing of a sling for the first 24 hours. When spasm persists, hot showers are beneficial; they relieve spasm, have a soothing effect and favor restoration of motion. Also, gentle massage together with radiant heat tends to reduce spasm and pain. Rehabilitation of the arm should be gradual and progressive, keeping the movements always within the tolerance of pain. Contused muscles usually respond promptly, and return to full activity in a matter of three or four days. Stretched muscle-tendon units may require a longer period of time, seven to ten days, before forceful movements of the arm can be executed.

**Acute Strains of the Rotatory Muscles.** The subscapularis is usually injured when the dynamic phase of throwing is initiated. At this point the arm is in extreme external rotation and abduction, and the subscapularis is at its maximum length. With forceful contraction of the muscle, tears may occur at or near its bony insertion.

On the other hand, the supraspinatus, infraspinatus and teres minor usually sustain injuries at their sites of insertion in the follow-through phase of throwing when the pitcher "throws his arm at the batter." The lesions are the result of severe overstretching of the muscles.

Rarely do the rotator muscles suffer complete tears of their tendinous insertions. If a complete tear should occur, it is linear in nature, involving the supraspinatus area.

Partial or incomplete tears of the cuff are more common.

By employing the method of examination and the performing of appropriate functional tests previously described, the extent and nature of the lesion of each of the rotator muscles can be determined. The initial treatment should be application of ice for 24 to 48 hours to the affected muscle and the wearing of a sling, followed by hot showers and motion of the arm within the tolerance of pain. Throwing is prohibited until all soreness disappears; then it is resumed but light throwing only is permitted. The tolerance and the strength of the unit must be checked constantly. Muscle effort must be increased by a graduated program. Return to full activity may require two to three weeks.

### Acute Partial and Complete Tears of the Cuff

In addition to the minor strains just described, more serious lesions, such as a partial avulsion of a portion of the cuff or even a complete tear of the cuff, may occur when a ball is being pitched hard. Partial avulsion causes immediate sharp pain, followed by an aching discomfort in the shoulder. Pain usually occurs at the end of the delivery after such an injury, and posterior tenderness is readily demonstrable. If these lesions are treated according to the method described for strains of the cuff and if hard pitching is eliminated until healing is complete, a satisfactory result can be anticipated.

When a complete tear occurs, the problem is entirely different. Clinically, the initial manifestations are the same. However, even with careful and conscientious management the pitcher tires after a few innings, and functional tests reveal some weakness of abduction against resistance. The diagnosis may be difficult to make but it can be established by an arthrogram. If a complete tear is present, surgical repair becomes mandatory. The tear, as a rule, is a linear defect in the supraspinatus region of the cuff and can be repaired with minimal trauma to the overlying structures. If a controlled and graduated rehabilitation program is instituted after the surgery, a complete recovery can be anticipated. For the technique of repairs of cuff tears see page 232.

### Injuries of the Biceps

It was previously noted that stretching and tearing of fibers of the tendon of the long head of the biceps muscle may occur in throwing. In baseball, when the arm is in extreme abduction and external rotation, great tension is imposed on the biceps tendon. Should a shallow bicipital groove be present the tendon may subluxate or even dislocate. Dislocation of the tendon is indeed rare in athletes, but it may occur. In sports using underhand delivery, the tendon may be injured by an entirely different mechanism. Underhand throwing requires powerful supination and flexion of the forearm, and both movements are performed by the biceps. In addition, vigorous internal rotation of the arm may occur in the throwing act. If overloading of the biceps occurs, strains may occur at either end of the muscle-tendon unit.

The acute injuries readily respond to a regimen comprised of ice to the affected area and rest of the arm in a sling for the first 24 hours, followed by radiant heat or hot showers and a graduated program of rehabilitation.

Conservative measures are futile for chronic dislocating tendons. In these instances the tendon should be anchored in the bicipital groove and that portion proximal to the site of attachment should be excised.

### Management of Complete Dissolution of Muscle-Tendon Units

Complete disruption of muscle-tendon units about the shoulder is rare. When such

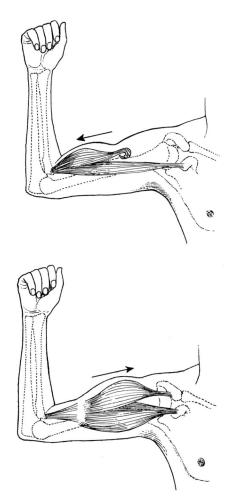

(*Top*) Fig. 8-3. Rupture of the tendon of the long head of the biceps. The muscle belly migrates distally; the deformity is readily seen when the arm is abducted, flexed at the elbow 90° and externally rotated.

(*Bottom*) Fig. 8-4. Rupture of the biceps at the distal musculotendinous juncture. The muscle mass migrates proximally.

a lesion does occur the integrity of the unit must be restored. This should be done as early as possible in order to avoid too much scar formation and retraction and shortening of the ruptured ends of the tendon. Prompt surgical repair is the only means of assuring restitution of normal continuity, length and strength of the unit.

I have never seen an acute massive avulsion of the rotator cuff in athletes except when it was associated with a dislocation of the shoulder. However, I have seen several small avulsions and complete linear defects resulting from strenuous abduction of the arm against resistance and from delivering a powerful pitch. The diagnosis may be difficult to make and at first the symptoms may simulate those of a subdeltoid bursitis. If evaluation of the patient definitely establishes a diagnosis of a complete lesion, surgical repair is indicated. As previously noted, the arthrogram is a valuable tool for confirming the diagnosis; it may be the only study that makes this diagnosis clear.

Acute rupture of the biceps tendon also is a rare lesion in young athletes, but it, too, may occur when the muscle contracts forcefully, especially against resistance. The rupture may occur at its insertion into the glenoid, at the musculotendinous juncture or at some point along the course of the tendon (Fig. 8-3 and 8-4). Pain is immediate and intense and is followed by an ache and tenderness along the course of the long head of the biceps. The muscle belly tends to migrate distally. This is readily demonstrable if the patient's arm is abducted, rotated externally and flexed at the elbow 90°; now, upon active contraction of the biceps the muscle mass moves towards the elbow.

Rupture of the long head of the biceps does cause some weakness of the shoulder; however, its effect on supination of the forearm is more important. It must be remembered that the biceps is a powerful supinator of the forearm. In young men the tendon should be anchored to the upper end of the humerus and the intracapsular portion of the tendon excised.

## CHRONIC STRAINS

Frequent repetition of the act of throwing may produce microscopic tears at the origin of insertion of the muscle-tendon units. Initially they may cause no pain or dysfunction, being subclinical in nature. However, with time, scarring and attritional changes occur at the sites of insult, resulting in chronic tendonitis. Essentially, these are chronic strains and may seriously impair the performance of the athlete. Examples of such lesions are the "tennis elbow," which is a chronic strain of the common extensor muscles of the forearm at their insertion into the lateral condyle, and the "pitcher's elbow," a chronic strain of the flexor muscles of the forearm at their insertion into the medial condylar area of the elbow.

In the shoulder similar lesions occur at the insertion of the rotator cuff into the tuberosities of the humeral head, at the insertion of the teres major into the scapula and at the site of the posterior attachment of the capsule into the glenoid. Scarring, thickening and roughening of the rotator cuff reduce the interval between its superior surface and the coracoacromial arch. When this circumstance exists the walls of the intervening subdeltoid bursa may become irritated and thickened, producing a bursitis (Fig. 8-5).

The biceps muscle may be similarly affected in the throwing arm; a tenosynovitis may be very disabling. In addition, constant irritation of the long head of the biceps tendon and its synovial sheath may produce a reactive process in the bony intertubercular sulcus. As a result, osteophytes and spurs form along the sides and on the floor of the groove. Excursion of the tendon in the groove is interfered with and the tendon may become firmly adherent in the groove. Such a lesion may be very disabling and may resist all forms of conservative treatment.

When the rotator cuff is involved, tenderness is localized along the line of its insertion into the tuberosities; if the bursa is involved the tenderness is more diffuse. Straining of the involved muscle units causes pain and this is even more evident if the unit is made to work against resistance. In mild forms there may be no loss

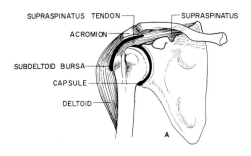

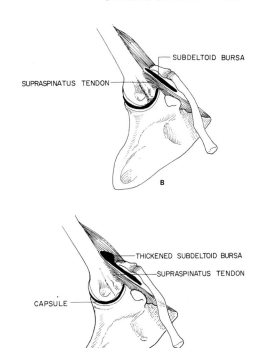

Fig. 8-5. Subdeltoid bursa. (A) With the arm at the side the greater part of the subdeltoid bursa lies under the deltoid. (B) With the arm abducted, the bursa migrates under the acromion; also note the narrow interval between the acromion and greater tuberosity through which the supraspinatus tendon must travel when the arm is widely abducted. (C) When the walls of the bursa are thickened, as in acute or chronic bursitis, its walls impinge against the edge of the acromion when the arm is abducted and restrict motion.

of functional power, but the pain associated with muscle effort may be significant enough to impair performance.

The logical and adequate management of all chronic strains comprises rest of the arm; application of heat, in the form of hot showers or radiant heat, to disperse the inflammatory products and enhance their absorption; local administration of steroids, to reduce the inflammatory reaction, and, most important, graduated rehabilitation of the arm. The reactivation of the affected unit or units must be slow, working up, step by step, to the anticipated demands. The doctor may have difficulty in enforcing such a graduated program, especially when a determined athlete is anxious to return to the sport and an impatient coach is "stewing" in the background.

It should be understood that chronic strains of long duration become refractory to conservative treatment. Undoubtedly this occurs because of the great amount of scar tissue at the site of the lesion, which

is associated with reduced vascularity of the area. As a result, repair is retarded or does not occur. Also, this circumstance may be accompanied by advanced attritional changes in the tendon which also reduces or does not respond to the repair process. In such instances, surgery may be sufficiently effective to return the athlete to full activity.

When in the rotator cuff a small partially avulsed portion of the cuff does not respond to conservative measures, it can be excised and the defect closed. Also, small complete tears can be repaired. This surgery can be performed through a small deltoid-splitting incision without detachment of any portion of the insertion of the deltoid and without doing an osteotomy of the acromion or resection of a portion of the acromion. It is my opinion that the less the normal anatomy of the shoulder girdle is disturbed the greater are the chances of full recovery. (For the technique of repairs of cuff tears see page 223.)

The same is true of chronic bicipital tenosynovitis. If conservative measures fail, the intracapsular portion of the tendon should be excised and the stump of the distal end should be anchored in the intertubercular groove. Some chronic strains do not respond to either conservative or surgical treatment. Now the athlete must face up to the situation and decide, either to reduce his total participation (if permitted) or to give up the sport.

## NERVE INJURIES ABOUT THE SHOULDER

Injuries to the neural elements of the shoulder are relatively common in athletes. They may be isolated lesions or they may be associated with fractures or fracture-dislocations of the bones and articulations comprising the shoulder girdle or the cervical spine. They are more common in sports in which the participant travels at high speeds, such as in skiiing, diving, automobile and motorcyle racing and horseback riding, than in contact or collision sports. Bateman has clearly and logically categorized nerve lesions about the shoulder according to the mechanisms of production and has also listed the clinical manifestations that are indicators of neural damage.

### Pertinent Symptoms of Neural Damage

The presence of the following symptoms should alert you to the possibility of nerve injury.

1. A sensation of burning and numbness in the shoulder, which may extend down the entire extremity;

2. A stunning sensation at the site of impact;

3. A feeling of heaviness and deadness of the extremity;

4. Sharp, lancinating pain in the shoulder, which may progress into the limb.

5. Loss of power in the muscles of the shoulder, arm, forearm, wrist and hand. It should be remembered that inability to move these parts may be owing to pain and not to injuries to nerves.

### Evaluation of Nerve Injuries

When any of the symptoms mentioned above are present, a careful history of the injury should be taken. This includes an accurate description of the mechanism of the injury, the area of impact and the amount of force applied. Clinical manifestations pointing to possible injuries to the cervical spine, such as a stiff neck, a fixed deformity of the neck, pain on motion of the neck or tenderness over the lateral masses or at the base of the neck, demand that the cervical spine be thoroughly examined clinically and rotentogenographically. The presence or absence of disruptive lesions of the cervical column must be established at once. By far the commonest lesions implicate the peripheral nerves; the roots and spinal cord are only rarely involved. The most informative clinical test is the evaluation of the motor power of the main muscles of the shoulder — trapezius, deltoid, serratus anterior, triceps, biceps, extensors and flexors of the wrist and the muscles of the hand. Changes in the sensory pattern about the shoulder are less informative, especially immediately after injury.

If an obvious deformity of the shoulder is present, such as a fracture of the clavicle or scapula, disruption of the acromioclavicular joint or fracture-dislocation of the glenohumeral joint, the identity of the nerve or nerves most likely to be injured, and the pattern of the neurological deficit are easily recognized.

Detailed roentgenographic examination must be made of the neck and shoulder in all suspected nerve injuries. Very often detection of a fracture of the first rib or of the scapula by roentgenographic examination may be the only clue to the severity of the neural damage.

Finally, electrical tests to determine the exact neural elements involved and the extent of nerve damage should be performed. Electromyographic evaluations should always be done, as should testing with the faradic (interrupted) current. A positive response of a nerve to faradic stimulation is a good prognostic sign. It indicates that continuity of the nerve is preserved, and recovery can be anticipated. A negative response is an ominous sign, indicating severe nerve damage and a poor prognosis.

## Principles of Treatment

In all peripheral nerve lesions the management is the same. If possible, the affected muscle or muscles should be supported. For example, the deltoid can be supported by a brace holding the arm in 45° of abduction. Some muscles, such as the trapezius and the spinati, cannot be supported adequately; however, a sling will give some support to the whole arm. Electrical stimulation of the paralyzed muscles on a regulated program tends to preserve muscle mass and prevents myostatic contractures.

Clinical and electrical evaluations should be made constantly to determine whether or not regeneration of the nerve is occurring. If there is no evidence of return of motor power in six to eight weeks, the nerve should be explored by a neurosurgeon. A properly performed and timely neurolysis may mean the difference between complete recovery and none at all. All nerves about the shoulder are accessible, as are the nerve roots and the brachial plexus.

## Brachial Plexus

The commonest causes of injury to the brachial plexus are projectile or headlong falls such as occur in diving, falling off a horse, skiing and football. Essentially the mechanism is elongation of the interval between the head and shoulder and stretching of the components of the plexus. The type of resulting lesion varies considerably, depending upon the exact areas of contact on the shoulder, the position of the head and neck (the neck may be flexed or extended) and the magnitude of the applied force. The nerve roots may be avulsed from the cord; more frequently, however, they are stretched over the adjacent transverse process.

## Avulsion of the Plexus

Fortunately this injury is rare. It is followed by paralysis of the entire extremity, with complete loss of sensation, especially from the elbow downward.

## Upper and Lower Nerve Roots

The upper roots—the fifth and sixth cervical nerve roots—are the most frequently implicated. The lesion occurs just distal to their exit from the intervertebral foramina. From these structures arise the suprascapular and axillary nerves which supply the spinati and deltoid. Therefore, paralysis of these muscles ensues. Because the suprascapular nerve occupies such a high position in the plexus it is the first to receive the brunt of a severe impact. In fact, it may be the only nerve involved.

The lower roots of the brachial plexus—the seventh and eighth cervical and the first thoracic nerve roots—are involved far less frequently than the upper roots; these are rare lesions. If the anterior aspect of the shoulder receives more of the impact, the inferior cord may be injured and fracture of the clavicle or the first rib may occur. As a rule, little or no motor damage results from these injuries; however, numbness, tingling in the whole limb and changes in the normal sensory pattern of the extremity point to lesions of the lower roots.

**Management.** The treatment comprises protection of the affected muscles and regular electrical stimulation of the muscles. The deltoid should be supported with a brace holding the arm in 45° of abduction. All joints of the limb should be put through their normal range of motion, actively (if possible) as well as passively. If after six or eight weeks clinical and electrical evaluation reveals no improvement in the extent of the paralysis, surgical exploration should be performed by a neurosurgeon.

### Posterior Cord

A driving, direct blow applied to the postero-inferior region of the axilla may severely injure the posterior cord of the brachial plexus. Essentially, the posterior cord is compressed against the inferior aspect of the glenohumeral joint. A similar injury may occur when, in a backward fall, the region of the quadrilateral space strikes the ground with a crushing impact or strikes a projecting object. These injuries occur in hockey, lacrosse, football and some of the riding sports. The neural elements of the posterior cord which are most likely to be injured are the nerve supply to the deltoid, triceps and the extensors of the wrist. The degree of involvement varies from weakness, of only one or of all of these mucles, to total paralysis.

**Management.** Protect the affected muscles—the deltoid with an abduction brace, the extensors of the wrist with a cock-up splint and the triceps with a sling. Daily electrical stimulation of the muscles is beneficial, as are active and passive movements of all the articulations of the limb. Failure to respond to this program in six to eight weeks is an indication for surgical exploration of the involved nerves.

### Axillary Nerve

Several mechanisms of trauma to the shoulder can injure the axillary nerve. As noted above, the nerve may be injured by a direct force to the postero-inferior aspect of the axilla. It is more frequently injured by direct violence to the anterior aspect of the shoulder when the arm is abducted and externally rotated. The structures in the anterior region of the axilla are compressed against the humeral head and glenoid. In football this is a common mechanism of injury. Also, the axillary nerve

may be injured by twisting injuries such as produce a dislocation of the shoulder when the arm is forced into extreme abduction and external rotation. Injuries to the axillary nerve by this mechanism occur more often than is generally appreciated. Whereas the two mechanisms involving direct force crush the nerve, the twisting mechanism stretches it; the latter injury is the more serious of the two.

In crushing injuries, if the nerve is only stunned, the arm feels numb and dead, with loss of abduction. These manifestations do not persist very long and, except for some weakness of abduction, they disappear within a matter of minutes. Persistent weakness and clinical evidence of loss of deltoid power indicates a more serious lesion and should be treated accordingly. Severe stretching of the nerve, such as occurs in dislocation of the glenohumeral joint, carries a more grave prognosis, because extensive damage may involve a large segment of the nerve.

**Management.** Treatment of these lesions includes adequate protection of the deltoid with an abduction brace and electrical stimulation of the deltoid. Active motion of all the other articulations of the limb and passive motion of the glenohumeral joint several times a day are very important parts of the program. If after six or eight weeks there is no return of power in the deltoid or the extent of improvement is insignificant, surgical exploration of the nerve should be performed.

### Accessory Nerve

The usual mechanism of injury is a direct, forceful blow in the interval between the neck and the shoulder and slightly posteriorly. Such mishaps occur in hockey, lacrosse and football, producing a crushing of the nerve just where the nerve passes under the upper border of the trapezius. Often the extent of the damage is not appreciated immediately. Later, the player is aware of a persistent, dull ache in the shoulder, weakness of abduction, drooping of the shoulder and inability to shrug the shoulder. Inspection of the shoulder reveals drooping of the shoulder and winging of the scapula, owing to loss of fixation of the scapula against the thoracic cage. Pressure over the site of penetration of the nerve into the trapezius produces local tenderness and a sensation of "pins and needles" which extends to the posterior aspect of the shoulder.

**Management.** As in other nerve injuries about the shoulder, the arm should be put to rest by placing it in a sling and the muscle should be electrically stimulated daily. If at the end of six or eight weeks the muscle fails to show any evidence of restoration of motor power, the nerve should be explored.

### Suprascapular Nerve

This nerve is injured by direct blows delivered to the area between the neck and shoulder and slightly posteriorly. Often the injury is associated with lesions of the upper roots of the brachial plexus, but it may present as an isolated lesion. A prompt diagnosis of involvement of this nerve is frequently not made and the patient may go on for months complaining of a dull ache in the posterior aspect of the shoulder, a feeling of heaviness, and weakened abduction of the arm. Although atrophy of the spinati may not be present immediately after the injury, later loss of mass of the spinati is apparent.

**Management.** It is difficult to put the spinati muscles at rest; however, the use of an abduction brace does provide considerable comfort. Daily electrical stimulation should be done. Failure to show any evidence of nerve regeneration in six to eight weeks is an indication for surgical exploration of the nerve.

### Long Thoracic Nerve

Injuries of the long thoracic nerve are

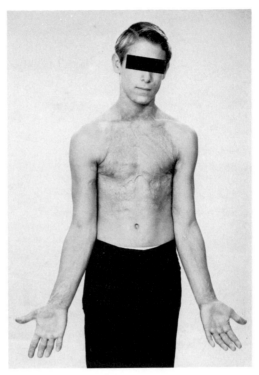

FIG. 8-6. Right hand pitcher with hypertrophy of the muscles of the right shoulder girdle, hypertrophy of the right forearm muscles and valgus deformity of the right elbow. (Courtesy of J. W. King)

relatively common and are usually the result of severe stretching of all the stabilizing muscles of the scapula. At the time of injury the player experiences a burning, numb feeling in the posterior aspect of the shoulder. Later the shoulder droops slightly and there is a sense of heaviness in the entire limb. Abduction is limited and weak and winging of the scapula is very apparent, especially so when the person performs the wall-crawling test.

Paralysis of the serratus anterior produces marked instability of the shoulder and hence much dysfunction. Fortunately, most lesions respond to conservative therapy; however, it may take many months to attain complete regeneration of the nerve. Stabilization of the scapula is difficult to achieve by any type of bracing. I employ an abduction brace with a pad over the

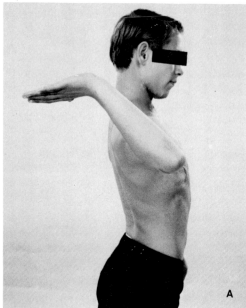

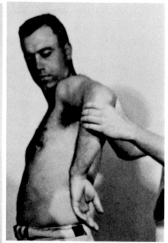

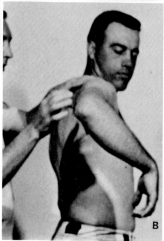

FIG. 8-7. (A) A pitcher with increased external rotation of the shoulder. (Courtesy of J. W. King). (B) A right hand pitcher showing decreased internal rotation in the pitching arm (*bottom*) as compared to the amount of internal rotation in the left arm (*top*).

lower angle of the scapula which is held in place by a strap encircling the thoracic cage. In addition, daily electrical stimulation of the muscle should be performed. Rarely is surgical intervention necessary.

### Musculocutaneous Nerve

Blows on the anterior aspect of the shoulder may contuse or crush the musculocutaneous nerve. As a rule, the injury is not severe. Local evidence of soft tissue trauma on the anterior aspect of the shoulder is present and burning, numb sensation extends distally along the outer border of the forearm to the thumb. The biceps mus-

cle is flabby because of loss of muscle tone, and contraction of the muscle is weak.

Most lesions respond to conservative management comprising rest of the arm with a sling, daily electrical stimulation and active motion of all the articulations of the limb. Only rarely is surgical intervention required; however, if in six to eight weeks the nerve shows little or no evidence of regeneration, exploration of the nerve should be performed.

### VASCULAR INJURIES

I have never seen a vascular injury in the arm caused by throwing. However, they may occur. Brewer reports a case of brachial artery thrombosis in a 24-year-old pitcher. Complete recovery in this case occurred with the establishment of an efficient collateral circulation.

## THE PITCHER'S ELBOW

In a discussion of affections of the throwing arm the elbow joint must be given due consideration. G. E. Bennett and more recently J. W. King have done much to clarify the mechanisms of injuries of the pitcher's elbow and the subsequent clinical syndromes associated with these mechanisms. A pitcher who cannot maintain a high level of performance is a financial liability to his team and a disappointment to the fans. The ability of a pitcher to perform consistently and effectively depends on the integrity of two structures, the shoulder and the elbow.

### External Appearance of the Pitcher's Arm

Pitching on a regular schedule (usually every fourth day) requires repeated extreme effort on the part of practically all the muscles of the limb, including the latissimus dorsi. All the muscles of the pitching arm become hypertrophied; in veteran pitchers the overdevelopment of the arm is apparent even to the casual observer. In the forearm, the flexor muscles stand out in marked contrast when compared with the flexors of the opposite forearm (Fig. 8-6).

Constant pitching exacts its toll from the elbow. As the result of repeated micro tears at the site of insertion of the flexors of the forearm, myostatic contractures occur in the muscle group, producing a fixed flexion deformity of the elbow. This amount of fixed flexion is accepted by pitchers and does not reduce the effectiveness of the pitch.

Most pitchers, especially the older ones, have a valgus deformity of the elbow, increased external rotation of the arm and decreased internal rotation (Fig. 8-7). The

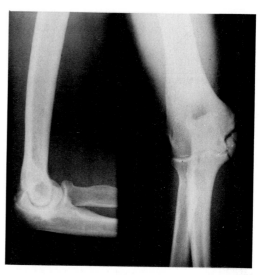

FIG. 8-8. Traction spurs on the medial side of the ulnar notch secondary to repeated chronic strains of the medial side of the elbow joint in older pitchers and fragmentation of the epicondyle. (Courtesy of J. W. King)

development of these deformities is directly related to the throwing act.

### Mechanism of the Development of Fixed Deformities

At the initiation of the dynamic phase of throwing, the arm is in extreme abduction and external rotation, the body moves forward and then the shoulder is thrust forward, leaving the arm and hand behind. In this act, great valgus stress is placed on the elbow, and the anterior structures of the glenohumeral joint are severely stretched. Repetition of this act results in a chronic strain of the attachment of the flexors of the forearm and a chronic sprain and attenuation of the capsule and ligaments on the medial aspect of the elbow. This explains the development of increased valgus of the elbow and increased external rotation of the shoulder. Repeated tearing and stretching of the muscles, capsule and ligaments of the medial side of the elbow may produce considerable pain and dysfunction, thereby reducing the efficiency

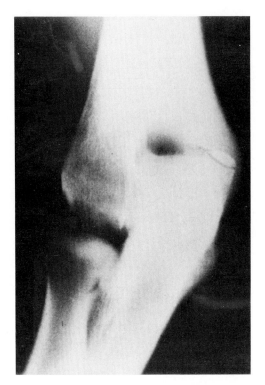

FIG. 8-9. Osteochondritis of the capitellum and a loose body on the tip of the olecranon. (Courtesy of J. W. King)

of the pitcher. This is the "medial stress syndrome" which may stubbornly resist any form of therapy and require giving up the sport.

In addition, the constant and repeated traumata to the soft tissue elements on the medial side of the elbow produce a reactive response at the site of attachment of the capsule and ligaments which initiates the formation of traction spurs. Such bony spurs are common findings in older pitchers. They usually occur on the medial aspect of the ulnar notch and project proximally (Fig. 8-8). The clinical pattern caused by implication of the joint differs from that produced by involvement of the flexor muscles alone. Joint involvement produces a deep-seated pain that is vague in its localization, and the maximum point of tenderness is over the joint line distal to the medial epicondyle.

Not infrequently the lateral side of the elbow joint is involved, and radiographic examination reveals free bodies within the radiohumeral side of the elbow joint. The most plausible explanation for the formation of the loose bodies is that repeated medial stresses applied to an elbow with great laxity and attenuation of the capsule and ligaments force the radial head to impinge against the capitellum, causing an osteochondritis (Fig. 8-9). Eventually, loose bodies are discharged into the joint.

Loose bodies are even more prevalent at the tip of the olecranon which lies intraarticularly. The exact mechanism responsible for the formation of the loose bodies is not clear. Usually a great number of free bodies tend to aggregate just proximal to the tip of the olecranon process (Fig. 8-9). This is one area where surgical intervention is very rewarding. Excision of the loose bodies can readily be achieved through a small lateral incision, and, as a rule, the pitcher will return to full activity.

Finally, the humerus of the pitching arm becomes markedly hypertrophied, a feature demonstrated by roentgenograms. Also, the olecranon process shows similar alterations which reduce the depth of the olecranon fossa. Therefore, the area of the articular surfaces of the humerus and the olecranon fossa are diminished.

## FRACTURE OF THE SHAFT OF THE HUMERUS IN THE THROWING ARM

During the act of throwing, a fracture of the shaft of the humerus may occur. This is a rare lesion. Usually a spiral fracture results. The greater number of such fractures in ball throwers have been reported to have occurred in softball players. Most of the literature on this subject cites as the cause of the fracture strenuous muscle contraction. More recently, however, Weseley and Barenfeld proposed that the lesion is the result of a violent torque applied perpendicular to the shaft of the humerus.

At the beginning of the dynamic phase of throwing, the arm is in extreme abduction and external rotation, and the shoulder is

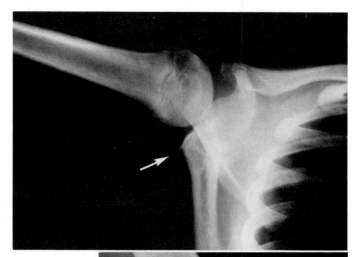

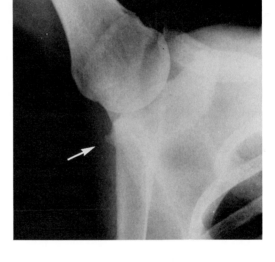

FIG. 8-10. (*Top*) An exostosis on the postero-inferior margin of the glenoid fossa in a young pitcher. (Courtesy of J. W. King. (*Bottom*) The same lesion in an adult pitcher.

extended. However, at the end of the follow-through phase the shoulder is adducted, internally rotated and flexed, the elbow remaining in some degree of flexion until the very end of the follow-through motion. Just before the ball is released the humerus is sharply rotated internally. This internal rotation is markedly accelerated by the torque produced by the weight of the ball at the end of the lever arm created by the flexed elbow. The intensity of the applied torque may be sufficient to produce a fracture of the shaft of the humerus.

## INJURIES TO THE PITCHING ARM OF YOUTHS

Interest in organized competitive sports for youngsters is steadily increasing from year to year. Many programs now enthusiastically sponsor and encourage these activities; among these are the Little League and Pony League Baseball Clubs; the Pop Warner Football Clubs, with their various divisions; wrestling and swim clubs, and the football, basketball, baseball and track teams of junior and senior high schools. As pointed out by Adams, youngsters participating in these organized programs are between 8 and 15 years of age. They are at a period of life when many variations in skeletal growth and maturity exist, and, because they normally are very active, they

are prone to skeletal injuries. In addition, they play the sport according to fixed rules laid down by adults who, in general, train and coach these youngsters to a level of performance equal to that of the professional athlete. Some guidelines have been laid down to regulate the age and size of the young athletes on a particular team; nevertheless, the participants labor under constant competitive pressures from the home, the school and the team. Furthermore, medical supervision in the selection of the participants is far from adequate. Except for major injuries, such as fractures and dislocations, proper medical care is denied these youngsters; it usually rests in the hands of the parents or trainers. Many

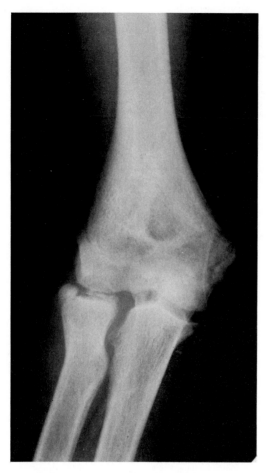

FIG. 8-11. Epiphysitis (aseptic necrosis) of the proximal radial epiphysis in an adolescent pitcher; also note the fragmentation of the medial epicondyle. (Courtesy of J. W. King)

young athletes are returned to the game long before they should be allowed to engage in full activity. The future promise of a brilliant athletic career is often destroyed in these early years.

On the other hand, there is a growing trend in this country among doctors, coaches and trainers toward better understanding of the problems of the youth athlete. In the near future, I am sure, more rigid rules of the game will be enforced to protect the young participants from injury caused by constant, repetitive effort. Medical supervision in the selection of young athletes for a particular sport will improve, as will the care and rehabilitation of the injured youngsters.

## Bone Injuries of the Shoulder

Injuries to the epiphyses of young athletes 15 years of age or younger is significantly high. Larson and McMahon in a study of 1,338 athletic injuries in this age range recorded an incidence of 6 percent. The shoulder is a frequent site of bone injury in young pitchers. These youngsters use their pitching arm in the same manner as their older counterparts, and the constant, repetitive, strenuous muscular effort of throwing may, in time, injure the upper humeral epiphysis and initiate a local inflammatory process. The changes that occur in the humerus are readily demonstrable by roentgenographic studies. They comprise accelerated growth of both the diaphysis and the epiphysis, and widening, demineralization and fragmentation of the proximal humeral epiphysis. This is not a true form of osteochondrosis, for, with rest, the process rapidly subsides and pain disappears. However, I have seen the roentgenograms of the shoulder of one 14-year-old pitcher whose proximal humeral epiphysis was deformed, widened, flattened and severely fragmented. It is difficult to conceive that such a severely affected epiphysis could ever return to normal regardless of the type of treatment instituted. Adams reported deformity and demineralization in the greater tuberosity of a 15-year-old pitcher; this same youngster also had an exostosis on the postero-inferior margin of the glenoid fossa (Fig. 8-10).

**Management.** Most epiphyseal injuries of the shoulder respond to a full rest from throwing. The local inflammatory process subsides and the arm becomes pain free. However, the process may be reactivated if hard pitching is resumed too soon. The wise course of management for young pitchers with sore arms and roentgenographic evidence of changes in the humeral epiphyses is to prohibit pitching until the epiphyses have united to the humeral shaft.

These youngsters may still play positions that do not require persistent, hard pitching.

## Bone Injuries of the Elbow

Persistent, repetitious, hard pitching subjects the immature elbow to repeated valgus strains that may severely affect the epiphyses of the elbow joint. Roentgenograms readily reveal the bony changes that are located primarily in two areas, the medial epicondylar and the radiohumeral. Usually the bony elements of the elbow exhibit varying degrees of accelerated growth. The medial epicondylar epiphysis may show demineralization, fragmentation and separation. In these cases, the symptoms come on gradually; they are relieved by rest from throwing and are aggravated by persistent pitching. The intensity of the symptoms generally increases from year to year. Sudden onset of pain during the act of pitching may be caused by a fracture through the medial epicondylar epiphysis.

Changes in the radiohumeral joint comprise: (1) osteochondritis of the capitellum of the humerus, and (2) osteochondritis of the head of the radius. These lesions are far less common than those affecting the medial epicondylar area. I have seen one young pitcher with involvement of the proximal radial epiphysis (Fig. 8-11). Adams reported one case in an 11-year-old pitcher. Trias and Ray reported one case, and, according to Adams, Ellman had collected four other cases, all in 11-year-old pitchers; these had not as yet appeared in the literature at the time of this writing.

**Management.** Treatment for epiphyseal lesions about the elbow is similar to that of lesions of the proximal humeral epiphysis. The arm should be rested from all throwing until the pain disappears. Hard pitching should be discontinued until the epiphyseal plates are closed; however, the youngster may play other positions.

## BIBLIOGRAPHY

Adams, J. E.: Injury to the throwing arm: a study of traumatic changes in the elbow joints of boy baseball players. Calif. Med., *102*: 127-132, 1965.
_____: Little league shoulder: osteochondrosis of the proximal humeral epiphysis in boy pitchers. Calif. Med., *105*:22-25, 1966.
_____: Bone injuries in very young athletes. Clin. Orthop., *58*:129-134, 1968.
Brewer, B. J.: The throwing arm — soft tissue injury. Am. Acad. Orthop. Surg., Symp. on Sports Medicine, St. Louis, C. V. Mosby, 1969.
Bateman, J. E.: Athletic injuries about the shoulder in throwing and body contact sports. Clin. Orthop., *23*:75-82, 1962.
_____: Nerve injuries about the shoulder in sports. Instruc. Course Lec., J. Bone & Joint Surg., *49A*:785-792, 1967.
Bennett, G. E.: Elbow and shoulder lesions of baseball players. Am. J. Surg., *98*:484, 1959.
_____: Shoulder and elbow lesions distinctive of baseball players. Ann. Surg., *126*:107, 1947.
_____: Shoulder and elbow lesions of the professional baseball pitcher. JAMA, *117*:510, 1941.
Brewer, B. J.: Athletic injuries; musculotendinous unit. Clin. Orthop., *23*:30-38, 1962.
Goff, C. W.: Legg-Perthes disease and related osteochondroses of youth. Springfield, Ill., Charles C Thomas, 1954.
Hale, C. J.: Injuries among 771, 810 Little League baseball players. J. Sports Med. Phys. Fitness, *1*:80-83, 1961.
Hirata, I., Jr.: The doctor and the athlete. Philadelphia, J. B. Lippincott, 1968.
King, J. W.: Analysis of the pitching arm of the professional baseball pitcher. Clin. Orthop., *67*:116-123, 1969.
Larson, R. L., and McMahon, R. O.: The epiphyses and the childhood athlete. JAMA, *196*: 607-612, 1966.
O'Donoghue, D. H.: Treatment of injuries to athletes. Philadelphia, W. B. Saunders, 1963.
Slocum, D. B.: The mechanics of some common injuries to the shoulder in sports. Am. J. Surg., *98*:394-400, 1959.
Trias, A., and Ray, R. D.: Juvenile osteochondritis of the radial head. J. Bone & Joint Surg., *45A*:576-582, 1963.
Weseley, M. S., and Barenfeld, P. A.: Ball throwers' fracture of the humerus. Clin. Orthop., *64*:153-156, 1969.

# 9

# Fractures, Sprains, Subluxations and Dislocations of the Shoulder Girdle

## FRACTURES OF THE CLAVICLE

Fractures of the clavicle are frequent injuries in athletes. The incidence of fractures of the clavicle in the general population is rising steadily, owing to the increasing number of accidents in high velocity vehicles. These are frequently associated with injuries of the neurovascular structures in the thoracic outlet. Therefore, it behooves the physician when he encounters a fracture of the clavicle to examine the patient thoroughly for injuries to the brachial plexus, the subclavian vessels, the lungs and pleura. Also, fractures of the clavicle may be associated with fractures and dislocations of other bones of the same extremity.

Clavicular fractures in children and those in adults are different lesions. In young children, the growth potential is such that some deformity and overriding can be accepted, with the expectation that, with growth, realignment and length of the bone will be restored. However, severe overriding and deformity in children should not be accepted, and, if correction is not obtained by manipulative closed methods, surgical intervention is justified. Severe deformities and shortening interfere with the normal crank-shaft function of the clavicle in the mechanics of the shoulder girdle. And, although in most situations this defect may not interfere with normal activities, in athletes it may be a serious handicap.

Before instituting treatment for fractures of the clavicle in children the state of skeletal maturation should be determined, for this differs in children of the same chronological age group. Those youngsters in whom skeletal maturation is nearly complete should be treated as adults. Clavicular fractures in children should be protected until healing is far enough advanced to meet the activities of the child. Refracture may occur if external fixation is removed too early. Although rare, delayed union and nonunion do occur in clavicular fractures in children; usually they are found in severely comminuted fractures or in fractures with wide separation of the fragments. These complications may occur in fractures that are poorly managed in respect to the method of external fixation (which may have been inadequate) or the period of immobilization (which may have been too short) or both.

Clavicular fractures in adults may be the cause of considerable concern. Delayed union and nonunion are not infrequent complications. Healing is slower than in children and, in some cases, it may require 4 to 6 months before union is achieved. Because remodeling of displaced fragments and spontaneous restoration of length in overriding fractures do not occur, it is imperative that realignment of the fragments and restoration of length be achieved. If conservative measures do not attain this goal, open reduction and fixation of the fragment should be performed. As pointed out by O'Donoghue, the athlete poses special problems. Time to him is of the essence, and restoration of a normal shoulder girdle is of utmost importance if he is to perform effectively. In line with this manner of thinking, I do not hesitate to operate on athletes. With internal fixation the rest of the girdle can be exercised, thereby preventing muscle atrophy, fibrosis and contractures of the ligaments and capsules of the other articulations of the girdle. This program returns the athlete to his sport much earlier than does conservative treatment.

Surgical management of clavicular fractures must not be taken lightly, especially when it is performed in athletes in preference to conservative treatment for the reasons just noted. The environment of the operating room should be such that sterility is assured and the operation should be performed by a competent surgeon. As for the surgical technique, the following surgical principles facilitate the operation and minimize the incidence of complications.

1. Fragments should be exposed with as little soft tissue stripping as possible; excessive stripping favors delayed union or nonunion.

2. For internal fixation (if it is used), an intramedullary pin provides the best type of fixation and ensures restoration of normal length of the clavicle. In comminuted fractures, the use of circumferential wires around displaced fragments together with the intramedullary pin provides excellent fixation. I prefer threaded wires of $7/64$ inch for intramedullary fixation.

3. Always pass the wire first into the medullary canal of the distal fragment and advance it until it pierces the skin medial to the acromioclavicular joint. Then insert and advance the wire into the canal of the proximal fragment.

4. Whenever possible add a few bone chips around the fracture site.

5. Always supplement internal fixation with some form of external fixation.

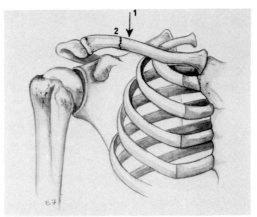

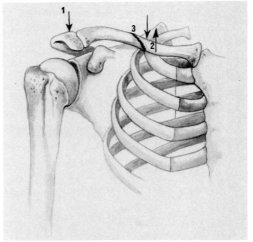

(*Top*) FIG. 9-1. Fracture of the middle third of the clavicle by a direct force (1) applied to the middle third of the clavicle. The fracture occurs at the juncture of the middle and outer thirds (2).

(*Bottom*) FIG. 9-2. Fracture of the middle third of the clavicle by a force applied to the top of the shoulder (1); the clavicle is forced against the first rib (2), and a spiral fracture of the middle third occurs (3).

### Fractures of the Middle Third of the Clavicle

This portion of the clavicle lies between the costoclavicular ligament medially and the coracoclavicular ligament laterally. Fractures in this region are common injuries in athletes, more so in the preado-

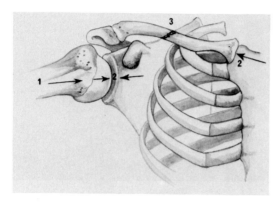

FIG. 9-3. Fracture of the middle third of the clavicle by an indirect force. The force travels along the shaft of the humerus (1); the counter points are the glenohumeral joint and the sternoclavicular joint (2); a spiral fracture of the middle third occurs (3).

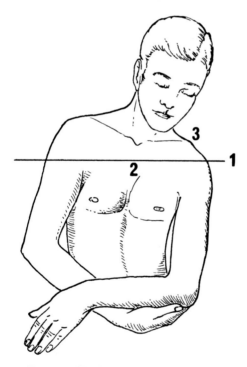

FIG. 9-4. Typical deformity of a complete fracture of the clavicle in its middle third. The affected shoulder is lower than the opposite side (1); the shoulder droops downward and forward and is closer to the middle line than the opposite side (2); there is swelling over the fracture site (3).

lescent and adolescent period of life than in the adult. On the other hand, fractures of the outer end of the clavicle are more likely to occur in the adult.

## Mechanisms of Fracture

Fractures of the middle third are produced by two kinds of mechanisms: direct, and indirect. In the direct mechanism the impact is directly on the bone. As a rule, the fracture occurs at the junction of the outer and middle thirds of the clavicle. The fracture may be segmental or transverse (Fig. 9-1). Another direct mechanism is application of a force to the top of the shoulder, forcing the clavicle against the first rib and producing a spiral fracture of the middle third of the clavicle (Fig. 9-2).

In the indirect mechanism, the patient falls with the arm abducted and flexed. The force generated travels along the shaft of the humerus and encounters two counterpoints, one at the glenohumeral joint and one at the sternoclavicular joint. This mechanism also produces a spiral fracture (Fig. 9-3). There may be no displacement of the fragments. If displacement does occur, the proximal fragment rides upward and the distal downward.

It should be noted that a direct impact on the top or the anterior aspect of the clavicle is often associated with contusion of the underlying soft tissues and hemorrhage into the tissues. X-rays may not reveal a fracture line. However, if after 10 to 14 days the patient still has pain on movements of the arm and tenderness over the shaft of the clavicle, a fracture must be suspected. X-rays at this time show either a line of bone absorption or the formation of callus at the fracture site.

## Diagnosis

Fractures with displacement offer no difficulty in the making of the diagnosis. There is always a history of violence to the shoulder either by a direct or an indirect mechanism. The affected shoulder is lower than the opposite shoulder and it droops downward and forward (Fig. 9-4). It may be difficult to make the diagnosis of incomplete fracture but X-rays taken 10 to 14 days later will resolve the problem. All movements of the arm cause pain when a fracture is present. Fractures close to the coracoclavicular and costoclavicular ligaments may simulate lesions of the ligaments of the adjacent joints. X-rays of the outer and inner ends of the clavicle should establish the diagnosis. Immediately after the injury the deformity at the fracture site is readily seen and is palpable. The proximal fragment is displaced upward and backward. Later, swelling of the soft tissues and hemorrhage obliterate the configuration of the deformity. However, by gentle manipulation, motion can be detected at the fracture site.

## Conservative Management

**For Infants and Small Children.** Fractures without displacement require nothing more than a posterior figure-of-eight bandage of muslin or flannel applied over large pads of cotton placed over the anterior aspect of the shoulders. The bandage must hold the shoulders up, outward and backward (Fig. 9-5). Maintain this postion for 3 to 4 weeks. After the bandage is removed the young patient is allowed free use of the extremity.

Greenstick fractures and fractures with displacement should be reduced and length of the clavicle restored by pulling the shoulders upward, backward and outward and by gentle manipulation of the fragments. If some difficulty is encountered or if the child is apprehensive, 5 ml. of 1 percent procaine injected into the hematoma will facilitate reduction. In some cases, general anesthesia may be necessary. After reduction is achieved a posterior figure-of-eight bandage of flannel or muslin maintains the reduction until the healing fracture becomes stable, usually in 3 to 4 weeks.

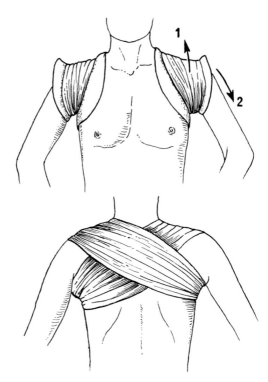

FIG. 9-5. Treatment for infants and small children: The figure-of-eight flannel bandage holds the shoulders up, outward and backward (1); the length and the alignment of the clavicle are restored and maintained by the weight of the arms over the axillary pads (2).

**For Adolescents and Adults.** If no displacement of the fragments is present a posterior figure-of-eight made of plaster bandages 5 inches wide and applied over four or five turns of cotton batting provides adequate immobilization of the fracture.

When there is displacement and overriding of the fragments, an attempt must be made to reduce the fracture and restore normal length of the clavicle. As in the case of young children, local or general anesthesia may be required.

A simple method of reduction (provided that the patient is awake) is to have the patient sit on a stool. The surgeon stands behind the patient and places one knee between the shoulder blades. Then, with a

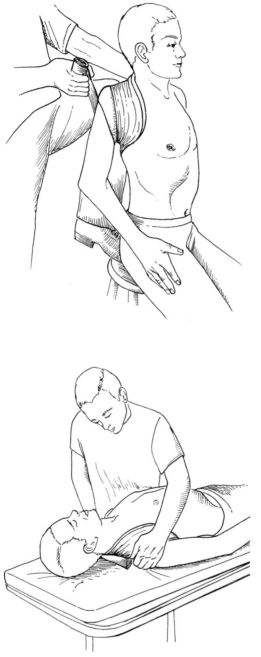

hand on each shoulder, he pulls the shoulders upward, backward and outward and at the same time makes counter-pressure on the mid scapular region with his knee. The patient holds this position while the operator applies four or five turns of cotton batting around the shoulders in the form of a posterior figure-of-eight. Then he applies 10 to 12 turns of plaster bandage, 5 inches wide. As the plaster bandage passes through the axilla on either side he makes firm tension on the bandage to elevate the shoulders while counter-pressure with the knee is maintained at all times (Fig. 9-6). This maneuver may be sufficient to attain normal alignment of the fragments. If not, while an assistant holds the shoulders in the elevated position the operator manipulates the fragments into place. This having been accomplished, the patient is placed in the supine position with a sandbag between the shoulder blades. Then the surgeon makes firm downward pressure over each shoulder, forcing the shoulders upward, backward and outward. He maintains this pressure until the plaster is firmly set (Fig. 9-7).

Immobilization should be maintained for 4 to 6 weeks until stability of the fragments is attained. Stability is determined better by clinical examination than by roentgenograms. During this period, free use of both extremities is encouraged within the limits of the fixation apparatus. Exercises must be performed on a regulated regimen, 5 to 10 minutes every hour. This is most important in adults, especially those beyond middle life, in order to preclude frozen shoulder.

(*Top*) Fɪɢ. 9-6. Application of posterior plaster figure-of-eight for displaced fractures of the middle third in adolescents and adults.

(*Bottom*) Fɪɢ. 9-7. Another method of reducing and maintaining the reduction of fractures of the middle third of the clavicle in adolescents and adults.

## Open Reduction

In children, open reduction is rarely indicated. However, if severe deformity or overriding cannot be reduced, surgical intervention is indicated in those fractures in which the resulting malunion of the clavicle is certain to interfere with the normal

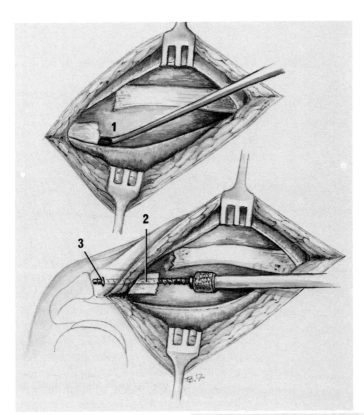

(*Left*) FIG. 9-8. Open reduction and internal fixation of fractures of the outer third of the clavicle: (1) Expose the site of fracture and deliver the lateral fragment into the wound; (2) pass a threaded Kirschner wire (5/64 inch in diameter) into the medullary canal of the lateral fragment and advance it until it pierces the skin medial to the acromioclavicular joint (3).

(*Below*) FIG. 9-9. Open reduction, continued: (1) Insert and advance the wire in the medullary canal of the medial fragment. Cut the wire so that it lies under the skin. (2) Add fine slabs of cancellous bone around the fracture site.

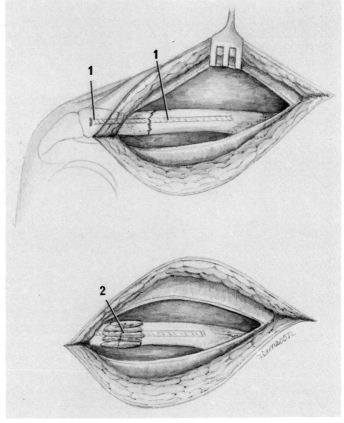

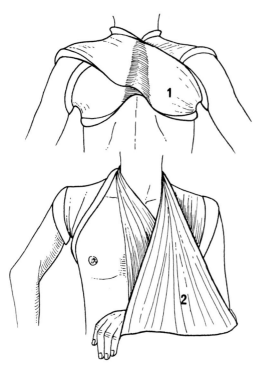

FIG. 9-10. Postoperative fixation. (1) Posterior figure-of-eight plaster cast. (2) A triangular sling supports the arm. (Note: in children apply a plaster shoulder spica.)

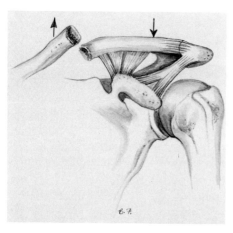

FIG. 9-11. Fracture of the outer end of the clavicle. The fracture is proximal to the coracoclavicular ligament which is intact; the medial fragment rides upward and backward.

mechanics of the shoulder. Also in adolescent athletes and in young adult athletes, to whom time is so vital, open reduction and internal fixation is justifiable. Finally, surgical methods should be used when conservative measures fail to restore an acceptable alignment of fragments and also, when compression of the structures in the thoracic outlet is present and is not relieved by closed methods.

**Operative Procedure.** Place the patient in the supine position with a sandbag under the shoulder. Make an incision parallel to and overlying the second rib, centered over the fracture site. Divide the platysma and, with the overlying tissues, reflect it upward. Expose the fracture site with minimal stripping of the fragments and deliver the distal fragment into the wound. Pass a threaded Kirschner wire ($7/64$ inch in diameter) into the medullary canal of the distal fragment and advance it until it pierces the skin medial to the acromioclavicular joint (Fig. 9-8). Insert the medial end of the wire into the medullary canal of the medial fragment and advance it for 1 or 2 inches. Cut the outer end of the wire so that it lies under the skin (Fig. 9-9). If available, add fine bone chips around the fracture site.

If the fracture is comminuted, in order to obtain good alignment of the displaced fragments, employ one or two wire loops around the fragments and anchor them to the intramedullary rod.

**Postoperative Management.** Following the operation apply a figure-of-eight plaster cast and support the arm in a sling (Fig. 9-10). After the operative reaction has subsided, usually in 10 to 14 days, the sling should be removed several times each day and the arm exercised within the limits of the plaster figure-of-eight. Stabilization of the fragments is usually attained in 4 to 6 weeks in children and in 6 to 8 or 10 weeks in adults. At this point the plaster cast is removed, the wire withdrawn and free use of the arm permitted.

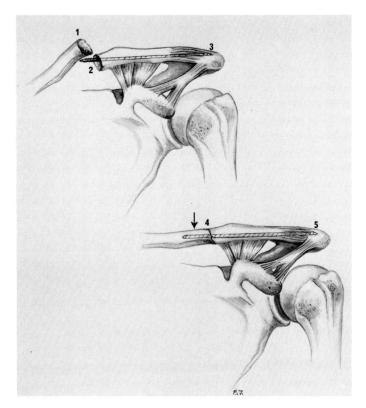

FIG. 9-12. Open reduction and internal fixation of the distal end of the clavicle: (1) Deliver the outer fragment. (2) Insert in its medullary canal one or two threaded Kirschner wires. (3) Advance the wires until they penetrate the acromion and the skin. (4) Reduce the fracture, and (5) insert and advance the wires into the medial fragment for a distance of 2½ inches.

## Fracture of the Outer End of the Shaft of the Clavicle

This fracture merits special consideration. It is produced by a direct blow on the top of the acromion. The force fractures the bone just proximal to the coracoclavicular ligament and the entire shoulder complex distal to the ligament—the coracoclavicular ligament, the distal end of the clavicle, the acromioclavicular joint and ligaments and the acromion—is driven downward. The proximal fragment rides upward, for it is no longer anchored to the scapula (Fig. 9-11). It is impossible to control the proximal fragment by close methods of treatment. The fragment tends to displace upward regardless of the type of external fixation used.

### Management

Open reduction and internal fixation by an intramedullary pin as previously de-

scribed is the treatment of choice. I no longer attempt to treat this fracture by external fixation and offer open reduction and internal fixation as the first choice in management (Fig. 9-12).

## Fractures of the Distal Third of the Clavicle

Essentially these fractures occur in the portion of the clavicle that lies between the acromioclavicular and the coracoclavicular ligaments. They may be produced by a direct or an indirect force and comprise approximately 10 percent of all clavicular fractures.

When the force is direct the impact is on the top of the shoulder, producing a fracture of the outer end of the clavicle lying between the two ligaments. The fracture may be transverse, spiral, oblique or comminuted in nature. Regardless of the type of fracture, both the acromioclavicular and

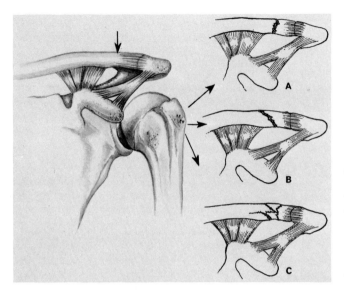

FIG. 9-13. A direct impact on the top of the shoulder may produce a fracture of the distal end of the clavicle distal to the coracoclavicular ligament; the fracture may be (A) transverse, (B) oblique, (C) comminuted (the comminution may extend into the acromioclavicular joint).

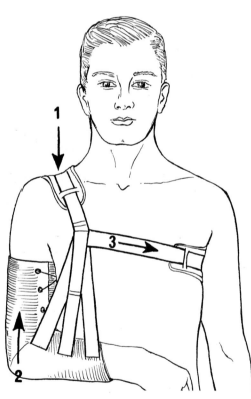

FIG. 9-14. Kenny-Howard sling: (1) The shoulder strap is applied over a piece of felt; it holds the ends of the clavicle down; (2) the sling supports the forearm and keeps the acromion in an elevated position; (3) the halter pulls both the shoulder strap and the sling inward.

the coracoclavicular ligaments remain intact and displacement of the fragments is minimal (Fig. 9-13).

Occasionally, in the absence of any displacement of the fragments, conventional roentgenograms may not reveal the fracture line. Roentgenograms in many planes, including the vertical plane, should be taken to avoid this oversight. In the event that all roentgenograms are negative, and pain persists, especially on movements of the arm, roentgenograms should be taken 10 to 14 days from the time of injury; these invariably reveal the fracture.

These fractures pose no difficulty in treatment. The Kenny-Howard sling provides excellent external support for these fractures (Fig. 9-14); the shoulder strap holds the fragments down and the sling supports the forearm and keeps the acromion elevated. The rate of healing varies from four to six weeks; the state of healing should be checked regularly both clinically and roentgenographically. In the meantime, the rest of the extremity should be regularly exercised. The patient should not return to full activity until union has been achieved.

Fractures produced by the indirect mechanism differ greatly from those just described. In the indirect mechanism the

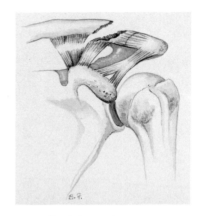

(*Top*) FIG. 9-15. Fracture of the distal end of the clavicle by an indirect mechanism. The fracture occurs distal to or through the coracoclavicular ligament. The distal fragment is anchored by the intact acromioclavicular ligament and the trapezoid portion of the coracoclavicular ligament. The proximal fragment rises upward and backward, owing to the action of the trapezius.

(*Bottom*) FIG. 9-16. Typical fracture through the distal end of the clavicle. Note that the distal fragment maintains its normal relation to the coracoid process and acromion; the proximal fragment is displaced upward and backward.

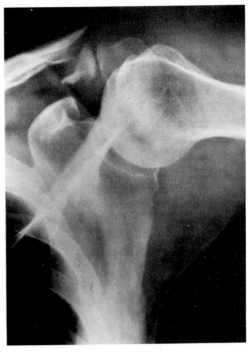

acromion is driven downward. The fracture occurs distal to or through the coracoclavicular ligament, and the distal fragment, which is securely anchored by the intact acromioclavicular ligament and capsule, follows the acromion. The coracoclavicular ligament ruptures completely from the proximal fragment which now loses its attachment to the scapula and rides upward and backward because of the action of the trapezius (Fig. 9-15). (According to Neer, the trapezoid portion of the coracoclavicular ligament remains attached to the distal fragment, but all portions of the ligament are torn from the proximal fragment.) The site and nature of the fracture vary greatly and it is this variation that, in a large measure, governs the treatment. The distal fragment may be small, involving only the outer inch of the clavicle; it may be comminuted, with or without involvement of the acromioclavicular joint; or it may be a sliver of bone attached to the acromioclavicular ligament (Fig. 9-16).

## Management

Regardless of the nature of the fracture, all fractures of the distal third of the clavicle associated with rupture of the coracoclavicular ligament should be treated surgically. Conservative management of this fracture frequently results in delayed union or nonunion. When healing does eventually occur, it is often associated with excessive callus and posterior angulation. Also, stiff-ness and soreness of the shoulder persist for many months. Rehabilitation is indeed slow. The age and the level of activity of the patient are good guides in choosing the type of surgical procedure.

In young patients, particularly athletes who need a strong shoulder girdle with normal and painless motion, I prefer to excise small and comminuted distal fragments and transfer the tip of the coracoid process, with the coracobrachialis and short head of the biceps attached, to the clavicle, as described by Bailey. Also, I reef the

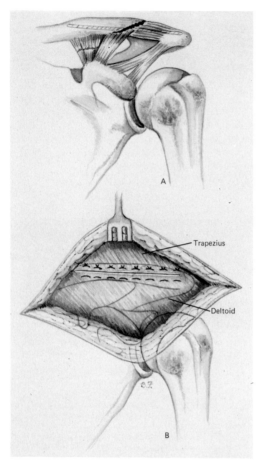

FIG. 9-17. Reduction and internal fixation of a fracture of the distal end of the clavicle: (A) The fracture is reduced and fixed with an intramedullary threaded wire (7/64 inch); (B) the edges of the trapezius and deltoid are lapped tightly over the clavicle by mattress sutures.

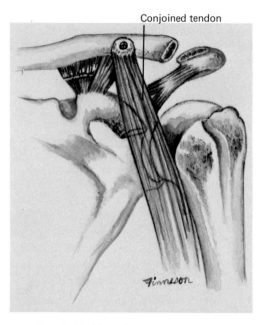

FIG. 9-18. The distal end of the clavicle is excised and the tip of the coracoid with the conjoined tendon of the short head of the biceps and the coracobrachialis is anchored to the clavicle with a screw.

tendinous origins of the trapezius and deltoid over the acromion and clavicle. If the distal fragment is large and not comminuted I strive to attain bony union between the fragments by fixing them with an intramedullary pin. In addition, I transfer the tip of the coracoid to the clavicle. It must be understood that removal of small distal fragments also implies excision of the articular surface of the clavicle. When this is done, in order to preclude future degenerative disorders of the acromioclavicular joint, I always remove the interarticular fibrocartilaginous disc.

In less active patients and in the elderly I simply excise the distal small or comminuted fragments and reef the origins of the trapezius and deltoid over the clavicle and acromion. If the distal fragment is large, I fix it to the proximal fragment with an intramedullary pin.

**Operative Procedure.** Expose the fracture site by a slightly curved 3-inch incision over the clavicle, terminating at the tip of the acromion. By sharp subperiosteal dissection reflect the attachments of the trapezius and deltoid but preserve the capsular ligaments of the acromioclavicular joint.

If the distal fragment is large, expose the ends of both fragments and deliver the outer one into the wound. Penetrate its fractured surface with a threaded wire $7/64$ inch in diameter and advance it so that it crosses the acromioclavicular joint, penetrates the acromion and pierces the skin. Now reduce the fracture and insert and advance the wire into the proximal fragment for a distance of 2 to 2½ inches. Cut the wire immediately below the skin. Finally, lap the tendinous origins of the trapezius and deltoid with mattress sutures tightly over the acromion process and the clavicle (Fig. 9-17).

Postoperatively, the arm is supported in a sling for 6 weeks. No shoulder motion is permitted during this period. The pin is removed after 6 weeks and rehabilitation of the shoulder begins.

If the decision is to remove the distal fragment or fragments and to transfer the tip of the coracoid process to the clavicle, extend the skin incision just medial to the tip of the coracoid process. Expose the fragments and, by sharp dissection, remove the distal loose bone or bones. Trim off any sharp edges of the proximal segment with a rongeur and excise the interarticular disc. Isolate the coracoid process and drill a hole in its center; then place a ¾-inch screw into the drill hole. Now osteotomize the coracoid process at its base just below the origins of the coracobrachialis and the short head of the biceps. Make a drill hole on the anterior surface of the clavicle ½ inch from its raw distal end and insert into it the screw, penetrating the tip of the coracoid process (Fig. 9-18). Finally, lap the insertions of the trapezius and deltoid tightly over the acromion and clavicle.

Postoperatively, the only external support for the arm is a sling, which is worn for 4 weeks. Then allow free use of the extremity.

In less active patients and the elderly perform the same procedure without transferring the coracoid process.

### Fractures of the Inner Third of the Clavicle

These are rare lesions and are the result of a direct force applied; at an angle, from the side (Fig. 9-19). Little or no displace-

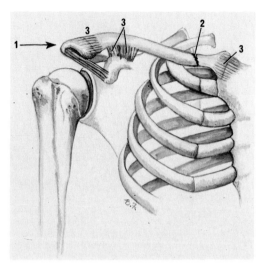

FIG. 9-19. Mechanism of fracture of the inner third of the clavicle. A direct force is applied from the side (1); a fracture of the inner third of the clavicle occurs (2); all ligaments are intact (3).

ment occurs because the costoclavicular ligament remains intact. Adequate treatment is the application of a plaster posterior figure-of-eight which is worn for 4 to 6 weeks.

### Complications of Fractures of the Clavicle

Complications associated with fractures of the clavicle are rare, but they occur occasionally. With the steady increase in the number of accidents caused by high velocity vehicles there is an increase in the incidence of complications. The most common are nonunion, excessive callus formation at the fracture site, and injuries to the neurovascular structures in the thoracic outlet.

### Nonunion of Fractures of the Clavicle

Certain circumstances predispose to nonunion. A common cause is too short an interval of immobilization of the fracture.

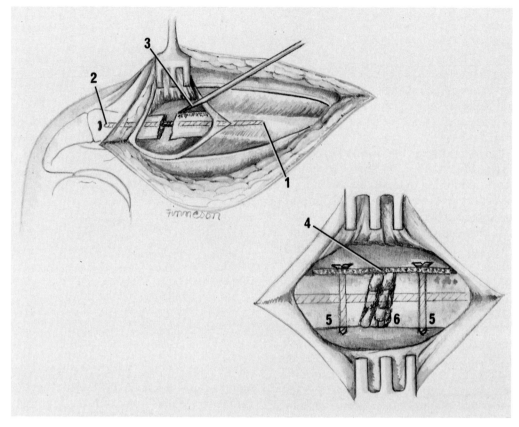

FIG. 9-20. Repair of nonunion of the clavicle: (1) Insert and advance the wire (7/64 inch) first into the medullary canal of the lateral fragment and then into the medial fragment; (2) cut the wire below the level of the skin; (3) with a fine osteotome shave the superior surface of each fragment to produce a flat, even surface; (4) apply a cortico-cancellous bone graft across the fracture site; (5) fix the graft with two screws; (6) pack the defect between the bone ends with cancellous bone chips.

Although most clavicular fractures heal in 4 to 8 weeks, some fractures require a longer period of immobilization. Severely comminuted fractures certainly must be immobilized for a longer period of time. When the fragments are widely separated, nonunion is likely to occur. Soft tissue interposed between widely separated fragments also plays a role.

Open reduction as the primary treatment favors nonunion. This is particularly true if the fragments are stripped excessively and unduly of surrounding soft tissue. Failure to supplement internal fixation of a fracture of the clavicle with adequate ex-

ternal support contributes to nonunion.

Once nonunion of the clavicle is established, it is the source of considerable pain and dysfunction of the shoulder girdle. Only rarely does this lesion produce no disability. I have seen nonunion of both clavicles in an elderly little woman. The lesions were seven years old and caused no pain or dysfunction, as far as she could determine.

In children with a history of trauma to the clavicle nonunion must be distinguished from a congenital pseudarthrosis. Congenital pseudarthrosis in children is neither a common lesion nor a rare finding. All cases of pseudarthrosis that I have en-

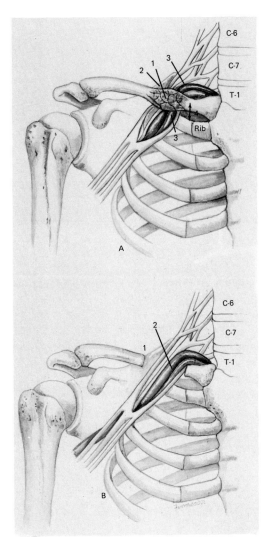

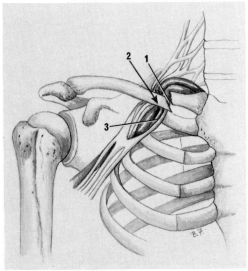

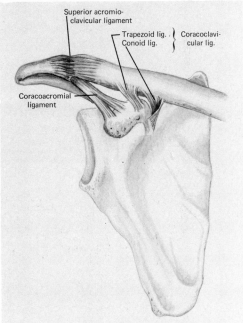

FIG. 9-21. (A) Comminuted fracture (1) of the middle third of the clavicle, with massive callus formation (2); The neurovascular structures (3) are compressed. The interval between the clavicle and the first rib (4) is markedly reduced. (B) The middle portion of the clavicle and callus (1) has been resected; the neurovascular structures (2) lie free in the supraclavicular space.

(Top) FIG. 9-22. Depressed fracture of the clavicle (1); lateral fragment is displaced downward (2); the neurovascular structures are compressed against the first rib (3).

(Bottom) FIG. 9-23. Acromioclavicular and coracoclavicular ligaments.

countered were associated with pain and dysfunction. All required surgical correction.

**Management.** The treatment for nonunion or a congenital pseudarthrosis is surgical repair of the defect. This is best achieved by first inserting an intramedullary pin or wire through the fragments. This provides some stability to the fragments and restores normal alignment. Next, span the defect with a corticocancellous bone graft and fix it to the clavicle with two screws. The graft is obtained from the anterior iliac

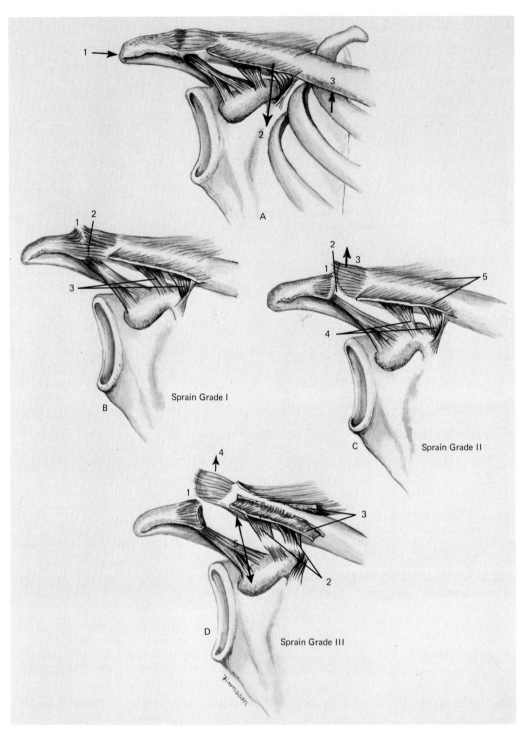

FIG. 9-24. Direct injury to the point of the shoulder. (A) The direct force is applied to the point of the shoulder (1), the scapula and the attached clavicle are forced downward and medially; the clavicle approaches the first rib (2). If the force continues, the first rib abuts against the clavicle, producing a counter force (3). Depending on the intensity of the force, a sprain grade I, II or III may occur. (B) Sprain Grade I: Few fibers of the acromioclavicular ligaments stretch or even (*cont'd on facing page*)

crest. Finally, pack the defect with cancellous bone chips (Fig. 9-20).

After the operation apply a plaster posterior figure-of-eight. External fixation must be maintained until bony union is achieved —12 to 16 weeks. During this period a regimen of exercises for the arm, hand and fingers should be enforced. Remove the intramedullary pin only after bony union is complete; never remove it earlier.

## Excess Callus Formation

Not infrequently massive callus forms at the fracture site, particularly if the fragments are comminuted or widely separated. Occasionally massive callus compresses the neurovascular elements in the thoracic outlet, although this is rare. The interval between the clavicle and the first rib varies considerably, and even a small space-taking lesion in this region in patients with a narrow costoclavicular interval may produce symptoms.

Symptoms of compression appear late. However, their intensity increases steadily with time. Management comprises excision of that portion of the clavicle and callus causing the compression. Excision of the bone may be very difficult because of the proximity of the vital structures beneath it. Also, the clavicle and callus should be exposed extraperiosteally in order to minimize the chances of recurrence of the callus (Fig. 9-21). The surgical procedure is described on page 236.

## Neurovascular Injuries

Injuries to the neurovascular structures are usually caused by displaced fragments of bone (Fig. 9-22). The type of injury varies from simple mild compression to laceration of the elements. The commonest of these injuries are compression or angulation of the subclavian vessels and brachial plexus. Injuries to the vessels may produce an aneurysm of the subclavian artery, thrombosis of the subclavian vein or an arteriovenous fistula.

Symptoms may vary, either at the time of injury or at a later date, depending upon the nature of the pathology. All available diagnostic aids should be used to establish the nature of the pathology, such as arteriograms, venograms and electromyographic studies. Following severe fractures it behooves the physician to make repeated checks on the neurovascular status of the limb. There should be no difficulty in recognizing immediately lesions associated with fresh fractures. As a rule, these usually respond to simple closed reduction and adequate immobilization of the fractures. In fresh lesions, if the manifestations are not relieved by closed methods, the displaced fragments must be exposed and elevated. Also, at this time, the fracture can be reduced and fixed by an intramedullary pin. The surgical technique is described on page 302.

In cases of longstanding compression caused by excessive callus, nonunion or malunion with great deformity, a portion of the clavicle should be excised extraperiosteally. If the complication occurs in a child, the clavicle should be excised subperiosteally, for, in children, reformation of the bone is desirable. In longstanding cases, excision of a portion of the clavicle

tear (1); the acromioclavicular joint is stable (2); the coracoclavicular ligament is intact (3). (C) Sprain Grade II (Subluxation): The capsule and the acromioclavicular ligaments rupture (1); the acromioclavicular joint is lax and unstable (2); the end of the clavicle rides upward, usually less than one half the width of the end of the clavicle (3); the coracoclavicular ligament remains intact (4); the attachments of the trapezius and deltoid to the clavicle are intact (5). (D) Sprain Grade III (Dislocation): The capsule and the acromioclavicular ligaments rupture (1); the coracoclavicular ligament ruptures (2); the insertions of the trapezius and the deltoid tear away from the clavicle (3); the clavicle rides upward (4); the interval between the clavicle and the coracoid process is greatly increased (5).

may have to be supplemented by lysis of the neurovascular structures, in order to relieve compression and angulation. The surgical procedure is described on page 236.

## ACROMIOCLAVICULAR JOINT

### Acute Sprain, Subluxation, Dislocation

*Pertinent Anatomical Features*

The acromioclavicular joint plays an important role in the functional mechanics of the shoulder girdle. It should be recalled that this joint, together with the sterno-clavicular joint, makes possible 60° of the 180° range of abduction of the arm. Also, it participates in protraction and retraction of the shoulder. The configuration of the joint and the arrangement of its ligaments make all this possible. The shape and size of the articular surfaces provide no stability; yet the arrangement of the ligaments of the joint are such that it is a very stable joint, and much force is required to disrupt its integrity.

The joint is formed by the flat, medial margin of the acromion and the distal end of the clavicle. The bone ends are encompassed completely in a weak, relaxed fibrous capsule which is reinforced above by the strong, tough superior acromio-clavicular ligament and below by the relatively weak inferior acromioclavicular ligament. Early in life, during the first decade, a fibrocartilaginous disc separates the two articular surfaces. However, this structure undergoes a rapid deterioration, so that in the second decade only remnants of the structure are present, in some joints. In other joints, it is totally absent. Because of this natural and rapid deterioration of the interarticular disc the erroneous concept that absence of the structure is a developmental defect has evolved. The superior acromioclavicular ligament is undoubtedly the most important single structure stabilizing the joint, but it receives help from other structures. The tendinous origins of the deltoid, particularly its an-

terior portion, and the trapezius help considerably in holding the clavicle in normal relation to the scapula. It is my belief that the superior acromioclavicular ligament, the trapezius and the deltoid are the prime stabilizers of the joint.

The coracoclavicular ligament comprises two fasciculi – the trapezoid and the conoid ligaments. It spans the interval between the clavicle and the coracoid process. Both fasciculi run from above, downward and medially. The direction of the fibers of both ligaments maintains a fixed relationship between the scapula and the clavicle by preventing medial displacement of the former on the latter (Fig. 9-23). The coracoclavicular ligament attaches to the clavicle where it curves posteriorly in its outer third. During elevation of the arm, outward rotation of the scapula displaces the coracoid process downward. In turn, the ligament, by virtue of its attachment on the posterior curve of the clavicle, causes the clavicle to rotate on its longitudinal axis. This, in my opinion, is the most important function of the coracoclavicular ligament. I am not in agreement with some workers, who hold that the stability of the acromioclavicular joint depends upon the integrity of the coracoclavicular ligament. In cadavers, severance of the ligament does not produce luxation of the acromioclavicular joint. Luxation occurs only when the superior acromioclavicular ligament and the coracoclavicular ligament are severed. I have made this observation many times on fresh cadavers.

*Mechanisms of Injuries*

The location of the acromioclavicular joint in the human skeletal frame and its superficial position render it vulnerable to many kinds of disruptive forces. These forces may be direct or indirect.

### Direct Injuries

Injuries to the capsule and ligaments of the joint may be the result of a direct downward blow on the tip of the shoulder or a fall on the point of the shoulder such as occurs when a rider falls off a horse and lands on the exposed shoulder. In these injuries the arm is usually at the side and perhaps even slightly adducted. The direct force drives the scapula and the attached clavicle downward and medially; the clavicle approaches the first rib. If the force continues, the first rib abuts against the clavicle, producing a counter force which, if sufficiently strong, may cause rupture of the acromioclavicular ligament, rupture of the coracoclavicular ligament and tearing of the insertions of the trapezius and of the anterior portion of the deltoid. Depending upon the intensity of the forces acting in this mechanism, one of three lesions may result (Fig. 9-24A): sprain grade I, sprain grade II, and sprain grade III.

**Sprain Grade I.** This lesion is caused by a relatively mild force which produces some stretching and even tearing of a few fibers of the acromioclavicular ligaments. The acromioclavicular joint remains stable, there is no laxity of the joint and the coracoclavicular ligament is intact (Fig. 9-24B).

**Sprain Grade II (Subluxation).** A grade II sprain is the result of a moderate force acting on the point of the shoulder. However, the force is great enough to rupture the capsule and the acromioclavicular ligaments and may tear a few fibers of the coracoclavicular ligament. As a result, the joint is unstable and exhibits obvious laxity. The end of the clavicle rides upward, usually less than one half the width of its outer end. Both the coracoclavicular ligament and the insertion of the deltoid and trapezius remain intact (Fig. 9-24C).

A grade II sprain may also be caused by a direct blow on the distal end of the clavicle, forcing the clavicle posteriorly, or from a fall on the posterosuperior aspect of the shoulder. In this lesion, elevation of the clavicle may not occur.

**Sprain Grade III (Dislocation).** This lesion

is caused by forces of great intensity. All the ligaments and capsule of the acromioclavicular joint are disrupted; these are the acromioclavicular ligaments, coracoclavicular ligament and the capsule of the joint. In addition, the insertions of the deltoid and trapezius are usually torn asunder (Fig. 9-24D). The clavicle rides upward and backward, and the clavicle and the coracoid process are widely separated. A direct blow on the outer end of the clavicle may drive it posteriorly without any upward displacement. This lesion may be difficult to diagnose because of the absence of an obvious deformity. Nevertheless, the capsule, the acromioclavicular and the coracoclavicular ligaments may be completely disrupted.

### Indirect Injuries

A great number of acromioclavicular sprains are caused by indirect mechanisms. This is particularly true in football; the player falls on the outstretched arm, the arm being in a position of abduction and slight flexion. From its point of application on the hand or arm, the force travels along the shaft of the humerus, crosses the stable glenohumeral joint and expends itself on the acromion, forcing the scapula upward and medially. In this mechanism the coracoclavicular ligament is seldom injured because it is forced into a relaxed position. Again depending on the intensity of the force, a sprain grade I or grade II may occur (Figs. 9-25 and 9-26).

### Diagnosis and Management of Sprains of the Acromioclavicular Joint

Generally, making the diagnosis of the various types of sprains is not difficult.

### Sprain – Grade I

The intensity of the pain in grade I sprains is not great, and normal motion of the arm causes no pain unless stress is applied. Local tenderness over the acromio-

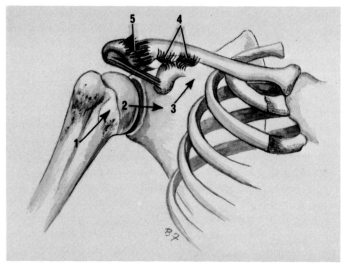

FIG. 9-25. Sprain Grade I produced by an indirect force. The force is transmitted along the shaft of the humerus (1); the force crosses the stable glenohumeral joint (2); the scapula is forced upward and medially (3); the coracoclavicular ligament is relaxed (4); few of the fibers of the capsule and the acromioclavicular ligaments stretch or tear.

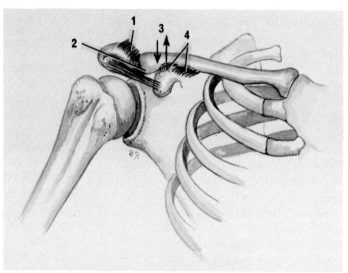

FIG. 9-26. Sprain Grade II produced by an indirect force. If the force is of sufficient intensity, the capsule and the acromioclavicular ligaments rupture (1), the acromioclavicular joint is unstable (2), and the clavicle is freely movable (3), but the coracoclavicular ligaments are relaxed and remain intact (4).

clavicular joint is always present and, because all ligaments are intact, no laxity of the joint is demonstrable. Roentgenograms of the joint taken immediately after injury exhibit no alterations in the configuration of the joint. However, those taken several weeks later may disclose some subperiosteal calcification surrounding the distal end of the clavicle.

Treatment of this lesion is relatively simple. The shoulder should be protected from further injury until it is pain free and until return of function and strength is complete. This is best accomplished by a sling. The application of ice immediately after injury tends to reduce swelling and to give comfort; later—in about 24 to 36 hours—heat should be applied. Recovery should be complete in 10 to 14 days.

### Sprains—Grade II

Pain in this lesion is of greater intensity than that in grade I sprains; also there is more localized tenderness and swelling over the acromioclavicular joint. All motions of the arm cause pain, especially if the arm moves against resistance. The de-

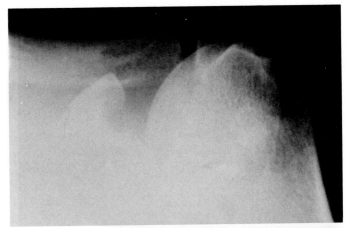

FIG. 9-27. This is a case of Grade II sprain with backward displacement of the clavicle. The only roentgenographic clue to the lesion is the widening of the joint space.

formity at this joint varies from the subtle to the obvious. The clavicle rides higher than the acromion but never more than 50 percent of the width of the outer end of the clavicle. The joint is unstable and ballottement of the end of the clavicle is readily performed. Stress roentgenograms of both shoulders should always be taken with a 10- to 15-pound weight suspended from each wrist. Such roentgenograms readily disclose the deformity at the acromioclavicular joint; however, there is no increase in the distance between the coracoid process and the clavicle. Backward displacement of the clavicle may produce no obvious deformity of the joint. However, careful palpation of the area reveals protrusion of the outer end of the clavicle posteriorly, and laxity of the joint. Roentgenograms, even those taken with stress on the arm, may fail to show any elevation of the clavicle, but there is, in all cases, widening of the joint space (Figs. 9-27 and 9-28).

There is general agreement that grade II sprains should be treated by closed methods. The subluxation is reduced and some form of external fixation is applied to maintain the reduction. There is no agreement on the most efficacious type of support. If you review the literature on this topic you will be amazed at the great number of different apparatuses that have been designed to fix the acromioclavicular joint. In one report, over fifty different modes of fixation

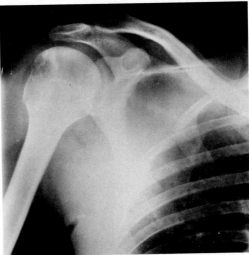

FIG. 9-28. Roentgenograph of a Grade II sprain. Note the slightly elevated clavicle and widening of the joint space.

were recorded. Today there is no need to use any form of adhesive dressing. These often may cause severe irritation of the skin. Also the patient can and often does change the position of the dressing, and rigid, constant immobilization of the joint in its anatomical position is virtually impossible. The Kenny-Howard sling halter overcomes all the disadvantages of adhesive dressings, and, in my opinion, it is far superior to any other form of immobilization so far designed.

Reduction of the subluxation is readily

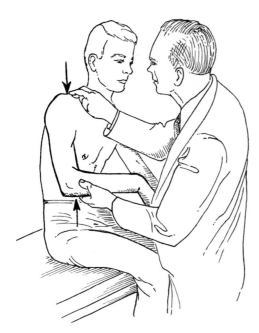

FIG. 9-29. Reduction of Grade II sprain of the acromioclavicular joint. Downward pressure on the clavicle and upward pressure on the forearm readily corrects the displacement.

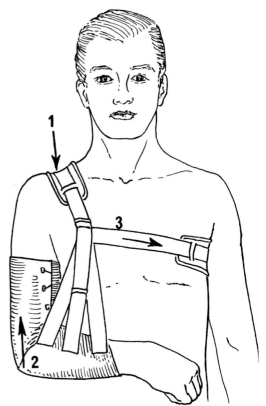

FIG. 9-30. Kenny-Howard sling. The shoulder strap is applied over a piece of felt; it holds the clavicle down (1). The sling supports the forearm and keeps the acromion in an elevated position (2). The halter pulls both the shoulder strap and the sling inward (3).

achieved by making downward pressure on the clavicle and upward pressure on the flexed forearm (Fig. 9-29). Now, apply the Kenny-Howard sling halter correctly. As demonstrated in Figure 9-30, the shoulder strap applied over a piece of felt holds the clavicle down; the sling supports the forearm and keeps the acromion in an elevated position, and the halter pulls both the shoulder strap and the sling inward. The apparatus is maintained in place for 3 to 4 weeks. The position of the sling should be checked frequently and under no circumstances should it be removed before the desired period of immobilization expires.

### Sprains — Grade III

A fresh, grade III sprain is usually associated with severe pain and marked dysfunction of the shoulder. Localized tenderness is pronounced over the joint, the outer

end of the clavicle and the coracoid process; upriding of the clavicle is obvious. All movements of the arm are painful, particularly if stress is applied. Stress roentgenograms reveal the clavicle riding high above the superior surface of the acromion and the interval between the coracoid process and the clavicle is extraordinarily wide (Figs. 9-31 and 9-32).

When the clavicle is displaced backward, the classic roentgenographic findings described above are not present. Instead, the width of the joint space between the acromion and clavicle is widened even when the superior surfaces of the acromion and clavicle are on the same horizontal plane. The

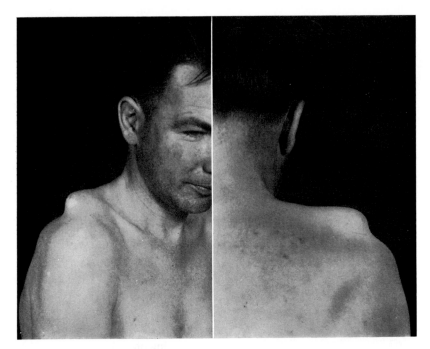

FIG. 9-31. Anterolateral and posterior views of a dislocated acromioclavicular joint. Observe the prominent outer end of the clavicle and drooping of the shoulder.

important clinical observations in this lesion are the palpable posterior displacement of the outer end of the clavicle, and the marked instability of the joint demonstrable by ballottement of the clavicle, even when clinically the acromion and clavicle appear to be in normal alignment.

No area in the field of orthopaedic surgery is more controversial than the treatment of complete disruption of the acromioclavicular joint. Essentially there are two camps: those who propose closed methods of treatment and those who advocate surgical methods. Furthermore, in each camp there is disagreement as to the type of closed method or surgical method producing the best results. Unfortunately, in the literature, there are no long-term end results of a significant number of cases treated by any single method, closed or open, which can be clinically evaluated as to its superiority over other methods of treatment. A thorough review of the literature suggests that good results are attain-

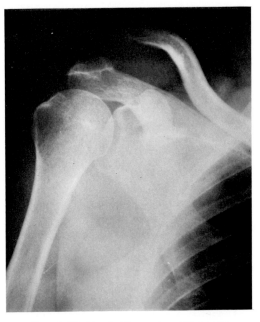

FIG. 9-32. Grade III sprain of the acromioclavicular joint. Note the elevation of the end of the clavicle and the wide interval between the clavicle and the coracoid process.

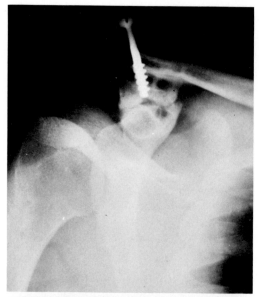

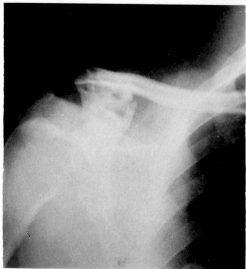

(*Top*) FIG. 9-33. This lesion was originally treated with a screw fixing the clavicle to the coracoid process. The screw worked out, the dislocation recurred and calcification and ossification of the coracoclavicular ligaments occurred. This was a painful joint.

(*Bottom*) FIG. 9-34. Same patient shown in Figure 9-33. The screw was removed and the outer end of the clavicle resected. This shoulder became pain free in spite of the ossification of the coracoclavicular ligament.

able by any method of treatment, and that all methods have their toll of unfavorable results, in regard to pain, dysfunction and residual deformity. It appears that the deciding factor as to whether a good or bad result is obtained is not the method but is, rather, how skillfully the method is employed. For example, Allman is a proponent of the closed method using the Kenny-Howard sling halter. His skillful and meticulous management of the patient during the period of immobilization produces results comparable to any operative method. On the other hand, few workers, including myself, have been able to attain the same results with the same method. But there are other factors governing the grade of end results such as damage to the articular surfaces of the acromion and clavicle: tearing and shredding of the interarticular disc; displacement of tabs of the acromioclavicular ligaments into the joint; pre-existing degenerative changes in the joint; avulsion and tearing of the insertions of the trapezius and the deltoid, and injury to the tendon of the long head of the biceps.

Also of interest is the total lack of correlation between the amount of residual deformity and dysfunction and pain in the shoulder girdle. In fact, I have yet to see an old, untreated, completely disrupted acromioclavicular joint that is symptomatic and interferes with normal function of the arm. This is the opinion of other workers also. Pain and dysfunction are more prevalent in shoulders with partial displacement of the clavicle than in those with complete displacement. This is undoubtedly due to internal derangement of the joint caused by damage to the interarticular disc or the articular surfaces of the joint or to tabs of the ligaments within the joint.

I prefer to treat surgically all fresh, complete lesions unless there are specific contraindications to surgical approach, such as advanced age. However, certain operative procedures, in my opinion, should not be performed and certain surgical steps en-

(*Right*) FIG. 9-35. Dislocation of the acromioclavicular joint treated by the insertion of
wires across the joint. The wires are not
threaded, their diameter is too small and the
patient was allowed free use of the arm. The
result is obvious. The wires broke and the
deformity recurred.

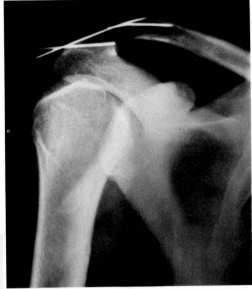

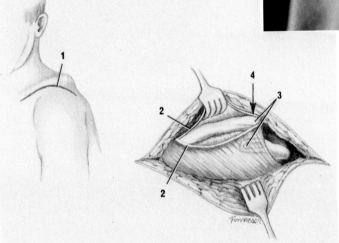

(*Left*) FIG. 9-36. Operative
technique: Make a slightly
curved 3-inch incision over
the clavicle, ending at the
tip of the acromion process
(1); reflect the attachments
of the deltoid and trapezius
by sharp subperiosteal dissection (2); remove all debris
and remnants of the interarticular disc from the joint
(3); reduce the dislocation
by downward pressure on
the clavicle and upward
pressure on the forearm (4).

hance the probability of attaining a favorable result.

Permanent, rigid fixation of the clavicle
to the coracoid process with a screw is unwise. It eliminates the rotatory function of
the clavicle and, hence, restricts abduction
of the arm. If this method is employed, the
screw should be removed after 6 weeks
(Figs. 9-33 and 9-34).

Anatomical reduction of the acromioclavicular joint is readily maintained by one
or two wires across the joint. However,
threaded wires should be used in order to
prevent their migration. After 6 to 8 weeks

the wires should be removed. During the
period of immobilization abduction movements of the arm must be restricted because the wires may break (Fig. 9-35).

All debris in the joint should be removed.
In fact, I do a complete débridement, removing the interarticular disc in toto. This
structure undergoes rapid attritional
changes even in the normal joint. It should
be removed to prevent trouble in the future.

The acromioclavicular ligaments, particularly the superior one, should be meticulously repaired. These are important stabilizing structures of the joint.

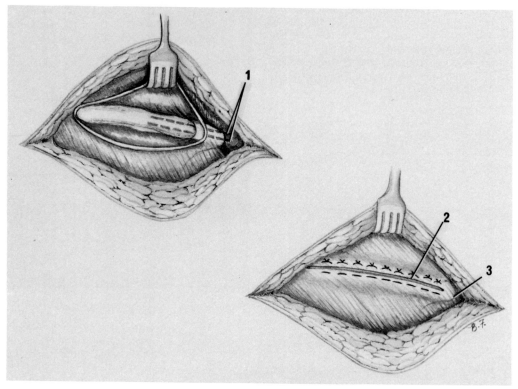

FIG. 9-37. Transfix the joint by two threaded wires (5/64 inch in diameter) passing through the acromion into the clavicle for a distance of one to 1½ inches; cut the wires below the skin (1); lap the margins of the trapezius and deltoid tightly over the clavicle and acromion by mattress sutures (2); approximate the edges of the superior acromioclavicular ligament (3).

The insertions of the anterior deltoid and trapezius should be explored, reflected subperiosteally and then reefed over the acromion and clavicle by mattress sutures. By so doing, tears of these structures are repaired; this alone may prevent pain in the future. Reefing the muscle insertions reinforces the stability of the joint.

As previously stated, my opinion is that the primary role of the coracoclavicular ligament is not to stabilize the joint but to guide the rotation of the clavicle. I ignore the state of this ligament.

In young athletes and in active adults in whom I strive for anatomical restoration of the joint, I prefer to transfer the tip of the coracoid process, with the coracobrachialis and short head of the biceps at-tached, to the clavicle. This tends to minimize any residual upward displacement of the clavicle.

**Operative Procedure.** Make a slightly curved 3-inch incision over the clavicle, terminating at the tip of the acromion process (Fig. 9-36). Dissect the skin and subcutaneous tissue from the insertions of the anterior deltoid on the acromion and clavicle and of the trapezius on the clavicle. Now, explore these muscles for any evidence of tears. By subperiosteal dissection reflect the insertions of both muscles. An effort must be made to avoid further damage to the superior acromioclavicular ligament.

The inside of the joint must be carefully inspected, noting any evidence of damage to the articular surfaces and the interarticular disc. Remove all debris and any remnants of the disc from the joint. The joint is now ready for reduction. This is readily achieved by downward pressure on the clavicle and upward pressure on the arm. While the reduction is maintained, transfix the joint by one or two threaded wires ($\frac{5}{64}$ inch in diameter) passing through the acromion into the clavicle for a distance of 1 to $1\frac{1}{2}$ inches. Cut the wires close to the skin and bury them under the skin (Fig. 9-37).

If it is decided that the tip of the coracoid process should not be transferred to the clavicle, simply lap the insertions of the trapezius and deltoid tightly over the clavicle and acromion by mattress sutures (Figs. 9-37, 9-38 and 9-39).

If the decision is to transfer the tip of the coracoid process, carefully isolate this bony prominence which lies in the extreme medial portion of the incision. Drill a hole in the cortex of the bony process and place a $\frac{3}{4}$-inch screw into the drill hole. Now, osteotomize the coracoid process at its base just below the origins of the coracobrachialis and the short head of the biceps. Make a drill hole on the anterior surface of the clavicle just medial to its outer articular surface and insert into it the screw penetrating the tip of the coracoid process (Fig. 9-40). Finally, lap tightly over the acromion and clavicle the insertions of the deltoid and trapezius by mattress sutures.

**Postoperative Management.** At the completion of the operation apply a sling, with a cotton pad in the axilla, and fix the arm to the chest wall with an elastic bandage 6 inches wide. Instead of a sling a collar and cuff may be used to support the arm. Encourage motion of the elbow and fingers within the limits of the dressing but do not allow abduction motion of the arm. After 6 to 8 weeks remove the wires and permit free use of the arm and shoulder. Also, institute a regulated regimen of physical therapy and exercises to restore normal motion in all joints of the extremity.

**Other Popular Surgical Procedures.** Cur-

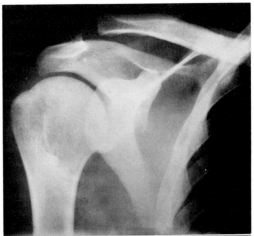

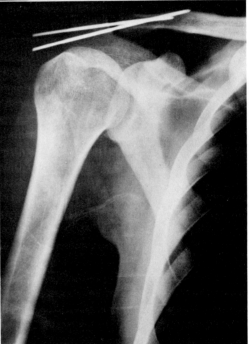

(*Top*) FIG. 9-38. Dislocation of the acromioclavicular joint.

(*Bottom*) FIG. 9-39. Dislocation in Figure 9-38, treated by two threaded wires crossing the joint and reefing of the insertions of the deltoid and trapezius.

rently other surgical procedures are favored by many competent orthopaedic surgeons. There is great variation in these different operations, and this is undoubtedly based on the philosophy of the individual sur-

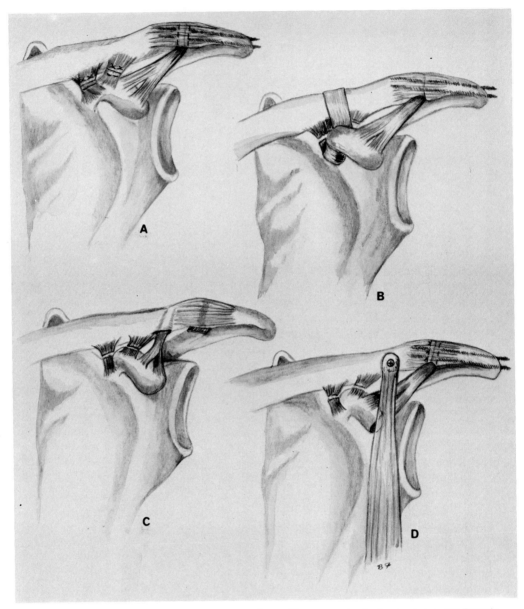

FIG. 9-40. Methods of repair of dislocation of the acromioclavicular joint: (A) Repair of the coracoclavicular ligament and the superior acromioclavicular ligament. (B) Reconstruction of the coracoclavicular ligament with fascia lata. (C) Reinforcement of the superior acromioclavicular ligament with the coracoacromial ligament (Neviaser). (D) Transfer of the coracoid process with the conjoined tendon to the clavicle (Bailey).

geon in regard to the role the superior acromioclavicular and the coracoclavicular ligaments play in the stability of the joint.

In some procedures the ligaments are not exposed or repaired; the dislocation is reduced and the normal interval between the clavicle and the coracoid is restored. The position is maintained by pins or wires across the acromioclavicular joint, or by a screw that fixes the clavicle to the coracoid, or by wires, braided silk or fascia, binding the clavicle to the coracoid process.

Other surgeons place great emphasis on the restoration of all ligaments. The superior ligament is meticulously repaired and both fasciculi of the coracoclavicular ligament are also exposed and repaired. Some reinforce the ligaments with fascia or some other structure. Neviaser has devised an ingenious operation in which he uses the coracoacromial ligament to reinforce the superior acromioclavicular ligament (Fig. 9-40).

**Complications.** Complications occur in both the conservative and the surgical treatment of severe sprains of the acromioclavicular joint.

COMPLICATIONS OF CONSERVATIVE THERAPY. The two most frequent complications are residual laxity or subluxation and pain in the joint. In the hands of most orthopaedic surgeons, the former complication is so common that they have discarded the conservative method and prefer the surgical approach to the problem. However, in the hands of some experts the incidence of subluxation is markedly reduced and compares favorably with the end results of some of the surgical methods now in use.

Pain is a common sequel and is not related to the degree of instability of the joint. Most likely it is the result of one lesion, or a combination of many, capable of producing pain and dysfunction in the acromioclavicular joint. Following trauma, degenerative changes may occur in the cartilaginous surface of the joint, or the interarticular disc may be disrupted or tabs of the capsule and ligaments may fall into the joint, producing an internal derangement. Any of these factors may produce an osteoarthritic process that is capable of causing pain.

Occasionally, calcification occurs in the coracoclavicular ligament; however, it occurs more frequently in the surgically treated cases. Fortunately, calcification of the ligament neither interferes with function nor causes pain.

COMPLICATIONS OF SURGICAL TREATMENT. These complications fall into two categories: those common to any surgical procedure and those peculiar to the acromioclavicular joint. The former group comprises infection, skin necrosis, postoperative hematoma and a painful scar. These complications can be reduced to a minimum by handling tissues gently, by avoiding unnecessary stripping of the acromion and clavicle, by obliterating dead spaces in the wound and by performing the operation with meticulous sterile technique.

Complications peculiar to the acromioclavicular joint are many, most of which are avoidable.

PROTRUDING PINS OR WIRES. The pins, if left protruding out of the skin, may produce considerable local irritation and may set the stage for a local infection. This is also true if the pins are buried under the skin but are too long, so that they may actually erode through the skin. The pins should be buried under the skin; they should be long enough to be accessible, but not so long as to put the overlying skin under tension.

*Migration and Breaking of Pins and Wires.* Migration of the pins and wires can be avoided if threaded wires or pins are used. If smooth pins are used, the outer ends should be turned up to avoid inward migration; however, this does not prevent outward migration of the pin. Breakage of the pins and wires across an acromioclavicular joint is a serious complication because it may require considerable surgery and exposure of the joint to remove the broken ends. Again, the incidence of this complication can be reduced by not permitting motion at the shoulder, particularly abduction, during the period of fixation.

*Complications Associated With Screw and Circumferential Wire Fixation.* Screws placed through the clavicle and into the coracoid process may pull out or break.

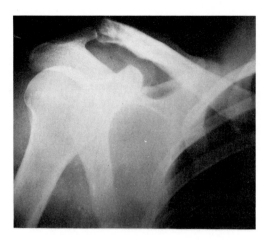

FIG. 9-41. Osteoarthritic changes in the acromioclavicular joint associated with a fracture of the distal end of the clavicle. The fracture-dislocation of the joint had been reduced openly and fixed by two threaded wires across the joint. This was a painful joint.

This occurs because motion of the clavicle is not eliminated completely during the period of fixation. The same is true when circumferential wires are employed. Clavicular motion may also cause bone absorption around the screw and fracture of the clavicle through the screw hole.

*Other Complications.* Calcification and ossification of the coracoclavicular ligament may occur in both conservative and operative methods of treatment, but it occurs more frequently when the ligament is exposed and repaired. As previously noted, this complication is relatively benign.

Osteoarthritis of the acromioclavicular joint is undoubtedly the commonest source of pain following surgical management of acromioclavicular dislocations. This complication also can be avoided in many instances. Careful debridement of the joint reduces the incidence and the intensity of this lesion. Also, residual subluxation should be avoided if possible, for incongruity of the articular surfaces favors development of degenerative changes. Piercing the articular surfaces with large pins or wires or making multiple punctures through the surfaces also enhances development of degenerative alterations.

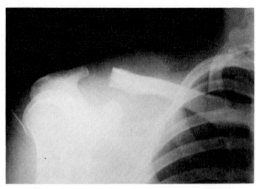

FIG. 9-42. Same joint as in Figure 9-41, after resection of the end of the clavicle; pain was relieved by this procedure.

In dislocations associated with fractures of the distal end of the clavicle osteoarthritis is particularly prone to develop if the fracture line traverses the articular surface of the clavicle or if the bone end is comminuted. In the initial management of these lesions the surgeon should give due consideration to the possibility of the development of osteoarthritis. Excision of the distal fragments and débridement of the joint at this time may spare the patient trouble in the future (Figs. 9-41 and 9-42).

## The Untreated Sprains

Both in sports and in the general population, many sprains of the acromioclavicular joint are not treated. Grade I sprains, unless re-injury occurs, cause no future trouble after the two- or three-week healing period following the injury. Grade II sprains are unpredictable; some may be the source of considerable pain and dysfunction of the shoulder girdle. However, the over-all disability resulting from this chronic state varies. In some patients the pain and weakness in the shoulder girdle may severely interfere with normal activities and in others it may cause no pain or perceptible dysfunction. It is not rare to find athletes performing effectively in their sports with an obvious subluxation of the acromioclavicular joint. In athletes and active young adults there is always the possibility of a grade II sprain being converted to a grade III sprain by repeated injury.

In general, after the initial pain and immediate impaired function caused by a fresh grade III sprain disappear, the patient has no pain; and, as far as he is concerned, he has no impairment of function. The only visible evidence of the lesion is the high-riding clavicle. In 1969 there were ten professional football players known to have grade III sprains who were performing without pain or impairment of function. Nevertheless, most orthopaedic surgeons knowledgeable in this lesion agree that complete disruption of the acromioclavicular joint does produce some weakness and discomfort in the shoulder girdle. This is readily appreciated in patients whose occupation demands that the arm function in the fully abducted position for long periods of time, such as painters, plasterers and paperhangers.

## Chronic Sprains of Grade II and Grade III

It should be remembered that not all grade II sprains are symptomatic. When they are and the pain and impairment of function are of such intensity that they interfere with normal living, then a program of treatment is indicated. The symptoms are usually the result of a traumatic arthritis characterized by erosion and fragmentation of the articular cartilage, local swelling of the capsule and even calcification of the ligaments and cartilage. Any movement of the arm that brings the articular surfaces of the joint into firm apposition, such as abduction of the arm, causes pain. Pressure over the joint line invariably produces pain, as do movements that put tension on the ligaments, such as traction on the arm.

A fair trial of conservative measures may be very rewarding in many of these cases. Rest to the shoulder girdle is most essential and can be provided by a sling. Radiant heat reduces local swelling; local injection of a corticoid preparation and the use of anti-inflammatory drugs are also beneficial.

If these measures fail, surgical intervention is indicated.

The surgical procedure should include two steps: débridement of the joint cavity, and resection of the distal $1/2$ or $3/4$ inch of the clavicle. As a rule, this procedure gives a painless shoulder with excellent function. If this procedure is correctly performed and the patient still has pain, it behooves the surgeon to look elsewhere for the etiology of the pain. One patient who had this operation performed continued to have pain in the shoulder; further investigations revealed that coronary heart disease caused his pain.

The management of old complete dislocations of the acromioclavicular joint remains controversial. It ranges from reconstruction of the ligaments to "do nothing." It should be remembered that these are painless lesions that do not interfere with function. When surgery is performed, its goal usually is to correct the deformity; only in rare instances is it performed to relieve pain. The age and the level of activity of the person should determine the nature of the operative procedure. I believe that if surgery is to be done in athletes and young adults, the operation should restore the anatomical configuration of the joint and $1/2$ to $3/4$ inch of the distal end of the clavicle should be removed. Removal of a portion of the distal end of the clavicle insures the patient against pain caused by degenerative changes which may develop in the joint when its articular surfaces are again in apposition. To hold the clavicle in normal relationship to the scapula I transfer the tip of the coracoid, with the short head of the biceps and the coracobrachialis attached, to the clavicle. Also, I reef the insertions of the deltoid and trapezius over the acromion and clavicle. If at the end of the operation the clavicle still rides high or anteriorly, I force it into normal alignment with the acromion and transfix both bones with one or two $5/64$ inch threaded wires. These are removed after 5 to 6 weeks, at which time the coracoid process is sufficiently anchored to permit the muscles

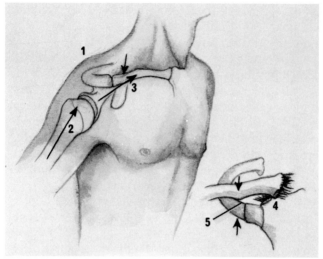

FIG. 9-43. Anterosuperior dislocation—mechanism of sprains of the sternoclavicular joint. The shoulder is depressed and extended (1); the impact is applied to the anterolateral aspect of the shoulder (2); the force is transmitted medially along the clavicle and posteriorly along the scapula (3); the product of these forces is expended at the sternoclavicular joint, producing an anterosuperior dislocation (4); if the force continues, the clavicle abuts against the first rib which acts as a fulcrum to lever the clavicle anteriorly and superiorly (5).

attached to it to hold the clavicle down (see Fig. 9-18).

In older persons, I urge acceptance of the deformity. However, if they refuse, I perform the simplest operation possible. I resect the distal 1/2 or 3/4 inch of the clavicle and reef the insertions of the deltoid and trapezius muscles.

Neviaser's operation is another excellent procedure for both the young and the old. He reinforces the superior acromioclavicular ligament by transferring to the clavicle the medial end of the coracoacromial ligament. He maintains the acromion and clavicle in normal alignment by transfixing them with a wire which he removes 5 weeks later (see Fig. 9-40C).

## STERNOCLAVICULAR JOINT

### Acute Sprain, Subluxation, Dislocation

### Pertinent Anatomical Considerations

The sternoclavicular joint is the only true articulation between the upper extremity and the trunk. It is formed by the inner end of the clavicle and the oblique outer surface of the manubrium and the cartilage of the first rib. Only a small portion of the articular surface of the clavicle (50%) is in contact with that of the manubrium. The joint is enveloped in a loose fibrous capsule which blends with the interarticular disc. The capsule is reinforced anteriorly and posteriorly by the sternoclavicular ligaments and superiorly by the interclavicular ligament. The joint contains an interarticular disc which in most instances divides the joint cavity into two compartments. Considerable incongruity exists between the articular surfaces of the clavicle and the sternum. However, this is compensated by the interposition of the disc, whose structural arrangement makes it an effective buffer to the stresses of function. The disc is convex-concave and has a broad, firm circular attachment on the upper and posterior aspects of the clavicle. Below, it blends with the cartilage of the first rib at its juncture with the sternum (*see* Fig. 4-6).

The costoclavicular ligament is a flat, strong structure, rhomboid in shape, which is attached below to the upper and medial portions of the cartilage of the first rib and above to the costal tuberosity on the under surface of the inner portion of the clavicle. The fibers of the ligament run obliquely upward, lateralward and backward from the rib to the clavicle (*see* Figure 4-6).

The bony anatomical configuration of the joint provides little stability. However, by virtue of the great strength of the interarticular disc and of the costoclavicular ligament the sternoclavicular joint is a very stable joint. It is essentially a plane joint but functions as a ball and socket joint permitting motion in all planes, including rotation of the clavicle. Every motion of the upper extremity is accompanied by some motion in the sternoclavicular joint in the form of rotation or glide, or impact. Yet, this articulation is capable of meeting the stresses of function with only minimal regressive changes.

The costoclavicular ligament plays an important role in the stability of the joint. It opposes upward displacement of the clavicle by the sternocleidomastoid and prevents upward and lateral displacement of the clavicle. In addition, it acts as the pivot during forward and backward motion and during elevation and depression of the shoulder. This ligament is extra-articular and corresponds to the coracoclavicular ligament.

The part that the interarticular disc contributes to the stability of the sternoclavicular joint is not generally appreciated. It is a tough, massive structure, and its upper attachment to the upper and posterior aspect of the end of the clavicle prevents upward and anterior displacement of the sternal end of the clavicle. The costoclavicular and the interarticular disc are undoubtedly the two structures responsible for the low incidence of disruptive lesions of the sternoclavicular joint.

Finally, it should be remembered that immediately posterior to the joint lie the main vessels of the neck, the dome of the pleura, the trachea and esophagus. The only barrier between the posterior capsule of the joint and the great vessels is that formed by the sternothyroid and sternohyoid muscles. Although rare, the vital structures may be injured by retrosternal displacement of the clavicle (see Fig. 4-7).

## Mechanisms of Injuries

Lesions of the sternoclavicular joint occur infrequently. The protected position of the joint and the strength of its ligamentous

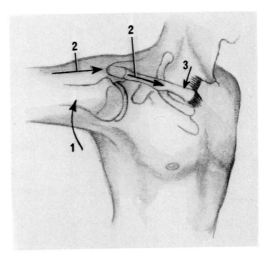

FIG. 9-44. Mechanism of sprains and anteroinferior dislocation of the sternoclavicular joint. The arm is abducted and the shoulder extended (1); the force travels along the humerus and medially along the clavicle (2); the force is expended at the sternoclavicular joint, producing an anteroinferior dislocation (3).

apparatus are responsible for this infrequency. Most injuries are the result of an indirect mechanism. The force is applied to the lateral aspect of the shoulder or along the abducted arm. It travels medially along the clavicle and expends itself at the sternoclavicular joint. The intensity of the force and the position of the arm in relation to the trunk govern the nature of the resulting lesion. By this mechanism the clavicle may be forced anteriorly, superiorly or posteriorly in relation to the sternum. Depending upon the intensity of the force, varying gradations of implication of the ligaments and interarticular disc occur; the lesions are classified as grade I, grade II and grade III.

**Anterosuperior Sprains.** These lesions are produced when the shoulder is depressed and extended and an impact is applied to the lateral aspect of the shoulder. The force travels medially along the clavicle and posteriorly along the scapula. The resulting force is expended at the sternoclavicular joint forcing the clavicle anteriorly and superiorly. When a great force is applied,

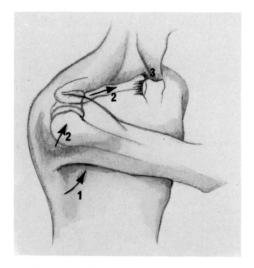

FIG. 9-45. Mechanism of sprains and posterior dislocation (retrosternal) of the sternoclavicular joint. The shoulder is elevated and flexed forward (1); the force travels along the humerus and medially along the clavicle (2); the force is expended at the sternoclavicular joint, producing a retrosternal dislocation (3). (The same lesion may be produced by a direct blow to the anterior aspect of the sternal end of the clavicle.)

the clavicle abuts against the first rib, which acts as a fulcrum to lever the clavicle anteriorly and superiorly (Fig. 9-43).

**Antero-Inferior Sprains.** These lesions occur when the arm is abducted and the shoulder is extended. The force travels along the humerus and medially along the clavicle. It expends itself at the sternoclavicular joint, forcing the clavicle into an antero-inferior position (Fig. 9-44).

**Posterior Sprains.** These lesions occur when the arm is elevated and flexed. The force travels along the humerus and medially along the clavicle. It expends itself on the posterior aspect of the sternoclavicular joint, forcing the clavicle into a retrosternal direction.

The same lesions may be produced by a direct blow on the anterior aspect of the sternal end of the clavicle, driving it posteriorly (Fig. 9-45).

**Sprain – Grade I.** The force producing this lesion is of minimal intensity. Some stretching and tearing of the fibers of the capsule and sternoclavicular ligaments occur; however, the integrity of the structures is preserved. The costoclavicular ligament and the interarticular disc remain intact (Fig. 9-46A).

**Sprain – Grade II.** In grade II sprains the force is sufficient to rupture the capsule and the sternoclavicular ligaments. In addition there may be some stretching and tearing of some of the fibers of the costoclavicular ligament and the fibers of attachment of the interarticular disc. This lesion permits partial displacement of the clavicle in relation to the sternum. The displacement may be anterosuperior, antero-inferior or backward, depending on the position of the arm and the direction of the force (Fig. 9-46B).

**Sprain – Grade III.** In this lesion the capsule and the sternoclavicular ligaments are completely ruptured; also, the costoclavicular ligament is torn completely and the attachment of the interarticular disc to clavicle is disrupted. Now, depending on the direction of the force, the clavicle lies anterosuperiorly, antero-inferiorly or posteriorly in relation to the sternum. As a rule, in anterior dislocations, the interarticular disc pulls off the sternum and follows the clavicle, whereas in posterior lesions it remains attached to the sternum (Fig. 9-46C).

Instead of a pure dislocation, a fracture-dislocation may occur. As the force drives the clavicle upward the strong costoclavicular ligament remains intact and avulses the inferior margin of the sternal end of the clavicle; the avulsed fragment may include the inferior portion of the head.

*Diagnosis and Management of Sprains*

**Sprain – Grade I**

Since all ligaments are intact, no deformity of the joint exists. There is some mild local swelling and local tenderness over the joint; pain is minimal.

Management is relatively simple. It comprises rest to the arm, best achieved with a sling; application of ice for the first 24 to 36

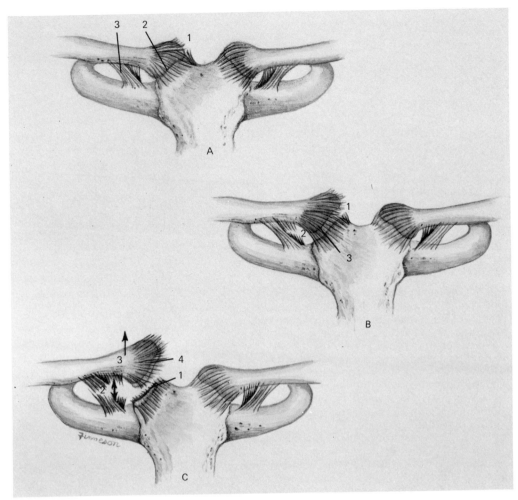

FIG. 9-46. Pathology of sprains. (A) Sprain Grade I: Some stretching and tearing of the sternoclavicular ligament (1); no disalignment of the articular surfaces of the clavicle and sternum (2). The costoclavicular ligaments are intact (3). (B) Sprain Grade II: The capsule and sternoclavicular ligaments rupture (1). Some tearing and stretching of the costoclavicular ligaments (2); partial displacement of the clavicle in relation to the sternum (3). (Note: The displacement of the clavicle may be anterosuperior, anteroinferior or backward, depending on the direction of the force.) (C) Sprain Grade III: Complete rupture of the capsule and sternoclavicular ligaments (1); complete rupture of the costoclavicular ligament (2); complete displacement of the clavicle in relation to the sternum (3). Usually in anterior dislocations the interarticular disc is avulsed from the sternum and follows the clavicle; in posterior dislocations it remains attached to the sternum (4). (Note: The displacement of the clavicle may be anterior or posterior, depending on the direction of the force.)

hours, followed by heat. Recovery is, as a rule, complete in 10 to 14 days.

### Sprain—Grade II

In this lesion, because the sternoclavicular ligaments and capsule are ruptured and some fibers of the interarticular disc detached, the joint exhibits some deformity. The sternal end of the clavicle is slightly displaced either anteriorly or posteriorly. There is mild laxity of the joint, local swelling and tenderness and moderate pain. All motions of the arm are somewhat pain-

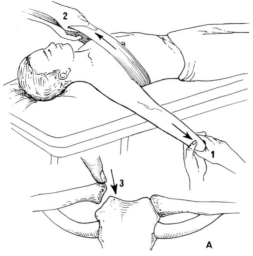

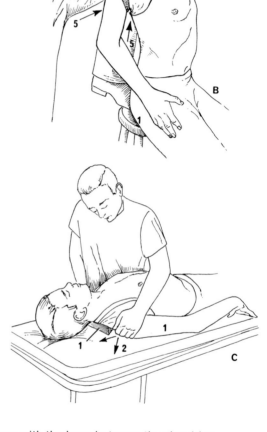

FIG. 9-47. Management of anterior sprains, Grades II and III, of the sternoclavicular joint. *Reduction:* (A) While an assistant makes steady traction on the abducted arm (1), a second assistant makes counter traction (2), the operator manipulates the sternal end of the clavicle (3). *Immobilization:* Maintain the reduction by pulling and holding the shoulders upward and backward; now apply a posterior figure-of-eight plaster of Paris bandage to hold this position. (B) Patient sits on a stool (1). Apply around the shoulders 4 or 5 turns of cotton batting in the form of a posterior figure-of-eight (2). The surgeon stands behind the patient and places one knee between the shoulder blades (3). Now apply 12 to 15 turns of plaster bandage 5 inches wide in the form of a posterior figure-of-eight (4). As the bandage passes through the axillae make tension on the bandage to elevate the shoulders and make counter pressure with the knee between the shoulder blades (5). (C) *Immobilization, continued.* Now place the patient in the supine position with a sandbag between the shoulder blades. Bring the arms to the sides (1); apply firm pressure over each shoulder forcing them upward and backward; maintain the pressure until the plaster is firmly set (2).

ful, and traction on the arm causes pain. Roentgenograms are not helpful in making the diagnosis. The diagnosis is made entirely on the clinical findings.

The local treatment comprises application of ice for 24 to 36 hours, then heat. The deformity must be reduced and the joint protected from further injury so that a grade II sprain is not converted to a grade III sprain by re-injury. Normal alignment of

the joint is readily attained by pulling the shoulders backward and outward and applying a plaster figure-of-eight bandage. The technique for the application of this form of external fixation is the same as that described for fractures of the clavicle (Fig. 9-47). Protection should continue for 6 weeks. During this period the arm should be in a sling and held to the side with a swathe. Active participation in any activity

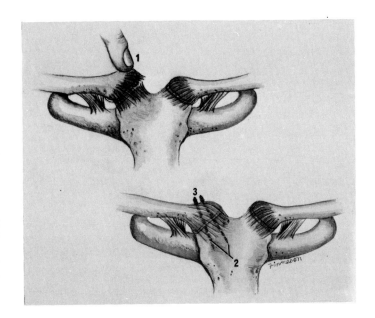

FIG. 9-48. Transfixation of sternoclavicular joint. This method is employed when reduction cannot be maintained by a plaster of paris figure-of-eight. Reduce the dislocation by direct pressure over the sternal end of the clavicle while the shoulders are pulled upward and backward (1); insert two threaded wires (5/64 inch in diameter) across the joint through the head of the clavicle into the sternum (2). Do not penetrate the posterior surface of the sternum.) Cut the wires below the level of the skin (3).

should not be allowed for 8 to 10 weeks. However, athletes rarely abide by this recommendation.

Most sprains grade II can be treated by the conservative method. Nevertheless, occasionally the sternal end of the clavicle cannot be held in its normal position regardless of the type of external fixation used. In this instance, open reduction is indicated. I prefer to expose the ligaments, to reduce the displacement and to maintain the reduction by two threaded wires ($^{5}/_{64}$ inch in diameter) inserted across the joint, first through the head of the clavicle and then into the sternum. The torn sternoclavicular ligaments should be repaired and external fixation by means of a plaster posterior figure-of-eight should be applied (Fig. 9-48). The wire and external support are removed after 6 weeks.

An alternate method is lateral traction, applied to the arm which is abducted 90°. I employ this method only if the operative method for some reason cannot be used (Fig. 9-49).

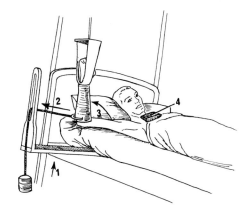

FIG. 9-49. Lateral traction. This method is employed if transfixing method is not acceptable to the patient and the first method (plaster of Paris posterior figure-of-eight bandage) fails. Elevate the side of the bed 4 to 6 inches (1); apply 8 to 10 pounds of traction on the abducted arm (2); the arm is abducted 90° to 120° (3). Place a small sandbag over the sternal end of the clavicle (4).

## Sprains — Grade III (Dislocation)

Characteristic of this lesion, in the fresh state, is severe local pain and tenderness and the presence of a deformity of the joint. Marked laxity of the sternal end of the clavicle is readily demonstrable. However, often the swelling obscures the deformity and pain may not permit manipulation of

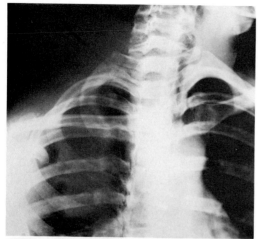

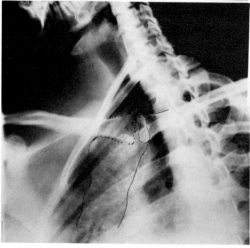

(*Top*) FIG. 9-50. Anterosuperior dislocation of the left sternoclavicular joint.

(*Bottom*) FIG. 9-51. Retrosternal dislocation of the right sternoclavicular joint.

the joint to reveal laxity. The diagnosis is difficult to establish. All movements of the arm cause pain, especially if stress is applied. Traction on the arm causes severe pain. It should be remembered that the clavicle may slip behind the sternum without complete disruption of the costoclavicular ligament. In this instance the end of the clavicle rides upward very little. Usually retrosternal dislocations occur, with complete disruption of all ligaments and detachment of the interarticular disc. The patients have severe pain at the base of the

neck and on deep breathing. There may be pressure on the trachea, the esophagus and the great vessels behind the sternum. Remember that retrosternal dislocations may be real emergencies! The patient may exhibit marked respiratory embarrassment, and even shock if the great vessels are injured.

Roentgenograms of the sternoclavicular joint, regardless of the views taken, are difficult to interpret, and, more often than not, the interpretation is wrong. Tomograms show the clavicles on different levels and this may be a clue to the diagnosis. Oblique views, as a rule, are of no value and it is impossible to obtain legible views at 90° to each other. Therefore, the diagnosis, in most instances, must be made on clinical manifestations (Figs. 9-50 and 9-51).

In adolescents a deformity of the sternoclavicular region simulating a dislocation of the joint may be caused by a fracture through the medial epiphyseal plate of the clavicle. The epiphysis remains in its normal anatomical position but the medial end of the clavicle rides upward. In this instance, roentgenograms reveal the true nature of the lesion.

Most complete dislocations, except retrosternal dislocations, can be reduced by traction on the abducted arm and manipulation of the sternal end of the clavicle. If the reduction remains stable, external fixation by a plaster posterior figure-of-eight holding the shoulders upward and outward may be adequate to maintain the correction. This should be worn for at least six weeks.

In some instances reduction cannot be attained by closed methods, or, following reduction, subluxation or dislocation recurs. These cases should be treated surgically. It should be mentioned that one cause of failure to reduce a dislocation is displacement of a portion of the interarticular disc.

**Operative Procedures.** Expose the joint through a 4-inch hockey stick skin incision and identify the ligaments and the interarticular disc. If a portion of the disc is

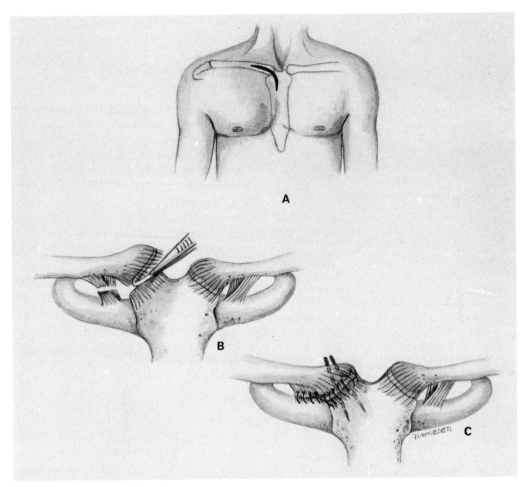

FIG. 9-52. Surgical reduction for anterior dislocations. (A) Expose the joint through a hockey stick incision 4 inches long. (B) Identify the detached portion of the inter-articular disc and restore it to its normal position. (C) Reduce the dislocation and maintain the position by two threaded wires transfixing the joint; suture the detached portion of the disc to the adjacent soft tissues of the sternum and first rib; cut the wires below the level of the skin.

detached and displaced, restore it to its normal position. Reduce the dislocation and maintain the position with two threaded wires (⁵/₆₄ inch in diameter) transfixing the joint as shown in the illustration (*see* Fig. 4-8). With interrupted sutures, anchor the detached portions of the disc to the clavicle or sternum or to the first rib. Repair, if possible, the sternoclavicular and costoclavicular ligaments. Cut the wires close to the skin and bury them under the skin (Figs. 9-52, 9-53 and 9-54).

If an avulsion fracture of the inferior margin of the sternal end of the clavicle (the costoclavicular region) accompanies the dislocation, reduce the displaced end of the clavicle and fix it to the unattached inferior fragment by stout sutures or even wire sutures; repair all torn ligaments.

Following the operation, supplement the internal fixation by a plaster of paris posterior figure-of-eight. The wires (if used) and the external fixation should be removed after 6 weeks. During this period the arm

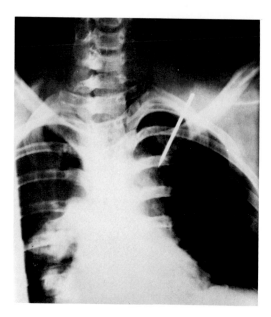

FIG. 9-53. An anterosuperior dislocation of the left sternoclavicular joint reduced openly. A threaded pin transfixes the joint.

should be supported in a sling and kept to the side with a swathe.

## Management of Retrosternal Dislocations

Although these lesions are rare, they deserve special consideration because of the serious complications that may accompany them. Manipulative reduction is rarely achieved, especially after 48 hours, and, if it is obtained, reduction if difficult to maintain. Generally, the interarticular disc remains attached to the sternum, but it is avulsed from the clavicle. Although difficult, manipulative reduction should be attempted in all fresh lesions (under 48 hours). If reduction cannot be achieved, or, if achieved, cannot be maintained, open reduction and internal fixation is indicated (Fig. 9-51.).

**Manipulative Reduction (Fig. 9-55).** Place a sandbag between the scapulae of the anesthetized patient. With the arm on the af-

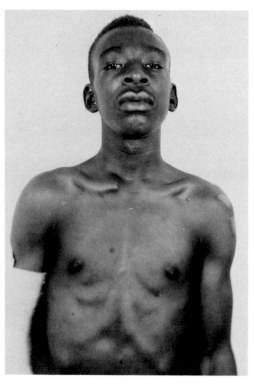
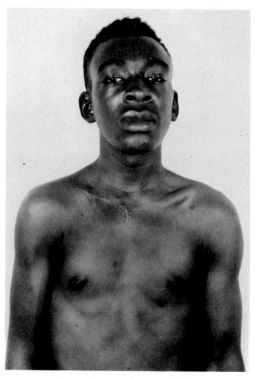

FIG. 9-54. (*Left*) Preoperative appearance of a dislocation of the right sternoclavicular joint. (*Right*) Postoperative appearance; the joint was transfixed with a threaded wire.

fected side hanging over the side of the table, an assistant makes steady traction downward. The operator grasps the clavicle; he places the fingers of both hands on the posterior-superior surface of the clavicle and the thumbs on the inferior surface. Then he pulls the sternal end of the clavicle upward, forward and laterally. The reduction is maintained by a plaster of paris posterior figure-of-eight for a period of six weeks.

**Operative Reduction (Fig. 9-56).** Drape the arm separately so that it can be manipulated during the operation. Expose the joint through a hockey stick incision four inches long. While an assistant makes lateral traction on the arm, with a blunt periosteal elevator lever the sternal end of the clavicle upward, forward and laterally. Take care not to injure the structures in the retrosternal space. If the interarticular disc is folded upon itself in the joint, restore it to its normal position.

By direct downward pressure on the head of the clavicle, reduce the dislocation. Maintain the position by two threaded wires ($^5/_{64}$ inch in diameter) transfixing the joint. Take care not to pierce the posterior cortex of the sternum with the wires. I have seen an aorta pierced by this method. Reattach the disc to the remaining soft tissues on the clavicle and repair all ligaments. Cut the wire close to the skin and pull the skin over the cut ends. At the completion of the operation apply a plaster of paris posterior figure-of-eight. Both pins and plaster are removed at the end of six weeks.

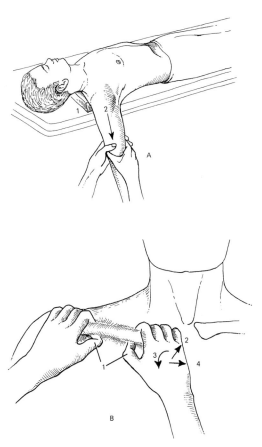

FIG. 9-55. Manipulative reduction of retrosternal dislocations. (A) Place a sandbag between the scapulae of the anesthetized patient (1); the arm on the affected side hangs over the side of the table and an assistant makes steady traction downward on it (2). (B) The operator grasps the clavicle; the fingers of both hands are placed on the posterior-superior surface of the clavicle and the thumbs on the inferior surface (1); the sternal end of the clavicle is pulled upward (2), forward (3) and laterally (4).

### Old Dislocations of the Sternoclavicular Joint

Many old lesions cause no pain or noticeable dysfunction. These lesions need no treatment except for cosmesis; however, cosmesis may be very important to some women. As a rule, if all ligaments are disrupted the lesions are asymptomatic. Pain and dysfunction are encountered more frequently when the costoclavicular ligament is intact. Operative measures are, as a rule, successful in fresh dislocations; in old dislocations the results are unpredictable. No study made of long term results of repair or reconstruction of the ligaments of old dislocations has sufficient statistical significance to permit prognostication of results. Clinical experience suggests that eventually, following surgery, the results are not good, particularly in athletes. After

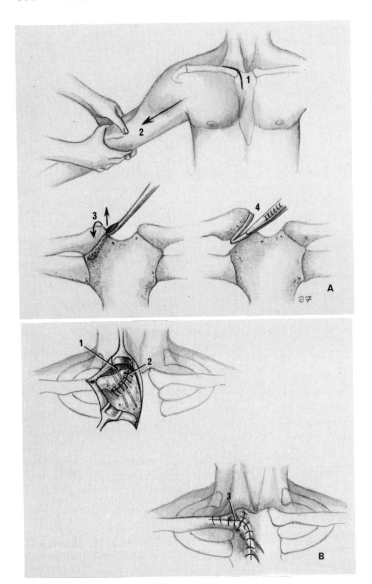

FIG. 9-56. Surgical reduction of retrosternal dislocations. (A) Expose the joint through a hockey stick incision 4 inches long (1). While an assistant makes lateral traction on the arm (2), lever the sternal end of the clavicle upward, forward and laterally (3). If the interarticular disc is folded upon itself in the joint, restore it to its normal position (4). (B) By direct pressure downward, reduce the dislocation and fix the end of the clavicle by two threaded wires, transfixing the joint (1). Suture the detached portion of the disc to the remaining soft tissues on the clavicle and, if possible, repair the sternoclavicular ligaments (2). Cut the wires close to the skin and then pull the skin over the cut ends (3).

several years of playing, the joint becomes painful and motion in the shoulder girdle shows varying degrees of restriction. Many athletes continue to play with a complete dislocation.

Also, the following observations and conclusions based on clinical experience are of practical importance in regard to surgery in chronic dislocations. Fusion of the joint must never be performed because the sternoclavicular joint participates in almost all movements of the arm. Fusion would reduce the overall performance of the extremity. Reconstruction of ligaments by fascia does not, in most instances, produce a painless, normal functioning joint. Fascia, with time, stretches and the joint loses stability. On the other hand, in cases with severe pain and marked restriction of movements of the arm, reconstructive procedures may decrease the discomfort, reduce the deformity and improve motion of the joint; therefore, it should be performed. The most gratifying procedure is excision of the medial end of the clavicle. The excision must always be done proximal

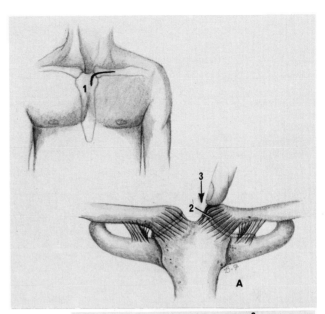

FIG. 9-57. Stabilization of the sternoclavicular joint. (A) Expose the joint through a hockey stick incision 4 inches long (1). Identify the detached portion of the disc (2). By direct downward pressure reduce the dislocation (3). (B) The position is maintained by two threaded wires transfixing the joint (1). The detached interarticular disc is sutured to the adjacent soft tissues of the sternum and rib (2), the wires are cut below the level of the skin (3) and a posterior plaster of Paris figure-of-eight is applied (4).

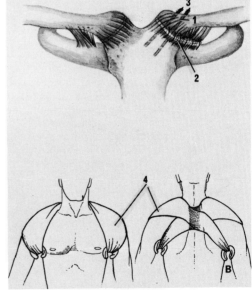

to the costoclavicular ligament. In anterior dislocations the interarticular disc remains attached to the clavicle and if it can be reattached to the sternum this may be sufficient to stabilize the joint.

## Operative Procedures

**Reattachment of the Interarticular Disc (Fig. 9-57).** The joint is exposed through a hockey stick incision four inches long. Identify the disc and inspect the sternoclavicular and costoclavicular ligaments. Remove by sharp dissection all debris in the joint which obstructs relocation of the head of the clavicle. Reduce the deformity by direct downward pressure on the head and maintain the position by two threaded wires transfixing the joint. By mattress sutures anchor the detached disc to the adjacent soft tissues of the sternum and first rib. If the costoclavicular ligament is torn or stretched, it should be reconstructed either by reefing the redundant ligament or encircling the clavicle and first rib with a strip of fascia.

**Resection of the Sternal End of the Clavicle (Fig. 9-58).** This procedure is performed when the disc is severely deteriorated so that it can no longer function as a stabilizer of the joint.

Expose the joint through a hockey stick incision four inches long. Then, by sharp subperiosteal dissection, reflect the clavicular head of the sternocleidomastoid upward and the insertion of the pectoralis major downward. Resect obliquely 1½ to 2 inches of the medial end of the clavicle.

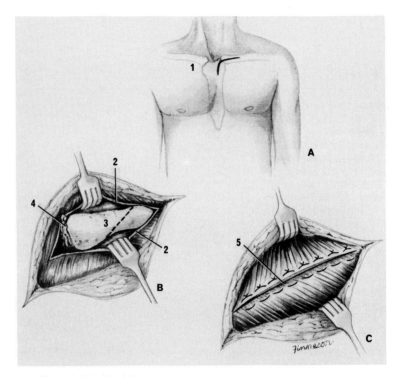

FIG. 9-58. Excision of the sternal end of the clavicle. (A) Expose the joint through a hockey stick incision 4 inches long (1). (B) By subperiosteal dissection, reflect the clavicular head of the sternocleidomastoid upward and the insertion of the pectoralis major downward (2); resect obliquely 1½ to 2 inches of the medial end of the clavicle (3); remove all remnants of the disc (4). (C) Carefully approximate the clavicular head of the sternocleidomastoid to the pectoralis major by mattress sutures (5).

The region of the clavicle where the costoclavicular ligament is attached must not be disturbed. Next, remove all remnants of the disc and other debris from the joint. Finally, by mattress sutures approximate carefully the clavicular head of the sternocleidomastoid and the pectoralis major. By so doing, the stability of the inner end of the clavicle is enhanced.

## GLENOHUMERAL JOINT

### Acute Sprain, Subluxation, Dislocation

### Pertinent Anatomical Features

The anatomy and the biomechanics of the shoulder girdle are discussed in detail in the appropriate chapters dealing with these subjects. However, at this point, certain anatomical and functional features of the glenohumeral region deserve re-emphasis so that the mechanism and nature of the acute injuries of the glenohumeral joint can be understood. The bony configuration of the glenohumeral joint provides no stability. The structures responsible for stability of the joint are the muscles that move it and a delicate neuromuscular balance, particularly of the rotator muscles. The location of this joint and its participation in almost every movement of the shoulder girdle render it vulnerable to many and diversified forms of trauma. Its proximity to the many large neurovascular structures

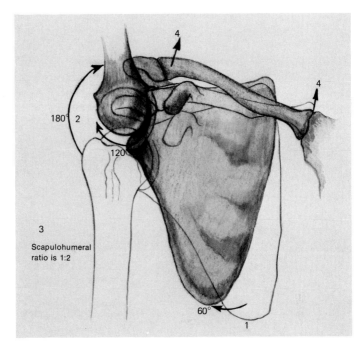

FIG. 9-59. Scapulohumeral motion. (1) The scapula has moved upward and forward on the chest wall 60°; (2) the humerus has reached 180° of elevation, having moved 120° in relation to the glenoid; (3) the scapulohumeral ratio is 1 to 2; (4) elevation of the clavicle at the sternoclavicular and acromioclavicular joints permits 60° of scapular motion (40° at the sternoclavicular and 20° at the acromioclavicular joint).

render these vital parts vulnerable to serious injuries when the joint is injured. Many variational abnormalities exist in this region, particularly on the anterior aspect of the joint. These involve primarily the glenohumeral ligaments and the subscapularis muscle; they play a major role in lesions of the glenohumeral joint, such as in recurrent dislocations. Finally, the soft tissues of this joint physiologically undergo rapid deterioration after the third decade; this, too, colors the nature of the lesions encountered in this region.

**Muscles.** Essentially, two layers of muscles envelop the joint, an outer and an inner layer that function in the manner of sleeves. The inner sleeve consists of the short rotators and the outer sleeve of the deltoid and teres major. Between the two sleeves lies an efficient gliding mechanism consisting of the subdeltoid bursa and a layer of fine, filmy areolar tissue. Abduction and flexion of the humerus is produced by the synchronous action of two groups of muscles: (1) the deltoid, the supraspinatus and the pectoralis major, and (2) the infraspinatus, the teres minor and the subscapularis. The latter group constitutes a functional

unit that depresses the humeral head and fixes it firmly against the glenoid cavity, enabling the former group to abduct and flex the arm. Without the stabilizing effect of the rotator muscles the deltoid would pull the humerus vertically under the acromion.

### Normal Motions of the Glenohumeral Joint

The upper arm possesses a range of motion of almost 360°. This comprises the summation of motion possible in the 4 articulations of the shoulder girdle: (1) the glenohumeral, (2) the sternoclavicular, (3) the acromioclavicular and (4) the thoracoscapular. Impairment of function in any of these four components is reflected in the total performance of the shoulder girdle. They function as a single unit; yet they are capable of independent motion. A special, constant, delicate, intrinsic relationship (scapulohumeral rhythm) exists between the humerus and the scapula during elevation and abduction of the arm. After the 30° of abduction and 60° of flexion (ranges in which the scapula finds a stable position

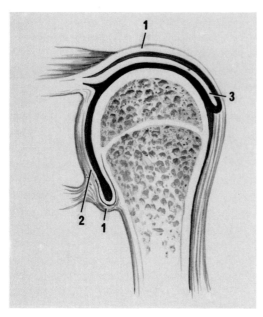

FIG. 9-60. Capsule of the glenohumeral joint. (1) Articular capsule; it is
spacious and redundant. (2) Labrum
glenoidale. (3) Biceps tendon.

in relation to the humerus), the ratio of
motion in the two joints is constant, being
2 (humeral) to 1 (scapular). For every 15°
of motion, 10° occurs at the glenohumeral
joint and 5° at the scapulothoracic joint.
Total glenohumeral motion is 120° and
scapulothoracic 60°. The glenohumeral
joint is capable of 90° of independent
motion. Normal scapular motion on the
chest wall depends upon normal motion at
either end of the clavicle. Any interference
of motion in the sternoclavicular or acromioclavicular joints compromises the total
range of elevation of the arm. The sternoclavicular joint contributes 40° and the
acromioclavicular 20° to the total range of
elevation (Fig. 9-59).

Regardless of the plane in which the arm
ascends to reach complete elevation, the
ultimate position of the humeral head in
relation to the glenoid cavity, the acromion
and the coracoid process is the same — the
pivotal position. In this position no internal
or external rotation of the arm is possible.

As the arm ascends, regardless of the horizontal plane in which it travels, the range of
rotation diminishes progressively until it
reaches the pivotal position; at which no
rotation is possible. During elevation, if
rotation of the humerus is in the proper
plane, the greater tuberosity slips under the
acromion and the motion is smooth and
rhythmical from beginning to end. If rotation of the arm in the right plane is obstructed, then the greater tuberosity abuts
against the acromion and locks in this position. Forcing the arm beyond the locked
position results in disruption of the soft
tissues of the joint or fracture of the
humerus or a combination of both.

Normally, to reach the pivotal position in
the sagittal plane the arm must rotate internally; in the coronal plane, it must rotate
externally. During elevation of the arm in
the sagittal plane, if internal rotation is
obstructed the humerus impinges upon the
acromion, which, acting as a fulcrum, may
lever the humeral head out of the glenoid
cavity or produce a break in the bone. The
same is true if external rotation is prevented
when the arm is elevated in the coronal
plane or the arm is hyperabducted beyond
the limits of the pivotal position.

The mechanism disrupting the glenohumeral joint (when the falling patient
applies force on the outstretched arm) is the
same as when leverage is applied to the arm
with the body in a fixed position. Anterior
or posterior lesions occur, depending upon
the direction of the disrupting forces. As a
rule, inferior dislocation occurs if hyperabduction is continued after the arm has
reached the pivotal position and an anterior
dislocation occurs if rotation is obstructed
after the arm has ascended to a point above
the horizontal plane. Posterior dislocation
occurs when the arm is below the horizontal, flexed and rotated internally beyond
limits of the locked position.

Other factors play a significant role in the
mechanism of disruption of the glenohumeral joint: (1) The impacting or telescoping force generated by a fall on the

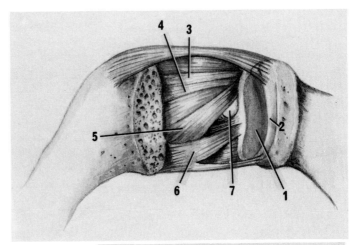

FIG. 9-61. Glenohumeral ligaments (from behind). (1) Glenoid fossa; (2) labrum glenoidale; (3) biceps tendon (long head); (4) superior glenohumeral ligament; (5) middle glenohumeral ligament; (6) inferior glenohumeral ligament; (7) subscapularis recess. Note that all three ligaments are directed toward the superior aspect of the glenoid fossa and that the subscapularis recess communicates with the inside of the joint cavity.

outstretched arm or on the partially abducted elbow, applied to the glenoid fossa through the bony axis of the humerus may disrupt the glenoid or the humeral head. (2) The position of the outstretched arm in relation to the trunk determines whether the forces act on the anterior or the posterior aspect of the joint. (3) With the arm abducted and externally rotated direct impacts on the posterior aspect of the shoulder can drive the humeral head anteriorly. This mechanism is rarely implicated.

The extent of implication of the capsule, ligaments, musculotendinous cuff and the bony elements of the joint depends upon the intensity of the forces involved in the various mechanisms. The soft tissue lesions vary from simple sprains to complete disruption of the tissues, permitting subluxation or dislocation of the head of the humerus.

**Ligaments and Capsule.** The capsule and the ligaments of the glenohumeral joint are intimately related and provide very little stability to the joint. The capsule is loose and redundant, especially its inferior portion, in order to permit the very wide range of motion the glenohumeral joint possesses (Fig. 9-60). Numerous variations of the glenohumeral ligaments are encountered. For a detailed discussion of the anatomy and function of these ligaments the reader is referred to Chapter 4 and Figure 9-61.

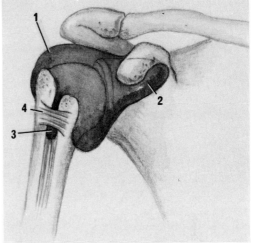

FIG. 9-62. Synovial capsule. (1) The synovial capsule is distended; (2) it is prolonged under the coracoid process to form the subscapularis recess; (3) it also extends along the bicipital groove and then onto the biceps tendon. (4) Transverse humeral ligament.

The synovial portion of the capsule extends under the coracoid process, forming the subscapularis recess, and along the bicipital groove and then is reflected over the biceps tendon (Fig. 9-62).

**Neurovascular Structures.** The proximity of these vital structures to the glenohumeral joint makes them vulnerable when the joint is injured. Also, they may be injured during reduction of a dislocation (Figs. 9-63 and

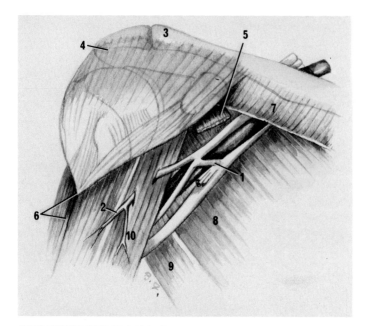

FIG. 9-63. Neurovascular structures in relation to the glenohumeral joint. (1) Axillary artery and brachial plexus; (2) musculocutaneous nerve; (3) clavicle; (4) deltoid; (5) pectoralis minor; (6) biceps; (7) pectoralis major; (8) subscapularis; (9) teres major; (10) coracobrachialis.

9-64). For a detailed account of injuries to these structures the reader is referred to Chapter 8.

### Mechanisms of Sprains, Subluxation, Dislocation

At this point it is necessary to review those features of the shoulder that protect the glenohumeral joint from disruptive forces. These are:

1. The prompt response of different muscle groups, working synchronously, which position the glenoid fossa squarely against the humeral head. This occurs regardless of the position of the arm in relation to the trunk at the time of injury.

2. The ability of the scapula to glide and recoil freely on the thorax on impact of a telescoping force.

3. The stabilizing influence of the rotator muscles, especially the subscapularis, and the triceps, biceps, deltoid and pectoralis major.

However, these protective mechanisms may be caught off guard or the force may be great enough to overcome them, thereby producing varying grades of sprains.

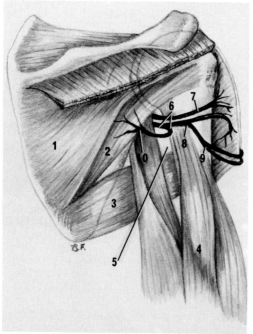

FIG. 9-64. Posterior aspect of the glenohumeral joint. (1) Infraspinatus; (2) teres minor; (3) teres major; (4) triceps; (5) quadrangular space; (6) axillary nerve; (7) anterior branch of the axillary nerve; (8) posterior branch of the axillary nerve; (9) cutaneous branch of the axillary nerve; (10) nerve to teres minor.

Other factors play a role in the causation of sprains. These are: (a) the physical condition of the person, (b) the degree of neuromuscular coordination and agility, (c) the presence of masked injuries that prevent normal motion, and (d) anatomical abnormalities of the anterior capsular and muscular buttress.

## Mechanism of Abduction and External Rotation of the Arm

**Sprain.** If the arm is locked in the position of external rotation and abduction and a mild force continues to act the humeral head is forced against the coracoacromial ligament and the anterior ligaments and capsule. The coracoacromial ligament does not yield but rather forces the head against the ligaments and capsule, some fibers of which stretch and tear. However, the integrity of the structures is intact and the stability of the joint is not impaired (Fig. 9-65).

**Subluxation.** If a greater force is acting, the acromion impinges against the tuberosity. The arm continues along its course of abduction and external rotation, and the rotator cuff rotates backward so that its superior portion slides posteriorly and the inferior portion of the capsule and ligaments lie anteriorly. As the head is levered over the rim of the glenoid it stretches and tears the capsule and ligaments, displacing the subscapularis upward. However, the force is such that it does not force the head out of the glenoid cavity; rather, it is readily reversed and the head slips back into the glenoid cavity. However, the anterior ligaments and the capsule stretch and tear sufficiently to permit subluxation of the head. The tears may occur anywhere in the capsule or at the attachment of the capsule along the glenoid rim. Tearing of the capsule and ligaments is incomplete and the greater portion of the capsule remains intact (Fig. 9-66). This is a severe sprain (grade II) and the mechanism is the commonest of those causing subluxation or

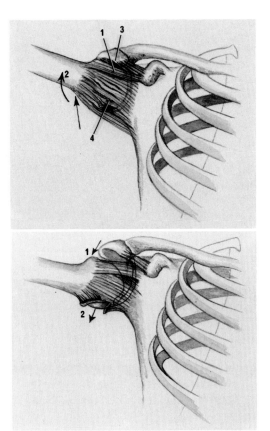

(*Top*) Fig. 9-65. Sprain Grade I produced by the abduction-external rotation mechanism. (1) The humeral head is in the locked position; (2) the arm is abducted and externally rotated; (3) the acromion impinges against the greater tuberosity; (4) the anterior ligaments and capsule are stretched; some fibers tear but the continuity of the structures remains intact.

(*Bottom*) Fig. 9-66. Subluxation— Sprain Grade II. (1) The acromion impinges against the greater tuberosity and levers it partially out of the glenoid fossa; (2) the anterior ligaments and capsule are stretched and torn sufficiently to permit a subluxation.

dislocation of the humeral head in young adults.

**Dislocation.** The mechanism is the same as that producing a subluxation except that a greater telescoping force is acting. The force is usually initiated at the hand, arm

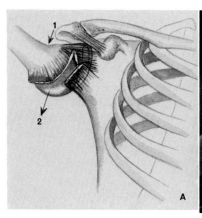
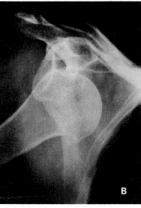
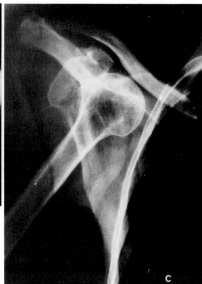

Fig. 9-67. Dislocation — Sprain Grade III. (A) (1) The acromion impinges against the greater tuberosity and levers the humeral head out of the joint anteriorly; (2) the anterior ligaments and capsule are severely stretched and torn, permitting a dislocation. (B) Roentgenogram of a subcoracoid dislocation. (C) Roentgenogram of a subclavicular dislocation.

or elbow. As it drives the arm into extreme abduction and external rotation, the humeral head is forced against the anterior capsular and the muscular buttress beneath the coracoacromial ligament. The neck of the humerus now impinges against the acromion. As the force continues, the tensile strength of the anterior buttress is overcome and the head is levered out of the glenoid fossa (Fig. 9-67A). The head now lies on the antero-inferior aspect of the neck of the scapula just under the coracoid. This is the commonest lesion in young adults (Fig. 9-67B). It is entirely a soft tissue lesion. Occasionally the head is driven into a subclavicular position (Fig. 9-67C).

Although rare, bone injuries do occur in

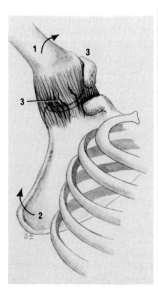
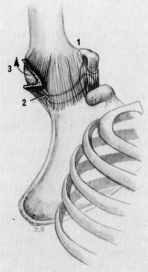

(Left) Fig. 9-68. Sprain Grade I by the hyperabduction mechanism. (1) The arm is in the locked (pivotal) position; (2) the scapula is completely rotated; (3) the acromion, acting as a fulcrum, impinges against the greater tuberosity, producing some stretching and tearing of the capsular fibers, but its continuity is intact.

(Right) Fig. 9-69. Subluxation — Sprain Grade II. (1) The acromion acts as a fulcrum, displacing the greater tuberosity downward and outward; (2) the inferior capsule is stretched and partially torn; (3) the humeral head subluxates.

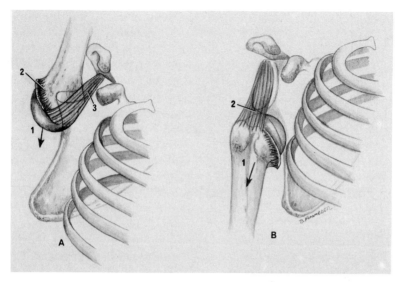

FIG. 9-70. Dislocation—Sprain Grade III (A) As the force continues, (1) the head leaves the glenoid fossa and is displaced directly downward, (2) the inferior capsule is completely torn, and (3) the rotator cuff stretches across the glenoid fossa. (B) (1) The arm drops to the side; (2) the head is in the subglenoid position, from which it usually migrates to a subcoracoid position.

young persons and involve the greater or lesser tuberosity, the coracoid process, the acromion and the anterior and inferior glenoid rims. In older persons fractures of the upper end of the humerus also may occur.

### Mechanism of Hyperabduction

**Sprain.** In this mechanism the arm is locked in the pivotal position, the scapula is rotated completely and the acromion abuts against the neck of the humerus. As the force continues, the inferior capsule and ligaments stretch and some of their fibers tear. Because the force is mild, continuity of the structures remains intact (Fig. 9-68).

**Subluxation.** When a greater force is acting in the mechanism described above, the head is displaced laterally and downward against the capsule and capsular ligaments. As these structures tear away from the glenoid rim, the head slides over the inferior glenoid rim (Fig. 9-69). This is a rare lesion because, if the force is sufficient to push the head over the inferior rim, it is also adequate to cause a dislocation. The latter injury is very serious, for invariably severe damage to the rotator muscles occurs. Complete avulsion of the rotator cuff may occur by this mechanism. Now when the arm returns to the side, the head hangs on the inferior lip of the glenoid. Since the suspensory function of the cuff is lost, the position of the head in relation to the glenoid fossa is maintained by strong contraction of the muscles of the outer muscular sleeve—the deltoid, biceps, triceps and pectoralis major. But these muscles are unable to maintain normal apposition of the head and glenoid; hence, the head actually hangs on the inferior rim of the glenoid.

This lesion occurs in young persons. It must not be confused with inferior subluxations seen following fractures of the upper end of the humerus in elderly persons, or with paralytic disorders of the shoulder. I have seen two inferior subluxations in

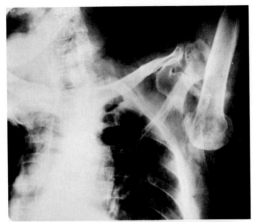

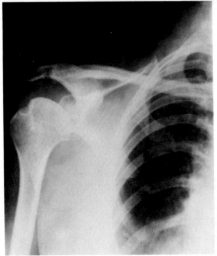

(*Top*) FIG. 9-71. Roentgenogram of luxatio erecta. The arm is in full abduction and the head is driven downward and lies far below the inferior glenoid rim. In this instance, the rotator cuff and capsule were completely detached from the head.

(*Bottom*) FIG. 9-72. Typical defect in superolateral aspect of the humeral head (Hill-Sache lesion) in a recurrently dislocating shoulder.

young people. Both were caused by violent automobile collisions and in both cases the victim was ejected from the automobile. A massive avulsion of the rotator cuff was found in the shoulder of both of these patients.

**Dislocation.** If the force in the mechanism just described for inferior subluxation is of great intensity, the head tears the capsule and capsular ligaments and slips over the inferior rim of the glenoid. As the arm is lowered it may remain in the subglenoid position, but usually it migrates anteriorly and assumes a subcoracoid position (Fig. 9-70).

**Luxatio Erecta.** This is a rare lesion and is caused by a variation of the hyperabduction mechanism described above. The acting force not only continues to abduct the arm but also drives the arm over the head and toward the midline. Complete detachment of all soft tissues from the humeral head occurs—capsule, capsular ligaments and rotator cuff. The head locks under the inferior lip of the glenoid and the shaft of the humerus points directly upward (Fig. 9-71). This is a serious injury and may be accompanied by damage to the great vessels and the brachial plexus.

### Pathology of Acute Anterior Dislocations

The pathology of these lesions shows much variation; and, because the nature of the pathology decides the treatment to be used, the different structures affected must be considered fully at this time.

### Capsular and Ligamentous Lesions

The extent of the injury to the anterior capsular and muscular wall varies greatly. The labrum may be torn, avulsed or shredded and detached with the capsule and periosteum from the neck of the glenoid. The capsule and periosteum may be detached but the labrum remains intact and firmly attached to the glenoid. Most dislocations are intracapsular (66%); however, the head may be driven through the capsule or it may pierce the subscapularis or tear it away from its bony insertion. In general, intracapsular dislocations with capsular and labral detachment occur in the young; dislocations with capsular ruptures and tears of the subscapularis occur in the elderly. In the latter group 33 percent of the dislocations are extracapsular. On the other hand, the head may dislocate with very little, if any, soft tissue damage.

### Fractures

Involvement of the osseous elements may occur on both the humeral and the glenoid side of the joint. A relatively common lesion in primary dislocations is a compression fracture of the superolateral aspect of the humeral head—the Hill-Sache lesion. It occurs in 35 to 40 percent of primary dislocations. The lesion may be difficult to recognize in primary dislocations even with special roentgenographic views. It is more readily seen in recurrent dislocations. Reeves, with his special technique, the notch view, has demonstrated the lesion in 90 percent of recurrent dislocations (Fig. 9-72).

Fractures of the anterior and inferior glenoid rim occur in 11 percent of all primary dislocations. Usually these are avulsion fractures, and the size of the fragments varies considerably. In most instances the fragment is attached to the capsule, but in some it lies free. These are serious lesions because they predispose to recurrent dislocations. In fact, I have never seen a primary dislocation with rim fractures that did not develop into a recurrent dislocation. However, there may be some that do not. In Rowe's series of primary dislocations, rim fractures were demonstrable in 5 percent of the cases; only 62 percent of these developed recurrent dislocations.

Fractures of the bony elements of the shoulder girdle occur in approximately 20 to 25 percent of all primary dislocations. The greater tuberosity is implicated more often than any other bony component of the girdle. These fractures occur in 12 to 15 percent of all primary dislocations with fractures. Usually they occur in older persons. Interestingly, the incidence of recurrent dislocations in this group of

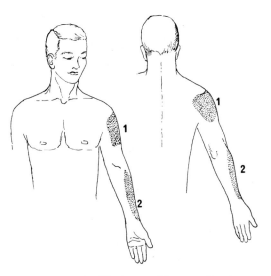

FIG. 9-73. (1) Area of hypoesthesia, or sensory loss, following injury of the axillary nerve. (2) Area of sensory loss associated with injury of the musculocutaneous nerve.

patients is indeed very small—and, if the fracture is through the upper end of the humerus, the incidence of recurrent dislocation is zero. I have never seen one. However, it should be remembered that these severe bony lesions accompanying a primary dislocation usually occur in older persons subjected to great violence.

### Injuries to the Rotator Cuff

Lesions of the rotator cuff occur more often than is generally realized. The lesion may vary from a small tear in the subscapularis tendon to complete avulsion of the cuff. Severe tears are more likely to occur in the elderly, but they may occur in the young, particularly when the dislocation is caused by the hyperabduction mechanism. Severe disruption of the cuff always occurs in luxatio erecta. I have seen two such lesions in young men. Both required surgical repair of the rotator cuff. In the series of acute dislocations that I explored, tears of varying degrees were found in 44 percent of the cases.

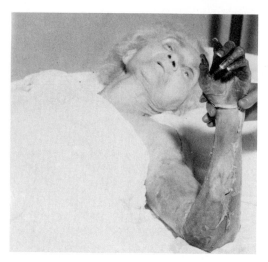

FIG. 9-74. Gangrene of the arm and hand, following an anterior dislocation of the shoulder. In this instance, the axillary artery and vein were severely traumatized and thrombosis of the vessels ensued. This was a fatal complication.

### Nerve Injuries

Nerve lesions also occur more frequently than generally appreciated. In the literature the incidence ranges from 5 to 30 percent. Many nerve lesions are not recognized. There are reasons for this. Many lesions are transient in nature, but, more important, the neurological deficit is not found because a neurological examination is not performed before the dislocation is reduced.

The axillary nerve may be contused or stretched at the time of the dislocation. The nerves of the median cord are frequently involved, especially the ulnar nerve. Next in order of frequency are the radial nerve and the axillary nerve from the posterior cord. Less frequently involved is the musculocutaneous nerve from the lateral cord. Generally, isolated nerve lesions are transient, but occasionally they are permanent. I have seen three patients with permanent paralysis of the deltoid. Combined nerve lesions are more likely to be permanent. A neurological examination of the entire extremity before and after reduc-

tion of a dislocation should be a "must"! It saves embarrassment and avoids malpractice suits (Fig. 9-73).

**Management of Nerve Lesions.** Management of most nerve lesions is watchful waiting. During this period maintain muscle tone by physical measures and electrical stimulation. Every day put the shoulder through a safe range of motion to prevent contraction and shortening of the adductor muscles. Encourage regular active exercises of the muscles of the elbow, wrist and fingers.

If return of function is progressive, continue with the above regimen. However, if after 3 months there is no improvement or there is progressive loss of muscle power, the nerve should be explored. Perform the exploratory operation with a neurosurgeon. He is better able to manage the nerve lesion.

### Vascular Injuries

Vascular injuries may occur at the time of the dislocation or during its reduction. Fortunately they are rare. They occur more frequently in the elderly in whom degenerative change in the vessel walls may exist. The vascular injuries are:

1. Rupture of the axillary artery. When this occurs the radial pulse is absent and a hematoma develops rapidly in the axilla or in front of the shoulder.

2. Rupture of the axillary vein. In this instance the hematoma develops slowly (Fig. 9-74).

3. Trauma to the vessel walls, followed by thrombosis of the vessels.

4. Aneurysm of the axillary artery.

5. Arteriovenous fistula.

**Arterial Injuries.** The chief arterial lesions that may occur are (a) rupture of the main trunk of the axillary artery, (b) avulsion of a large branch from the artery, usually the subscapularis or the circumflex artery, and (c) internal damage of the walls of the axillary artery, followed by thrombosis. Regardless of the management insti-

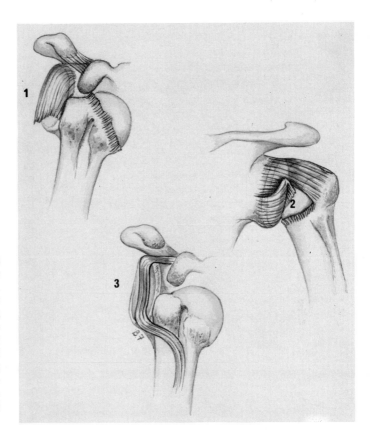

FIG. 9-75. Some causes for failure to reduce an acute anterior dislocation. (1) The rotator cuff lies in front of the glenoid fossa like a curtain. (2) The inferior capsule is interposed between the humeral head and the glenoid fossa. (3) The biceps tendon is displaced posteriorly, preventing apposition of the head to the glenoid fossa.

tuted, the prognosis is poor; 60 percent of such injuries are fatal and, of the remainder, very few patients have a useful extremity.

Theoretically, ligation of the artery should not cause any circulatory embarrassment because the collateral circulation is adequate. However, in traumatic dislocation, soft tissue trauma may be severe and the collateral circulation may be impaired at the time of the dislocation or during forceful reduction. Also, the vessels may be arteriosclerotic and narrow or a large hematoma may obliterate the lumens of the anastomotic vessels. Many patients exhibit profound shock and hypotension; these circumstances do not favor opening up of the collateral vessels.

MANAGEMENT. If vascular embarrassment is present before the shoulder is reduced, reduce the dislocation immediately but gently. If the embarrassment is not relieved by the reduction, explore the vessels. When vascular impairment occurs following reduction, explore the axillary artery immediately. Hemorrhage is controlled by compressing the subclavian artery against the first rib. Whenever possible, after resection of the traumatized ends of the vessels, do an end-to-end anastomosis. If this is not possible, ligate the artery. Ligation is more likely to be successful in young persons. If time and circumstances permit, the vascular surgery should be performed by a vascular surgeon.

### Irreducible Dislocation

Once the muscle spasm about the shoulder is overcome, it should be possible to reduce the dislocation with minimal traction and manipulation, In fact, when the muscles are relaxed, the dislocation may reduce spontaneously. When there is resistance to reduction, something is wrong. Of the

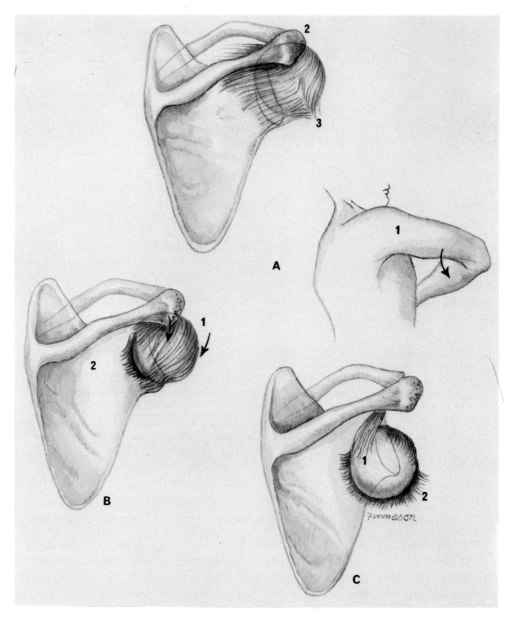

FIG. 9-76. Mechanism of posterior lesions — Sprains Grade I, II, III. (A) Sprain Grade
I. The arm is flexed and internally rotated (1); the head is locked under the acromion
(2); the posterior capsule is stretched; some fibers tear but the continuity of the
capsule remains intact (3). (B) Subluxation — Sprain Grade II. If the above force continues, the acromion levers the humeral head backward and outward partially out
of the glenoid fossa (1); the posterior capsule is partially torn, thus permitting a subluxation (2). (C) Dislocation — Sprain Grade III. If the above force continues further,
the acromion levers the humeral head completely out of the glenoid fossa (1); the
posterior capsule is severely torn, thus permitting a dislocation (2).

causes of resistance to reduction the commonest are the following:

1. The cuff may lie in front of the glenoid like a curtain; this occurs in elderly people usually, and rarely in the young (Fig. 9-75).

2. The inferior portion of the capsule may be sucked into the joint. This usually occurs in dislocations produced by the hyperabduction mechanism (Fig. 9-75).

3. The biceps tendon may be avulsed from its groove and lie between the glenoid and the humeral head (Fig. 9-75).

4. The greater tuberosity may be fractured and the biceps tendon may lie between it and the head of the humerus.

5. Fragments of bone may be interposed between the head and the glenoid. The fragments may come from the humeral head, the glenoid brim or the lesser tuberosity.

*Mechanism of Flexion and Internal Rotation (Posterior Sprains)*

### Sprains

Sprains of the posterior capsule usually occur during the follow-through phase of pitching. These lesions are discussed in Chapter 8. However, they may occur when a backward force is applied to the lower end of the humerus, with the arm flexed and internally rotated. In this position, the head is locked under the acromion and the force tends to lever the head over the posterior rim of the glenoid. The capsule stretches and some of its fibers tear. Since the force is minimal, it is quickly reversed before subluxation or dislocation occurs (Fig. 9-76A).

### Subluxation

If the force is of greater intensity than that producing a simple sprain of the posterior capsular tissues, the head may be driven over the posterior lip of the glenoid. Again, the mechanism is quickly arrested and the subluxation is reduced spontaneously. It is impossible to make a positive diagnosis of subluxation, for the clinical

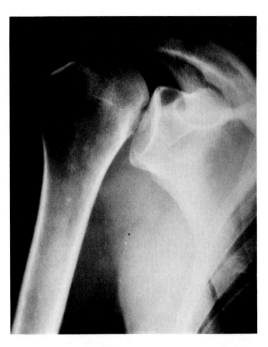

FIG. 9-77. Fracture of the humeral head associated with a posterior dislocation of the glenohumeral joint.

manifestations are those of a sprain of the posterior elements. Of some help may be the patient's statement that he felt the joint slip out and in. The basic pathology is partial rupture of the capsule and stretching and tearing of some of the fibers of the posterior rotators. However, the integrity of the capsule and rotator cuff is still sufficiently preserved to prevent dislocation of the head (Fig. 9-76B).

### Dislocation

With the same mechanism that produces a subluxation a greater force drives the head posteriorly out of the glenoid fossa. The head lies in one of three positions: subglenoid (rare), subacromial (93%) or subspinous (6%). The labrum may be torn or avulsed. The capsule is severely torn and the posterior rotators are greatly stretched or even torn. A fracture of the head or the posterior rim of the glenoid or the lesser tuberosity may occur. The greater

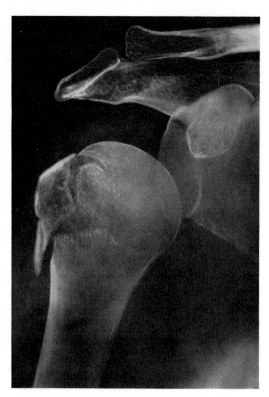

FIG. 9-78. Fracture subluxation of the glenohumeral joint. Note that the humeral head is teetering on the inferior glenoid rim.

tuberosity may fracture. In one instance the biceps tendon slipped between the greater tuberosity and the head of the humerus, preventing manipulative reduction. The subscapularis tendon may tear over the anterior glenoid rim or may be avulsed from the lesser tuberosity (Figs. 9-76C and 9-77).

Arterial and nerve lesions complicating acute posterior dislocations are rare, but they have been reported. I have seen one dislocation complicated by a transient paralysis of the deltoid. Acute posterior dislocation is not a common lesion in sports. I encounter it more frequently in the general population. The lesion frequently is not recognized immediately after the injury (60%). In most instances, the diagnosis is made long after the injury.

*Diagnosis and Management of Anterior Sprains, Subluxations, Dislocations*

### Anterior Sprains

**Diagnosis.** At the time of injury, the patient experiences sudden, severe pain along the anterior aspect of the shoulder. The pain is relieved if he holds the arm at his side. He indicates positively how he sustained the injury; the arm was forced backward and upward. In severe sprains, even with the arm at the side, some soreness persists along the anterior aspect of the shoulder. The patient resists any attempt to rotate the arm externally; this aggravates the pain.

Careful palpation delineates the area of tenderness on the shoulder. It is along the anterior aspect of the shoulder medial to the bicipital groove. Also, tenderness is present just medial to the coracoid process but not along the bicipital groove. Any attempt to rotate the arm externally intensifies the spasm of the internal rotators and the adductors. This lesion is difficult to differentiate from strains of the subscapularis or the pectoralis major. However, adduction and internal rotation of the arm should cause no pain if the lesion is a capsular sprain. On the other hand, when a strain of the internal rotators and adductors exists, these movements cause pain.

**Management.** Any dressing that prevents external rotation and abduction is adequate. The capsule must be kept in a relaxed state until healing is complete. I prefer the following dressing. Place a cotton pad in the axilla and encircle the arm and chest with a 6-inch elastic bandage. Support the forearm in a sling. The arm is immobilized for 2 to 3 weeks. During this period encourage active use of the fingers, hand and elbow, provided that the patient experiences no pain. After the dressing is removed institute pendulum exercises. Increase the range of exercises gradually in range and frequency, but always within the tolerance of pain.

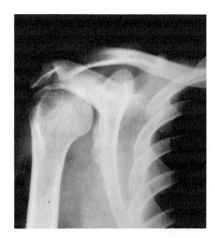
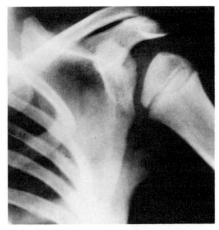

FIG. 9-79. (*Left*) Congenital malformation of the glenoid. This 22-year-old man developed recurrent dislocations of this shoulder at the age of 11 years. (*Right*) Congenital malformation of the glenoid and flattening of the humeral head, resulting in habitual dislocation.

## Anterior Subluxation

**Diagnosis.** At the time of injury the patient feels severe pain on the anterior aspect of the shoulder. The pain is immediately relieved when the arm is brought to the neutral position at the side. As in anterior sprains, the patient says that the arm was forced upward and backward; and, he adds, he felt the joint slip out and in. Palpation along the anterior aspect of the shoulder and medial to the coracoid process causes pain. Attempts to abduct or rotate the arm externally initiates spasm of the internal rotators and adductor muscles, muscle spasm and a feeling that the shoulder is going to slip out. It must be emphasized that it is virtually impossible to distinguish clinically a subluxation from a spontaneously reduced dislocation. Both lesions must have vigorous and meticulous management to prevent recurrent dislocations.

**Management.** The aim in the management of this lesion is to attain healing of all disrupted tissues with minimal scar formation and without elongation of the structures. All movements of abduction and external rotation, passive or active, must be avoided during the healing period. The healing time must not be compromised. It takes at least 6 weeks and no less to get firm healing. Only by adhering to these principles can healing of the disrupted tissues be achieved without overlength. Overlength means weak structures and instability of the joint. With overlength the stage is set for recurrent subluxation, and finally recurrent dislocation.

The treatment is simple and is the same as that for sprains. The difference lies in the period of immobilization—6 weeks for subluxations. Place a cotton pad in the axilla and fix the arm to the side with a 6-inch elastic bandage encircling the trunk. Support the forearm with a sling. Do not permit any abduction or external rotation of the arm during the 6-week period. At no time permit anyone to test the state of healing by active or passive movements of the arm that bring the extremity from the trunk in any direction. At the end of the six weeks, remove the dressing and permit pendulum exercises which increase progressively in range and frequency, but also within the patient's tolerance of pain. Full activity is allowed only when the arm has a full range of painless motion.

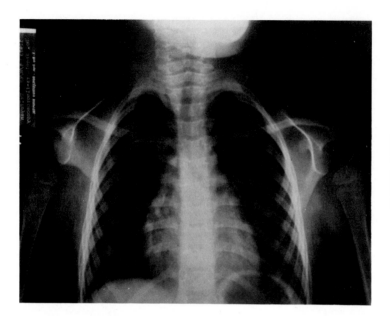

FIG. 9-80. Bilateral congenital dislocations of the glenohumeral joints. This child could voluntarily dislocate both joints inferiorly at will and without pain or discomfort.

## Inferior Subluxation

**Diagnosis.** As previously noted, massive avulsion of the cuff may occur in young people. It is caused by forcing the arm into severe hyperabduction. There always is a history of some violent trauma, following which the patient is unable to move the arm. At the time of injury the patient feels a wrenching, tearing, painful sensation in the shoulder.

The one patient I saw shortly after the injury had occurred was very apprehensive, almost in shock. He held his injured arm close to his body with his other hand placed under the elbow of the affected extremity. Because of pain, he was unable to move the arm in any direction. He resisted any passive motion because of pain. Any attempts at passive movements evoked pronounced spasm of all the muscles about the shoulder.

Roentgenograms taken at this time gave no information. However, those taken the following day, under the influence of an analgesic and with the arm hanging at the side, showed the humeral head teetering on the inferior glenoid rim. Also, the interval between the acromion and the top of the head was widened. Arthrograms at this time confirmed the diagnosis of a rupture of the cuff.

**Management.** Once the diagnosis is established surgical repair of the cuff becomes mandatory.

SURGICAL PROCEDURE. With the patient in a semi-sitting position and the arm at the side of the chest, locate the anterior crease of the axilla. Make an incision over the top of the shoulder in line with the anterior axillary crease and just lateral to the acromioclavicular joint. Extend the incision downward on the anterior aspect of the deltoid for 2 to 2½ inches. Then extend the incision posteriorly as far as the posterior margin of the acromion. By sharp dissection, develop the lateral skin flap by cutting the subcutaneous tissue from the top of the acromion and the tendinous origin of the deltoid. In like manner develop the medial skin flap. Separate vertically the anterior fibers of the deltoid for a distance not exceeding 2 inches below the edge of the acromion. Now the subacromial bursa comes into view; divide this in line with the muscle split. Do not resect the walls of the bursa.

Inspect the damage to the rotator cuff by rotating the arm externally and internally. If wider exposure of the cuff is needed to facilitate the repair, excise three eighths of an inch of the clavicle or of the acromion, depending upon the direction in which more

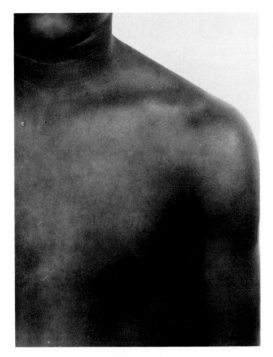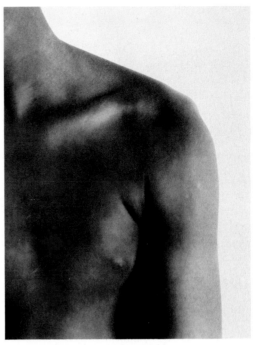

FIG. 9-81 (*left and right*). Bilateral congenital recurrent dislocation of the gleno-humeral joints. This child (12 years old) could voluntarily dislocate both shoulders anteroinferiorly. (*Left*) Left shoulder in normal position; (*Right*) shoulder held in dislocated position.

exposure is desired (see Fig. 7-63A).

Identify the torn edge of the cuff, pull it over the head and reattach it to the head of the humerus by mattress sutures passing through drill holes in the bone (see Fig. 7-63B and 7-63C).

For postoperative immobilization fix the arm to the chest with a swathe and support the forearm with a sling. Maintain the immobilization for 6 weeks.

### Inferior Fracture Subluxation

The lesion usually occurs in the older people and is caused by an abduction-external rotation mechanism. At the time of injury, partial detachment of the inferior portion of the cuff occurs. The head hangs on the inferior glenoid rim and usually is displaced slightly anteriorly. Roentgenograms taken with the patient standing and the arm unsupported readily show the lesion (Fig. 9-78). Surgery is not needed for this lesion. Reduction usually occurs spontaneously within 6 to 8 weeks.

**Management.** Never use a hanging cast to immobilize this lesion. The reason for this is obvious. All that is needed is a swathe around the chest and a sling. Keep the arm immobilized for 2 or 3 weeks. Remember you are dealing with people in the older age bracket! During the period of fixation encourage motion of the elbow, hand and fingers. After two or three weeks discard the sling, except at night. Institute an active program of exercises, beginning with pendulum exercises every hour for 5 or 10 minutes, always within the tolerance of pain. Radiant heat and gentle massage are comforting. Allow free use of the arm within the limits imposed by pain.

### Acute Anterior Dislocation

**Diagnosis.** Whenever the diagnosis of a primary dislocation must be made it is important to remember that, from an etio-

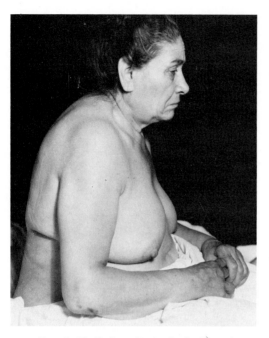

FIG. 9-82. Deformity typical of a sub-coracoid dislocation. Note that the arm is fixed in slight abduction and directed upward and inward; the shoulder is flattened, the acromion process is unduly prominent, the elbow is flexed, the forearm is internally rotated and there is an abnormal prominence in the subcoracoid region.

logical viewpoint, there are two groups. The characteristic features of each group differ greatly. The two groups are: (1) the traumatic anterior dislocation, and (2) the atraumatic dislocation. The former is caused by severe telescoping forces applied to the hand, forearm or elbow. The force travels up the shaft of the humerus and expends itself at the glenohumeral joint.

The atraumatic dislocations may occur with only little force or may occur spontaneously. The causes vary. Congenital malformations of the glenoid or of the humeral head may be the underlying cause (Fig. 9-79), or there may be some congenital dysplasia of the connective tissues of the person. In the latter, all the connective tissues show great elasticity and all the joints are hypermobile, or only the shoulder tissues may be hyperelastic. Individuals so

afflicted frequently can voluntarily subluxate or even dislocate the shoulder joint anteriorly, posteriorly and inferiorly. Both joints may be affected (Fig. 9-80). For some unknown reason, the intricate neural co-ordinating system of the muscles of the shoulder may be out of balance. This, too, may predispose to anterior dislocation.

Finally, in the atraumatic group is the young adolescent female, with none of the above stigmata, who is able to dislocate her shoulder at will by activating some muscles and depressing others. Be wary of these young ladies! Usually some psychological disturbance lies beneath this behavior. They need psychological guidance; without it any surgical procedure is doomed to failure (Fig. 9-81).

**Statistical Data Related to Acute Anterior Dislocations.** Many long-term end-result studies of acute anterior dislocations have appeared in the literature in the past two decades. They give us some very pertinent information. Primary dislocations occur as frequently before the age of 45 as after 45 years. The ratio between males and females is two to one, and the right shoulder is involved as frequently as the left. Of all dislocations, 96 percent are anterior dislocations. Of interest and importance is the recurrence rate in the different categories of anterior dislocations. Recurrences occur in 55 to 60 percent of traumatic dislocations as compared to 85 to 90 percent of those of congenital origin. In persons under 20 years of age the incidence of recurrence is 83 to 90 percent, whereas in those between 20 and 40 it is 60 to 63 percent. On the other hand, the incidence in persons over 40 is 10 to 16 percent.

Interestingly the recurrence rate of dislocations is markedly reduced in the presence of fractures. When the greater tuberosity is fractured, recurrences occur in only 7 percent of the cases, and, when the anatomical or surgical neck of the humerus is implicated, the recurrence rate is zero. It should be remembered that fractures of the upper end of the humerus associated with dislocations occur in the elderly. In contrast to these low recurrence rates, brim fractures have a high rate of recurrences. I, myself, have never seen an anterior dislocation associated with a fracture of the anterior or inferior glenoid lip that did not recur. In one study the incidence of recurrence was 62 percent. Bilateral dislocations occur in 2 to 3 percent of all dislocations and carry a recurrence rate of 80 to 85 percent. Depending upon the mechanism producing the dislocation, there are three types: subglenoid, subcoracoid and subclavicular (see Fig. 9-67, B and C).

**Clinical Picture of an Anterior Dislocation.** In thin persons the diagnosis is readily made by the appearance of the shoulder and the position of the arm in relation to the trunk. However, this is not true for athletes or any muscular person. Characteristically, the prominence of the acromion is striking and, below it, there is a visible and palpable depression. The roundness of the shoulder is lost. The arm is held away from the trunk and it appears longer than the opposite arm. Careful and gentle palpation of the anterior aspect of the shoulder reveals a rounded mass—the humeral head—lying between the inner edge of the deltoid and the outer margin of the pectoralis major (Fig. 9-82).

The arm is held abducted and rotated internally. Although the patient may permit a few degrees of abduction and external rotation he resists any attempts to adduct or internally rotate the arm.

Remember that nerve injuries frequently occur in anterior dislocation. Therefore, no examination is complete unless a thorough neurological examination of the entire extremity is done before reduction and after reduction of the dislocation. Do not fail to evaluate the vascular status of the extremity before and after reduction.

Also, roentgenograms should be taken before and after reduction. In addition to the conventional views an axillary view should be taken, and a careful search should be made for fractures on the glenoid or humeral side of the joint.

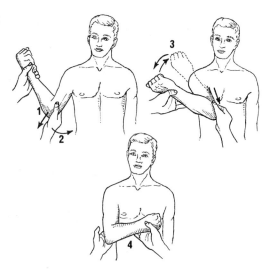

FIG. 9-83. Reduction of anterior dislocations. Patient should be completely relaxed with a general anesthetic, preferably intravenous Pentothal sodium. (1) Make steady traction on the arm in the plane in which it lies in relation to the trunk; (2) then, with traction maintained, swing the arm to the adducted position. This usually effects a reduction. If not, (3) gently rotate the arm externally and internally while traction is maintained. (4) After reduction, lay the arm across the chest.

All primary anterior dislocations must be treated as emergencies. Reduction should be performed as soon as possible. If the patient is first seen in the emergency room or in an infirmary, certain pertinent information should be obtained before treatment is instituted. How did the injury occur and what was the position of the arm at the time of impact? Is this the first time the shoulder dislocated? How long is it since the injury?

**Management.** ANESTHESIA. If the patient is seen within a few minutes of the injury, before pain and muscle spasm set in, a skillful surgeon may reduce the dislocation on the spot without relaxants or anesthesia by simply pulling on the arm in the line of the trunk. Leverage should never be used and forceful manipulation has no place in the reduction of dislocations. Once muscle spasm sets in, no attempt should be made to reduce the dislocation without anesthesia.

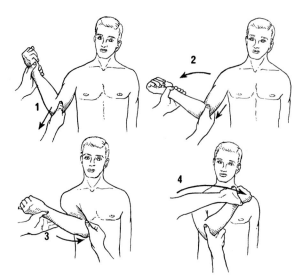

FIG. 9-84. Kocher's Method. This is used only if the method shown in Figure 9-83 fails. It should be performed in one smooth gliding maneuver. (1) Preliminary stretching in line of the long axis of the shaft of the humerus. (2) While maintaining steady traction, rotate the arm externally and very gently until 80° of external rotation is achieved. (3) With the arm externally rotated bring the elbow forward to a point near the midline of the trunk. (4) Rotate the arm internally and place the hand on the opposite shoulder.

Relaxation of the muscles of the shoulder girdle is the key to a successful atraumatic reduction. If the patient is seen shortly after the injury occurred, analgesia may suffice to relax the muscle. Usually ¼ grain or ⅓ grain of morphine is adequate. However, I believe that if the patient is first seen after several hours injury, general anesthesia should be employed. A few ml. of Pentothal will produce the desired relaxation.

METHODS OF REDUCTION. A simple atraumatic method is steady, gentle traction on the arm, made against countertraction. The patient is in the supine position and traction is maintained for 60 to 90 seconds. If only an analgesic is being used, the traction must not produce pain, for this only stimulates the muscles into a state of spasm. If more traction is desired, the operator places his foot against the patient's chest wall—*never* in the axilla.

Another very effective method when only an analgesic is given is the Stimson method. The patient is in the prone position, with the affected arm hanging over the edge of the table. Tie a weight to the wrist so that it hangs free. Muscle relaxation usually occurs within a few minutes and the dislocation reduces spontaneously. This is an excellent atraumatic method and should be used more often.

If the above methods fail, manipulative methods are indicated. These, too, must always be performed gently and with the use of as little leverage as possible. The following methods are used for all three types of anterior dislocations. The patient is always under general anesthesia.

With the patient in the supine position, make steady traction on the arm (with the elbow flexed) in that plane in which it lies in relation to the trunk. Then, while traction is maintained, adduct the arm. This maneuver usually reduces the dislocation. If it does not, while traction is maintained, gently rotate the arm externally and internally to disengage the head. Now the free head slides into the glenoid fossa. After reduction, relax the traction and lay the arm across the chest (Fig. 9-83). If this method fails, I employ the Kocher's method. This method uses leverage and, if used forcefully, can produce severe soft tissue damage. Perform it as one smooth, gliding maneuver.

*Kocher Method.* The patient lies in the supine position with the elbow flexed. Grasp the wrist and lower end of the humerus and make steady traction on the slightly abducted arm. Hold this position for 60 to 90 seconds, for it stretches the muscles and tissues of the shoulder girdle. Next, rotate the arm externally very gently and smoothly until the arm reaches 80° of external rotation. Now bring the elbow forward to a point near the midline of the trunk. Finally, rotate the arm internally and place the hand on the opposite shoulder (Fig. 9-84).

WARNING: Again, it should be remembered that this method uses the arm as a lever to put the head of the humerus through a series of rotatory movements. Great force can be expended on the soft tissues of the shoulder joint, vessels and brachial plexus if the maneuvers are performed forcefully or improperly. Fractures of the shaft of the humerus, avulsions of the rotator cuff and injuries to the circumflex nerve may ensue.

If the Kocher method fails to achieve a reduction, this should be taken as a warning signal that some complication exists that is preventing reduction.

IMMOBILIZATION. Postreduction immobilization for young patients should be adequate, and long enough in duration to allow soft tissues to heal with minimal scar formation and without overlength. Immobilize the extremity for at least 3 weeks. There is much disagreement in regard to the period of immobilization; some advocate no immobilization, others as much as six weeks. In view of the disruptive nature of most primary dislocations, I feel that a period of immobilization sufficient to allow firm tissue healing should reduce the incidence of recurrent dislocations.

I prefer the use of the Nicola sling (Fig. 9-85); it restricts abduction, extension and all rotatory motions, but it allows motion at the elbow, wrist and fingers. An alternative dressing is a swathe encircling the chest, with the forearm supported by a sling.

REHABILITATION OF THE SHOULDER GIRDLE. After 3 weeks discard the dressing and allow free use of the extremity. Institute a program of graduated exercises within the limits of pain, beginning with pendulum exercises every hour for 5 to 10 minutes. Later, add crawling and pulling

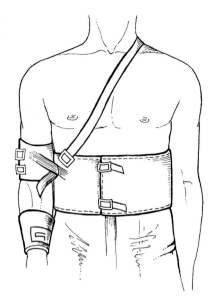

FIG. 9-85. Postreduction immobilization for young patients. Nicola sling: it restricts abduction, extension and all rotatory motions. It allows motion at the elbow, wrist and fingers.

exercises. The daily application of radiant heat and gentle massage are useful. Do not permit strenuous activity or sports for at least 3 months. While the dressing is still in place encourage the patient to do muscle setting exercises and to use muscles against resistance. This develops muscle tone and power and prevents contractures.

Postreduction immobilization for patients beyond middle life and expecially for the elderly should not be rigid. Some motion is beneficial, for it prevents adhesions about the shoulder and staves off a frozen shoulder. A collar and cuff is adequate. This limits abduction and external rotation sufficiently to prevent redislocation and at the same time permits some motion at the shoulder joint and free motion of the elbow, wrist, hand and fingers.

Pendulum exercises are started within two or three days, for 10 minutes 4 or 5 times each day. Encourage the use of the limb within painless arcs of motion. For the first 2 weeks restrict movement in ab-

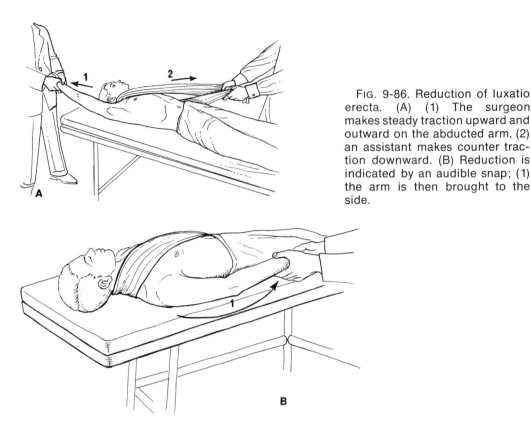

FIG. 9-86. Reduction of luxatio erecta. (A) (1) The surgeon makes steady traction upward and outward on the abducted arm, (2) an assistant makes counter traction downward. (B) Reduction is indicated by an audible snap; (1) the arm is then brought to the side.

duction to 45°. After 2 weeks permit movement to 90°. Discard the dressing at the end of 3 weeks. Now, allow free use of the arm and intensify the program of exercises. During this period daily radiant heat and gentle massage give much comfort to the shoulder.

### Luxatio Erecta

Again remember that in young people this is a serious lesion and may be associated with a massive tear of the cuff. If after reduction an inferior subluxation persists, surgical repair of the cuff is mandatory. An arthrogram at this time will establish the diagnosis (see Fig. 9-71).

**Reduction.** With the patient on his back make steady traction upward and outward on the abducted arm while an assistant makes countertraction downward (Fig. 9-86A). Reduction occurs with an audible snap; now bring the arm to the side (Fig. 9-86B). A Nicola sling provides excellent fixation or a swathe encircling the chest and a sling for the forearm may be used. The postreduction management is the same as for anterior dislocation. Immobilize the arm for 3 weeks.

### Management of Irreducible Fresh Dislocations

When the roentgenograms reveal no fracture of the humeral head, the glenoid or the coracoid process, assume that failure to reduce a dislocation is due to soft tissue lying between the head and the glenoid. (In young people bony lesions are rare, but they do occur.) Reduction is obstructed when: (1) the rotator cuff lies in front of the glenoid like a curtain, (2) the inferior capsule lies in the joint between the head and the glenoid, or (3) the biceps tendon lies posterior to the head preventing its relocation (see Fig. 9-75). There is still another cause of failure to reduce a fresh anterior dislocation. The anterior rim may fit into a defect on the posterolateral aspect of the head so tightly that the head cannot be dislodged by manipulative maneuvers. In this lesion the subscapularis stretches in front of the head like a tense, wide rubber band, preventing internal rotation of the arm. Before reduction can be achieved the tendon of the subscapularis must be divided. These are indeed rare lesions. I have seen two and have read an account of two others in the literature. These complications can be corrected only by exploration of the joint and removal of the obstruction.

### Operative Procedure (Fig. 9-87)

Make an incision over the top of the shoulder in line with the axillary crease and just lateral to the acromioclavicular joint. Extend the incision downward on the anterior aspect of the shoulder for 2 to 2½ inches; then extend it backward as far as the posterior margin of the acromion. Split the anterior fibers of the deltoid vertically for 2 inches below the edge of the acromion. Open the subacromial bursa in line with the muscle split. Do not excise the walls of the bursa. By rotating the arm internally and externally inspect the subacromial area and identify the pathology preventing reduction.

If more exposure is desired to facilitate repair of the disrupted tissues, excise ⅜ inch of the clavicle or the acromion adjacent to the acromioclavicular joint, depending upon the direction in which more exposure is desired.

**When the Cuff Lies in Front of the Humeral Head.** Remove the cuff from the joint and reduce the dislocation. Reattach the edges of the cuff to the greater tuberosity with mattress sutures passing through drill holes in the bone (Fig. 9-87C).

**When the Biceps Tendon Lies Behind the Head.** Replace the tendon in its normal position and reduce the dislocation. Cut the tendon at its insertion into the superior glenoid rim. Excise the intracapsular portion of the tendon and suture the proximal end of the remaining tendon in the intertubercular groove. First, with a sharp curette, scarify the floor of the groove; then fix the tendon in the groove with interrupted sutures passing through the transverse ligament overlying the groove (Fig. 9-87D).

**When the Capsule Lies in the Joint.** Remove the capsule from the joint and reduce the dislocation. No suture of the capsule is necessary (Fig. 9-87E).

### Diagnosis and Management of Posterior Sprain, Subluxation, Dislocation

### Posterior Sprain and Subluxation

These lesions are the result of a backward force applied to the humerus with the arm flexed forward. The patient has immediate pain in the posterior aspect of the shoulder and, if a subluxation occurred, he may feel the joint slip out and in. Also, if the arm is placed in extreme internal rotation and the humerus is thrust backward, the patient experiences intense pain and a feeling as if the head were going to slip out. Pressure over the posterior aspect of the humerus beneath the acromion elicits much tenderness. The symptoms may simulate those of strain of the posterior muscle units of the shoulder. These lesions do not occur frequently and rarely does recurrent posterior dislocation follow.

**Management.** Usually a swathe encircling the chest and a sling provide sufficient immobilization. If this position is uncomfortable or painful, apply a plaster of Paris

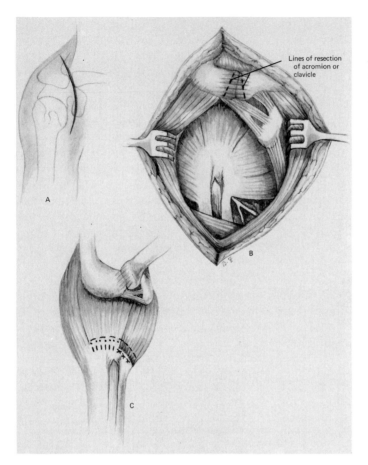

Lines of resection
of acromion or
clavicle

Fig. 9-87 (A-E). Operative procedure for unreducible fresh anterior dislocations. (A) Make an incision over the top of the shoulder lateral to the acromioclavicular joint and extend it downward on the anterior aspect of the shoulder for 2 to 2½ inches. (B) Split the fibers of the deltoid vertically for 2 inches below the edge of the acromion. Open the subacromial bursa but do not excise the walls of the bursa. If more exposure is needed resect ³/₈ of an inch of either the clavicle or the acromion. Now explore the subacromial region and identify the cause preventing reduction. (C) When the torn cuff lies in front of the glenoid, remove the cuff from inside the joint cavity, reduce the dislocation and then reattach the cuff to the greater and lesser tuberosities by mattress sutures passing through drill holes in the bone.

shoulder spica which holds the arm in 30° to 35° of abduction, slight external rotation and slight extension. Three weeks immobilization ensures good healing. At that time institute a program of shoulder exercises to restore normal motion and good muscle tone and power. Permit full and unrestricted activity after 4 to 6 weeks.

## Posterior Dislocation

This lesion is frequently overlooked; 60 percent of the cases are missed. They occur more frequently than is generally realized. Posterior dislocations comprise from 0.9 to 4.3 percent of all acute dislocations. In the reported cases, the age ranges from less than 2 years to 82 years. However, most occur in the first two decades. The ratio of males to females is approximately three to one. Bilateral cases are rare but they do occur. The incidence of recurrences following a primary dislocation is not known. In Rowe's series, 6 of 10 acute dislocations developed recurrences.

Anatomically, there are three types of acute posterior dislocation: the subglenoid, the subacromial (or retroglenoid), and the subspinous. In addition to the mechanisms associated with trauma (which were discussed in a preceding section), posterior dislocations may occur during epileptic seizures and shock therapy.

In making the diagnosis the clinical findings are most important. The limb is locked in adduction and internal rotation, making the coracoid process prominent. With the arm flexed forward a round

FIG. 9-87 (Cont'd) (D) When the biceps tendon precludes reduction: Replace the tendon in its normal position and reduce the dislocation. Next cut its attachment to the superior glenoid rim and excise the intracapsular portion of the tendon. Finally, suture the proximal end of the remaining tendon in the intertubercular groove by sutures anchoring it to the transverse ligament. (E) When the capsule lies in the joint, remove the capsule and reduce the dislocation. No suturing of the capsule is necessary.

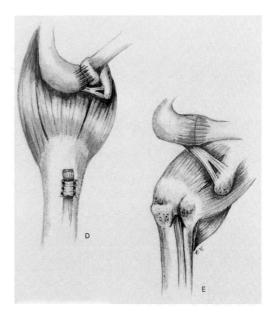

prominence can be felt posteriorly under the acromion. Abduction is greatly restricted and no internal rotation is possible actively or passively. In fresh injuries, reduction is accomplished easily and the prognosis good.

Roentgenograms taken in the anteroposterior view are frequently interpreted as negative. Axial, tangential and transthoracic views are more reliable and clearly show the lesion. However, if studied carefully, the anteroposterior view reveals some characteristic features of the posterior dislocation. The shaft of the humerus is rotated internally and the shadow of the glenoid overlaps that of the articular surface of the humeral head. Also, the head is displaced upward in relation to the glenoid (Fig. 9-88). Likewise, the axial view shows the head behind the glenoid and the head displaced slightly upward. All the above findings are slightly accentuated if the different views are taken with the arm internally rotated as far as possible. These roentgenographic features are not entirely reliable. However, an avulsion fracture of the lesser tuberosity is very suggestive of a posterior dislocation. This lesion is best seen in the axillary view. Another suggestive feature is the vacant appearance of at least the anterior half of the glenoid. In all fractures of the upper end of the humerus posterior dislocation of the head must be ruled out. Axillary views should be taken in all these fractures to confirm or rule out posterior dislocation of the humeral head. All views taken on the injured side must be compared with similar views of the normal shoulder.

The transthoracic view of the normal shoulder shows the axillary border of the scapula and the inferior portion of the medial wall of the neck and shaft of the humerus forming a smooth arch (Moloney's line). In posterior dislocations, the arch is interrupted (Fig. 9-89). This line is comparable to Shenton's line in the hip joint.

**Reduction.** The reduction should be done with the patient under general anesthesia. Make steady traction on the arm in the long axis of the humerus with the elbow flexed. An assistant assists mobilization of the head by pressing downward on the head with his thumb. While traction is maintained, adduct the arm. When the head reaches the glenoid rim, rotate the arm externally, then rotate it internally. This reduces the dislocation (Fig. 9-90).

The best form of immobilization is a plaster of Paris shoulder spica which holds the arm in 30° to 35° of abduction, in slight rotation and slightly behind the plane of the trunk. Discard the spica after 3 weeks and then institute a program of exercises designed to restore normal motion

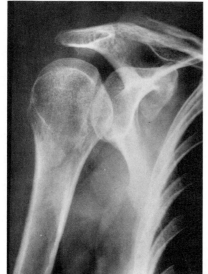

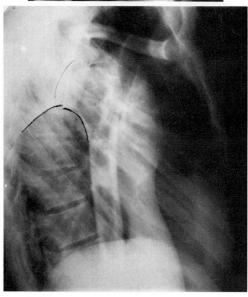

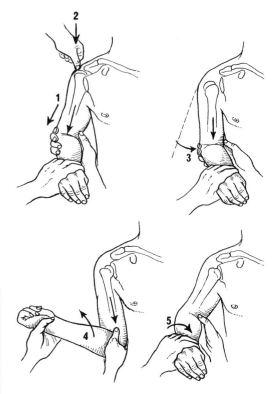

FIG. 9-90. Reduction of posterior dislocation. (1) Make steady traction on the arm, with the elbow flexed, in the long axis of the humerus. (2) An assistant helps in mobilization of the head by pressing downward on the head. (3) Adduct the arm with traction maintained. When the head reaches the glenoid rim effect the reduction by first (4) rotating the arm externally and then (5) gently rotating the arm internally.

(Top) FIG. 9-88. Anteroposterior view. Roentgenogram of a posterior dislocation of the glenohumeral joint. Note that the humeral shaft is rotated internally, the shadow of the glenoid overlaps that of the articular surface of the humeral head and the humeral head is displaced upward in relation to the glenoid.

(Bottom) FIG. 9-89. Thoracic view. Moloney's line is broken, indicating a posterior dislocation of the humeral head.

of the shoulder and normal muscle power and tone. Do not permit strenuous activity or sports for at least 3 months.

If recent posterior dislocations (less than 2 weeks old) cannot be reduced, open reduction must be performed.

## Management of Complications of Fresh Dislocations

**Rupture of the Rotator Cuff.** As noted previously, this is not a common lesion in young persons but it occurs more frequently

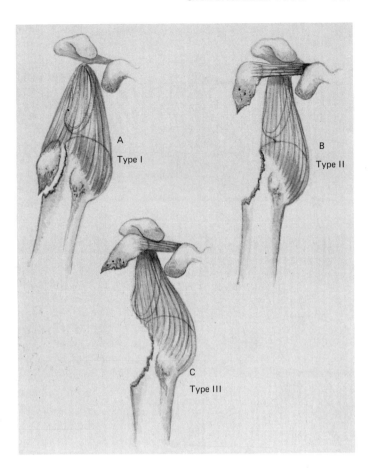

A
Type I

B
Type II

C
Type III

FIG. 9-91. Types of fractures of the greater tuberosity associated with anterior dislocations: (A) Type I, (B) Type II, (C) Type III.

than is generally realized. After middle life and in the elderly it does occur frequently. After reduction of the dislocation pain and muscle spasm may obscure the lesion. If the patient can forcefully abduct the arm after reduction, no serious injury to the cuff is present. On the other hand, no active abduction or weak abduction indicates a complete tear of the cuff or an injury to the axillary nerve. Absence of sensory loss over the course of the sensory branch of the axillary nerve rules out an injury to the axillary nerve. When the patient attempts to abduct the arm, he shrugs his shoulders instead of elevating the arm. This happens because the disrupted cuff is unable to fix and depress the head against the glenoid cavity when abduction is attempted. Therefore, the deltoid pulls the

humerus straight upward. An arthrogram of the shoulder joint taken at this time can definitely establish or eliminate the diagnosis of a complete tear of the rotator cuff.

In the young, massive avulsion of the cuff may occur with a severe hyperabduction mechanism. After reduction, an inferior subluxation of the humeral head should make one suspicious of such a lesion. This injury has been discussed previously (pp. 347, 348, 349).

Once the diagnosis of a complete, massive tear of the cuff is made, surgical repair should not be delayed. A freshly torn cuff is readily pulled down to the greater tuberosity of the humerus. If the repair is delayed, the cuff retracts and its margins become fibrotic, thickened and friable. Still later, it becomes sclerotic and it may then

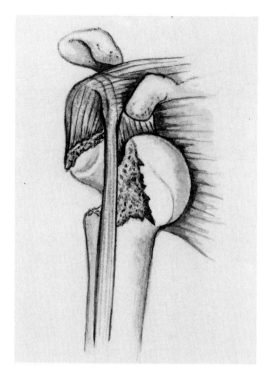

FIG. 9-92. Complication of Type I fracture of the greater tuberosity. The dislocation is complicated by avulsion of a portion of the cuff. This always includes the supraspinatus tendon.

be impossible to approximate the torn edges of the cuff to the greater tuberosity. In very old cases degeneration of the cuff may occur as far proximal as the muscle bellies of the rotator muscles. This circumstance leaves only one alternative arthrodesis of the shoulder.

Surgical management of partial and complete tears of the rotator cuff is described in Chapter 7.

### Fractures Complicating Dislocations

Fractures of the bony elements of the glenohumeral joint occur in approximately 25 percent of all dislocations. The mechanism responsible for the fracture is the same as that producing the dislocation. To this must be added the strong pull of certain muscle groups, producing avulsion of bone fragments such as avulsion of the greater or lesser tuberosities. Recurrence of dislocation does not occur frequently in patients with fractures. The exception to this is fracture of the anterior and inferior glenoid rim.

### Greater Tuberosity Fractures

Fracture of the greater tuberosity occurs in 25 to 30 percent of all dislocations. There are three types (Fig. 9-91): in Type I the tuberosity follows the head: in Type II the tuberosity remains in its normal relation to the scapula, and in Type III the tuberosity retracts under the acromion. In Type I, the cuff is severely stretched but generally remains intact. However, a complete tear of the cuff may occur (Fig. 9-92); check later for this complication. In Type II, there is wide separation between the greater tuberosity and the upper end of the humerus. In the event that reduction cannot be achieved by conservative methods, suspect posterior displacement of the biceps tendon and interposition of the cuff and tuberosities between the glenoid and the head (Fig. 9-93). Type III lesion is best treated by open reduction.

**Management of Types I and II Fracture-Dislocations.** Uncomplicated Type I and Type II lesions can easily be reduced by the methods employed to reduce anterior dislocations without fracture of the tuberosity. First, make steady traction on the flexed arm in the plane that the arm lies in, in relation to the trunk. Then, while traction is maintained, adduct the arm. This usually reduces the dislocation. If not, gently rotate the arm internally and externally to disengage the head. After dislocation is reduced lay the arm across the chest (see Fig. 9-83).

If the above method fails, use Kocher's method of reduction (see Fig. 9-84). Again, beware of the dangers of this method; if used forcefully, much damage can be done to the rotator cuff, the great vessels and the circumflex nerve. The shaft of the humerus may fracture.

The postreduction management is the same as that described for uncomplicated anterior dislocations.

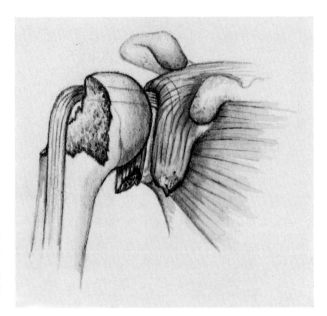

FIG. 9-93. Complication of Type II fracture of the greater tuberosity. The biceps tendon is displaced behind the humeral head, and the tuberosities and cuff drop in front of the glenoid cavity.

Failure to reduce the dislocation by the methods indicated above means that one of the complications associated with these fracture-dislocations is present. If so, the joint must be explored and the obstruction to reduction removed.

**Management of Complications.** In Type I fracture-dislocations it may be impossible to recognize a massive tear of the cuff after reduction. However, if the patient is unable to abduct the arm three or four weeks after reduction and if there is no evidence of injury to the axillary nerve, then it must be assumed that the cuff is completely torn. An arthrogram of the shoulder taken at this time will confirm the diagnosis. Once the diagnosis of a complete tear is made, the cuff tear should be repaired immediately (see pp. 229 to 233).

**Surgical Management of Complications in Type II Fracture-Dislocation.** The superior approach provides the best exposure of this lesion. After the subacromial region is exposed, the nature of the pathology is readily seen. Then the tuberosities, with the cuff attached, must be removed from the joint, and the biceps tendon disengaged from the posterior aspect of the humeral head. Now the head can readily be manipulated into its normal position. Excise the intracapsular portion of the biceps tendon and anchor the proximal end of the remaining tendon into the bicipital groove. Finally, reattach the tuberosities with the cuff to the humerus with interrupted sutures passing through drill holes in the bone. The surgical technique of this procedure and the postoperative management are described on page 238.

**Surgical Management of Complications in Type III Fracture-Dislocation.** In this instance, the rotator cuff pulls the greater tuberosity under the acromion. This lesion cannot be treated by abducting the arm. Abduction does not approximate the greater tuberosity to the site of the fracture on the humerus, and it favors redislocation. There is only one treatment: do an open reduction and reattach the tuberosity with the attached cuff to the humerus (see page 239).

## Fractures of the Head and Neck of the Humerus with Dislocation

Fractures of the head and neck complicating a dislocation are caused by the same force and mechanism which produce the dislocation. They usually occur after middle

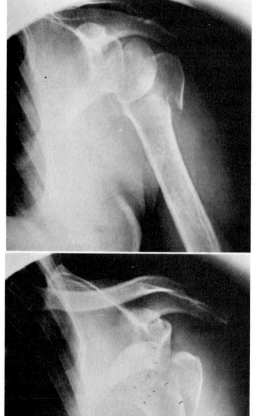

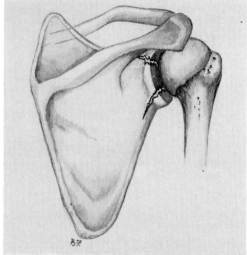

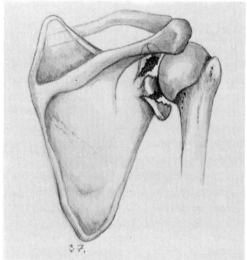

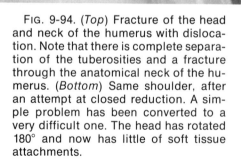

FIG. 9-94. (*Top*) Fracture of the head and neck of the humerus with dislocation. Note that there is complete separation of the tuberosities and a fracture through the anatomical neck of the humerus. (*Bottom*) Same shoulder, after an attempt at closed reduction. A simple problem has been converted to a very difficult one. The head has rotated 180° and now has little of soft tissue attachments.

(*Top*) FIG. 9-95. Stellate fracture of the glenoid with minimal displacement.

(*Bottom*) FIG. 9-96. Stellate fracture of the glenoid with wide separation of the fragments.

life and in the elderly in whom the cancellous bone of the upper end of the humerus is weak and brittle, hence permitting severe comminution to occur. The pathology comprises pronounced disorganization of the bony and soft tissue elements of the joint. The jagged ends of the fragments may injure the brachial plexus or the great vessels at the time of the dislocation. But most injuries to these structures occur during closed reduction. Closed methods may convert a simple impacted fracture-dislocation into one with wide separation of the fragments. Methods of reduction employing abduction and strong traction are dangerous and should be condemned (Fig. 9-94A and B).

The most logical approach to this problem is to visualize the pathology and to reduce the dislocation under direct vision. Reduce the dislocation gently, preserve all soft tissue attachments and avoid any unnecessary stripping of the fragments. Usually the fragments can be reassembled and fixed to one another and to the shaft of the humerus by wire or stout Nylon sutures. All free pieces of bone devoid of soft tissue should be removed.

Occasionally, the head lies free, without any soft tissue attachments, or it is so comminuted that aseptic necrosis of the head is certain to follow. In such instances, the head fragment or fragments can be removed and replaced by a metallic prosthesis. The results of this procedure are far superior to a flail shoulder, which follows resection of the head, or to a painful arthritic shoulder, which occurs when the head fragments undergo aseptic necrosis.

The superior approach to the shoulder joint provides the best exposure of fracture-dislocations. Surgical management of these lesions is described on page 240.

### Fractures of the Glenoid

Rim fractures may be produced by direct and indirect forces applied to the glenoid through the head of the humerus. Often indirect mechanisms also produce a dislocation of the joint. Generally, direct forces do not, but, since the resultant rim fracture predisposes to recurrent subluxation or dislocation of the joint, they also are considered here.

### Stellate Fractures of the Glenoid

Force applied directly to the lateral side of the humerus usually produces a stellate type fracture of the glenoid (Fig. 9-95). The

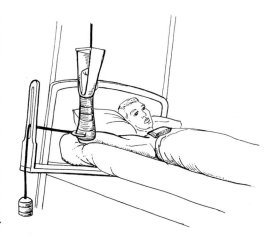

FIG. 9-97. Lateral traction for stellate fractures of the glenoid.

amount of displacement of the fragments depends on the severity of the force. Most stellate fractures require no reduction, for the articular surface of the glenoid can tolerate much incongruity and still function normally. The glenohumeral joint is not a weight-bearing joint. However, in severely displaced stellate fractures an attempt should be made to approximate the fragments (Fig. 9-96).

**Management of Fracture with Minimal Displacement.** These fractures require nothing more than a sling to support the arm. For the first 24 or 36 hours apply ice to the shoulder and later heat. After 10 to 14 days permit active graduated pendulum exercises within the tolerance of pain. Also, apply daily radiant heat and gentle massage to all the soft tissues of the shoulder. After 3 or 4 weeks discard the sling and increase the range and frequency of the exercises.

**Stellate Fractures with Wide Separation of the Fragments.** Since these fractures are caused by a direct force, the capsule and ligaments remain intact. Traction on the structures causes the displaced fragments to approximate one another to a considerable degree. Skeletal traction is the best form of traction for these fractures.

LATERAL TRACTION (Fig. 9-97). With

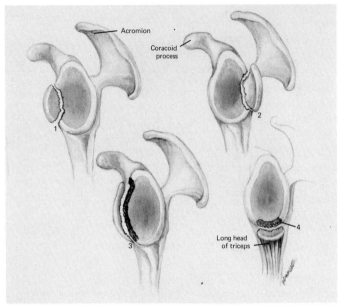

Acromion

Coracoid process

1

2

3

Long head of triceps

4

FIG. 9-98. Types of fractures of the glenoid. (1) Fracture of the anterior portion of the glenoid with minimal displacement. (2) Fracture of the posterior portion of the glenoid with minimal displacement. (3) Avulsion fracture of the glenoid rim (usually associated with dislocations of the glenohumeral joint). (4) Avulsion fracture of the inferior glenoid rim caused by severe contracture of the triceps.

the patient in the supine position and a board under the mattress, elevate the side of the bed about 4 inches. Insert a threaded wire through the base of the olecranon and apply about 6 to 12 pounds of traction. Also apply 3 to 6 pounds of traction to the forearm. The extremity in traction should be maintained in a position of 90° of abduction of the arm and 90° of flexion of the forearm. Maintain the traction for 3 weeks, then remove the wire and place the arm in a sling for 2 weeks. Immediately after the traction apparatus is removed institute progressive shoulder exercises on a regulated program (5 or 10 minutes every hour). Gradually increase the range and frequency of the exercises until normal motion is attained.

### Rim Fractures Produced by a Direct Mechanism

A direct impact on the flexed elbow (such as occurs in a fall) may drive the head of the humerus against the anterior or posterior rim of the glenoid. The force may be sufficient to shear off a portion of the rim. These fractures are not the same as the rim fractures that occur in anterior and posterior dislocations. The latter fractures are true avulsion fractures and often are associated with pronounced disruption of the capsule.

If the displacement is not great, no treatment is necessary other than the application of a sling. The sling is worn for 3 or 4 weeks, but active pendulum exercises begin after 10 to 14 days.

If the fragments show wide separation (over $3/8$ inch), and particularly if they are large fragments, they must be restored to their anatomical position on the glenoid. The surgical procedure is an easy one to perform in fresh lesions but very difficult in cases of long standing. In fact, replacement of the fragments may be impossible in old lesions. Failure to replace the fragments invariably is followed by recurrent subluxation or dislocation of the joint.

The surgical techniques for replacement of anterior and posterior rim fractures are described on page 240 to 243.

### Rim Fractures Produced by Indirect Mechanism

These rim fractures occur when the shoulder joint dislocates anteriorly, posteriorly or inferiorly, as in luxatio erecta

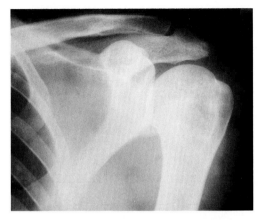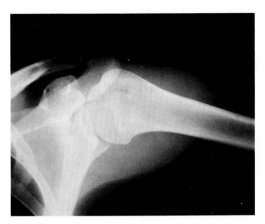

FIG. 9-99. (*Left*) Fracture of the posterior rim complicating a posterior dislocation; this patient developed recurrent posterior dislocation of the shoulder. (*Right*) Note that the fragment changes position when the arm is elevated, indicating that it is attached to the capsule.

(Fig. 9-98). As the head is driven over the glenoid rim, the capsule tenses and may pull off a portion of the glenoid rim to which it is attached. These are true avulsion fractures and they are always associated with extensive stretching and tearing of the capsule and ligaments. In most instances the fragments are small but they may be one third or one quarter of the width of the glenoid fossa; such joints are difficult to hold in the reduced position. I recall one patient with a subcoracoid dislocation that was complicated by a fracture of the antero-inferior rim. The dislocation reduced easily with simple traction on the arm, but, when the traction was released, the head slipped off the glenoid. Only after the glenoid fossa was explored did I appreciate the size of the defect in the glenoid, for the roentgenograms failed to show the true nature of the lesion. The roentgenograms of a patient who presents with a shoulder injury caused by an indirect mechanism show only a rim fracture; the head is in its anatomical position. In such cases, it is best to assume that the patient had either a subluxation of the joint or a dislocation that reduced spontaneously. Further, it should be assumed that the capsule, the ligaments and even the rotator cuff may be severely injured. This patient is as likely to develop recurrent

subluxation or dislocation as is the patient with a complete dislocation (Fig. 9-99).

When the fragments are small and not greatly displaced, the treatment is the same as for uncomplicated dislocations except that movements of the arm that put the capsule on the stretch are avoided for five or six weeks.

Large rim fragments (anterior, posterior or inferior fragments) with wide separation should be replaced surgically. Also, I treat all cases requiring open replacement of rim fragments as recurrent dislocations. In addition to replacing the rim fragment I also perform an operation to cure recurrent dislocation. For example, in cases with anterior and inferior rim fractures I always transfer the tendon of the subscapularis to the lateral side of the bicipital groove. Unfortunately, there are very few dislocations with rim fractures that require open reduction. I say unfortunately, because I have never seen such a fracture-dislocation that did not develop recurrent dislocation regardless of the type of conservative treatment instituted.

## Avulsion of the Inferior Glenoid Rim by the Triceps

A common rim fracture in athletes is avulsion of the inferior glenoid rim by powerful contraction of the long head of the triceps. Baseball pitchers and tennis players sustain this fracture more often than do participants in other sports. The size of the fragment varies considerably and may be nothing more than a sliver. In such an instance, it may be impossible to make the diagnosis by roetgenographic study.

At the time of the injury the patient feels severe pain deep in the axilla. Pressure over the inferior rim elicits tenderness, and active stretching of the triceps accentuates the pain.

Treatment consists of putting the arm at rest in a sling for three to five weeks and preventing any movements which stretch the triceps. Progress in the rehabilitation period should be deliberately slow, because—for example—one hard overhead

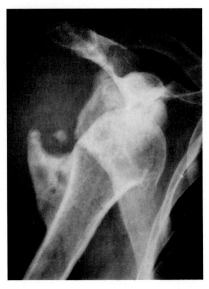

FIG. 9-101. Old anterior dislocation of 7 years duration. Note the extensive hypertrophic bony changes of the glenoid and humeral head, and the mass of new bone along the outer surface of the shaft of the humerus. This patient had a fair range of motion and little pain in the shoulder.

pitch may undo the entire healing process. Return to full participation too early is undoubtedly the commonest cause for recurrence of the injury.

As a rule, healing by fibrous union occurs between the glenoid and the avulsed bony fragment, and this healing is usually adequate to meet the demands of normal activity. Occasionally, strenuous demands on the arm cause pain when the triceps

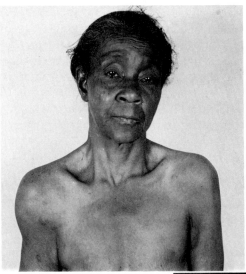

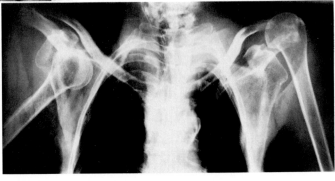

FIG. 9-100. (Top) Elderly patient with bilateral dislocations of 10 years duration. This patient had a fair range of motion and little pain in either shoulder. (Bottom) Roentgenogram of patient shown above.

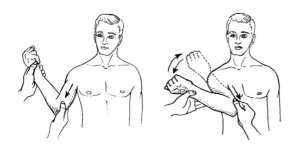

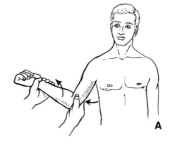

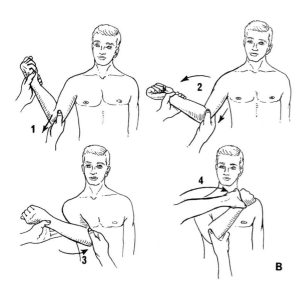

FIG. 9-102. Closed reduction of old anterior dislocation. Employ general anesthesia for the reduction of all old dislocations. (A) Make steady traction on the arm with the elbow flexed. This maneuver tends to mobilize the head. Next, rotate the arm inwardly and outwardly, slowly and forcefully. Then stretch the adductors and internal rotators by abducting and rotating the arm externally. Follow this with the Kocher maneuvers. (B) Kocher Maneuvers: Make steady traction in the line of the long axis of the shaft of the humerus in slight abduction (1); while maintaining steady traction, rotate the arm externally 80° (2); with the arm externally rotated, bring the elbow forward to a point near the midline of the trunk (3); finally, rotate the arm internally and place the hand over the opposite shoulder (4).

contracts forcefully. If the arm must be used in this fashion, the bony fragment can be excised and the tendon sutured to the inferior aspect of the glenoid.

Chronic strains of the triceps muscle-tendon unit are discussed in Chapter 8.

## Other Fractures Complicating Dislocations

Fracture of the coracoid process or the acromion may occur with dislocations; these are indeed rare lesions. Generally there is little or no displacement. In the treatment, the fracture is disregarded. The patient is treated in the same manner as in uncomplicated dislocation.

**Fracture of the Acromion, Complete**

**Dislocation of the Acromioclavicular Joint and Posterior Dislocation of the Glenohumeral Joint.** This is a rare lesion; I have seen only six cases. It is a serious injury and its treatment is difficult. It is the result of great violence. Not only does the acromion fracture at its base and the head dislocate posteriorly but also there is a complete dislocation of the acromioclavicular joint. The treatment is surgical. First, reduce the posterior dislocation, then reduce the fracture of the acromion and fix the fragments with threaded wires; and finally, reduce the dislocation of the acromioclavicular joint, transfix the joint with threaded wires and repair, if possible, the superior acromioclavicular ligament. In two cases, because of the severity of disruption of the acromioclavicular joint, I resected the distal ¾ inches of the clavicle.

## Old Anterior Dislocations

These are serious lesions and reduction by closed methods is virtually impossible after six weeks. I believe all anterior dislocations of over six weeks duration and those of less than six weeks that cannot be reduced by closed methods should be reduced by surgical methods. Closed methods in longstanding cases may cause tragic complications such as rupture of the axillary artery, injury to the brachial plexus and fracture of the humerus. These disasters may also occur in operative reduction, but to a lesser degree. In some instances, longstanding dislocations are painless and permit a fair range of motion. In the elderly, such lesions should be left undisturbed. In young persons and in those with pain and vascular impairment reduction of the dislocation must be done (Fig. 9-100).

Regardless of the methods of reduction, open or closed, the shoulder rarely achieves complete restoration of function. However, the results are better in those dislocations reduced by closed methods than in those treated by open methods. Also, the results are better in recent injuries than they are in dislocations of long standing. After six months the chances of getting a serviceable shoulder are poor. Unless other complications exist it may be better to accept the dislocation. It is clear that the prognosis in longstanding anterior dislocations should always be guarded.

## Pathology

In addition to the soft tissue and bone damage occurring at the time of injury, secondary changes, related to healing and degeneration of tissues, set in. Depending on the duration of the lesion, varying degrees of fibrosis, contracture and shortening of all the soft tissues occur. This process involves in particular the capsule, ligaments and musculotendinous cuff. Dense scar tissue fixes the humeral head in the displaced position to the surrounding structures. The long adductors and internal rotators also become fibrotic and shortened (pectoralis major, teres major and latissimus dorsi). Tough, inelastic scar tissue fills and obliterates the joint cavity.

In very late cases, extensive degeneration of the articular cartilage of the glenoid fossa and humeral head occurs. Loose bony fragments become embedded in fibrous tissue. The osseous elements— glenoid, humeral head and shaft—show profound demineralization. Along the glenoid rim and at the point of contact of the head against the scapula, cartilaginous and bony proliferations appear (Fig. 9-101).

In most instances, the biceps tendon shows evidence of severe trauma and secondary degenerative changes. It may be thickened, injected and fibrotic, and embedded in scar tissue; in some cases it ruptures completely and the distal end reattaches itself to the shaft of the humerus below the lesser tuberosity. In several cases the tendon was displaced posteriorly, thereby preventing reduction.

## Management

**Closed Method.** Complete relaxation is needed and this is best attained by general anesthesia. Before definitive manipulative maneuvers are used, the humeral head is mobilized by steady traction on the arm with the elbow flexed and by rotating the arm internally and externally (Fig. 9-102A). Perform this step slowly but forcefully, in the hope that the head will free itself from surrounding adhesions. Next, while traction is maintained, slowly abduct and externally rotate the arm (Fig. 9-102A). The purpose of this maneuver is to overcome the contractures and shortening of the long and short adductors and internal rotators, particularly the pectoralis major and the subscapularis. Next, attempt to reduce the dislocation by the Kocher method (Fig. 9-102B). If this fails, a second attempt is justifiable. Remember that every attempt causes more soft tissue damage and increases the risk of severe complications. My opinion is that if the shoulder is not reduced by the second effort, further attempts are futile and dangerous. Two choices remain: (1) accept the dislocation and, by physical measures, try to regain as much motion as possible, or (2) at a later date, perform open reduction.

**Postreduction Management.** After the dislocation is reduced place a cotton pad in the axilla, encircle the arm and chest with a swathe and support the forearm with a sling. The arm should be fixed to the side for 3 to 4 weeks. During this period permit no abduction or external rotation movements of the arm. However, encourage motion at the elbow, wrist and fingers. After the sling is discarded start the patient on pendulum exercises, always within the limits set by pain. He performs the exercises every hour for 5 to 10 minutes. Later, add wall crawling and pulley exercises. Physical therapy in the form of heat and massage is beneficial. Do not permit strenuous activity or sports for at least 3 months.

The surgical technique and postoperative management of open reduction of old anterior dislocations is described on page 243.

### Old Posterior Dislocations

In the discussion of fresh posterior dislocations it was pointed out that the lesion is relatively rare, occurring in 2 to 3 percent of all dislocations. Also, because the deformity of the shoulder is not striking, many posterior dislocations are not recognized for weeks or even months. In some instances, longstanding posterior dislocations masquerade as frozen shoulders and are treated as such. Most of the longstanding cases that come to my attention were not recognized at the time of the injury. This lesion, although uncommon, may

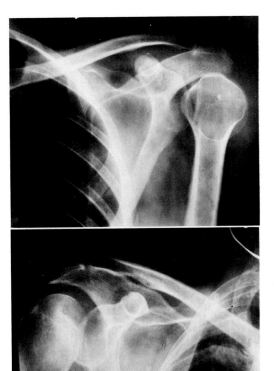

(*Top*) FIG. 9-103. Roentgenogram, anteroposterior view, of old posterior dislocation of the shoulder. Note that the humerus is rotated internally and the shadow of the glenoid overlaps that of the articular surface of the humeral head. The head is displaced slightly upward in relation to the glenoid fossa.

(*Bottom*) FIG. 9-104. Roentgenogram, anteroposterior view, of an old posterior dislocation of the shoulder. This head was firmly locked in the dislocated position. Note the large defect in the humeral head.

occur in young people. Awareness of the lesion is most important in making the diagnosis.

Careful examination of the shoulder reveals some characteristic features of the lesion. The deformity is not obvious, but there is increased prominence of the coracoid process; the humeral head is less prominent anteriorly than usual but more prominent posteriorly in the subacromial region. Motion at the glenohumeral joint

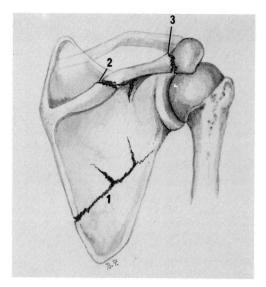

FIG. 9-105. Types of fractures of the scapula produced by violent direct trauma: (1) Fracture of the body. (2) Fracture of the spine. (3) Fracture of the acromion.

is greatly restricted; very little abduction is possible and no external rotation.

Roentgenograms of these cases frequently are read as negative. Yet there are certain features characteristic of the lesion. First, each view taken of the dislocated shoulder must be compared with a similar view of the normal shoulder. In the anteroposterior view the shaft of the humerus is rotated internally and the shadow of the glenoid overlaps that of the articular surface of the humeral head. Also the head is displaced slightly upward in relation to the glenoid cavity. The axial view shows the head behind the glenoid and displaced slightly upward (Fig. 9-103).

### Pathology

The extent of disorganization of the joint depends upon the duration of the dislocation. The basic pathology includes: (1) the presence of a defect in the head just medial to the lesser tuberosity, into which the posterior rim of the glenoid engages; (2) avulsion of the posterior capsule from the labrum and scapula; (3) stripping of the infraspinatus from the posterior surface of the neck of the scapula and erosion of the posterior rim of the glenoid. Not infrequently the posterior rim or the rim together with a large portion of the posterior glenoid is sheared off. This lesion renders the joint extremely unstable. In longstanding lesions the head is firmly locked in the dislocated position by dense scar tissue. Also, as in anterior dislocations of longstanding, all the muscles, especially the short rotators contract, shorten and become fibrotic; and the articular cartilage of both the glenoid and the humeral head undergoes profound degenerative changes (Fig. 9-104).

### Management

Reduction by closed methods is virtually impossible in dislocations over two weeks old and often fails even in more recent ones. This is in contrast to fresh lesions which readily reduce by closed manipulation. If the dislocation is not more than two weeks old, an attempt should be made to reduce it by closed methods, with the patient under general anesthesia. I use the same manipulative maneuvers described for reduction of fresh posterior dislocations except that heavier traction and more force is required to reduce old dislocations. The postreduction management also is the same as for fresh lesions (p. 364).

For all dislocations over two weeks old open reduction should be the first choice of treatment; however, as in longstanding anterior dislocations, in posterior dislocations of over six months duration and reduced by surgery, the chances of obtaining a painless, functioning shoulder are indeed slim. If no other complications are present, it is better to accept the dislocation. The shoulder then functions as an arthrodesed shoulder joint.

The technique for operative reduction of old posterior dislocations is described on page 245.

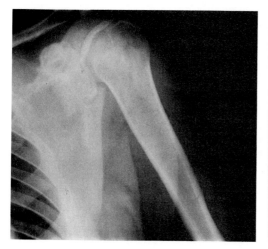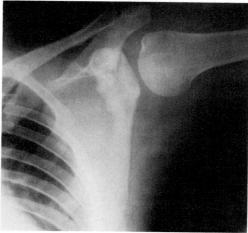

FIG. 9-106. (*Left*) Fracture of the neck of the glenoid; the glenoid is displaced medially and tilted upward. This amount of displacement is not acceptable. (*Right*) Same lesion, after the application of lateral traction (12 pounds). The position of the glenoid has improved considerably.

### Intrathoracic Dislocation of the Humeral Head

This rare lesion may have serious consequences. The acting force drives the humerus between the ribs of the upper thorax, and, as the arm descends to the side, the head snaps off inside the thoracic cage. The entire cuff tears off the humerus and fragments of the greater and the lesser tuberosity may remain attached to it. The patient may or may not exhibit signs of respiratory embarrassment. The wide interval between the upper end of the humerus and the humeral head, as seen on roentgenograms, is the clue to the nature of the lesion.

#### Management

The head must be removed from within the thoracic cage. The reconstructive measures performed to give the patient a useful limb depend on the amount of comminution of the upper end of the humerus and whether or not the rotator cuff can be reassembled. The operative procedure should always be performed in cooperation with a thoracic surgeon.

### FRACTURES AND DISLOCATIONS OF THE SCAPULA

These fractures are the result of a violent force applied directly to some portion of the scapula. However, occasionally severe muscle contraction may cause a fracture of the body or avulse a segment of bone from the spine of the scapula. Not infrequently, fractures of the ribs and those of the spine are associated lesions. In crushing injuries, fractures of the scapula are frequently overlooked (Fig. 9-105).

#### Fractures of the Body

Fractures of the body need no reduction. Large muscle masses invest the scapula, preventing wide separation of the fragments. Often the body is comminuted. Moreover, complete anatomical alignment of the fragments is not necessary for the scapula to function normally.

**Management.** For the first 24 or 48 hours apply ice to the traumatized area, then follow this with heat. Also, during this time apply a firm compression bandage over the scapula, using moleskin. Suspend the arm in a sling.

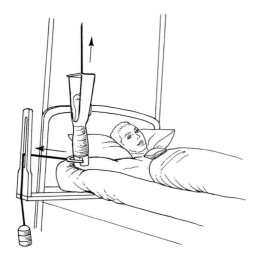

FIG. 9-107. Type of lateral traction employed to reduce fractures of the neck of the scapula with severe displacement.

After 10 to 14 days remove the sling and encourage the use of the shoulder girdle within the tolerance of pain. Also, start pendulum exercises, increasing progressively in range of motion and frequency. Although the patient usually regains full range of motion of the shoulder girdle, he feels some discomfort for several weeks, especially when he forces the arm.

## Fractures of the Neck of the Scapula

Fractures of the neck of the scapula occur as the result of direct impact on the anterior or posterior region of the shoulder. In this lesion the articular surface of the glenoid remains intact and the capsule and ligaments are not involved.

Anatomical restoration of the fragments is not necessary. The scapula can function normally with some disalignment of the neck. However, any severe angulation of the articular surface of the glenoid must be corrected. Such deformities restrict motion in the glenohumeral joint or may predispose to subluxation or dislocation of the joint. Most fractures respond to closed methods; the need for surgical intervention is rare.

**Fractures With Minimal Displacement.** Minimal displacement of the glenoid fragment is acceptable.

For the first 24 or 48 hours apply ice to the part, then apply heat. Support the extremity in a sling. After 10 to 14 days begin graduated active exercises of the shoulder within the tolerance of pain. Physical therapy in the form of heat and gentle massage gives comfort to the patient and is beneficial to the tissues; it helps absorption of blood and tissue exudates and restores elasticity to the soft parts. After three or four weeks discard the sling and increase progressively the range and frequency of the pendulum exercises. Then add wall crawling and pulley exercises.

**Fractures with Marked Displacement.** Fractures with severe angulation of the articular surface of the glenoid or with marked displacement respond to lateral traction (Fig. 9-106). The patient assumes the supine position, with a board under the mattress and the side of the bed elevated about 4 inches. Apply skeletal traction through the base of the olecranon and add 6 to 12 pounds. Always use a threaded wire through the olecranon. Apply skin traction to the forearm, using 3 to 6 pounds. The position of the arm in traction is 90° of abduction and 90° of flexion at the elbow (Fig. 9-107).

Maintain the traction for 3 weeks, then place the arm in a sling for two more weeks. After the traction is removed, institute a program of progressive shoulder exercises and physical therapy in the form of heat and massage.

### Dislocation of the Scapula

This is indeed a rare lesion, but it occasionally occurs. It responds to manipulative reduction; surgery is never indicated. The entire body of the scapula is displaced forward and outward and its lower angle is locked between the ribs (Fig. 9-108).

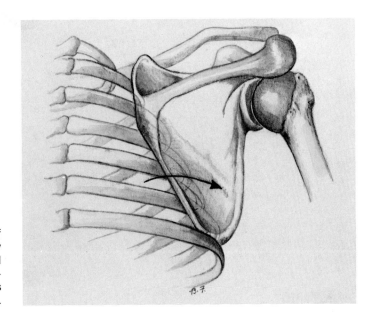

FIG. 9-108. Dislocation of the scapula: the entire body of the scapula is displaced outward and rotated outward, the lower angle is wedged between the ribs.

**Management.** While an assistant makes steady traction on the hyperabducted arm, grasp the axillary border of the scapula and in one movement rotate the bone forward and push it backward (Fig. 9-109).

After reduction, fix the scapula to the chest wall with eight or ten lengths of 3-inch adhesive tape. Place a pad of cotton in the axilla, apply a swathe around the arm and chest and support the arm with a collar and cuff sling. After 7 to 10 days, reinforce the dressing. Discard the dressing after 2 weeks and permit free use of the arm.

## FRACTURES OF THE UPPER END OF THE HUMERUS

Fractures of the upper end of the humerus include fracture through the surgical neck, which is the area between the tuberosities and the insertion of the pectoralis major and the triceps area.

### Mechanism of Fracture

A direct blow to the top of the shoulder rarely causes a fracture of the upper end of the humerus, which is protected by the overhanging acromion. The exception is a direct blow to the point of the shoulder while the arm is in backward extension.

Most fractures in this region are the result of an indirect mechanism—the same forces that produce dislocation of the humeral head. The patient falls on the outstretched arm, but the arm fails to rotate quickly enough to reach the safety of the

FIG. 9-109. Reduction of dislocation of the scapula. While an assistant makes steady traction on the hyperabducted arm (1), the surgeon grasps the axillary border of the scapula and, in one movement, rotates the bone forward and pushes the scapula directly backward (2).

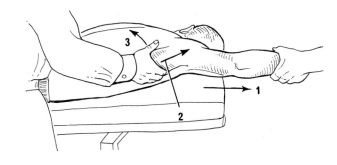

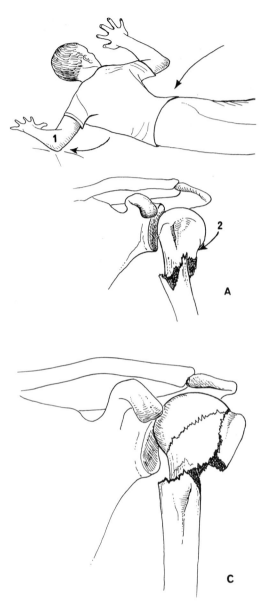

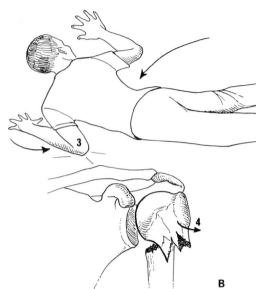

FIG. 9-110. Mechanism of fractures of the upper end of the humerus. (A) Abduction fractures. In this mechanism the arm strikes the ground as it moves away from the body (1); the acromion locks under the greater tuberosity, producing an abduction fracture (2). (B) Adduction fractures. The arm strikes the ground as it moves toward the body (3); the acromion locks under the tuberosity, producing an adduction fracture (4). (C) In the elderly, this mechanism may produce comminution of the upper end of the humerus through the planes of the lines of epiphyseal union, resulting in four main fragments or any combination of these fragments.

pivotal position or is forced beyond it. When this happens, the acromion abuts against the humeral head and acts as a fulcrum at the base of the greater tuberosity while the humerus becomes the long arm of the lever. If the force continues, either a dislocation or a fracture, or a combination of the two ensues.

The mechanism produces different lesions in different age groups. In children it produces an epiphyseal separation, the epiphyseal plate being the weakest point. In youths and young adults, it may cause dislocation or, occasionally, a fracture of the greater tuberosity or of the surgical neck. In the older group, in which the cancellous bone is weak and brittle, the result may be comminution of the upper end of the humerus. This may or may not be associated with dislocation of the head.

The type of lesion resulting from the mechanism described above is governed by many other circumstances: the severity of the force; the exact point on the humerus at which the force is expended; the degree of rotation of the humerus; the weight and

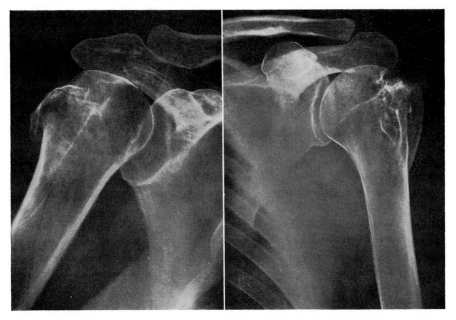

FIG. 9-111. Compression fractures of the greater tuberosity. The normal configuration of the bicipital groove is frequently disrupted in this type of fracture, resulting in bicipital tenosynovitis.

velocity of the falling body and the direction the arm takes on striking the ground. If the arm moves toward the body, adduction fractures result; if the arm moves away from the body, abduction fractures result. The former are the commonest in children and the latter in adults. The force of contraction of the rotator muscles at the time the force expends itself may avulse the greater or lesser tuberosity or the rotator cuff (Fig. 9-110).

### Anatomical Classification

The mechanism just described produces the following types of fractures:
1. Fracture of the greater tuberosity
2. Fracture of the lesser tuberosity
3. Fracture of the anatomical neck
4. Fracture of the surgical neck
5. Separation of the upper humeral epiphysis
6. Fracture of the head of the humerus
7. Any combination of the preceding six types

8. Comminution of the entire upper end of the humerus, and
9. Fracture-Dislocations; any of the above types may occur with a dislocation of the head.

### Considerations in the Management of Fractures of the Upper End of the Humerus

Ideally, the objectives in the treatment of fractures of the upper end of the humerus are: (1) restoration of all involved tissues to their normal anatomical state, and (2) restoration of a completely functional limb to the individual in the shortest time possible. However, in this region, clinical experience reveals that the first objective is not always possible and, fortunately, it is not essential to achieve the second.

An understanding of the anatomical peculiarities of the upper end of the humerus is helpful in planning the treatment of fractures in this region. It should be remembered that the stability of the

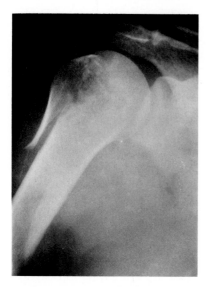

FIG. 9-112. Fracture of the greater tuberosity with minimal displacement. Generally, this fracture needs no reduction and the prognosis is good, except in very young people, particularly athletes, in whom surgical replacement of the tuberosity is justified.

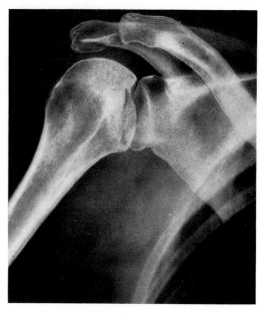

FIG. 9-114. Fracture of the head of the humerus with impaction of the fragments. This fracture carries a poor prognosis.

glenohumeral joint depends not on the bony configuration of the joint but on the muscle groups that move it, especially the rotator muscles. Within reasonable limits, incongruity of the articular surfaces is compatible with good function because the muscle apparatus can readjust itself to changes in the configuration of the bony elements. Hence, considerable deformity can be accepted with the assurance that

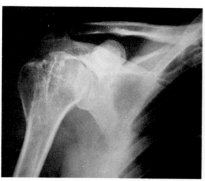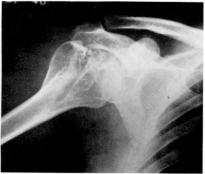

FIG. 9-113. (Left) Fracture of the greater tuberosity, with pulling away of the fragment from the humerus. If this fracture is allowed to heal with displacement of the tuberosity, severe impairment of abduction invariably ensues. (Right) Note that when the arm is abducted about 60° the displaced tuberosity impinges against the acromion.

the joint will have a good range of motion. This is particularly applicable to impacted fractures of the upper end of the humerus.

Motion in the glenohumeral joint is produced by muscles working as a single unit. The overall performance of the group is not seriously affected if one component of the unit fails to function normally. For example, complete tears of the cuff, within certain limits, do not preclude good function. On the other hand, massive disruption of the cuff seriously impairs function.

Bony union occurs in most fractures and it is not greatly influenced by the method of treatment. Impacted fractures always heal; unimpacted fractures heal provided that there is some contact of the fragments.

Displacement of the fragment, in most instances, is never great. There are reasons for this. The soft tissues of the upper end of the humerus are so arranged that they hold the fragments together. The musculotendinous cuff has a strong, broad insertion into the tuberosities, the subacromial bursa adheres closely to the tuberosities, the periosteum prevents wide separation of the fragments and the tendon of the long head of the biceps aligns the fragments. Fractures of the tuberosities with wide separation of the fragments indicate extensive tearing of the musculotendinous cuff. On the other hand, no soft tissues attach to the anatomical neck. If a violent, dislocating force causes a fracture in this area, the fragments may be widely separated.

Most essential to a complete and rapid recovery is preservation of the gliding mechanisms between the soft tissue layers of the shoulder. To attain this, motion must start early. This is especially true in patients over 40 years of age.

On the basis of the special features of the upper end of the humerus, fractures in this region may be placed into two groups:

(1) fractures requiring no reduction, and

(2) fractures requiring reduction.

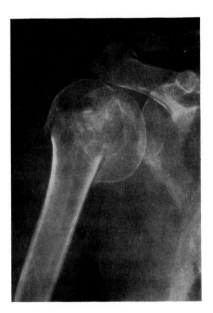

FIG. 9-115. Impacted adducted fracture. This fracture needs no reduction; the head-neck angle measures 120°.

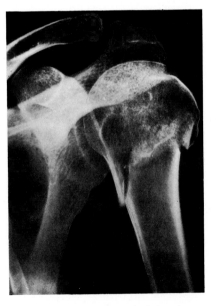

FIG. 9-116. Impacted abduction fracture. This fracture needs no reduction: the head-neck angle measures 160°.

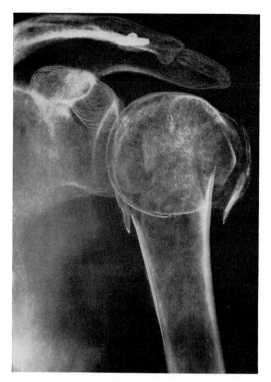

FIG. 9-117. Impacted fracture of the neck, with extensive comminution of the head of the humerus.

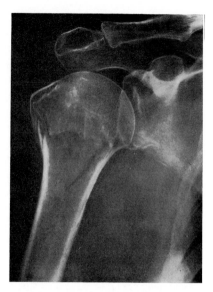

FIG. 9-118. Fracture through the anatomic neck of the humerus with mimimal displacement. Some comminution of the tuberosities is present.

### Fractures Requiring No Reduction

### Compression Fracture of the Greater Tuberosity

Except for the depression of the greater tuberosity the general configuration of the upper end of the humerus is good. Unfortunately, this fracture often implicates the bicipital groove. Bicipital tenosynovitis or a frozen shoulder are frequent complications. I doubt whether any form of treatment would change the prognosis of this fracture (Fig. 9-111).

### Fracture of the Greater Tuberosity with Minimal Displacement

The tuberosity is avulsed from the humerus; the amount of displacement is very small. Most of these fractures need no reduction and the prognosis is good. However, when such a fracture occurs in very young men, particularly athletes, who cannot afford to compromise the functioning of the shoulder, replacement of the tuberosity by surgery is indicated (Fig. 9-112).

In other cases, there may be little or no upward displacement of the tuberosity; rather, the tuberosity pulls away from the humerus like an opened book. Most of these fractures are still accepted as they are (Fig. 9-113). However, in my experience, if these fractures are not reduced, the result is invariably poor regardless of the age of the patient. The intertubercular sulcus may be involved, causing bicipital tenosynovitis. Also, the fracture may heal with an excessive amount of new bone. Consequently, when the arm is elevated the tuberosity impinges on the coracoacromial arch. I believe that this fracture should be explored and the tuberosity replaced in its normal position on the humerus.

### Fracture of a Portion of the Head with Impaction (Fig. 9-114)

A portion of the humeral head with its articular surface is driven into the re-

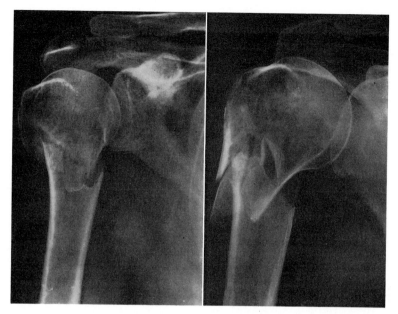

FIG. 9-119. (*Left*) Abduction fracture of the surgical neck of the humerus. The amount of displacement is acceptable and needs no reduction. (*Right*) Adduction fracture of the surgical neck. This amount of displacement is compatible with good function and needs no reduction.

mainder of the humeral head. This fracture frequently occurs during electric shock therapy. It needs no reduction. The prognosis is poor regardless of the treatment used. In my experience, all patients with this fracture developed severe pain and frozen shoulder. I do not believe surgical management can improve the results.

## Impacted Fracture of the Neck of the Humerus

The normal head-neck angle of the humerus is 140°. An increase of 25° above or below this angle does not interfere with good function. An impacted fracture of the neck of the humerus, such as is shown in Figure 9-115, does not need reduction. The head-neck angle measures 120°. This fracture occurs frequently in the elderly.

In Figure 9-116, the impacted upper fragment is in valgus; the head-neck angle is 160°. Again, this fracture needs no reduction.

Another fracture commonly seen in older persons is an impacted fracture of the head and neck with severe comminution of the upper fragment (Fig. 9-117). This fracture needs no reduction, but mobilization must start early, for the patients frequently—in fact, too often—develop frozen shoulders. This lesion carries a poor prognosis.

Fractures through the anatomical neck of the humerus without impaction and with minimal displacement require no reduction or internal fixation (Fig. 9-118). This is also true of valgus fractures through the surgical neck, provided that the head-neck angle does not exceed 160°.

Comminuted fractures through the surgical neck of the humerus with moderate deformity are acceptable and need no reduction. Even greater deformities need no reduction so long as the fragments are in contact. Head-neck angles greater than 160° and less than 115° can be brought to acceptable angles very easily. The weight of the arm corrects most or all of the deformity and also most of any rotatory displacement (Fig. 9-119).

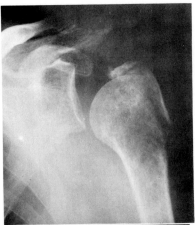

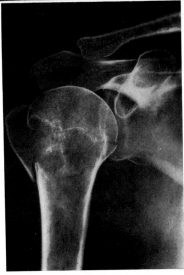

(*Top*) FIG. 9-120. Fracture of the greater tuberosity, with upward displacement of the fragment. This fragment must be replaced by surgery.

(*Bottom*) FIG. 9-121. Fracture of the greater tuberosity, with downward and outward displacement of the fragment. This fragment can be approximated to the humerus only by surgery.

## Management of Fractures Requiring No Reduction

There is no need to treat any of the fractures discussed above by cumbersome apparatuses such as plaster casts, hanging casts, abduction braces or splints. A simple collar and cuff is adequate.

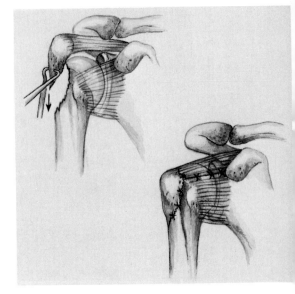

FIG. 9-122. Reduction and fixation of a fracture of the greater tuberosity with retraction toward the acromion.

**Impacted Fractures.** Because the fragments are stable, motion of the arm can be started early. First institute pendulum exercises for 3 to 5 minutes every hour; then, as pain subsides, increase slowly and progressively the range of motion and the time periods. Discard the collar and cuff after 3 weeks; however, during sleeping hours the patient wears a sling. Wall-crawling exercises can be started as early as the second or third day; as the patient gains confidence and has less pain, add pulley exercises. Encourage free use of the arm within the limits set by pain at all times. Physical therapy—heat and gentle massage—is comforting and beneficial; it should be given daily. Return of the greatest amount of function possible may require 10 to 12 weeks. The prognosis, as a rule, is good, except in depressed fractures of the greater tuberosity and depressed fractures of the articular surface of the head.

**Unimpacted Fractures.** The treatment is the same as that of impacted fractures except that the arm must stay at the side for at least 3 weeks before allowing motion at the glenohumeral joint. During this time

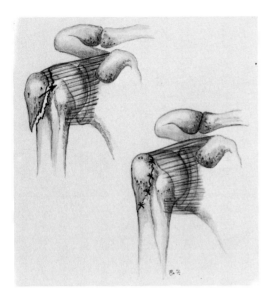

FIG. 9-123. Reduction and fixation of a fracture of the greater tuberosity with downward and outward displacement.

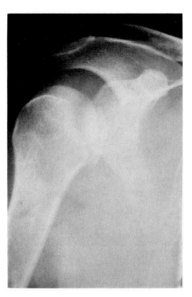

FIG. 9-124. Fracture of the lesser tuberosity. This is an avulsion fracture; the fragment is displaced medially by the subscapularis.

healing will have progressed far enough to allow the proximal and distal fragments to move in unison.

## Fractures Requiring Reduction

### Fractures of the Greater Tuberosity

Fractures of the greater tuberosity may occur with or without dislocation; the former have already been considered. When the tuberosity is displaced, it may be pulled under the acromion by the rotator muscles. This lesion is comparable to a rupture of the cuff. Closed methods of treatment fail to reduce this fracture. The fragments can be approximated only by surgery (Fig. 9-120).

The tuberosity may be displaced laterally or it may be displaced downward and outward. In most instances the tuberosity should be replaced, except in the elderly. If it is not replaced, the tuberosity heals in malposition and marked limitation of motion ensues. Occasionally, the displaced fragment may be only a sliver of bone; in this instance excise it and reattach the cuff to the bone. Not infrequently these fractures occur in combination with fractures of the anatomical neck of the humerus (Fig. 9-121). This associated fracture does not change the method of treatment.

**Operative Technique (Fractures Depicted in Figs. 9-120 and 9-121).** Make a 3- to 4-inch incision over the top of the shoulder, in line with the axillary crease and just lateral to the acromioclavicular joint. Extend it over the anterior part of the deltoid for 1½ to 2 inches below the edge of the acromion. By sharp dissection, develop the lateral skin flap by cutting the subcutaneous tissue from the top of the acromion and the tendinous origin of the deltoid on the lateral edge of the acromion. Next divide the acromion with a sharp osteotome in line with the skin incision about ⅜ to ½ inch from its outer edge. The cut extends the entire length of the acromion. Retract laterally the cut portion of the acromion with the attached portion of the deltoid. If more exposure is needed,

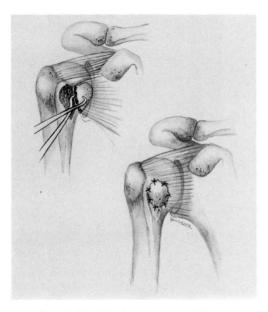

FIG. 9-125. Replacement and fixation of the lesser tuberosity.

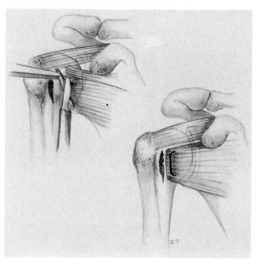

FIG. 9-126. If the lesser tuberosity fragment is small, it can be excised and the tendon can now be either sutured or stapled to the humerus.

detach the anterior longitudinal fibers of the deltoid from the outer portion of the clavicle as far medially as necessary. Now the entire middle and anterior portions of the deltoid may be retracted laterally and inferiorly without danger to the axillary nerve, and the tuberosities and cuff are clearly seen.

If the tuberosity lies under the acromion, grasp it with a towel clip and pull it down to its natural position. Fix it to the adjacent soft tissues by interrupted sutures or to the humeral head with a screw (Fig. 9-122).

If the tuberosity is displaced downward and outward, replace it in its normal position. Fix it to the humerus with interrupted sutures or a screw. Occasionally, it may be necessary, in both lesions, to drill holes in

the humerus to hold the sutures (Fig. 9-123). Inspect the rotator cuff for tears; if any are found, repair them.

The deltoid is anchored in place by passing two or three threaded wires through the cut end of the acromion into its base.

When the tuberosity fragment is small or just a sliver of bone, excise it. Remember that it may be pulled under the acromion. After the bone is excised reattach the cuff to the head by interrupted sutures passing through drill holes in the bone.

**Postoperative Management.** I like the use of an abduction brace holding the arm in about 45° of abduction. This takes the weight of the arm off the site of reattachment of the deltoid. The brace is worn for 5 to 8 weeks or until the patient

FIG. 9-127. (*On facing page*) Fractures of the anatomical and surgical neck of the humerus with marked displacement. (A) Fracture through the anatomical neck; the head is widely separated from the shaft which is displaced inward and abducted. (B) Fracture through the surgical neck; there is usually some comminution of the neck of the humerus, the shaft is displaced inward and abducted. (Parts (A) and (B) from DePalma, A.F.: The Management of Fractures and Dislocations, Ed. 2, Philadelphia, W. B. Saunders, 1970) (C) Typical fracture of the surgical neck of the humerus: a nonimpacted abduction fracture with marked angular deformity. In this case repositioning of the fragments is necessary. (D) Typical fracture of the anatomical neck; this required open reduction and internal fixation (E).

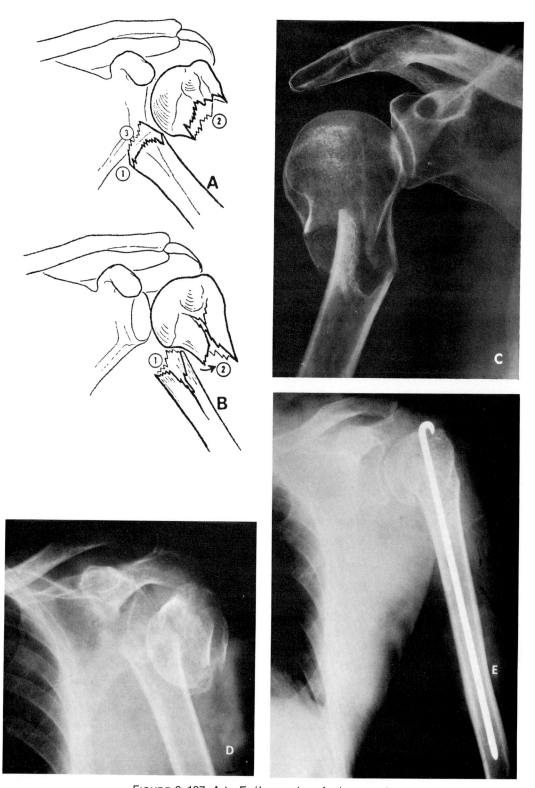

FIGURE 9-127, A to E. (*Legend on facing page*)

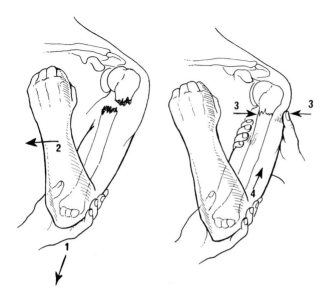

FIG. 9-128. Manipulative reduction of fractures of the anatomical and surgical neck of the humerus. Maneuvers (1) and (2) restore length while (3) and (4) align and engage the fragments.

is able to actively abduct the arm. Attempts at active abduction should start at the end of the fourth week. During this time encourage motion at the elbow, wrist and fingers and apply heat and massage to the entire shoulder daily.

After removal of the brace start the patient on an intensive program of pendulum exercises and later add wall crawling and pulley exercises.

### Fractures of the Lesser Tuberosity (Requiring Reduction)

The subscapularis may avulse the lesser tuberosity from the humerus, although this is rarely found as an isolated lesion. It is more frequently seen in comminuted fractures of the upper end of the humerus and in dislocations. When it does occur as an isolated fracture, the fragment usually lies between the coracoid process and the head of the humerus. In this position it blocks certain motions of the arm. If the fragment is large, it should be reattached to the humerus; if small, it should be excised. In the latter instance, the subscapularis tendon must be reattached to the humerus (Fig. 9-124).

**Operative Technique.** In men, the area can be approached by an anterior incision; for women I prefer the axillary incision. The anterior incision starts in line with the acromioclavicular joint and in line with the axillary crease. Mobilize the medial and lateral flaps, and then develop the incision through the anterior fibers of the deltoid for 2 inches below the edge of the acromion.

Retraction of the muscle fibers exposes the subacromial bursa; divide it in line with the muscle split (do not resect the walls of the bursa). Rotate the arm externally so that the subscapularis muscle with the attached bony fragment can be seen. Grasp the fragment with a towel clip, and, with the arm rotated internally, pull it into its normal position (Fig. 9-125). Anchor the fragment in place by interrupted sutures passing through drill holes made in the fragment and in the edges of the defect in the humerus. If the bone fragment is small, excise it. Reattach the subscapularis tendon to the shaft of the humerus with interrupted sutures passing through drill holes in the bone or with a staple (Fig. 9-126).

**Postoperative Management.** Apply a collar and cuff. On the second day start pendulum exercises for 3 to 5 minutes every hour. Do not permit external rotation of the arm for 3 weeks. At the end of three weeks discard the collar and cuff; however, a sling is needed at night. Now add wall crawling and pulley exercises and encourage free use of the arm within the tolerance of pain. Usually it takes 8 to 10 weeks to regain full function.

### Fractures of the Anatomical and Surgical Neck with Marked Displacement (Requiring Reduction)

These fractures are common in adults and are rarely found in children. Reduction is required in those with marked separation of the fragments. Fractures such as those depicted in Figure 9-127 show wide separation of the fragments and no contact between the fragments. Often muscle tissue or the biceps tendon is interposed between the fragments, making closed reduction impossible. Characteristic of these fractures is the inward displacement of the distal fragment and the abducted position of the proximal fragment. Not infrequently considerable comminution of one or both fragments is present.

**Management.** Many of these fractures can be reduced by closed methods. They should never be treated in abduction splints. Such a position makes tension on the pectoralis major which pulls the distal fragment, so that the fracture heals with a severe valgus deformity which impairs function.

Complete relaxation is necessary to reduce the fractures. This is best attained with general anesthesia.

With the patient on his back make steady traction on the arm in line with the long axis of the body. While traction is maintained, bring the arm across the chest toward the midline; and at the same time, flex the arm in relation to the frontal plane of the body. These maneuvers, together with the traction, restore the length of the arm.

Now place the other hand in the axilla. While firm pressure is made on the head

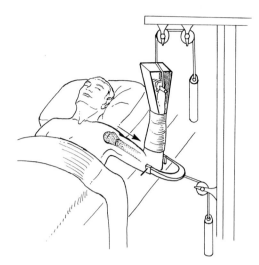

FIG. 9-129. Skeletal traction used to maintain reduction in unstable fractures of the neck of the humerus.

fragment with the thumb, push the shaft fragment outward with the fingers encircling the arm. The fragments should now be aligned. Finally, release the traction gradually and allow the fragments to engage (Fig. 9-128).

POSTREDUCTION MANAGEMENT. A collar and cuff provide adequate immobilization. With the arm hanging at the side of the trunk, the weight of the arm maintains length and alignment. No motion is allowed for 3 weeks; at that time, healing should be such that both fragments move in unison. Start pendulum exercises, followed by wall crawling and pulley exercises. The arm should be protected with a sling during sleeping hours. Allow free use of the arm within the patient's tolerance of pain. Usually it takes 8 to 12 weeks to attain good function.

**Alternate Method—Skeletal Traction.** In some fractures of the neck of the humerus that can be reduced by closed methods the correction is lost just as soon as traction is released. These are unstable fractures. They need continuous traction until sufficiently healed to allow the traction to be removed without loss of the reduction.

Make traction on a threaded wire passed

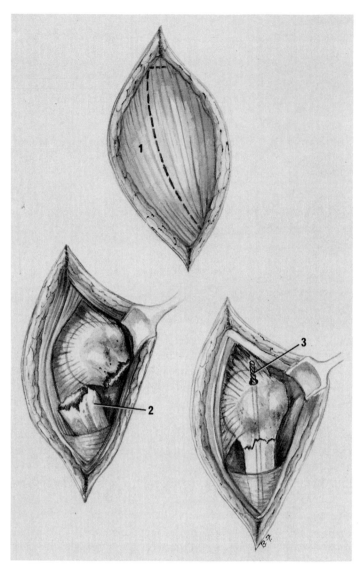

FIG. 9-130. (1) Exposure of the region through an anterior deltoid splitting incision. (2) Visualization of the position of the fragments. (3) After reduction, the fragments are held in position with a stout threaded wire or a Rush nail.

through the base of the olecranon. Place the arm in 45° to 60° of abduction (never exceed 60°). Apply just enough weight to hold the desired alignment; too much weight causes distraction of the fragments. This must be avoided (Fig. 9-129).

Usually after 2½ to 3 weeks the traction can be removed without fear of losing the reduction. Now apply a collar and cuff which is worn for approximately three weeks. After the traction apparatus is removed the postreduction management is

the same as that described for stable fractures of the humeral neck.

**Open Reduction.** This is reserved for those fractures of the neck that cannot be reduced by closed reduction.

Expose the fracture site through an anterior deltoid-splitting incision. Inspect the pathology at the fracture site, remove interposed tissue if present or loose pieces of bone. With both fragments in clear view lever them into normal position. To maintain alignment, pass a stout threaded wire or a Rush nail through the head and into the medullary cavity of the distal fragment (Fig. 9-130). Cut the end of the wire so that it lies beneath the skin.

POSTOPERATIVE MANAGEMENT. After the operation apply a collar and cuff. Start pendulum exercises immediately. Discard the collar and cuff at the end of 3 weeks. Protect the arm with a sling during sleeping hours. Steadily increase the exercises and general activity of the patient; but always stay within the tolerance of pain. Remove the wire or pin after 4 to 6 weeks. It usually takes 8 to 12 weeks to achieve full activity of the extremity.

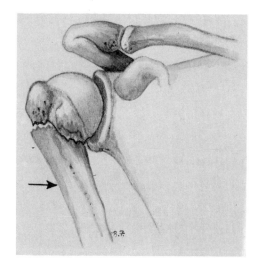

## Impacted Adduction Fractures of the Neck with Severe Angulation

In the aged, do not disturb this lesion; the impaction must not be broken down. On the other hand, in young persons the deformity must be corrected because, if it heals without correction, restriction of motion would be too great. Many can be reduced by closed methods; if not, surgical reduction is necessary. In a child, the impaction is on the inner side of the fragments and the distal shaft fragment is adducted in relation to the proximal fragment (Fig. 9-131).

**Closed Reduction.** The affected arm is abducted 70°, and an assistant makes steady traction on the arm. While traction is maintained, stabilize the upper fragment with the thumb of one hand; with the other hand, abduct further the lower fragment (Fig. 9-132).

Postreduction immobilization in children must be rigid. Apply a plaster of Paris shoulder spica which holds the arm in 45° to 60° of abduction. Remove the spica after four or five weeks and support the arm in a sling for two more weeks. Start exercises for the shoulder after the spica is removed, and allow full use of the arm after the sling is discarded.

In young adults use a collar and cuff to

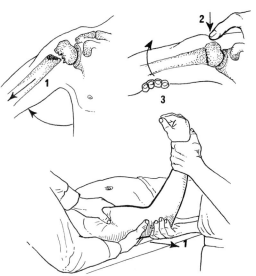

(*Top*) FIG. 9-131. Type of adduction deformity usually seen in children; the inner side of the neck is impacted.

(*Bottom*) FIG. 9-132. Maneuvers to reduce severe impacted adduction fractures: (1) restoration of length by traction; (2) stabilization of the head with the operator's thumb and (3) alignment of the lower fragment with the upper.

support the arm. The patient starts immediately to exercise the shoulder with pendulum exercises. After 3 weeks remove the

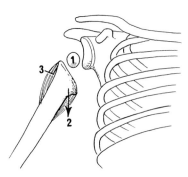

FIG. 9-133. Roentgenographic feature of separation of the proximal humeral epiphysis at birth. (1) The ossification center of the epiphysis has not appeared. (2) The metaphysis of the humerus is displaced downward in relation to the glenoid. (3) Callus formation is evident (10 days after injury).

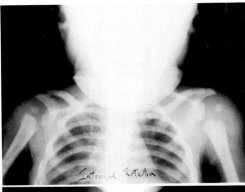

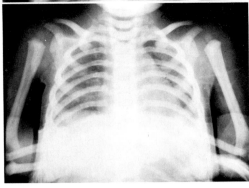

FIG. 9-134. (*Top*) Roentgenographic features of separation of proximal humeral epiphysis in early childhood. The epiphysis is centered in the glenoid cavity, and the metaphysis is displaced downward in relation to the glenoid fossa. (*Bottom*) Roentgenogram showing reduction of the humeral epiphysis.

collar and cuff; at night replace it with a sling. Now, also institute a full program of rehabilitation and allow free use of the arm. Full recovery is achieved in 8 to 12 weeks.

**Open Reduction.** When closed methods fail to reduce the fracture, or the fracture is so unstable that without continuous traction the reduction cannot be held, surgical reduction and internal fixation are necessary.

Expose the fracture site through an anterior deltoid-splitting incision. Inspect the nature of the pathology; then carefully lever the fragments into normal alignment. Next, transfix the fragments with either a stout threaded wire or a Rush nail (see Fig. 9-130). Remove the wire or nail after four or five weeks.

For children, fix the arm in a plaster of Paris shoulder spica holding the arm abducted 45° to 60°. For adults a collar and cuff are adequate. The postreduction management in each instance is the same as that described above for fractures treated by the closed method.

## SEPARATION OF THE UPPER EPIPHYSIS OF THE HUMERUS

In order to attain the best results in epiphyseal injuries of the upper end of the humerus, certain characteristics of all epiphyseal injuries must be respected. Treatment of these lesions must never be taken lightly, for growth disturbances may occur under the most favorable conditions. It behooves the surgeon to warn parents of such possibilities, but it is not necessary to alarm them. Growth disturbances may not be apparent for 6 to 12 months; therefore, all epiphyseal injuries must be observed for at least one year.

The healing process at the site of epiphyseal injury is very active, and reduction of a fracture becomes more difficult with every day's delay. Reduction of these lesions is an emergency; it should be done the same day the injury occurs. After ten

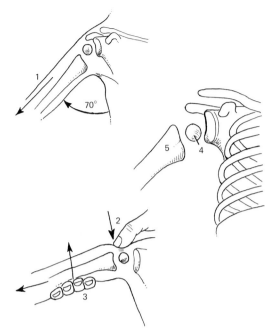

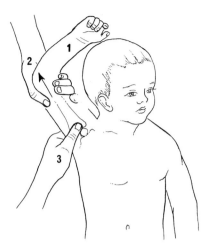

FIG. 9-136. Alternate method of reduction. (1) With the forearm flexed 90° abduct the arm completely; (2) while an assistant makes steady traction upward, (3) place the thumb in the axilla over the upper end of the shaft and push it backward.

FIG. 9-135. Manipulative reduction of separated proximal humeral epiphysis. (1) Make steady traction on the arm abducted 70°; (2) stabilize the epiphyseal fragment with the thumb, and (3) bring the arm into further abduction.

days it is virtually impossible to manipulate the fragments unless great force is applied. Such treatment injures the epiphyseal plate.

If the epiphyseal plate is not severely disrupted and its alignment is intact, such as in Type I and Type II lesions, considerable displacement of the epiphysis can be accepted. Subsequent remodeling will eventually restore the normal position of the epiphysis. This is particularly true in young children and less true in children approaching adolescence. On the other hand, if the segments of the epiphyseal plate are not in normal alignment and the articular surface of the epiphysis is incongruous, as in Type III and Type IV epiphyseal fractures, it is necessary to restore normal alignment even if open reduction must be performed.

Epiphyseal lesions of the upper end of the humerus can be divided into three groups: (1) those occurring at birth and in infants under one year of age, (2) those occurring in children under ten years of age and (3) those occurring after the age of ten.

## Epiphyseal Separation at Birth and in Infants Under One Year of Age

At birth, the separation may be accompanied by a dislocation that generally reduces spontaneously. Frequently the wrong diagnosis of brachial palsy is made and an abduction splint is applied. This abduction position favors redislocation. Before applying an abduction splint be sure your diagnosis is correct. Because in children under one year the humeral epiphysis is entirely cartilaginous, it may be impossible to make the diagnosis by roentgenograms. However, the relationship of the metaphysis to the center of the glenoid fossa may be a clue (Fig. 9-133). Also, lateral views of the shoulder may be helpful.

The diagnosis of epiphyseal separation in the infant must be made on the clinical signs and symptoms. There is local swelling

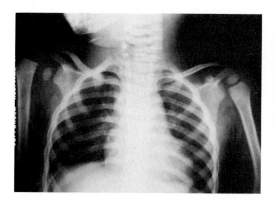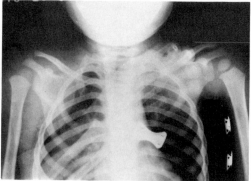

FIG. 9-137. (*Left*) Separation of the proximal humeral epiphysis with upward and outward displacement of the humeral shaft. (*Right*) This reduction was achieved by traction and abduction of the arm.

and any motion of the arm causes pain. The infant does not move the arm so that it hangs at the side, simulating a paralyzed limb. However, within 5 days roentgenograms show callus formation at the site of injury. This confirms the diagnosis.

These lesions in infants are usually Type I; they need no reduction, and growth will correct any displacement of the epiphysis.

**Management.** Nothing more than fixing the arm to the chest is required. Place a cotton pad in the axilla and fix the arm to the chest with an encircling cotton elastic bandage; support the forearm with a collar and cuff. Remove the dressing after 2 to 3 weeks and allow free use of the arm.

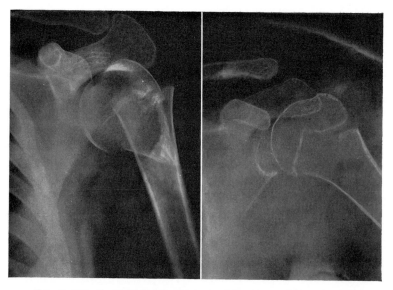

FIG. 9-138. (*Left*) Type II epiphyseal fracture of the proximal humeral epiphysis. Note the triangular piece of metaphysis still attached to the epiphyseal plate. (*Right*) This reduction was obtained by closed manipulation.

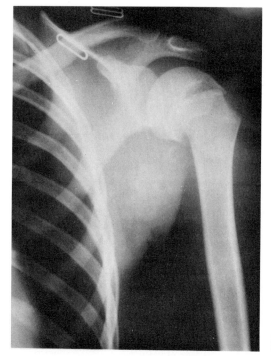 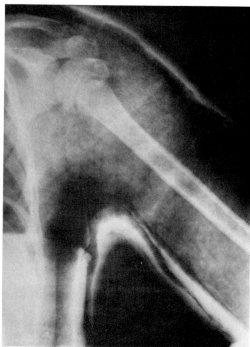

FIG. 9-139. (*Left*) Typical Type I epiphyseal fracture of the proximal humeral epiphysis. (*Right*) This reduction was obtained by closed manipulation.

## Epiphyseal Separation in Early Childhood (Under Ten Years)

Marked displacement in this age group should be corrected. As in infants, the lesion is usually Type I. Surgery is never indicated, for the deformity can be corrected by closed methods. Figure 9-134 illustrates the usual roentgenographic features. The epiphysis is centered in the glenoid cavity and the metaphysis is displaced downward in relation to the glenoid cavity.

**Closed Reduction.** The child must be completely relaxed, under general anesthesia. While an assistant makes steady traction on the arm abducted 70°, stabilize the epiphyseal fragment with the thumb of one hand and with your other hand further abduct the shaft of the humerus (Fig. 9-135).

After reduction apply a shoulder spica which holds the arm in 45° to 60° of abduction. Remove the spica after four or five weeks and apply a sling for another week. Now allow full use of the arm. No other supplementary treatment is needed in these children.

**Alternate Method.** The following is an excellent method to reduce the epiphyseal separation, and should be used when the method described above fails.

The child is in the recumbent position. Abduct the arm completely to the overhead position and flex the forearm 90°. While an assistant makes upward traction place your thumb in the axilla immediately over the upper end of the shaft of the humerus and push it directly backward. This usually reduces the separation (Fig. 9-136).

After reduction apply a shoulder spica which holds the arm in 145° to 160° of abduction. Remove the spica after 3 weeks and apply a sling for two more weeks. Now allow free use of the arm.

Occasionally the shaft of the humerus may be displaced upward and outward, as

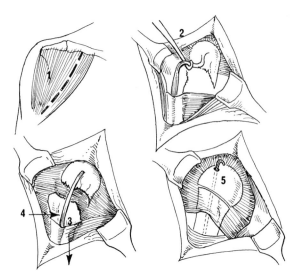

FIG. 9-140. Open reduction of unreducible or unstable fracture of the proximal humeral epiphysis. (1) Incision; (2) exposure of the fragments and interposed biceps tendon, (3) and (4) reduction of the fragments. (5) If the reduction is not stable, use internal fixation—a stout threaded wire or a Rush nail.

shown in Figure 9-137A. In these instances, simple abduction of the arm will effect a reduction (Fig. 9-137B).

## Epiphyseal Separation After the Age of Ten

In this age period, Type II lesion occurs most frequently. The epiphysis does not need to be reduced completely to attain a good result. During growth, remodeling corrects the deformity unless the deformity is unusually severe or the patient is approaching the end of the growth period.

As a rule, manipulative methods attain an acceptable reduction. If the displacement is severe and closed methods of reduction applied early fail, it must be as-

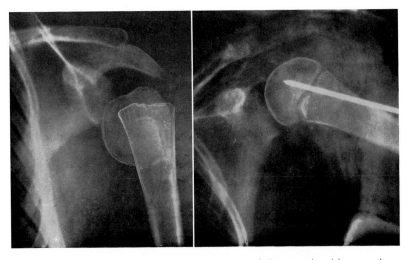

FIG. 9-141. (*Left*) Unreducible fracture of the proximal humeral epiphysis (Type II). Reduction was precluded by interposition of the biceps tendon between the fragments. (*Right*) Reduction obtained after removing the obstruction (biceps tendon) to reduction; in this instance, the fragments were transfixed by a stout wire.

sumed that there is an obstruction to the reduction. In such instances, the biceps tendon lies between the fragments. This is an indication for surgical reduction.

Figure 9-138 reveals the fractures of Type II lesions seen on roentgenograms. A triangular piece of metaphysis remains attached to the epiphyseal plate; the shaft of the humerus rides upward in relation to the glenoid fossa, and the continuity of the epiphyseal plate is not broken, for the separation occurs through the hypertrophic layer of cells of the plate. Figure 9-139 reveals a Type I epiphyseal fracture with the same typical deformity seen in Figure 9-138.

**Management.** Reduce this lesion by the same manipulative method described for epiphyseal separations in children under 10 years of age.

### Irreducible Epiphyseal Separations

In these lesions there is wide separation of the fragments, and, as I stated above, interposition of the biceps tendon between the fragments prevents reduction in most instances.

Expose the fracture site through an anterior deltoid splitting incision and evaluate the local pathology. Locate the biceps tendon and disengage it from between the fragments. Next, pull the arm downward to restore length, then push the shaft under the epiphysis. Never use an instrument between the fragments to pry them apart and to lever them into place. This may result in severe damage to the epiphyseal plate.

Now test the fracture for stability. If the fracture is unstable and the fragments tend to displace when traction on the arm is released, internal fixation is needed. I use a threaded wire through the epiphysis and into the medullary cavity of the shaft. Cut the wire below the level of the skin (Fig. 9-140 and 9-141). Remove the wire after 4 weeks.

The postoperative management is the same as that described for epiphyseal separations reduced by closed methods.

## BIBLIOGRAPHY

Allman, F. L., Jr.: Fractures and ligamentous injuries of the clavicle and its articulations. A.A.O.S. Instructional Course Lecture, J. Bone & Joint Surg., 49-A:774-784, 1967.

Arner, Or., Sandahl, U., and Ohrling, H.: Dislocation of the acromioclavicular joint. Review of the literature and a report on 50 cases. Acta chir. scand., 113:140-152, 1957.

Badgley, C. E.: Sports injuries of the shoulder girdle. JAMA, 172:444-448, 1960.

Baker, D. M., and Stryker, W. S.: Acute complete acromioclavicular separation. Report of 51 cases. JAMA, 192:689-692, 1965.

Bateman, J. E.: Athletic injuries about the shoulder in throwing and body-contact sports. Clin. Orthop., 23:75-83, 1962.

Cerney, J. V.: Athletic Injuries. pp. 718-719. Springfield, Illinois, Charles C Thomas, 1963.

Colson, J. H. C., and Armour, W. J.: Sports Injuries and Their Treatment. p. 187. Philadelphia, J. B. Lippincott, 1961.

DePalma, A. F.: Surgery of the Shoulder. Philadelphia, J. B. Lippincott, 1950.

————: Degenerative Changes in the Sternoclavicular and Acromioclavicular Joints in Various Decades. Springfield, Illinois, Charles C Thomas, 1957.

DePalma, A. F., and Cautilli, R. A.: Fractures of the upper end of the humerus. Clin. Orthop. Rel. Res., 20:73-93, 1961.

Ferguson, A. B., Jr., and Bender, J.: The ABC's of Athletic Injuries and Conditioning. p. 53. Baltimore, The Williams and Wilkins Co., 1964.

Greenlee, D. P.: Posterior dislocation of the sternal end of the clavicle. JAMA, 125: 426-428, 1944.

Gurd, F. B.: The treatment of complete dislocation of the outer end of the clavicle. An hitherto undescribed operation. Ann. Surg., 113:1094-1098, 1941.

Hall, R. H., Isaac, F., and Booth, C. R.: Dislocations of the shoulder with special reference to accompanying small fractures. J. Bone & Joint Surg., 41-A:489-494, 1959.

Hill, H. A., and Sachs, M. D.: The grooved defect of the humeral head. A frequently unrecognized complication of dislocations of the shoulder joint. Radiology, 35:690-700, 1940.

Hoyt, W. A., Jr.: Etiology of shoulder injuries in athletes. A.A.O.S. Instructional Course Lecture. J. Bone & Joint Surg., *49-A*:755-766, 1967.

Inman, V. T., Saunders, J. B. de C. M., and Abbott, L. C.: Observations on shoulder joint. J. Bone & Joint Surg., *26*:1-30, 1944.

Jacobs, B., and Wade, P. A.: Acromioclavicular joint injury. J. Bone & Joint Surg., *48-A*: 475-486, 1966.

Lam, S. J. S.: Irreducible anterior dislocation of the shoulder. J. Bone & Joint Surg., *48-B*: 132-133, 1966.

Kennedy, J. C., and Cameron, H.: Complete dislocation of the acromioclavicular joint. J. Bone & Joint Surg., *36-B*:202-208, 1954.

Key, J. A., and Conwell, E. H.: The Management of Fractures, Dislocations and Sprains. Ed. 2. p. 437. St. Louis, The C. V. Mosby Co., 1937.

Kremens, V., and Glauser, F.: Unusual sequela following pinning of medial clavicular fracture. Am. J. Roentgenol., *76*:1066-1069, 1956.

Lazcano, M. A., Anzel, S. H., and Kelly, P. J.: Complete dislocation and subluxation of the acromioclavicular joint. End-result in seventy-three cases. J. Bone & Joint Surg., *43-A*: 379-391, 1961.

Litton, L. O., and Peltier, L. R.: Athletic Injuries. p. 94. Boston, Little, Brown and Co., 1963.

Mazet, R., Jr.: Migration of a Kirschner wire from the shoulder region into the lung. Report of two cases. J. Bone & Joint Surg., *25*:477-483, 1943.

Moseley, H. F.: Athletic injuries to the shoulder region. Am. J. Surg., *98*:401-422, 1959.

Mumford, E. B.: Acromioclavicular dislocation. A new operative treatment. J. Bone & Joint Surg., *23*:799-802, 1941.

Neer, C. S., II: Nonunion of the clavicle. JAMA, *172*:1006-1011, 1960.

————: Fracture of the distal clavicle with detachment of the coracoclavicular ligaments in adults. J. Trauma, *3*:99-110, 1963.

————: Fractures of the distal third of the clavicle. Clin. Orthop. & Rel. Res., *58*: 43-50, 1968.

Neviaser, J. S.: Acromioclavicular dislocation treated by transference of the coracoacromial ligament. Bull. Hosp. Joint Dis., *12*:46-54, 1951.

————: Injuries in and about the shoulder joint. A.A.O.S. Instructional Course Lecture, J. Bone & Joint Surg., *13*:187-216, 1956.

Norrell, H., Jr., and Llewellyn, R. C.: Migration of a threaded Steinman pin from an acromioclavicular joint into the spinal canal. A case report. J. Bone & Joint Surg., *47-A*:1024-1026, 1965.

O'Donoghue, D. H.: Treatment of Injuries to Athletes. p. 123. Philadelphia, W B. Saunders, 1962.

Quesada, F.: Technique for roentgen diagnosis of fractures of the clavicle. Surg., Gynec., Obstet., *42*:424-428, 1926.

Quigley, T. B., and Banks, H.: Progress in Treatment of Fractures and Dislocations, 1950-1960. p. 13. Philadelphia, W B. Saunders, 1960.

Reeves, B.: Experiments on the tensile strength of the anterior capsular structures of the shoulder in man. J. Bone & Joint Surg., *50-B*:858-865, 1968.

Ryan, A. J.: Medical Care of the Athlete. p. 168. New York, McGraw-Hill, 1962.

Sage, F. P., and Salvatore, J. E.: Injuries of the acromioclavicular joint. A study of the results in 96 patients. Southern Med. J., *56*: 486-495, 1963.

Savastano, A. A.: Athletic injuries to the upper extremity. Rhode Island Med. J., *42*:807-811, 1959.

Thorndike, A.: Athletic Injuries. p. 152. Philadelphia, Lea and Febiger, 1956.

Tucker, W. E., and Armstrong, J. R.: Injury in Sports. p. 402. Springfield, Illinois, Charles C Thomas, 1964.

Urist, M. R.: Complete dislocations of the acromioclavicular joint. The nature of the traumatic lesion and effective methods of treatment with an analysis of forty-one cases. J. Bone & Joint Surg., *28*:813-837, 1946.

————: Complete dislocation of the acromioclavicular joint (follow-up note). J. Bone & Joint Surg., *45-A*:1750-1753, 1963.

# 10

# The Unstable Shoulder

In this chapter I shall discuss recurrent anterior and posterior subluxations and recurrent anterior and posterior dislocations of the glenohumeral joint. Inferior subluxations have already been discussed in Chapter 9. The pathology of recurrent subluxations and that of recurrent dislocations differ only in degree of the same lesions; therefore, both are considered under the heading "Pathology of the Unstable Joint." The causes and treatment of the unstable joint have been and still are areas replete with disagreement.

## HISTORICAL SKETCH OF RECURRENT DISLOCATIONS

The current concepts of the causes and the principles of treatment have an interesting evolution.

We must have a beginning for our story, and I can find no better period than that of Hippocrates when the attitude toward medicine, for the first time, discarded the religious basis for suffering and disease and began to grope for a scientific basis. Hippocrates in his writings "On the Articulations" reveals that he had firm convictions in regard to the different types of recurrent dislocations, the seriousness of the lesions and the methods that should be employed to cure the disorders. He wrote:

In cases of dislocations those persons who are not attacked with inflammation of the surrounding parts [he means here atraumatic dislocations (Au.)] can use the shoulder immediately without pain, and do not think it necessary to take precautions with themselves; it is therefore the business of the physician to warn them beforehand that dislocation is more likely to return in such cases than when the tendons have been inflamed [i. e., traumatic dislocations (Au.)]. It deserves to be known how a shoulder which is subject to frequent dislocations should be treated. For many persons owing to this accident have been obliged to abandon gymnastic exercises, though otherwise qualified for them, and from the same misfortune have become inept in warlike practices and have thus perished. And this subject deserves to be noticed because I have never known any physician treat the case properly; some abandon the attempt altogether and others hold opinions and practice the reverse of what is proper. For many physicians have burned the shoulders subject to dislocations at the top of the shoulder, at the anterior part where the head of the humerus protrudes, and a little behind the shoulder; these burnings, if the dislocation of the arm were upward or forward or backward would have been properly performed; but now, when the dislocation is downward they rather promote than prevent dislocation, for they shut out the head of the humerus from the free space above.*

It is obvious from Hippocrates' words that the problems of his day are still with us; though I must concede that since his era we have learned much about the biomechanics of the shoulder and about the mechanisms that produce injuries of the shoulder. Also, our methods of treatment are more refined. But I doubt if the principles of treatment have changed much and if we have really identified the causes responsible for recurrent dislocations.

There is no doubt that the progress of surgery in general, which made possible exploration of the shoulder, and the X ray

* The Genuine Works of Hippocrates. Translated by Francis Adams. Vol. 2. pp. 553-654. London, Sydenham Society, 1849.

Fig. 10-1. Tenosuspension operations for recurrent dislocation of the shoulder: (A) Henderson operation. (B) Nicola operation.

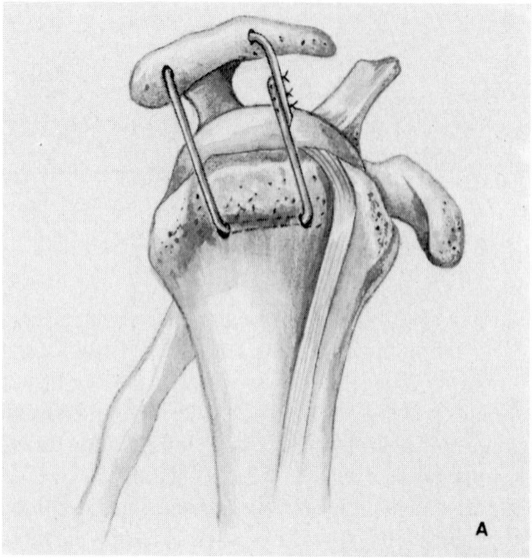

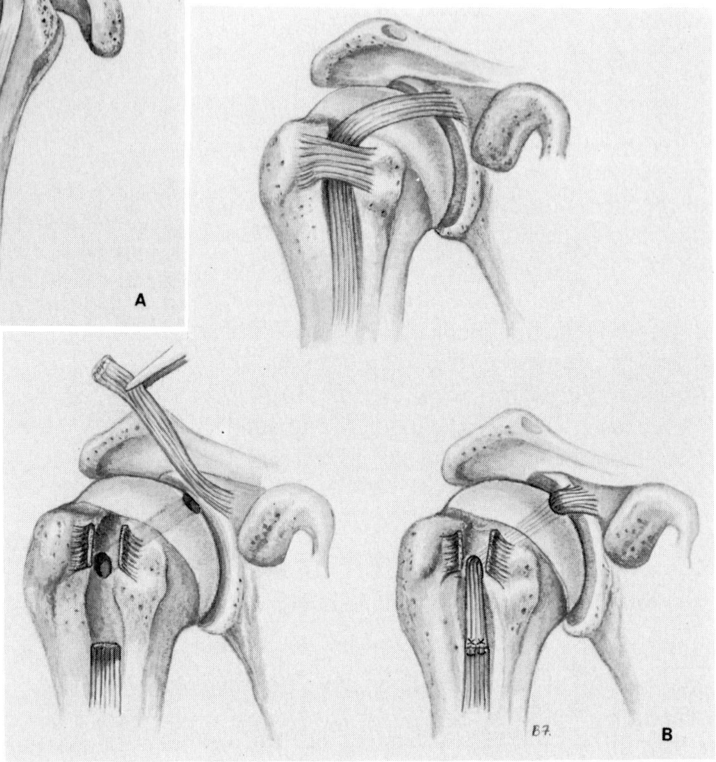

have opened new fields of investigation that have added considerably to our knowledge of the normal, variational and abnormal anatomy of the shoulder. However, many of the abnormalities of tissues associated with recurrent dislocations were observed and recorded many decades ago. Unfortunately, many of these findings were forgotten and had to be rediscovered.

Late in the nineteenth century many sharp investigators recorded accurately their observations on recurrent dislocation of the shoulder. Time has not invalidated them. Jossel in 1880 accurately described his observations made on four patients with known recurrent dislocations upon whom he performed autopsies. He found disruption of the rotator tendons. From this he

concluded that following dislocation of the shoulder the rotator muscles do not reattach to the greater tuberosity, and that the weakened rotator muscles predispose the shoulder to recurrent dislocations. He also observed that the volume of the joint capsule was increased. This, too, he reasoned, made the shoulder vulnerable to recurrent dislocations. Finally, he found fractures of the glenoid and of the head of the humerus which produced incongruity of the articulating surfaces. This incongruity, he believed, was capable of causing recurrences.

The posterolateral defect in the head of the humerus, which most of us believe to be a constant lesion in recurrent dislocations, was observed and recorded long

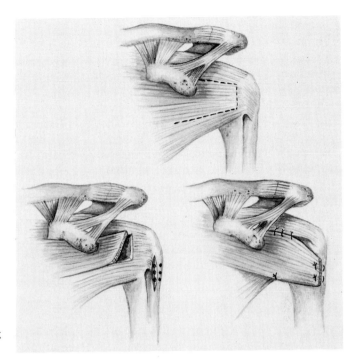

FIG. 10-2. Magnuson-Stack operation.

before the report of Hill and Sacks in 1940. Cramer, Kuster and Volkman independently described the lesion in 1882. And, in 1887, Caird stated that a posterolateral compression fracture of the humeral head always occurred in subcoracoid dislocations. Furthermore, he produced the lesion experimentally in cadavers. Broca and Hartmann in 1890 described in detail detachment of the labrum, stripping of the periosteum from the anterior surface of the neck of the scapula and the posterolateral defect in the humeral head.

Perthes, in 1906, was the first to hold that recurrent dislocation could be cured only by correcting the basic pathology by surgery. He believed that the basic lesion was either separation of the capsule and the rotator tendons from the greater tuberosity or tearing away of the labrum from the glenoid rim, with the formation of a pouch under the subscapularis. He described the operations he performed for these lesions. His repair for detachment of the labrum was the same as the Bankart operation except that he used staples to anchor the labrum to the glenoid.

In 1909 Clairmont and Ehrlich and in 1917 Finisterer performed myoplasties to cure recurrent dislocations. These operations failed and are no longer performed.

For a time, various suspension operations were very popular. In 1927 Gallie and LeMesurier attempted to stabilize the joint by constructing a new ligament from fascia lata. The ligament passed through drill holes in the scapula and the humeral head, tying one to the other. The operation is very effective and is still used by some surgeons. On the other hand, the teno-suspension operation of Nicola (1929) and that of Henderson (1949) did not fare well. Nicola suspended the head of the humerus from the superior glenoid rim by passing the tendon of the long head of the biceps through the humeral head. Henderson, using a portion of the peroneus longus tendon, suspended the head from the acromion (Fig. 10-1). Later, Nicola modified his technique; he combined his operation with either the Bankart or the Putti-Platt operation.

To Bankart must go the credit for focusing attention on the pathology present in the anterior aspect of the glenohumeral joint in recurrent dislocations; and, as a result of the emphasis he placed on the importance of repairing the so-called *essential lesion* many operations to achieve this goal have been developed. On the other hand, some investigators place more importance on the posterolateral defect in the humeral head as the cause of recurrences than on the pathology present on the anterior aspect of the joint. Ivor Palmer (1948) believes the posterolateral defect is the "essential lesion." Eden in 1918 and Hybbinette in 1932 had come to the same conclusion; both attempted to cure recurrences by placing a bone graft on the anterior aspect of the glenoid.

In 1943 Magnuson proposed another theory for the cause of recurrences. He stated that the stability of the shoulder depends on the integrity of the anterior muscular wall, the subscapularis. At the time of the initial dislocation the anterior wall is stretched, causing neuromuscular imbalance. This, in turn, diminishes the protective mechanism of the subscapularis, thereby making the shoulder subject to recurrent dislocation. On the basis of this premise, Magnuson transferred the tendon of the subscapularis to a more lateral and distal position on the humerus (Magnuson-Stack operation) (Fig. 10-2).

Victorio Putti and Sir Harry Platt also used the subscapularis to construct an anterior barrier to dislocation. In 1948 Osmond-Clarke described the operation and called it the Putti-Platt operation.

More recently, another concept of recurrent dislocation has appeared. Saha (1967) lists four predisposing factors, any of which may cause recurrences: (1) Congenitally altered relationship between the humeral head and the glenoid fossa. Since the radius of the head is greater than that of the glenoid fossa, the head rides high on the glenoid margin and labrum in all positions of movement. (2) Increased retroversion of the upper end of the humerus. (3) Reduced retrotilt or anterior tilt of the glenoid. This may fail to protect the head as the arm is elevated to the vertical position. (4) Weakness of the subscapularis, infraspinatus and teres minor, owing to congenital weakness, paralysis or elongation from previous trauma.

Depending on the predominance of one or more of the causes, Saha proposes several operations for the cure of recurrences: (1) Osteotomy of the neck of the scapula to restore the normal tilt of the glenoid; (2) rotation osteotomy of the upper end of the humerus to reduce the relative anteversion effect when the arm is in complete elevation; and (3) transference of the latissimus dorsi to the posterior and inferior aspects of the greater tuberosity. The last mentioned operation enhances the power of the infraspinatus and the teres minor to rotate the head posteriorly when the arm is elevated.

In a brief historical sketch such as this it is impossible to include the many contributions on recurrent dislocations, especially in the past several decades. Among the contributors, to mention just a few, are McLaughlin, Moseley, Neviaser, Bateman, Rowe, Lequit and Dickson.

## CLINICAL TYPES OF UNSTABLE GLENOHUMERAL JOINT

Both recurrent subluxations and dislocations fall into two groups: traumatic and atraumatic. In the traumatic group are shoulders that develop recurrences after a specific traumatic episode. The atraumatic group comprises shoulders that develop instability spontaneously or after insignificant trauma. In the latter group, the cause of the instability may lie in some congenital malformation of the humeral head or glenoid or some dysplastic disorder of the connective tissues of the joint that makes the joint hypermobile. This disorder may involve all the joints of the body; on the other hand, it may be limited to one or both shoulders. In rare instances, it is limited to one or both shoulders and another large joint. I have seen two cases of posterior recurrent dislocation of the shoulder associated with bilateral subluxating patellae. Spontaneous shoulder instability may develop early in life and may not cause any impairment of function or pain until early adulthood. One patient in my series demonstrated instability of the right shoulder at the age of seven, but it caused no disability until she was seventeen years old; at that time the recurrent dislocation interfered with her gymnastic activities. In some shoulders no abnormalities of the joint can be found to explain the disorder. In these some neuromuscular imbalance must be considered. That there is a familial predisposition to develop recurrent dislocations of the shoulder is an established fact. I have as patients one family in which the father and two sons developed recurrent dislocations. Also, in my series is a set of twins, both with recurrent dislocations of the left shoulder. All in the first-mentioned family developed recurrences without specific trauma. In the second, both boys suffered a severe traumatic initial dislocation while playing football. One of the twins had an operation to stabilize the shoulder before I saw him; the operation had failed.

Whereas in traumatic recurrences the shoulder displaces either anteriorly or posteriorly, in the atraumatic group some shoulders may displace in any direction—anteriorly, posteriorly and inferiorly. A patient may have the inherent potential instability in both shoulders but actual displacement may occur in only one; occasionally it occurs in both, usually first in one and then the other. Bilateral recurrences are rare, but they do occur frequently enough, and the physician should be on guard when operative repair of one shoulder is considered.

Finally, in the atraumatic group is the "queer adolescent female" who can at will displace the humeral head in one or more directions with little or no discomfort. She may do this many times in one day. Yet, no traumatic or anatomical basis can be found to explain this shoulder behavior. Many of these children have psychological problems which need more attention than their shoulder disorder. Before attempting any surgical repair in these patients, it behooves the physician to analyze and evaluate carefully not only the local problem but also the total patient. Operative intervention may cause much embarrassment. After an excellent anterior repair, the patient still develops a posterior recurrent dislocation. This has happened to me on two occasions. Or, the anterior or posterior repair may not cure the disorder. This, too, has happened to me with two patients.

The maneuvers that voluntary subluxators or dislocators employ to achieve displacement of the humeral head are interesting to observe. In order to produce a posterior displacement they place the arm at the side slightly elevated; then they adduct and internally rotate the arm. They reduce the displacement by merely relaxing all the muscles. The head slides out and into the glenoid with an audible thud. It appears that these patients are able simultaneously to activate some muscles of the shoulder girdle and repress the normal synchronous action of others. In the above example, the internal rotators are forcefully activated and the external rotators are repressed. Those patients capable of producing voluntary anterior displacement of the head reverse the process while holding the arm slightly abducted and externally rotated.

Some patients in the atraumatic category suffer displacement of the humeral head only when the arm executes some specific movement. This may be performed voluntarily or involuntarily. Some shoulders whose initial dislocation was definitely traumatic suffer so many recurrences that the patient can displace the head at will. Thus, some traumatic dislocations take on the features of atraumatic lesions.

There is still another interesting group of atraumatic subluxators or dislocators. These persons can displace the humeral head at will, but they never suffer involuntary displacements. We must concede that these shoulders have the inherent potential factor capable of producing luxations, but the neuromuscular apparatus is so well coordinated and balanced that luxations can occur only when they are willed.

There are other differences between the two groups. In general, the frequency of recurrences in the traumatic group is lower than that of the atraumatic. Also the incidence of recurrences is lower after a primary traumatic dislocation (55 to 60%) than in the atraumatic (85 to 90%).

## PATHOLOGY OF THE UNSTABLE JOINT

In the past few decades many reports concerned with the pathology of the unstable joint have appeared in the literature. In general, most investigators agree in their descriptions of the lesions found on the anterior and posterior aspects of the joint in anterior and posterior recurrences. However, there is disagreement on which of the lesions is primarily responsible for the recurrences, and there is another group of observers who believe that none of the so-called essential lesions is the primary cause. (I shall say more about causation later.)

The abnormalities may be grouped according to whether they are associated most frequently with traumatic or with atraumatic recurrences. However, many atraumatic recurrences, if they go untreated for a long time, eventually develop lesions similar to those in the traumatic group. Essentially the lesions found in subluxating shoulders are comparable to those encountered in dislocating shoulders. The difference between the two lies in the magnitude of the abnormalities. Over the past ten years, I recorded the pathological lesions present at the time of operative repair in 28 cases of recurrent anterior subluxation. The age of the patients ranged from 10 to 26 years. In 20 patients the first subluxation was produced by trauma;

all were males and 17 of the 20 were injured while playing football. The remaining 8 patients had no history of a traumatic subluxation; there were 5 females and 3 males.

## Pathology of Anterior Recurrent Subluxation

During the operative repair of subluxating joints initiated by a traumatic episode I have observed at least one of the following abnormalities or a combination of them.

All exhibited attenuation of the anterior capsulomuscular wall and pouching of the anterior capsule and ligaments. In some ($\frac{1}{3}$) the antero-inferior portion of the labrum was avulsed from the glenoid rim in varying degrees; and in about $\frac{1}{4}$ of the shoulders there was a defect in the anterior capsule. It appeared as if the capsule had been torn from its attachment to the labrum and neck of the scapula. In several instances, the capsular defect was associated with tears in the subscapularis tendon. In instances of long duration erosion of the anterior glenoid rim was a common finding; and in some of these, small osseous-cartilaginous nodules formed on the irregular glenoid rim. In a few shoulders, the nodules had separated from the glenoid and were in the joint as loose bodies.

A defect in the posterolateral aspect of the humeral head was identified in approximately 25 percent of the shoulders. It is difficult to explore this region of the humeral head so that I am sure some small defects were missed. In only 2 humeral heads was the defect a well defined punched out area of bone. In most, the defects resembled a leveling off rather than an excavation of bone.

Five shoulders in this traumatic group showed none of the above lesions except attenuation and pouching of the anterior capsulomuscular wall.

The number of shoulders in the atraumatic group is small; yet, the operative findings are significant. Four showed no lesions except attenuation and distention of the anterior capsule, ligaments and muscular wall. The remainder disclosed lesions similar to those found in the traumatic group. Two humeral heads revealed well defined defects in their posterolateral aspects.

### Pathology of Posterior Recurrent Subluxations

Recurrent subluxation following atraumatic subluxation is exceedingly rare; I have encountered only three. I have explored 7 posterior recurrent subluxations, 3 of which were atraumatic subluxations. The age of the patients ranged from 14 to 24; there were 5 males and 2 females. In both groups the pathological findings on the posterior aspect of the joint were similar to those in anterior recurrent subluxations. The outstanding feature of the atraumatic group was the lack of labral or capsular tears and the attenuation and pouching of the posterior capsulomuscular wall in all cases. Only one of the 3 shoulders in this group showed a small detachment of the posterior labrum. In the traumatic group all 4 shoulders exhibited either a defect in the posterior capsule or a detachment of the labrum. The posterior rim in 3 was irregular and slightly eroded. A defect in the anteromedial aspect of the humeral head was noted in 5 of the 7 shoulders.

### Pathology of Anterior Recurrent Dislocation

I explored 38 anterior recurrent dislocating shoulders at the time an operative repair was performed. There were no females in this series; the age of the patients ranged from 14 to 38; the average age was 22 years. In 36 patients the primary lesion was produced by trauma and in the remaining two the initial dislocation was spontaneous. All the joints were explored through an adequate anterior incision. But, before doing an arthrotomy, the humeral head was dislocated by abducting and externally rotating the arm. This brought into clear view the relationship of the anterior capsulomuscular wall to the dislocated humeral head. The following abnormal changes were found.

### Laxity of the Subscapularis Muscle

The subscapularis in all shoulders was lax and its tone was decreased. This feature was readily demonstrated by making tension on two towel clips, one placed in the muscle belly and the other in the tendon of the muscle. This abnormality became even more apparent when the tension and tone of the subscapularis was compared with the tension and tone of the supraspinatus tested in a similar manner. I must concede, however, that this is a clinical impression.

Several shoulders revealed a defect along the inferior margin of the subscapularis tendon. It appeared as if the tendon had been partially torn from its bony attachment and separated from those muscle fibers of the subscapularis that normally insert just below the lesser tuberosity. This laxity of the subscapularis has been observed by other investigators.

### Hypermobile Subscapularis Muscle and Tendon

In 3 shoulders, upon dislocating the head of the humerus, the subscapularis muscle and tendon shifted upward and over the advancing humeral head. Also, in these shoulders, the capsule below the inferior margin of the tendon appeared redundant and saccular.

### Anterior Pouch With Redundancy of the Anterior Capsule

In 13 shoulders, the dislocated humeral head settled in a large pouch on the anterior aspect of the neck of the scapula. The pouch extended medially as far as the

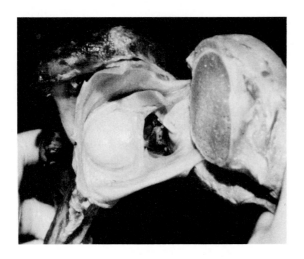

FIG. 10-3. Part of the humeral head had been removed, the better to visualize the inside of the joint. Note that in this shoulder the middle glenohumeral ligament is absent.

coracoid process. Essentially the pouch comprised a distended subscapularis recess (or recesses). No tears were found in the anterior capsular walls. In each joint the labrum was frayed, and in 6 shoulders the labrum was partially detached from the glenoid rim.

Of special interest was the anatomy of the middle glenohumeral ligament in this group of shoulders. In 6 the ligament was present but underdeveloped. The medial end of the ligament did not extend to the labrum but blended with the periosteum on the anterior aspect of the neck of the scapula. In 3 the ligament was absent, and in 4 it was a well developed structure with its medial end torn from the labrum.

I should like to point out that the abnormalities described above have their counterparts in the variational anatomy that is normally found on the anterior aspect of the glenohumeral joint. It is obvious to me — and, I hope, to the reader — that underdeveloped or absent middle glenohumeral ligaments can offer no resistance to a dislocating humeral head (Fig. 10-3). Also, in many instances, a well formed ligament can offer only token resistance; in so doing it may tear from its attachment and allow the head to settle in the enlarged subscapular cavity (Fig. 10-4). It appears that shoulders with the above variational patterns dislocate with less

force than those possessing a strong capsulomuscular wall (Fig. 10-5).

### Detachment of Soft Tissues From the Glenoid Rim

In 5 shoulders a rent was found in the capsule just lateral to the glenoid labrum. The size of the rent varied from 2 cm. to the entire length of the anterior portion of the capsule. In all shoulders the labra were attached to the rims, but they showed advanced changes such as small tears, fraying, thinning and lamination. (Incidentally, detachment of the capsule from the labrum was the first lesion Bankart described (1923). The so-called Bankart lesion was not described by Bankart until 1938.)

In 10 shoulders, both the labrum and the capsule were sheared off the glenoid rim. The extent of the detachment varied from 2 cm. to the entire length of the anterior half of the glenoid margin. Some labra had deteriorated so much that they could barely be identified. It appeared that all the soft tissue structures except the periosteum were sheared off the glenoid rim.

In addition to separation of the capsule and labrum from the glenoid rim, in 7 shoulders the periosteum was also elevated from the neck of the scapula. It appeared that the capsule and its ligaments, the labrum and the periosteum separated in one mass from the glenoid and neck of the scapula.

## Loose Bodies

In 12 joints loose debris was found in the joint cavity. Some of the material resembled pieces of degenerated labrum, some had fibrocartilaginous features, and some were osteocartilaginous. In 2 joints the loose bodies, which were pieces of bone covered with degenerated cartilage and fibrous tissue, were weakly attached to the capsule. Both of these shoulders showed much erosion and irregularity of the anterior glenoid rim. It appeared that the loose bodies were pieces of bone and cartilage sheared off the anterior rim of the glenoid.

## Erosion of the Glenoid Rim

All the joints that had some degree of detachment of the labrum showed some reactive changes on the glenoid rim. In most the rim was eroded, and, in some, small osteocartilaginous nodules had formed on the eroded surface of the rim. In 4 shoulders the entire antero-inferior rim was absent and the remaining surface of the glenoid was studded with irregular osteocartilaginous nodules.

## Humeral Defects

All the humeral heads showed some abnormality of the posterolateral surface. In about 75 percent of the heads the defect was an angular excavation into which the anterior rim of the glenoid fitted when the head· was dislocated. The defect in the remaining heads was either a flat surface or a smooth concavity; it appeared as if the bone in this region of the head had worn away.

## Pathology of Posterior Recurrent Dislocations

Like posterior recurrent subluxation, posterior recurrent dislocation following a primary traumatic posterior dislocation

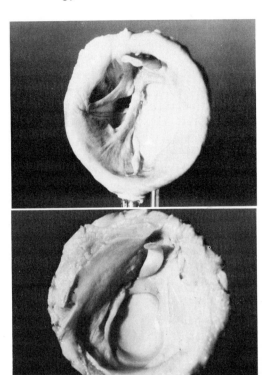

(*Top*) FIG. 10-4. In this specimen the middle glenohumeral ligament is well formed; however, it is doubtful that it could offer much resistance to a dislocating humeral head.

(*Bottom*) FIG. 10-5. Note that the subscapularis recess is small and the middle and inferior glenohumeral ligaments together with the capsule form an effective passive barrier to forces tending to dislocate the humeral head.

is rare. I have explored and recorded the pathology in 15 patients with recurrent posterior dislocations. In 7 patients the initial dislocation was produced by trauma, and in 8 patients the dislocations were spontaneous. The age range was from 11 to 29 years, the average age was 23 years. There were 5 females in this series and in none was the initial dislocation traumatic. Two patients had bilateral recurrent dislocations—a male 11 years old and a female 14 years old.

All the shoulders in the traumatic group revealed marked laxity of the posterior capsulomuscular wall. When the head was in the dislocated position it was apparent that the posterior structures were so attenuated that they offered no resistance to the head. This was even more apparent in the shoulders in the atraumatic group.

The labrum was partially detached in 3 of 5 shoulders in the traumatic group, and the capsule was torn and detached in the other two. But all 5 shoulders showed advanced degenerative changes in the labrum; the labra were frayed, laminated and, in two instances, worn so thin that they were barely identifiable. On the other hand, in the atraumatic shoulders no labral or capsular detachments were present, but the labra did show some evidence of wear and tear in 3 shoulders. In these the disorder had been present for a long time—2, 4, and 5 years.

All the shoulders with labral detachments also showed erosion in varying degrees of the posterior glenoid rim, and in 2 shoulders several loose bodies were found.

A defect on the anteromedial aspect of the humeral head was present in all shoulders except those of the 11-year-old patient who had bilateral dislocations. The size of the defect in general was much larger in the traumatic than in the atraumatic shoulders.

## CAUSE OF RECURRENT SUBLUXATION AND DISLOCATION

It is my belief that none of the different lesions described above, such as separation of the labrum, tears in the fibrous capsule, disruption of the glenohumeral ligaments, pouching of the anterior or posterior capsule, erosion of the glenoid rim and defects in the humeral head, singly or in combination, is the cause of recurrent subluxation or dislocation. But I do concede that some of these abnormalities, such as humeral head defects, extensive erosion of the glenoid rim and attenuation and tears of the capsule, facilitate recurrences.

## Dynamic Stabilizers of the Joint

The bony architecture of the glenohumeral joint provides no stability. Only a small area of the humeral head articulates with the glenoid fossa while the arm is at rest at the side or in motion. The shoulder possesses almost a global range of motion. No other articulation in the human frame is capable of the motions performed by the glenohumeral joint.

What makes such versatility possible in the glenohumeral joint? First, the joint possesses a very loose capsule. Second, the constant relationship between the head and the glenoid fossa, at rest and during motion, is maintained by a delicate coordinated balance between the scapulohumeral, axioscapular and axiohumeral muscles.

The most important of these are the scapulohumeral muscles. These are so arranged about the humeral head that they form both an anterior and a posterior capsulomuscular wall. During elevation of the arm they depress and fix the head in the glenoid fossa, thus establishing a fulcrum. In addition, the subscapularis in front and the infraspinatus and teres minor behind roll the head posteriorly. This posterior roll of the head opposes any tendency toward anterior displacement of the head. Saha has shown by electromyographic studies that the power of the subscapularis rises from 120° of elevation to its maximum at 150°. Then it drops steadily. At 150° of elevation the infraspinatus takes over and its power rises steadily, reaching its maximum at 180°. The crucial range is between 150 and 180°, when the relative anteversion of the humerus is at its highest point; but it is in this range that the powerful action of the infraspinatus comes into play. From the electromyographic studies it appears that the teres minor supplements the power of both the subscapularis and the infraspinatus. It shows a plateau curve from 60 to 180°.

It is clear, then, that the rotator muscles

work synergistically and that the anterior and posterior capsulomuscular walls are really dynamic buttresses opposing forces that tend to displace the humeral head posteriorly or anteriorly. Therefore, it is reasonable to assume that if the power of the muscular walls is diminished, recurrent luxations will occur. This occurs with paralysis or congenital weakness of tissues, or after trauma that produces elongation, slackness and weakness of the capsulomuscular walls.

## Anatomical Features Predisposing to Recurrences

In addition to those causes mentioned above, which produce weakness of the anterior and posterior capsulomuscular walls that predispose to recurrence, there are other anatomical causes that render the joint vulnerable to recurrent luxations. Among these are the congenital malformations of the head of the humerus or of the glenoid. Although rare, when they do occur they may so disturb the normal mechanics of the joint that it becomes unstable. Essentially, these comprise flattening of the humeral head, flattening or rounding of the glenoid fossa, and diminution or obliteration of the normal retrotilt of the glenoid.

The other anatomical predisposing causes are confined to the anterior portion of the joint where on the inner aspect of the joint, are found the glenohumeral ligaments — superior, middle and inferior. In general, they are thickened portions of the capsule and arise from the anterior portion of the glenoid labrum; they insert into the lesser tuberosity of the humerus. If they are substantial structures, together with the capsule they act as check reins to extension, abduction and external rotation of the arm. These, together with the subscapularis, comprise the anterior capsulomuscular wall. The detailed variational anatomy of glenohumeral ligaments has been described in Chapter 4. This information was obtained from an investigation made on 96

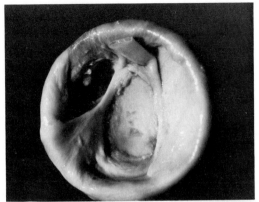

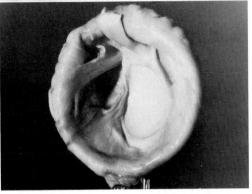

(*Top*) FIG. 10-6. The bursal recess in this specimen occupies about one half the glenoid margin; only the lower half of the capsule and the inferior glenohumeral ligament are attached to the labrum. This is a very deficient "anterior capsular mechanism."

(*Bottom*) FIG. 10-7. Note that the bursal recess is bridged by a poorly developed middle glenohumeral ligament. This arrangement unsupported could never effectively oppose an advancing humeral head.

shoulders obtained from cadavers. In a later study of 122 shoulders, the above information was reconfirmed and the role of the subscapularis muscle in the anterior part of the shoulder was also studied. In the following discussion it will be necessary to restate some of the pertinent observations made in both studies.

The relationship of the capsule, the glenohumeral ligaments, the tendon of the subscapularis and the glenoid labrum to

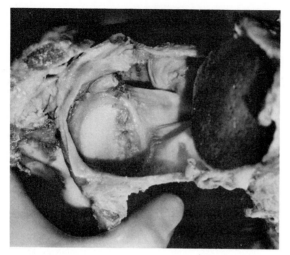

Fig. 10-8. Note that when the anterior capsular mechanism is stretched the ligaments, capsule and labrum appear as one continuous structure; also note the degenerative changes in the labrum and along the anterior glenoid rim. This is a specimen from the fifth decade.

one another shows many variations. Although no two shoulders look alike, the variations fall into six specific patterns. These types and their frequency are depicted in Figure 4-27. Of important clinical significance is the observation that in 88.6 percent of the shoulders dissected (there were 96 shoulders in this study) a bursal recess of varying size was present. In these shoulders the anterior portion of the fibrous capsule is not continuous with the labrum. Instead, it continues to the root of the coracoid process, swings around and continues laterally on the neck of the scapula as far as the glenoid rim. The reflected portion of the capsule is very thin. Thus, a recess is formed in the capsule which extends from the glenoid rim to the base of the coracoid process, the subscapular bursal recess. As seen in the different arrangements of the glenohumeral ligaments (Fig. 4-27) this recess may be subdivided into two bursal recesses by the position of the middle glenohumeral ligament.

If the bursal recess occupies one third or less of the anterior glenoid margin, the remaining capsule together with the middle and inferior glenohumeral ligaments comprise an effective passive barrier to forces tending to dislocate the humeral head (Fig. 10-5). Moreover, in the circumstances described above, the subscapularis muscle and tendon are firmly attached to the cap-

sule and hug the neck of the scapula very closely. In this position the subscapularis acts as a dynamic buttress and also reinforces the inelastic capsule and ligaments immediately in front of the joint.

On the other hand, in 32.6 percent of the joints studied, the bursal recess occupies more than one third of the anterior glenoid margin. In these joints the middle glenohumeral ligament is deficient or absent and, if present, is not attached to the glenoid labrum. Hence, a very large pouch exists on the anterior neck of the scapula; it extends medially as far as the base of the coracoid process. The capsule forming the pouch is very thin. In these joints, the subscapularis muscle and tendon lie at a distance from the neck of the scapula. They can readily be displaced from the neck of the scapula because of their extreme hypermobility. The subscapularis tendon is adherent only to a thin, redundant capsule which lines its posterior surface. From a practical viewpoint, these joints have no anterior capsular mechanism. The only structure capable of stabilizing the joint is the muscular apparatus working in a coordinated manner. Also, in these joints the subscapularis is the only active or passive barrier on the anterior aspect of the joint capable of counteracting dislocating forces (Figs. 10-6 and 10-7). Presumably, the force required to dislocate a joint with

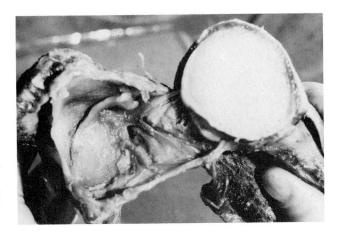

FIG. 10-9. This is a specimen from the seventh decade; note the extensive degeneration of the labrum and the alterations along the anterior glenoid rim. Also note the marked thickening of the ligaments and synovial membrane.

such an inadequate anterior capsulomuscular wall would be less than that required to dislocate a joint with an intact thick capsulomuscular wall.

Repair of recurrent dislocation in a joint with a large defect in the anterior capsule by the Bankart operation or one of its modifications is virtually impossible because there is no capsular tissue to attach to the glenoid rim. In these instances, the posterior portion of the tendon of the subscapularis must be used to obtain an adequate repair.

### The Role of Degenerative Changes in Recurrent Dislocation

The other observations germane to this discussion concern the degenerative changes that occur in the labrum as the result of normal function. As previously shown, all gradations of degenerative alterations occur, ranging from minimal fraying and small separations to gross maceration and complete separation of the labrum from the glenoid rim. The abnormalities are more severe after the fourth decade. The reason for these changes is clear. In joints having the capsule and ligaments firmly anchored to the labrum, when the ligaments and capsule are stretched, strong traction is placed on the anterior labrum. In fact, when severely stretched, the ligaments, capsule and labrum appear grossly as one continuous structure (Fig. 10-8). Therefore, it is clear that during normal function the ligaments and capsule exert varying degrees of traction on the labrum. Over many years, this mechanism causes degenerative changes in the labrum and also may pull it away from the glenoid rim. In the latter decades the degenerative changes induce a reparative process in the subsynovial tissues. This produces, in some instances, profound proliferative changes in the labrum which appears thickened and studded with numerous synovial villi (Fig. 10-9).

Those decades of life (after forty) when the labrum and capsule show the greatest degree of degeneration and may be completely separated from the glenoid rim comprise the same period in which recurrent dislocations rarely occur. This observation does not support Bankart's premise that the labrum must be attached to the rim to insure stability of the joint. In fact, in some of the shoulders in the later decades there is no labrum on the anterior rim.

### WHAT IS THE CURE FOR RECURRENT SUBLUXATIONS AND DISLOCATIONS?

It is my belief that neuromuscular coordination and balance of the rotator muscles must be restored in order to cure recurrent subluxations and dislocations. If the disorder affects primarily the anterior components of the joint, the subscapularis must be dealt with; if it affects the posterior elements, the infraspinatus must be dealt with. This is true only if the bony elements of the joint have a normal or nearly normal configuration. For example, if the glenoid fossa shows a large anterior defect caused by erosion or fracture, it may be virtually impossible to restore muscle balance. In this instance, the size and configuration of the glenoid fossa must first be restored by an anterior bone graft before the rotator muscles can work efficiently. The same is true if the posterior portion of the glenoid fossa is involved. Also, in those recurrences associated with inherent muscle weakness or dysplasia of the connective tissues, such as is seen in some voluntary subluxators or dislocators, muscle balance and efficiency is enhanced by buttressing the anterior or posterior glenoid margin with a bone graft. The increased mechanical stability provided by the bone grafts reduces the demands made on the rotator muscles in stabilizing of the joint.

It is clear then that the choice of operation must be made on an individual basis. A patient must not be fitted to any one operation; rather, the operation must fulfill those requirements that will effect a cure.

Based on my reasoning of the cause of recurrences, in uncomplicated anterior recurrent dislocations and subluxations I disregard all the soft tissue abnormalities in the joint. I attempt to restore neuromuscular balance by performing a modified Magnuson-Stack operation.

Simply stated, in this operation, the tendon of the subscapularis is transferred to the lateral side of the bicipital groove and below the greater tuberosity. However, other requirements must be fulfilled if the operation is to be successful. The tendon must be transferred laterally far enough to put the muscle under moderate tension while the arm is in the position of internal rotation. This takes up all the slack in the

muscle and brings the muscle and tendon closer to the neck of the scapula. The tendon must be anchored far enough below the greater tuberosity so that it forms a cup around the inferior surface of the humeral head. This achieves three goals: (1) Being attached to the shaft below the tuberosity, the tendon cannot slip over the head when the arm is abducted and externally rotated. (2) When dislocating forces are applied to the arm, the subscapularis pulls the head upward and backward into the glenoid fossa and resists the downward and forward pull of the pectoralis major, latissimus dorsi and teres major. (3) In its new position, when the arm is elevated, the tendon can more effectively roll the head posteriorly and oppose any forces displacing the head anteriorly.

This operation is simple to perform and it produces results comparable to any other operation used today. Much is said about the amount of residual limitation of external rotation it produces. It is true that some degree of limitation is present in many shoulders following this operation, but it is also true that as time passes the amount of limitation steadily decreases. Also, the limitation, even immediately after surgery, in no way handicaps the overall performance of the shoulder, not even in the football quarterback or the baseball pitcher. This objection to the Magnuson-Stack operation that many observers raise is entirely overdone and invalid.

To cure recurrent posterior subluxations and dislocations, something more than advancement of the tendon of the infraspinatus is needed. Still, the principles of treatment for both anterior and posterior lesions are the same. Nevertheless, it has been my experience and the experience of others that too many failures follow this simple operation. It appears that in order to restore neuromuscular balance, the posterior rotator muscles need more help than that provided by simple advancement of the infraspinatus tendon. Therefore, in all posterior recurrences, I supplement the muscle operation with a posterior bone graft. The operative techniques to cure anterior and posterior instability of the shoulder are described in Chapter 7.

The question that naturally arises is: How does the Bankart operation and its numerous modifications and the Putti-Platt operation effect a cure of recurrent anterior dislocation? That these operations have a low incidence of failure is now generally accepted; the incidence ranges from 1 to 6 percent and, in the hands of the skillful orthopaedic surgeon, it is less than 1 percent. Let us first consider the Bankart operation. It is my belief that this operation corrects the same essential defect that the Magnuson procedure does. It restores the neuromuscular balance of the rotator muscles by bringing the subscapularis in close opposition to the neck of the scapula and glenoid rim. Also, the slackness of the muscle is reduced; this must naturally follow the separation of the subscapularis tendon and muscle from the underlying capsule and the subsequent healing of these structures.

In some instances this operation actually tethers the muscle to the glenoid rim; this occurs when the anterior capsular wall is deficient or absent. In these instances, the surgeon knowingly or unknowingly closes the defect by suturing a portion of the subscapularis tendon to the glenoid rim. Townley, in describing the operation he performs, makes the following statement: "After injury to the subscapularis tendon has been ruled out, the structure is dissected from the capsule starting near the tendon insertion and leaving much of the thickness of the tendon on the capsule side."* Bost and Inman wrote: ". . . relatively poor and thinned out capsular structures are sometimes found at the site of resuture. This condition has been circumvented by suturing some of the posterior surface of the subscapularis to the glenoid rim."†

* Townley, C. O.: J. Bone & Joint Surg., *32A*:370, 1950.
† Bost, F. C., and Inman, V. T.: J. Bone Joint Surg., *24*:595, 1942.

The Putti-Platt operation actually shortens the subscapularis muscle; in addition, by suturing the lateral edges of the cut tendon to the glenoid rim it creates a firm anterior capsulomuscular wall. These features of the operation take up all of the slack in the subscapularis muscle and hence improve its efficiency.

I must admit that these operations, theoretically, should be the procedures of choice. They reconstruct a passive barrier that contains the humeral head and opposes those forces tending to displace the head forward. Also, the operations restore neuromuscular balance to the rotator muscles. However, evaluation of long term results of these operations and the results of the Magnuson-Stack procedure reveals that the incidence of failure is about the same. I prefer the Magnuson-Stack procedure because it is a simpler procedure to perform than the Bankart or the Putti-Platt.

## CLINICAL PICTURE OF RECURRENT SUBLUXATION OF THE GLENOHUMERAL JOINT

### Recurrent Anterior Subluxations

Acute anterior subluxation is the most common injury of the shoulder in athletes, especially football players, but it may occur spontaneously. Recurrences follow initial traumatic subluxations if adequate treatment is not instituted immediately. The arm must be fixed to the side for at least 6 weeks. During this period, the arm must never be abducted or externally rotated. Nor must the arm ever be manipulated to test its range of free motion or the state of healing. Should recurrent subluxation follow an initial subluxation, in many instances, the lesion will progress to recurrent dislocation.

In my series of 28 shoulders, the age ranged from 10 to 26 years; there were 23 males and 5 females. Of the 23 males, 20 had sustained an initial traumatic subluxation. All 5 females had spontaneous subluxations. In the traumatic group, the time between the first subluxation and the first recurrent subluxation ranged from 4 months to 3½ years.

**Symptoms and Signs.** The symptoms are fairly characteristic of the lesion. Upon abduction and external rotation of the arm, in some instances against resistance and in others without resistance, the patient's shoulder slips out, often with an audible click. On reversing the movements the shoulder slips in. As a rule, after each subluxation there remains some residual soreness in the shoulder, and often a feeling of numbness down the length of the limb. In the interval between subluxations, and particularly immediately after a subluxation, the arm feels weak and the patient avoids motions that would precipitate a subluxation.

Between subluxations, the shoulder exhibits no deformity except in longstanding cases. There may be a slight atrophy of the deltoid, supraspinatus and infraspinatus. The patient resists any attempt to rotate the arm externally, and when the arm is passively rotated externally, he experiences a feeling of imminent slipping of the shoulder. Generally some tenderness is present along the anterior aspect of the shoulder. Also, upon passively rotating the arm internally and externally, in some shoulders crepitus and clicking can be elicited.

If the shoulder is examined when the head is in the subluxated position, the head can be palpated in the anterior position, and there is some prominence of the anterior aspect of the shoulder. The arm is slightly abducted and externally rotated and no motion is possible. When the head slips back into the joint, if the hand is placed on the humeral head, it can be felt to slip into the glenoid.

**X-Ray Findings.** If roentgenograms are taken while the head is in the subluxated position, the anteroposterior and axial views readily show the lesion. However, the opportunity to x-ray a subluxated joint is rare. The patient usually presents himself in an interval between subluxations. Nevertheless, roentgenograms may show certain bony changes which may occur in recurrent subluxation. If views are taken in different positions of internal rotation (50 to 70°) and if the "notch view" of Reeves is included, many humeral heads will show a posterolateral defect similar to that seen in recurrent dislocation. In my series, 36 percent showed such a defect. Also, erosion and irregularity of the rim and exostoses on the rim were observed in 33 percent. Small loose bodies were noted in 3 shoulders.

Recently the Orthopedic Service at West Point, the United States Military Academy, has developed a new technique to bring into view the anteroinferior aspect of the glenoid brim. Essentially it is a postero-anterior view taken with the patient lying in the prone position and the arm extended laterally from the trunk. This view shows lesions of the glenoid rim and capsule in over 90 percent of patients with recurrent subluxations. The lesions noted are erosions of the antero-inferior rim of the glenoid and irregular areas of calcification in the capsule. Figure 10-10 clearly shows the lesions. These findings were confirmed when the glenohumeral joints were explored during operative repair of the unstable joints.

Arthrography may be useful in detecting some of the changes associated with this lesion. It may show a recess on the anterior aspect of the joint and irregularities of the glenoid rim. If the subluxation can be produced passively or voluntarily, cineradiography will show the head slipping out and in the joint.

**Management.** The management of recurrent subluxations is an individual problem. The lesion should be treated conservatively and by careful watchful waiting in those persons who have frequent subluxations and do not engage in sports or other strenuous activity. This is also true for those who have only an occasional subluxation with no increase in frequency. On the other hand, in a young athlete who desires to

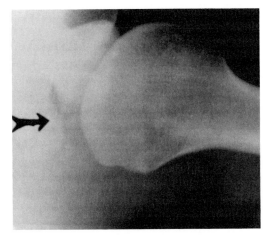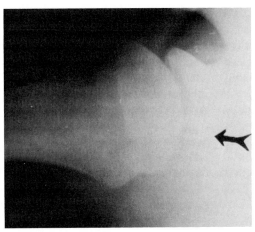

FIG. 10-10. West Point views of two recurrent subluxating shoulders. Note the erosions of the antero-inferior rim and of the glenoid and the areas of calcification in the capsule just below the rim.

continue to play but cannot trust the shoulder, surgical repair should be performed. Also, surgical intervention is indicated in those with frequent subluxations, whether they be traumatic or spontaneous in origin.

For the usual uncomplicated subluxation I perform a Magnuson-Stack operation. For spontaneous subluxation with an abnormal glenoid fossa (the fossa may be shallow, the glenoid may be antetilted or the anterior rim may be defective) I supplement the Magnuson-Stack operation with an anterior bone graft. (See Chapter 7.)

At this point, a word of caution: Before any surgery is attempted be sure the diagnosis is correct. Too many posterior recurrent lesions have been missed, and the surgery performed on the anterior side of the joint. Subsequent posterior subluxations may bring not only embarrassment to the surgeon but also a law suit. I know of one such incident.

## Posterior Recurrent Subluxations

Posterior recurrent subluxation is a rare lesion. Undoubtedly many so-called snapping shoulders are recurrent subluxations, but by the time the patient seeks medical aid they have progressed to recurrent dislocations. Also, the diagnosis of posterior recurrent subluxation is difficult to make from the patient's history alone. It can be made only if the patient is examined when the subluxation is present (for most of the lesions reduce spontaneously) or if the patient is able to produce the subluxation voluntarily. Most patients can produce the subluxation voluntarily.

I have explored 7 posterior recurrent subluxations. The age ranged from 14 to 24 years; there were 5 males and 2 females. Three patients had a definite history of trauma that produced the initial displacement of the humeral head. In one patient the initial lesion was a true posterior dislocation, as proved by roentgenograms taken at the time of the injury. Subsequently he developed recurrent subluxation. One sustained the initial injury while playing football and the other while wrestling. In the remaining four the subluxation occurred spontaneously—in one patient while he was swimming. All of these patients were able to subluxate the shoulder voluntarily; therefore, the diagnosis was made without difficulty.

Thus, there are two types of posterior recurrent subluxation: the traumatic and the atraumatic. In the former, the primary subluxation is caused when a backward force is applied to the lower end of the humerus, with the arm flexed, internally rotated and adducted. Most of these patients are treated initially for a sprain of the shoulder. Subsequently the patient develops snapping of the shoulder when the arm is flexed and internally rotated, with or without adduction. They volunteer the information that the shoulder slips out and in. Also, in some instances, the same thing happens when the arm carries weight while it is in the forward and overhead position.

Most patients can reduce the subluxation by simply relaxing the muscles or forcing the arm into abduction and external rotation. As time goes on the subluxations become more frequent and, in most instances, can be produced voluntarily.

In the atraumatic group, there is no history of severe trauma causing the subluxations. Three patients in the atraumatic group informed me they could snap their shoulders when they were children. These patients have marked laxity of the capsulomuscular walls and require minimal force to subluxate the shoulder. These are the habitual subluxators.

**Symptoms and Signs.** As a rule, the patients in the traumatic group have more disability and discomfort when the subluxations first occur than do those in the atraumatic group. But as the subluxations become more frequent the intensity of the pain decreases. Not infrequently the patient will try to avoid those positions of the arm that cause it to subluxate.

When the shoulder is in its normal position there are few signs that point to recurrent subluxation. In most instances, if the arm is flexed, adducted and internally rotated the patient has an imminent feeling that the shoulder is about to slip out. However, if the patient can be persuaded to subluxate the arm voluntarily, the head can be seen to slip posteriorly, and when the muscles are relaxed, to slip anteriorly.

Roentgenograms taken with the arm subluxated confirm the diagnosis. Cineradiography is a useful tool to establish the diagnosis. The head of the humerus can be seen moving first downward and then backward into a position of subluxation. It stops just short of a complete dislocation.

The cause and the pathology of recurrent posterior subluxations have been described on page 411.

**Management.** As in recurrent anterior subluxation, the management of recurrent posterior subluxation is determined by the individual features of each subluxating shoulder. Patients who suffer only an occasional subluxation need no treatment if the disorder does not interefere with normal activity. On the other hand, frequent subluxations, especially those that seriously handicap the patient's normal way of living, must be treated surgically. I know of no effective conservative methods of treatment. Exercises designed to improve the tone and power of the shoulder muscles, in my experience, have never cured a recurrent subluxating or dislocating shoulder.

Although the type of operation performed depends on the nature of the disorder, I do not place much reliance on soft tissue repairs for posterior subluxation or dislocation. No doubt some of these procedures succeed in some instances, such as the Bankart or Putti-Platt operation performed on the posterior side of the joint. On the other hand, too many fail. I disregard capsular tears and labral detachments. My preference is to buttress the posteroinferior glenoid rim with a bone graft, and, in addition, I advance the tendons of the infraspinatus and teres minor. I have had no failures since doing this combined operation.

## Anterior Recurrent Dislocation

Anterior recurrent dislocations fall into two groups: traumatic and atraumatic. It is important to make this distinction in any

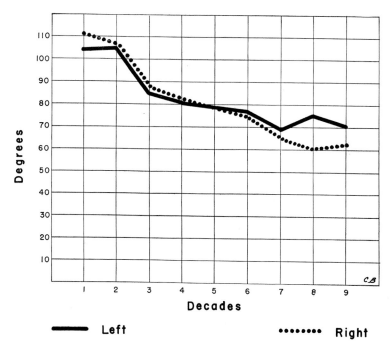

FIG. 10-11. The average range of external rotation at each decade. The graph shows a gradual decrease in the range of external rotation with advancing age. This study was made on 800 persons, 100 in each decade from the first to the eighth. Only persons who never had suffered a dislocation or who had never had severe injuries to the shoulder joint were selected for this study.

consideration of anterior recurrent dislocation, for the two differ in prognosis and treatment. The traumatic group includes recurrent lesions that initially occurred as the result of severe violence. The atraumatic group comprises recurrent dislocations that initially occur without trauma or with only minor trauma.

In the atraumatic group are the shoulders with congenital anomalies of the glenoid or the humeral head and shoulders with marked laxity of the capsulomuscular walls. Also in this category are patients with various forms of dysplasia of all the elastic tissues of the body such as are found in Ehlers-Danlos syndrome, Marfan's syndrome, syringomyelia and arthrochalasis. Although the last group is rare, when one is seeking the cause of atraumatic recurrent dislocations, especially in children, these syndromes should be considered. Most

bilateral recurrent dislocations fall in the atraumatic group. Finally, patients with familial predisposition to recurrent dislocation belong in the atraumatic group.

Although primary anterior dislocations occur as frequently under the age of 45 years as after 45, there is a great difference in the rate of recurrence in the two groups. Under the age of 45 years the recurrence rate is between 85 and 90 percent whereas after the age of 45 years it is from 10 to 15 percent. The recurrence rate in the traumatic group is high—about 55 to 60 percent; it is still higher in the atraumatic group— 85 to 90 percent. Over 80 percent of bilateral dislocations develop recurrences. The ratio of recurrence in the male to recurrence in the female is two to one.

Why are recurrences less frequent after the age of 45 years? In my opinion, the decreased incidence of recurrence is due to two changes that occur in the aging shoulder: (1) With increasing age there is a general increase in fibrous tissue in the shoulder joint. This is the natural process associated with the degenerative changes that occur with aging and function. (In Chapter 6 the degenerative alterations are discussed in detail.) (2) The resulting loss of elasticity produces a progressive reduction of motion of the shoulder, especially external rotation. Fig. 10-11 clearly shows the loss of external rotation from decade to decade. Note that in the third decade the average range of external rotation is between 105 and 108°, whereas in the fifth decade it is 80°. Clearly, these older shoulders are better able to resist dislocating forces than are shoulders with marked laxity and a wider range of external rotation.

Seventy percent of all recurrences occur in the first two years after the primary dislocation, only 20 percent occur between the second and the fifth year. Not infrequently fractures of the upper end of the humerus or of the glenoid complicate primary traumatic dislocations. When fractures occur the incidence of recurrence is greatly reduced. In dislocations with fractures of the greater tuberosity the recurrence rate is about 7 percent; when fractures of the anatomical neck or comminuted fractures of the upper end of the humerus complicate the dislocations the rate of recurrence is zero. On the other hand, fractures of the anterior glenoid rim carry a poor prognosis. I have never seen dislocations complicated by fractures of the rim that did not develop recurrences. However, in one series only 60 percent went on to recurrent dislocations.

In regard to prognosis of a primary dislocation it is safe to state that, in general, the older the patient, the greater the initial trauma, and the more difficult the reduction, the lower is the rate of recurrence. Also, initial dislocations that are self reduced or easily reduced have a much higher incidence of recurrence than those that are difficult to reduce or cannot be reduced. In the former group the rate of recurrence is over 90 percent.

What is the effect of adequate treatment of primary dislocations on the rate of recurrence? Most orthopaedic surgeons are of the opinion that: (1) the arm should be immobilized at the side for a period of at least 3 weeks, (2) longer periods of immobilization do not significantly reduce the incidence of recurrence and (3) periods under 3 weeks increase the recurrence rate. On the other hand, some surgeons are so convinced that the die is cast at the time of the primary dislocation that they do not immobilize the arm, and they return the patient to full activity just as soon as the muscle soreness and other local symptoms about the shoulder subside. As for athletic injuries, there has been no significant long-term study on which to evaluate either method of treatment.

I am of the opinion that the die is cast at the time of the first dislocation, but I am not ready to concede that a period of immobilization, which allows soft tissues to heal without increase in length, does not in some instances influence the future of the joint. Until there is more proof that "no treatment" produces results comparable to those of "treatment," I shall continue to immobilize the arm for at least 3 weeks.

**Clinical Picture.** The pathology, cause and mechanism of the different varieties of recurrent anterior dislocations have been discussed in the preceding section. The dislocation following a primary traumatic dislocation occurs as the result of a less violent force, but there is aggravation of the pathology—that is, the capsule tears or the labrum detaches from the rim just a little more, the posterolateral defect in the head may become a little deeper, more erosion of the anterior rim may occur, and the anterior capsulomuscular wall becomes more stretched. With each successive dislocation, the intensity of the pathology is increased, and, if healing occurs, the tissues heal with increased length. Finally, dislocation occurs by merely placing the arm in abduction and external rotation. Force is no longer needed to produce the dislocation. In some instances, the patient can produce the dislocation at will.

There are all gradations of this clinical picture. Dislocations may occur only at intervals or they may occur frequently and at the slightest provocation. When they attain the latter pattern they assume the features of habitual dislocations characteristic of spontaneous recurrent dislocations.

The first recurrent dislocations may evoke sufficient pain and muscle spasm to require reduction with analgesics or even anesthesia. Later, very little effort is required to reduce the dislocation, and the patient may be able to reduce the dislocation himself.

In young people, when dislocations are the result of force, as with the primary dislocation, always bear in mind the possibility of an injury to the proximal humeral epiphysis. This lesion can be ruled out only by x-ray examination. Axillary views show the lesion best.

The atraumatic dislocations present a clinical pattern entirely different from that of the traumatic recurrent dislocations. In this group the initial dislocation occurs without trauma or with only minor trauma. Many of these persons report that they could snap their shoulders when children. The frequency of the dislocations is greater than that of the traumatic variety, and, in many instances, the patient can dislocate the shoulder at will from the very onset of the disorder. The lesion may be bilateral.

Remember also that dislocation in more than one direction is a common feature in this group. Awareness of this is most essential when surgical repair is contemplated. In all these patients, the capsulomuscular walls are markedly attenuated, and, with time, some of the shoulders develop pathology in the joint not unlike that observed in the traumatic group. On the other hand, such pathology, except for relaxation of the capsulomuscular walls, may be absent.

In this group is found the "queer adolescent female" who can dislocate the shoulder at will and, in some instances, in more than one direction. Beware of this child! She needs psychiatric help in addition to stabilization of the shoulder. It may be better not to perform any surgery on these children. The results are often failures, and many operations may be required before the shoulder is stabilized.

**X-Ray Examination.** Every shoulder in which a dislocation is suspected should have an adequate x-ray examination. This means that a number of different views should be taken so that no local osseous pathology is missed. Posterolateral defects of the head are best seen in views with the arm in moderate abduction and in 50 to 80° of internal rotation. Also, the "notch view" often shows the lesion when other views do not. In some humeri the posterolateral defect is delineated by a sharp vertical line of sclerosis. In others, the notch is indicated by some flattening of the head; no well defined groove or notch is present. Remember that any flattening of the humeral head is abnormal, and in dislocating shoulders it invariably means a traumatic defect produced either by one or more severe traumas or by repeated minor trauma. The axillary view not only shows the relation of the head to the glenoid but also clearly reveals the outline of the anterior rim. As I noted previously, this is an excellent view for detecting any epiphyseal lesions.

An adequate x-ray examination should also detect or rule out fractures of the rim and loose bodies, and congenital malformations of the humeral head and glenoid.

If the patient is cooperative and will allow the examiner to dislocate the joint, or in the case of voluntary dislocators, by means of serial radiographs or cineradiography the head can actually be seen to slip out of and into the joint.

Arthrograms show the large pouch in the anterior capsulomuscular wall.

**Management.** Most traumatic anterior recurrent dislocations can be cured by one of the plastic procedures done on the capsule, labrum or subscapularis tendon. The exception to this is a fracture of the anterior rim or erosion of the rim involving a large segment of the glenoid fossa. In these, I believe the soft tissue operation should be supplemented by a bone graft on the anterior surface of the neck of the scapula. My preference is the Magnuson-Stack operation and I have given my reasons for this preference.

Results comparable to the Magnuson-Stack operation are obtained by the Bankard, Putti-Platt, Dutoit, Bristow and Eden-Hybbinetti operations. The techniques are described in Chapter 7.

Of course, not all recurrent anterior dislocations must be subjected to surgery. The choice of treatment for these lesions depends upon the specific circumstances of each case. I previously stated that a dislocation that recurs at long intervals—once or twice a year—in a person who does not engage in athletics or other strenuous activities and is not handicapped by the disorder should be treated conservatively (i. e., watchful waiting). As a rule, these persons learn to use their arms in the safe arcs of motion and avoid those movements or activities that favor dislocation. Remember that as the person gets older the recurrences decrease. They are rare after 50 years of age. Exercises of any form, in my experience, have never prevented or cured recurrences.

On the other hand, let us suppose that the patient is an athlete, or a youngster with extraordinary potential in sports, who has suffered only one or two recurrences, and because of the fear of another episode or a feeling of instability in the shoulder, his performance has suffered considerably. In such situations, operative repair is justified and should be done immediately.

A different case would be the athlete with one or two recurrences whose level of performance before the primary dislocation was always at the "bottom of the ladder": the best course here would be to direct the young man into another field of activity.

A familial predisposition to develop recurrent dislocations, in my opinion, rules out any thought of conservative treatment. In fact, much time, money and anxiety would be saved if the shoulder is stabilized after the primary dislocation.

Timing of an operation should be given some consideration. I do not believe that the time interval between the last recurrence of dislocation and operation is of any significance in those recurrences that occur spontaneously, are self reduced and, after reduction, give rise to little or no pain or dysfunction. As a matter of fact, I should not hesitate to operate immediately after the last dislocation. On the other hand, a dislocation that was produced by considerable force and resists reduction indicates disruption of tissues and hemorrhage. In this instance, operation immediately after the dislocation would encounter frayed, fragile tissue infiltrated with blood and tissue fluid. These circumstances would make approximation of capsular or tendon flaps difficult. A wait of 6 to 8 weeks would remove these obstacles and make the operation relatively simple.

Again, I cannot emphasize too much the need to be sure of the direction in which the head dislocates before performing an anterior repair. The best way to determine this is to see the head in the anterior position. This can often be accomplished with a cooperative patient who will allow the head to be dislocated. Should this not be possible, the direction of the pathway of the head should be determined at the time of operation before the joint is exposed. The direction the head takes can be readily determined when the patient is under anesthesia and all muscles are relaxed. With very relaxed and attenuated capsulomuscular walls in habitual dislocations the surgeon can determine whether the head dislocates anteriorly and posteriorly with the same amount of force and ease. If so, the patient needs both an anterior and posterior repair.

## OPERATIVE PROCEDURES FOR RECURRENT ANTERIOR DISLOCATIONS

The surgical procedures used to cure recurrent anterior dislocations can be grouped into four categories: (1) Plastic operations on the anterior capsule, anterior labrum or tendon of the subscapularis; (2) a bone block operation on the anterior aspect of the neck of the scapula; (3) transfer of the subscapular tendon or the tendon of the latissimus dorsi, and (4) suspension operations, using either tendon or fascia lata.

All these operations except the suspension operations have achieved their goal, and, in the last group, the Gallie-Le-Mesurier operation still has its supporters. The surgical techniques for most of these operations are described in Chapter 7.

### Plastic Procedures on the Capsule, Labrum and the Subscapularis Tendon

**Bankart Operation.** In 1923 Bankart described his operation to stabilize shoulders with recurrent anterior dislocation. He considered detachment of the labrum or tearing of the capsule from the anterior rim of the glenoid as the "essential lesion" responsible for recurrences. He advocated reattachment of the labrum or capsule to the glenoid rim. He held that, by restoring what he believed to be the normal anatomy of the anterior aspect of the joint, the restored soft tissue barrier consisting of the anterior capsule would be effective in preventing recurrences. Although I believe that the premise on which Bankart evolved this procedure is wrong, nevertheless, if properly performed, this operation cures 96 to 99 percent of recurrent anterior dislocations.

This is a difficult surgical procedure. Be-

cause of this, many modifications of the operation have been developed.

**Johannesburg Stapling Operation.** In this procedure the goal is again to correct the "essential lesion" and to restore the normal anatomy of the anterior aspect of the joint. The detached labrum or the torn capsule is reattached to the rim of the glenoid with staples. The advantage of this operation is that the period of postoperative disability is greatly decreased. As a rule, the patients return to work two weeks after the operation. Also, there is supposed to be no residual restriction of external rotation. The staple may be inserted extracapsularly or intracapsularly, depending on the nature of the pathology.

This operation was first performed by Fouche in 1931. Dutoit and Roux reported the results of a series of cases performed by this method in 1955. They advise against the use of this procedure in recurrences associated with congenital abnormal mobility of the shoulder. Dutoit reported 7 failures in a series of 150 shoulders operated on by this method.

**Putti-Platt Operation.** The operation was first performed by Valtancoli in 1925; later Putti and Platt independently performed the same procedure. Osmond-Clarke reported on the operation in 1948. Essentially it reconstructs the anterior capsulomuscular wall by dividing the subscarpularis vertically; then with the arm rotated internally, the lateral flap of the muscle is sutured to the glenoid rim or the labrum. The medial flap is double breasted over the lateral flap. The aim of the operation is to restrict external rotation. This is a very popular and effective operation.

Many surgeons combine this procedure with the Bankart operation—a combination that is most effective.

### Tendon Transfers

**Magnuson-Stack Operation.** This procedure was designed in 1941 by Magnuson and Stack. Its goal was to reconstruct a capsulomuscular barrier in front and below the humeral head, and also to provide a dynamic force which, on elevation of the arm, pulls the head of the humerus upward and backward into the glenoid fossa. The subscapularis tendon is transferred to the lateral side of the bicipital groove at a site on the shaft below the head of the humerus. In this position, when the arm is elevated, the tendon forms a cup under the head. Fastened in this position, the tendon cannot slip up between the head and the coracoid process. But, what is even more important, by transferring the tendon to the outer side of the bicipital groove all slack in the muscle is taken up. This increases the efficiency of the muscle and restores neuromuscular balance to the rotator muscles.

There are reasons why, following a primary dislocation, the subscapularis so readily loses its effectiveness in preventing recurrent dislocation. Because of evolutionary changes in the bones and muscles of the shoulder the subscapularis works at a great disadvantage, whereas the advantage of the external rotators is enhanced. This results from the shift of the insertion of the pectoralis minor from the greater tuberosity to the coracoid process. In the Bantu, this primitive insertion is found in 17 percent of specimens. Another change is the torsion of the humerus, which carries with it the tuberosities and the bicipital groove to a more medial position. This decreases the rotatory potential of the subscapularis. Although the mass of the subscapularis is equal to that of the external rotators, its mechanical disadvantage reduces its efficiency. Now, in order to maintain coordinated muscle action about the shoulder, the subscapularis must do more work than the external rotators.

**Transfer of the Latissimus Dorsi.** The objective of this operation is to enhance the power of the infraspinatus and teres minor which help roll the head of the humerus posteriorly when the arm is elevated. This movement counteracts the tendency toward anterior displacement of the humeral head.

The tendon of the latissimus dorsi is transferred to the lower posterior aspect of the greater tuberosity. Saha, who designed this operation and reported it in 1963, has had no recurrences in a series of 45 patients. The operation was performed for both traumatic and atraumatic recurrences.

## Bone Block Operation

These operations are very effective in curing recurrences. The two most popular are the Eden-Hybbinetti and the Bristow operations. They are excellent operations to stabilize the head in the glenoid fossa when the glenoid is malformed or when the rim has a large defect caused by erosion or fracture. Also, they are used with much success when there is much laxity of the capsulomuscular walls such as seen in some spontaneous recurrences. Also, the Bristow operation is widely used to stabilize the traumatic recurrent anterior dislocation.

**Bristow Operation.** Bristow designed this operation in the late thirties and Helfet reported on it in 1958. The distal $1/2$ inch of the coracoid process, to which are inserted the conjoined tendons of the short head of the biceps and the coracobrachialis, is transplanted through a vertical slit in the subscapularis to a raw surface on the anterior aspect of the neck of the scapula just medial to the antero-inferior lip of the glenoid rim. The transplanted bone and tendons reinforce the weak inferior capsule. Also, when the arm is abducted and externally rotated, the buttressing effect is enhanced by the slinglike action of the muscles as they are pulled across the antero-inferior portion of the capsule.

**Eden-Hybbinetti Operation.** Eden and Hybbinetti designed this operation independently; the former made his report in 1918 and the latter in 1932. A bone graft is placed against the anterior aspect of the neck of the scapula and glenoid rim. The graft is so placed that it forms a bony buttress against anterior dislocation of the head. Palmer and Widen reported their modification of this operation in 1948. They insert an iliac graft 1 inch long and ½ inch wide in a subperiosteal pocket at the inferior part of the anterior lip of the glenoid.

## Suspension Operations

The objective of these operations was to create a suspensory ligament for the humeral head which would hold the head in the glenoid fossa. The ligament was made from tendon or fascia. The principal ones are the Nicola, the Henderson and the Gallie-LeMesurier operations. I report on these procedures more for historical reasons than for any other. Both the Nicola and the Henderson operation resulted in too many failures and have been discarded. However, the Gallie-LeMesurier operation has been more successful and has some very strong supporters.

**Nicola Operation.** In the Nicola operation the long head of the biceps tendon is used as the suspensory ligament. The tendon is divided at the distal end of the bicipital groove. Then the proximal end is passed through a tunnel in the humeral head. Finally, the two ends are united by interrupted sutures.

**Henderson Operation.** Henderson employed a portion of the peroneus longus tendon. This was passed through two transverse and parallel drill holes, one through the acromion and the other through the greater tuberosity; then the two ends were joined together.

**Gallie-LeMesurier Operation.** In this operation a fascial sling is used to tie the neck of the scapula and the head of the humerus. The operation was reported in 1948. In a series of 175 operations there were only 7 recurrences. As stated previously, this operation still has some ardent supporters.

## Recurrent Posterior Dislocation

**Clinical Picture.** As stated previously, recurrent posterior dislocations are rela-

tively rare lesions. The lesions fall into two groups: the traumatic and the atraumatic. In the former, the initial lesion is always produced by trauma. The subsequent dislocations may occur spontaneously at varying intervals. In some instances, the arm dislocates every time it is placed in a position of flexion, slight adduction and internal rotation. These recurrences have assumed the characteristics of the habitual type of recurrence.

In the atraumatic group the joint dislocates spontaneously without trauma. In some patients the cause may be a congenital anomaly of the glenoid or humeral head or some generalized dysplastic disorder of the connective tissues associated with laxity of the joint capsule and ligaments. In others, no local congenital malformations or any stigmata of connective tissue disorders may be present. The only positive finding in the latter patients is increased laxity of the posterior capsulomuscular wall. In the atraumatic group are the habitual dislocators; the shoulder dislocates every time it is brought up to a determined position, usually the position of flexion and internal rotation. Many in the atraumatic group can voluntarily dislocate the shoulder. The 11-year-old boy in my series could voluntarily dislocate both shoulders. Most spontaneous dislocations are self reduced.

Unless the patient is seen with the shoulder dislocated it is difficult to make a positive diagnosis on the physical findings. One must depend, in a large measure, on the patient's description of the disorder. If there has been trauma, knowing the position of the arm when the force was applied to it may provide a clue; also, if the patient is able to place the arm in the position that precipitates spontaneous dislocation, it is helpful.

On the other hand, if the patient can dislocate the shoulder at will, one can see the head snap posteriorly, and often hear a thud. A concavity or depression appears below the acromion and the clavicle and the coracoid becomes prominent. Posteriorly, under the acromion, a bulge appears that is readily palpable.

The usual story is that when the arm is placed in certain positions, especially against resistance, the shoulder "slips out." In most instances, the patient can reduce the dislocation by bringing the arm into slight abduction and external rotation; then the shoulder "slips in." One of my patients sustained his first posterior dislocation swinging a golf club and another serving a tennis ball.

In the series I explored, the age ranged from 11 to 29 years; the mean age was 23 years. There were 5 females and 10 males. In 7 shoulders, the initial dislocation was produced by trauma and in 8 it occurred spontaneously. Two patients in the atraumatic group had bilateral dislocations.

**X-Ray Examination.** With the humeral head reduced there is little to see on routine x-ray examination. In axial views, a defect may be seen in the anteromedial portion of the head, or some irregularity of the posterior rim may be seen. In the dislocated position, the axillary view confirms the position of the head. Arthrograms invariably show a distended posterior pouch.

**Management.** As in recurrent anterior dislocations, the treatment of posterior dislocations depends upon the nature of the disorder in the person affected. It is an individual matter. In persons past the third decade who have only occasional dislocations and are not restricted in their activities, the treatment should be "watchful waiting." These patients learn to live with their disability and need no surgical repair.

On the other hand, younger persons with frequent recurrences and, also those with infrequent dislocations whose athletic activities are seriously curtailed by the mere possibility of a dislocation need surgical correction of the disorder.

The choice of operation depends upon the nature of the pathology. However, I have never been satisfied with plastic operations on the infraspinatus and teres minor, and on the posterior capsule or labrum. I have seen too many repairs of this nature fail. There are reasons why this is so.

Many of us fail to appreciate how many times during normal daily activity we bring the arm into a position of flexion, adduction and internal rotation. Considerable force is used to execute these movements in certain activities such as swimming, throwing and tennis. In fact, this act is reported more frequently in everyday living than is that of abduction and external rotation. Apparently, the constant, forceful repetition of the act of flexion, adduction and internal rotation of the arm places considerable tension on any soft tissue repair and weakens the capsulomuscular wall. Finally, the repair stretches sufficiently to cause complete loss of muscle balance between the posterior and anterior rotator muscles. This permits dislocation to occur.

In all posterior dislocations I advance the insertions of the infraspinatus and teres minor, and, in addition, place an iliac bone graft on the posterior aspect of the neck of the scapula. I have never had a failure with this combination. When the glenoid is very shallow or the neck of the scapula has an increased retrotilt, instead of using a posterior bone graft, I do an osteotomy on the posterior neck of the scapula and rotate the posterior part of the glenoid anteriorly. The techniques for these operations are described in Chapter 7.

## BIBLIOGRAPHY

Abbott, L. C., Saunders, J. B., Hagey, H., and Jones, E. W., Jr.: Surgical approaches to the shoulder joint. J. Bone & Joint Surg., *31-A*: 235, 1949.

Adams, J. C.: Recurrent dislocation of the shoulder. J. Bone & Joint Surg., *30-B*:26, 1948.

Albee, F. H.: The bone graft wedge. Its use in the treatment of relapsing, acquired, and congenital dislocation of the hip. N. Y. Med. J., *102*:433, 1915.

Arden, G. P.: Posterior dislocation of both shoulders. Report of a case. J. Bone & Joint Surg., 38-B:558, 1956.

Asplund, G.: Ein operierter Fall von willkürlicher (habituellwillkürlicher) hinterer Schultergelenkluxation. Acta chir. scand. 87: 103, 1942.

Badajoz, E. J.: Posterior dislocations of the humerus from trauma. Rev. Ortop. Traum. (Brazil), 2/1:61, 1958.

Badgley, C. E.: Sports injuries of the shoulder girdle. JAMA, 172:444, 1960.

Bennett, G. E.: Shoulder and elbow lesions of the professional baseball pitcher. JAMA, 117: 510, 1941.

Bailey, R. W.: Acute and recurrent dislocation of the shoulder. J. Bone & Joint Surg., 49-A: 767, 1967.

Bankart, A. S. B.: Recurrent or habitual dislocation of the shoulder joint. Brit. Med. J., 2:1132, 1923.

————: Dislocation of the shoulder-joint. In Robert Jones Birthday Volume 307-314. London, Oxford Univ. Press, 1928.

————: The pathology and treatment of recurrent dislocation of the shoulder-joint. Brit. J. Surg., 26:23, 1938.

Bateman, J. E.: The shoulder and environs. St. Louis, C. V. Mosby, 1955.

————: Gallie technique for repair of recurrent dislocation of the shoulder. Surg. Clin. N. A., 43:1655, 1963.

Bibley, D. L.: Posterior dislocation of the shoulder joint. Brit. M. J. 5031:1345, 1957.

Biebl, R.: Behandlung und Prognose frischer Schulterluxationen. Arch. Orthop., 35:381, 1935.

Bonadeo Ayrolo, A.: Sobre un caso de luxación posterior recidivante de la articulación escápulohumeral. Rev. Ortop. Traum., 3:188, 1933.

Bost, F. C., and Inman, V. T.: The pathological changes in recurrent dislocation of the shoulder. A report of Bankart's operative procedure. J. Bone & Joint Surg., 24:595, 1942.

Broca, A., and Hartman, H.: Contribution à l'étude des luxations de l'épaule (luxations dites incomplète, décollements périostiques, luxations directes et luxations indirectes). Bull. Soc. Anat. de Paris, 65:312, 1890.

————: Contribution à l'étude des luxations de l'épaule (luxations anciennes, luxations recidivantes). Bull. Soc. Anat. de Paris, 65: 416, 1890.

Brow, W. H., Dennis, J. M., Davidson, C. N., Rubin, P. S., and Fulton, H.: Posterior dislocation of the shoulder. Radiology, 69:815, 1957.

Caird, F. M.: The shoulder joint in relation to certain dislocations and fractures. Edinburgh Med. J., 32:708, 1887.

Cameron, B. M.: Recurrent posterior dislocation of the shoulder. Texas J. Med., 51:33, 1955.

Carter, C., and Sweetman, R.: Recurrent dislocation of the patella and of the shoulder. Their association with familial joint laxity. J. Bone & Joint Surg., 42-B:721, 1960.

Clairmont, P. and Ehrlich, H.: Ein neues Operationsverfahren zur Behandlung der habituellen Schulterluxation mittels Muskelplastik. Verhandl. Deutsch. Ges. Chir., 38:79, 1909.

Codman, E. A.: The Shoulder. p. 12. Boston, The Author. 1934.

Cooper, Astley: On the dislocations of the os humeri upon the dorsum scapulae, and upon fractures near the shoulder joint. Guy's Hosp. Rep., 4:265, 1839.

Coover, C.: Double posterior luxation of the shoulder. Penn. Med. J., 35:566, 1932.

Copenhaver, W. M., and Johnson, D. D. (eds): Bailey's Textbook of Histology. Ed. 16. Baltimore. Williams & Wilkins, 1972.

Cowan, D. J., and Shaw, P. C.: Two cases of anterior subluxation of shoulder locking in abduction, J. Bone & Joint Surg., 46-B:108, 1964.

Cramer, F.: Resection des Oberarmkopfes wegen habitueller Luxation. (Nach einem imarztlichen Verein zu Wiesbaden gehaltenen Vortrage.) Berliner klin. Wschr., 19:21, 1882.

De Anquin, C.: A reliable operative procedure for recurrent dislocation of the shoulder. Scientific Exhibit, The American Academy of Orthopaedic Surgeons, Miami Beach, Florida, January 8-13, 1961.

Delorme, E.: Die Hemmungsbänder des Schultergelenks und ihre Bedeutung für die Schulterluxationen. Arch. klin. Chir., 92:79, 1910.

Denegri, L.: Sulla lussazione posteriore della spalla. Minerva ortop. (Torino), 8:383, 1957.

DePalma, A. F.: Surgery of the shoulder. Ed. 1. Philadelphia, J. B. Lippincott, 1950.

————: Results following a modified Magnuson procedure in recurrent dislocation of the shoulder. Surg. Clin. N. Am., 43:1651, 1963.

DePalma, A. F., Callery, G., and Bennett, G. A.: Variational anatomy and degenerative lesions of the shoulder joint. American Academy of Orthopedic Surgeons Instructional Course Lectures, 6:255, 1949.

Dickson, J. W., and Devas, M. B.: Bankart's operation for recurrent dislocation of the shoulder. J. Bone & Joint Surg., 39-B:114, 1957.

Dorgan, J. A.: Posterior dislocation of the shoulder. Am. J. Surg., *89*:890, 1955.

DuToit, G. T., and Roux, D.: Recurrent dislocation of the shoulder (A twenty-four year study of the Johannesburg stapling operation). J. Bone & Joint Surg., *38-A*:1, 1956.

Eden, R.: Zur Operation der habituellen Schulterluxation unter Mitteilung eines neuen Verfahrens bei Abriss am inneren Pfannenrande. Deutsch. Z. Chir., *144*:269, 1918.

Eyre-Brooks, A. L.: Recurrent dislocation of the shoulder. J. Bone & Joint Surg., *30-B*:39, 1948.

Fèvre, M. M., and Mialaret, J.: Indications et technique des butées rétroglénoidiennes dans les luxations postérieures de l'épaule. J. Chir., *52*:156, 1938.

Fick, R.: Handbuch der Anatomie und Mechanik der Gelenke. *In*: von Bardeleben: Handbuch der Anatomie des Menschen. Vol. 2. Sect. 1, Part 1, pp. 163-187. Jena, Gustav Fischer, 1910.

Finerty, J. C., and Cowdry, E. V.: A Textbook of Histology. Fifth edition. Philadelphia, Lea & Febiger, 1960.

Finsterer, H.: Die operative Behandlung der habituellen Schulterluxation. Deutsch. Z. Chir., *141*:354, 1917.

Fried, A.: Habitual posterior dislocation of the shoulder joint. Acta. orthop. scand., *18*:329, 1949.

Galli, H.: Habitual posterior shoulder dislocation. Z. Orthop., *92*:97, 1959.

Gallie, W. E., and LeMesurier, A. B.: An operation for the relief of recurring dislocation of the shoulder. Trans. Am. Surg. As., *45*:392, 1927.

———: Recurring dislocation of the shoulder. J. Bone & Joint Surg., *30-B*:9, 1948.

Gardner, E., and Gray, D. J.: Prenatal development of the human shoulder and acromioclavicular joints. Am. J. Anat., *92*:219, 1953.

Giannestras, N. J.: Discussion of traumatic posterior (retroglenoid) dislocation of the humerus by J. C. Wilson and F. M. McKeever. J. Bone & Joint Surg., *31-A*:172, 1949.

Glasser, O.: Cinematography in Roentgenography. Medical Physics, vol. 3. Chicago, Year Book Publishers, 1960.

Gomez Barneuvo, L.: Posterior luxation of the shoulder. Rev. ortop. traum., *2/1*:54, 1958.

Greep, R. O.: Histology. Ed. 2. New York, Blakiston, 1966.

Haines, R. W.: The development of joints. J. Anat., *81*:33, 1947.

Ham, A. W.: Histology. Ed. 6. Philadelphia: J. B. Lippincott, 1969.

Harmon, P. H.: The posterior approach for arthrodesis and other operations on the shoulder. Surg., Gynec., Obstet., *81*:266, 1945.

Hass, J. and Hass, R. Arthrochalasis multiplex congenita. Congenital flaccidity of the joints. J. Bone & Joint Surg., *40-A*:663, 1958.

Helfet, A. J.: Coracoid transplantation for recurring dislocation of the shoulder. J. Bone & Joint Surg., *40-B*:198, 1958.

Henderson, M. S.: Tenosuspension operation for recurrent or habitual dislocation of the shoulder. Surg. Clin. N. Am., *29*:997, 1949.

Hermodsson, M. S.: Röentgenologischen Studien über die traumatischen und habituellen Schultergelenkverrenkungen nach vorn und nach unten. Acta. radiol., Suppl. 20, 1934.

Hill, H. A., and Sachs, M. D.: The grooved defect of the humeral head. A frequently unrecognized complication of dislocations of the shoulder. Radiology, *35*:690, 1940.

Hindenach, J. C. R.: Recurrent posterior dislocation of the shoulder. J. Bone & Joint Surg., *29*:582, 1947.

Hindmarsh, K., and Lindberg, A.: Eden-Hybbinetti's operation for recurrent dislocation of the humeroscapular joint. Acta. orthop. scand., *38*:459, 1967.

The Genuine Works of Hippocrates. Translated by Francis Adams. Vol. 2. pp. 553-654. London, Sydenham Society, 1849.

Hybbinette, S.: De la Transplantation d'un fragment osseux pour remédier aux luxations récidivantes de l'épaule; constatations et résultats opératoires. Acta chir. scan., *71*:411, 1932.

Ilfeld, F. W., and Holder, H. G.: Recurrent dislocation of the shoulder joint. J. Bone & Joint Surg., *25*:651, 1943.

Inman, V. T., Saunders, J. B., and Abbott, L. C.: Observations on the function of the shoulder joint. J. Bone & Joint Surg., *26*:1, 1944.

Jens, J.: The role of the subscapularis muscle in recurring dislocation of the shoulder. J. Bone & Joint Surg., *46-B*:780,

Joessel: Ueber die Recidive der Humerusluxationen. Deutsche Z. Chir., *13*:167, 1880.

Jones, V.: Recurrent posterior dislocation of the shoulder. Report of a case treated by posterior bone block. J. Bone & Joint Surg., *40-B*:203, 1958.

Judet, J., Judet, R, Lagrange, J., and Moreau, C.: A propos des luxations postérieures de l'épaule. Mém. Acad. Chir., *83*:30, 1957.

Keiser, R. P., and Wilson, C. L.: Bilateral recurrent dislocation of the shoulder (a traumatic) in a thirteen year old girl. J. Bone & Joint Surg., *43-A*:553, 1961.

Key, J. A., and Conwell, H. E.: The management of fractures, dislocations and sprains. Ed. 6. p. 383. St. Louis, C. V. Mosby, 1956.

Kocher, T.: Eine neue Reductionsmethode für Schulterverrenkung. Berliner Klin. Wschr., 7:101, 1870.

————: Textbook of Operative Surgery. Ed. 3. Translated from the fourth German edition by Harold J. Stiles. London, Adam and Charles Black, 1911.

Kuster, E.: Ueber habituelle Schulterluxation. Verhandl. deutschen Ges. Chir., 11:112, 1882.

Landsmeer, J. M. F., and Meyers, K. A. E.: The shoulder region exposed by anatomical dissection. Arch. Chir. Neerl., 11:174, 1959.

Leguit, P.: Habituelle Schoulderluxatie. Thesis. Assen, Van Grocum and Co., 1942.

McLaughlin, H. L.: Discussion of acute anterior dislocation of the shoulder by Toufick Nicola. J. Bone & Joint Surg., 31-A:172, 1949.

————: Posterior dislocation of the shoulder. J. Bone & Joint Surg., 34-A:584, 1952.

————: Recurrent anterior dislocation of the shoulder. Morbid anatomy. Am. J. Surg., 99:628, 1960.

McLaughlin H. L., and Cavallero, N. U.: Primary anterior dislocation of the shoulder. Am. J. Surg., 80:615, 1950.

Magnuson, P. B.: Treatment of recurrent dislocation of the shoulder. Surg. Clin. N. Am., 25:14, 1945.

————: Discussion of paper of Brau, E. A.: Evaluation of the Putti-Platt reconstruction procedure for recurrent dislocation of the shoulder. J. Bone & Joint Surg., 37-A:731, 1955.

Magnuson, P. B., and Stack, J. K.: Recurrent dislocation of the shoulder. JAMA, 123:889, 1943.

Malgaigne, J. F.: Traité des Fractures et des Luxations. Paris, J.-B. Ballière, 1855.

Manzoni, A.: Lussaizione posteriore della spalla; Arch. Ortop. (Milan) 71:631-638, 1958.

May, H.: Nicola operation for posterior subacromial dislocation of the humerus. J. Bone & Joint Surg., 25:78, 1943.

Michaelis, L. S.: Internal rotation dislocation of the shoulder. Report of a case. J. Bone & Joint Surg., 32-B:223, 1950.

Miller, E. R.: X-Ray movies—Editorial radiology, Radiology, October, 1954.

————: Cinefluorography in practice. Radiology, 73:560, 1959.

Miller, E. R., and Lusted, L. B.: Progress in indirect cineroentgenography. Am. J. Roentgenol., 75:56, 1956.

Miller, E. R., Nickel, and Lusted, L. B.: Cineradiography. Inst. of Radio Engineers National Convention, March 1955. Convention Record, Part 9.

Möllerud, A.: A case of bilateral habitual luxation in the posterior part of the shoulder joint. Acta. chir. scand., 94:181, 1946.

Moseley, H. F.: The use of a metallic glenoid rim in recurrent dislocation of the shoulder. Canad. M. A. J., 56:320, 1947.

————: An Atlas of Shoulder Dislocations. North Chicago, Abbott Laboratories, 1951.

————: Shoulder lesions. Ed. 2. New York, Paul B. Hoeber, 1953.

————: Athletic injuries to the shoulder region. Am. J. Surg., 98:401, 1959.

————: Recurrent Dislocation of the Shoulder. Montreal, McGill University Press, 1961.

Moseley, H. F., and Overgaard, B.: The anterior capsular mechanism in recurrent dislocation of the shoulder (Morphological and clinical studies with special reference to the glenoid labrum and the glenohumeral ligaments). J. Bone & Joint Surg., 44B-913, 1962.

Moullin, C. W. M., and Keith, A.: Notes on a case of backward dislocation of the head of the humerus caused by muscular action. Lancet, 1:496, 1904.

Mynter, H.: Subacromial dislocation from muscle spasm. Ann. Surg., 36:117, 1902.

Nicola, Toufick: Recurrent dislocation of the shoulder. Am. J. Surg., 86:85, 1953.

————: Recurrent dislocation of the shoulder. Its treatment by transplantation of the long head of the biceps. Am. J. Surg., 6:815, 1929.

Nobel, W.: Posterior traumatic dislocation of the shoulder. J. Bone & Joint Surg., 44-A: 523, 1962.

O'Conner, G. A., and Badgley, C. E.: Combined procedure for the repair of recurrent dislocation of the shoulder (to be published).

Olsson, O.: Degenerative changes of the shoulder joint and their connection with shoulder pain, Acta chir. scand., Supp. 181, 1953.

Ombredanne, L.: Butée ostéoplastique pour luxation congenitale de l'épaule en arriére. J. chir., 43:481, 1934.

Osmond-Clarke H.: Habitual dislocation of the shoulder. J. Bone & Joint Surg., 30-B:19, 1948.

Palmer, I., and Widén, A.: The bone block method for recurrent dislocation of the shoulder joint. J. Bone & Joint Surg., 30-B:53, 1948.

Perkins, G.: Rest and movement. J. Bone & Joint Surg., 35-B:521, 1953.

Perthes, G.: Über Operationen bei habitueller Schulterluxation. Deutsch. Z. Chir., 85:199, 1906.

Peycelon, R., Replumas, P., and Michel, C. R.: Les luxations postérieures traumatiques de l'épaule, Rev. chir. orthop., 42:630, 1956.

Popke: Zur Kasuistik und Therapie der habituellen Schulterluxation. Inaug. Dissert., Halle, 1882.

Preston, M. E.: Fractures and Dislocations: Diagnosis and Treatment. p. 62. St. Louis, C. V. Mosby, 1915.

Rendlich, R. A., and Poppel, M. H.: Roentgen diagnosis of posterior dislocation of the shoulder. Radiology, *36*:42, 1941.

Robertson, R., and Stark, W. J.: Diagnosis and treatment of recurrent dislocation of the shoulder. J. Bone & Joint Surg., *29*:797, 1947.

Rocher, H. L.: Butée glénodienne postérieure par greffon costal dans une subluxation habituelle de l'épaule due a une paralysie obstrétricale. Rev. Tech. Chirurg. (Paris Chirurg.), *23*:33, 1931.

Rowe, C. R.: Prognosis in dislocations of shoulders. J. Bone & Joint Surg., *38-A*:957, 1956.

———: The surgical management of recurrent dislocation of the shoulder using a modified Bankart procedure. Surg. Clin. N. Am., *43*:1663, 1963.

Rowe, C. R., and Sakellarides, H. T.: Factors related to recurrences of anterior dislocations of the shoulder. Clin. Orthop., *20*:40, 1961.

Rowe, C. R., and Yee, L. B. K.: A posterior approach to the shoulder joint. J. Bone & Joint Surg., *26*:580, 1944.

Saha, A. K.: Anterior recurrent dislocation of the shoulder. Acta. orthop. scand., *68*:479, 1967.

Samilson, R. L., and Miller, E.: Posterior dislocations of the shoulder. Clin. Orthop., *32*:69, 1964.

Schlemm, F.: Ueber die Verstarkungsbänder am Schultergelenk. Arch. Anat., Physiol., wissenschaftliche Med. p. 45, 1853.

Scott, D. J., Jr.: Treatment of recurrent posterior dislocations of the shoulder by glenoplasty. J. Bone & Joint Surg., *49-A*:471, 1967.

Scougall, S.: Posterior dislocation of the shoulder. J. Bone & Joint Surg., *39-B*:726, 1957.

Sharkawi, A. H.: Posterior dislocation of the shoulder. J. Egypt Med. A., *4*:22, 1958.

Sjovall, H.: A case of spontaneous backward subluxation of the shoulder, treated by the Clairmont-Ehrlich operation. Nord. med. *21*:474, 1944.

Sutton, J. B.: On the Nature of Ligaments (Part II). J. Anatomy & Physiol., 19:27, 1884.

Taylor, R. G., and Wright, P. R.: Posterior dislocation of the shoulder. Report of six cases. J. Bone & Joint Surg., *34-B*:624, 1952.

Thomas, M. A.: Posterior subacromial dislocation of the head of the humerus. Am. J. Roentgenol., *37*:767, 1937.

Toumey, J. W.: Posterior recurrent dislocation of the shoulder, treated by capsulorraphy and iliac bone block. Lahey Clin. Bull., *5*:197, 1948.

Townley, C. O.: The capsular mechanism in recurrent dislocation of the shoulder. J. Bone Joint Surg., *32A*:370, 1950.

Warrick, C. K.: Posterior dislocation of the shoulder joint. J. Bone & Joint Surg., *30-B*: 651, 1948.

Watson-Jones, R.: Recurrent dislocation of the shoulder. Editorial, J. Bone & Joint Surg., *30-B*:6, 1948.

Weissman, S. L., and Torok, G.: Bilateral recurrent posterior dislocation of the shoulder. J. Bone & Joint Surg., *40-A*:479, 1958.

Welcker, H.: Ueber das Huftgelenk, nebst Bemerkungen über Gelenke überhaupt, insbesondere über das Schultergelenk. Z. Anat. Entwicklungsges., *1*:41, 1876.

Wickstrom, J.: Birth injuries of the brachial plexus: treatment of defects in the shoulder. Clin. Orthop., *23*:187, 1962.

Wilson, J. C., and McKeever, F. N.: Traumatic posterior (retroglenoid) dislocation of the humerus. J. Bone & Joint Surg., *31-A*:160, 1949.

Wood, J. P.: Posterior dislocation of the head of the humerus and diagnostic value of lateral and vertical views. U. S. Navy Med. Bull., *32*:532, 1941.

Zadik, F. R.: Recurrent posterior dislocation of the shoulder joint. J. Bone & Joint Surg., *30-B*:531, 1948.

# 11

# Shoulder Lesions Associated with Degenerative Changes

The degenerative changes that occur with aging in the different articulations of the shoulder were discussed in Chapter 6. These are the result of wear and tear in normal physiological function. However, they may be influenced by other circumstances: trauma, occupation, disease and even congenital factors; the building blocks in some people are made of better material than in others. In most people, the degenerative alterations are compatible with satisfactory function. Nevertheless, these abnormalities are the foundation for the development of many disorders about the shoulder. Some of these can be the source of pain and dysfunction.

Since aging is the prime factor in the development of degenerative changes, disabling lesions associated with these changes occur after the fourth decade of life, but there are exceptions to this time table.

The syndrome, including pain, muscle spasm and restriction of motion of the glenohumeral joint, may arise from many sources. In fact, it may be impossible to pinpoint the exact cause of the syndrome by clinical and x-ray examinations. Only exploration of the area reveals the responsible pathology. Bosworth designated this all-inclusive clinical picture "the supraspinatus syndrome," and, because the treatment of many of the lesions causing this clinical pattern is the same, the designation is an appropriate one. However, since the time Bosworth wrote of the supraspinatus syndrome and McLaughlin of the "internal derangement of the subacromial joint" we have learned much about the pathological processes that affect the shoulder joint. Also, new diagnostic tools are at our disposal, so that many of the lesions that could not at one time be recognized, except by exploration of the shoulder, can now be diagnosed. X-ray shows the calcific deposit, and arthrograms establish the diagnosis of an incomplete or a complete tear of the cuff and of a frozen shoulder.

The chief obstacle to a specific diagnosis is the compactness of the subacromial region of the shoulder. The intimate relation of the many structures in this small area makes it almost impossible to detect clinically the source of trouble. In this compact area are the musculotendinous cuff, the subacromial bursa, the coracoacromial ligament, the biceps tendon and the bicipital groove. Also, although not in the subacromial region, lesions of the acromioclavicular joint may confuse the picture.

## THE SUBACROMIAL REGION

The interval between the undersurface of the acromion and its extension, the coracoacromial ligament, and the musculotendinous cuff and tuberosities is indeed a narrow one. In this space lies the subacromial bursa. This is the largest bursa in the body; its roof is attached to the undersurface of the acromion, to the underside of the coracoacromial ligament and to the fibers of the deltoid arising from the edge of the acromion. Its base is firmly adherent

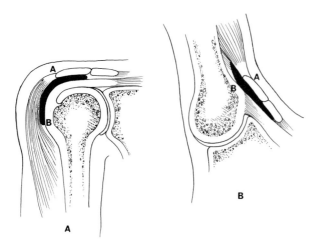

FIG. 11-1. Coronal section through the right shoulder. (A) The roof of the bursa is attached to the undersurface of the acromion, the undersurface of the coracoacromial ligament and the subdeltoid fascia. Its base is firmly attached to the outer ¾ inch of the greater tuberosity and to the distal ¾ inch of the musculotendinous cuff. The periphery of the bursa lies beyond the sites of anchorage above and below. (B) During elevation of the arm the periphery folds on itself or travels, as its fixed base assumes different positions in relation to the fixed roof. Note that during elevation the tuberosity passes under the acromion and point Ⓑ passes to point Ⓐ.

to the upper and outer ¾ of an inch of the greater tuberosity and to about ¾ of an inch of the musculotendinous cuff where it attaches to the tuberosities. The periphery extends distally under the deltoid, posteriorly and laterally under the acromion and medially under the coracoid. Here it lies between the coracoid and the subscapularis and under the conjoined tendon of the short head of the biceps and the coracobrachialis. It is clear that the so-called subdeltoid bursa and subcoracoid bursa are nothing more than extensions of the subacromial bursa. In the normal state the bursa is really a collapsed sac made of a fine, delicate membrane whose inner surface is lined by a delicate layer of synovial cells and whose walls are separated by nothing more than a film of synovial fluid.

From a functional point of view, the subacromial bursa can be considered a *secondary scapulohumeral joint*. During motion, one surface moves on the other in any direction, but they never separate from one another, even on rotation. In order to adjust itself to the wide range of motion of the arm, the periphery of the bursa folds on itself as its fixed base assumes different positions in relation to the fixed roof (Fig. 11-1). The bursa is concave-convex in shape and lies slightly obliquely. When the

bursa is distended it forms a concavoconvex sac under the deltoid and lies in an anterolateral position (Fig. 11-2).

In the normal shoulder the floor of the bursa is smooth, glistening and symmetrical. The musculotendinous cuff completely fills the sulcus at the junction of the head and neck of the humerus. Then, it is continuous with the outer surfaces of the tuberosities. The surface looks like that of a true articular joint.

It is apparent that any alterations in the floor or roof of the bursa that reduce the interval between the coracoacromial arch and the head of the humerus or any incongruity of the opposing surfaces of these structures inflict trauma on the walls of the bursa, which in turn initiates an inflammatory, proliferative process. Consequently, on motion of the arm, the bursal walls buckle and impinge on the edge of the acromion or coracoacromial ligament when the arm is elevated. Furthermore, adhesions firmly binding the roof to the floor of the bursa restrict motion of the arm.

What are some of the lesions that might disturb the normal mechanics of the joint by implicating the subacromial bursa? There are several, all producing similar signs and symptoms, and at one time all were included in the supraspinatus syndrome. They are degeneration of the tendons of the musculotendinous cuff, chronic strains of these tendons (tendonitis), incomplete tears of the cuff, bicipital tenosynovitis and calcific deposits. Although rare, lesions that primarily affect the bursa should also be considered in the differential diagnosis of this region. These include such lesions as villonodular synovitis, osteochondromatosis, tuberculosis and rheumatoid arthritis.

## SUPRASPINATUS SYNDROME

In my opinion, there are really only two lesions that can be included in the supraspinatus syndrome: (1) degeneration of the tendons of the rotator cuff, and (2) chronic sprains of the tendons from repetitive trauma. In both, the subacromial bursa is involved secondarily and, hence, a subacromial bursitis always accompanies these lesions.

At this point, it should be emphasized that a primary subacromial bursitis does not occur in people past middle life. However, a bursitis almost always occurs secondary to other pathology in the subacromial area. The exceptions to this are such lesions as osteochondromatosis, villonodular synovitis, rheumatoid arthritis and tuberculosis. The last entity is indeed rare but I have seen two instances without implication of the shoulder joint. On the other hand, a primary bursitis does occur in young athletes such as baseball pitchers. In the act of throwing they may repeatedly jam the head of the humerus against the coracoacromial arch. This maneuver traumatizes the subacromial bursa which may become acutely inflamed. But even in these athletes the bursitis may be secondary to a severe strain of the muscle-tendon units of the rotator muscles.

### Clinical Picture

The clinical manifestations of the supraspinatus syndrome are pain, muscle spasm, atrophy of the spinati muscles and tender-

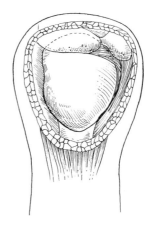

FIG. 11-2. The supralateral view of the right shoulder. Note that the bursa is concave-convex and lies in the anterolateral position.

ness over the site of insertion of the musculotendinous cuff. Usually the maximum site of tenderness is over the supraspinatus tendon. When the cause is degeneration of the cuff, the tendons may be frayed, laminated and torn from their insertion into the head of the humerus. The tears are usually incomplete and may be on the deep or the superficial surface of the tendon. Those on the deep surface can be visualized by arthrography, those on the outer surface cannot. As stated previously, complete tears should not be included in the supraspinatus syndrome, because they can be diagnosed by arthrography. Unfortunately, this tool is still not used as often as it should be in the diagnosis of shoulder lesions; and, since small complete tears produce the same clinical picture as that described above, although without loss of muscle power, they often are never recognized. Also, they respond to the treatment used for degeneration and chronic strains of the cuff.

The degenerative process in the tendons is aggravated by repetitive minor trauma; more tendon fibers tear, old tears become larger, and fraying and lamination of the fibers increase. Degenerative alterations are more severe in the region of the supraspinatus tendon than elsewhere on the outer side of the cuff. I have made this observation many times at the operating table. But, more important, this same finding was emphasized in the record of the observations made on 100 shoulders in our investigation on the bursal side of the cuff (*see* p. 117). It appears that the supraspinatus region of the cuff is an area of greater stress and strain than the other areas. The secondary changes that follow make the supraspinatus tendon more likely to impinge against some point on the coracoacromial arch than the other tendons of the cuff.

Degenerated tissue is avascular tissue; therefore, adequate healing never occurs. The cuff tendons become permeated with friable scar tissue, and abortive attempts in healing only produce much poorly organized granulation tissue. The accumulative result of this process is the "piling up" of scar tissue and degenerated tendon fibers which reduce the interval between the coracoacromial arch and the tuberosities. This space is further compromised by the secondary inflammatory response of the subacromial bursa. The bursal walls become thickened and edematous and the synovial lining forms villi of varying sizes and shapes.

Under these circumstances the patient may be unable to abduct the arm completely, or he feels that the arm locks at certain positions of abduction, or he feels a jog or snap before he can complete the abduction movement. All this means that the degenerated and inflammatory tissue in the cuff tendons and subacromial bursa rolls up in front of the edge of the acromion when the patient attempts to abduct the arm. If he is successful in forcing this tissue under and beyond the edge of the acromion he feels a snap or jog.

Chronic strains of the rotator tendons may occur in any age group. In the athlete, frequent repetitions of the act of throwing may produce microscopic tears at the insertion of the muscle-tendon units of the rotator muscles. Initially they may cause

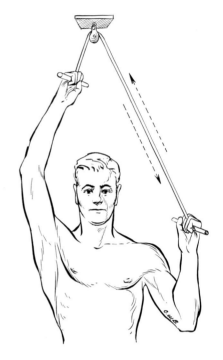

FIG. 11-3. (Continued on facing page) Exercises for shoulder

no dysfunction, but, with time, scarring and attritional changes occur at the sites of insult, resulting in chronic tendonitis. Swelling and proliferation of the injured tissues follow; also, the bursal walls become secondarily involved. The thickened tissues reduce the size of the interval between the coracoacromial arch and the tuberosities. Consequently, motions of abduction are restricted because of pain when the inflamed bursa is squeezed under the arch or by an actual mechanical block.

The same mechanism of injury to the muscle-tendon units occurs in people past middle age. The repeated trauma to the cuff may occur during occupational activities. The chronic strains aggravate the existing degenerative process in the cuff tendons and induce secondary inflammatory changes in the walls of the subacromial bursa.

Tears on the synovial side of the rotator cuff and small complete tears represent advanced stages of the degenerative alterations normally found in this region, and

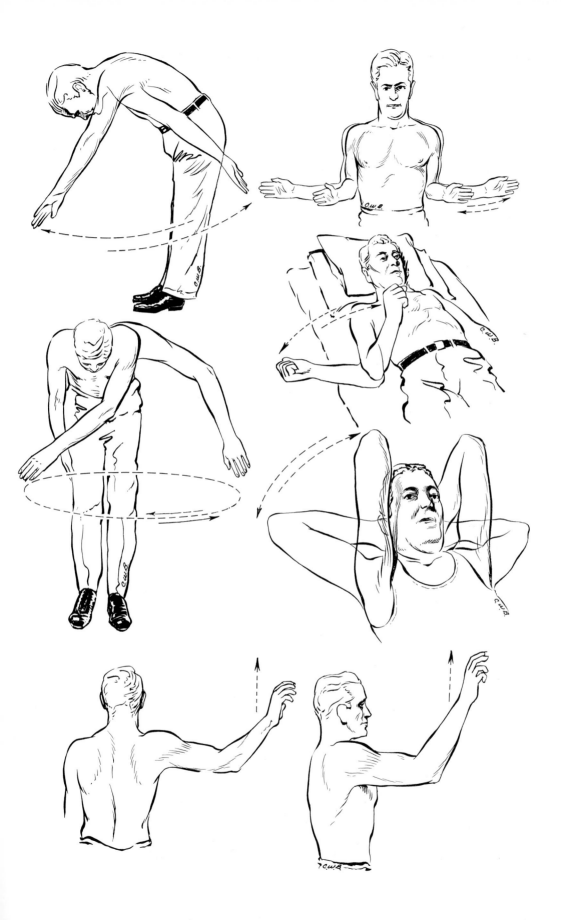

they may be readily extended by repeated minor trauma. It should be remembered that the degenerative changes render the cuff, at its insertion, avascular, inelastic and weak. This is now the weakest portion of the muscle-tendon unit and hence the most vulnerable. The clinical picture of these lesions and their treatment are the same as those of the other entities in the supraspinatus syndrome.

## Management

In most instances, conservative management relieves pain and muscle spasm and restores function. Since a specific diagnosis is often not made, the treatment is directed toward the relief of symptoms and restoration of function. The most essential feature of the program is rest to the shoulder. If the shoulder is put at rest, the inflammatory process in the cuff and bursa will subside. This relieves pain and muscle spasm and restores motion. Rest does not mean complete immobilization of the limb; rather, permit the use of the arm only within the painless arcs of motion. Only in acute episodes is enforcement of total rest justified; and this must not be prolonged, for people in this age group are prone to develop frozen shoulders. Usually the use of a sling in between exercise periods suffices. Abduction splints should never be used.

Physical therapy in the form of radiant heat and gentle massage is beneficial. Mild pendulum exercises are most important. They preserve muscle tone and prevent formation of adhesions in the bursa and capsule of the joint. The exercises should always be performed within painless arcs of motion and, at first, in the stooped position. This position permits the patient to abduct the arm by gravity without the need of a fulcrum against the glenoid. Indeed, in this position the rotator muscles are relaxed; very little muscular effort is necessary to move the arm, and the weight of the arm stretches the contracted capsular, bursal and cuff tissues (Fig. 11-3).

Often the local injection of steroids relieves pain and reduces the local inflammation and swelling. Remember that any injection into the tissues of the shoulder joint (as in any other joint) must be done with strict aseptic technique. I have seen too many suppurative shoulder joints following injections; these are avoidable tragedies.

Unless there is a serious cuff lesion, the patient shows considerable improvement in 2 or 3 to 6 weeks. If the syndrome does not respond to adequate treatment, it must be assumed that a serious cuff lesion exists, and exploration of the joint is indicated. However, before surgery is performed, the shoulder should again be examined carefully and an arthrogram should be done. The arthrogram will establish the diagnosis of a partial tear on the inside of the cuff and also of a complete tear of the cuff. Although I avoid excision of any part of the acromion, in cases of chronic tendonitis of the rotator muscles acromionectomy has a place and should be done (*see* Chapter 7).

## INCOMPLETE TEARS OF THE ROTATOR CUFF

### Types of Incomplete Tears

It should be remembered that incomplete tears of the rotator cuff occur after the fourth decade from normal wear and tear of the shoulder. These lesions may produce no pain or restriction of motion. Incomplete or partial tears involve only a portion of the cuff, so that the continuity of the cuff remains intact. There is no communication between the joint cavity and the subacromial bursa. The lesions may occur on the synovial side of the cuff, on the bursal side or deep within the substance of the musculotendinous cuff, or the tears may run parallel with the cuff fibers. The nature of this pathology differs from that found in complete tears in that in the complete tears the entire thickness of the cuff undergoes degeneration. Consequently, the joint cavity communicates with the subacromial bursa.

## Pathology of Incomplete Tears on the Synovial Side of the Cuff

I shall discuss primarily lesions on the synovial side of the cuff, for these are the tears that are most frequently responsible for pain and restriction of motion of the arm. With aging, some of the innermost fibers of the cuff tear from their insertion into the humeral head. With each successive decade the severity of the lesions rises, and the most profound lesions are found in the sixth and seventh decades. The characteristic features of these lesions (which have been pointed out previously) are as follows: (1) As a rule, tears in the supraspinatus tendon extend into the infraspinatus tendon for varying distances; (2) suprainfraspinatus tears occur in 37.3 percent and subscapularis tears in 20 percent of the patients; (3) the lesions vary from small tears to extensive tearing, fraying and thinning of all regions of the cuff (*see* Fig. 6-20); (4) in moderate or severe lesions the torn fibers and the synovial membrane just proximal to the tears are hypertrophied and thickened (*see* Fig. 6-18).

It is clear that when the pathology described above is present, excessive use of the arm, minor injuries and, certainly, severe injuries may extend the existing tears. Such extension of the lesions is invariably accompanied by local hemorrhage and edema of the affected tissues and irritation of the overlying bursa. The walls of the bursa then become swollen and hypertrophied and the space between the coracoacromial arch and the tuberosities is reduced in size. The stage is now set for development of the symptoms of the supraspinatus syndrome described above.

Although incomplete tears of the subscapularis tendon are relatively common in the aging shoulder (20%), they rarely give rise to pain and restriction of motion. This is not true of the supra-infraspinatus region of the cuff, which is a common source of trouble.

Symptomatic incomplete tears occur not only after the age of 40 years. They can occur in young people also—especially athletes. Also, they not infrequently occur in dislocations of the shoulder. Because these lesions are not suspected in the young, frequently the diagnosis is never made.

## Mechanisms of Injury to the Cuff

Direct injuries to the shoulder never cause an extension of existing tears or produce fresh tears of the cuff. This region is adequately protected by the overhanging acromion which receives all impacts delivered to the point of the shoulder. Rather, the lesions are produced by indirect mechanisms that impose on the cuff strains beyond its functional capacity. This is particularly true of the supraspinatus region of the cuff.

In the older age group, the usual history of injury is of a fall on the outstretched arm or of sudden forceful abduction of the arm while grasping a heavy object. When the degenerative changes in the cuff are profound, the simple act of picking up some object or suddenly elevating the arm may be all that is necessary to extend the existing lesions.

However, in young people, much greater force is required to produce a primary tear of the cuff fibers. The baseball pitcher may sustain a partial or complete tear of the cuff when delivering a powerful pitch. Also, strenuous abduction of the arm against resistance may produce tears of the cuff such as occur when a defensive football player tries to block an onrushing ball carrier with his outstretched arm.

## Clinical Picture

The clinical manifestations of incomplete tears on the synovial side of the cuff are the same as those described for the supraspinatus syndrome. Routine x-ray examination cannot establish the diagnosis of this lesion; however, arthrograms will do so. Arthrograms clearly visualize a lesion on

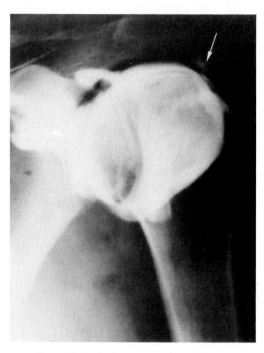

FIG. 11-4. Arthrogram visualizing an incomplete tear (arrow). (Courtesy of R. H. Freiberger)

the inner side of the cuff and should be performed routinely in all patients with a supraspinatus syndrome (Fig. 11-4). It should be remembered that, although incomplete tears may restrict abduction of the arm because of the associated pain, muscle spasm, or even mechanical blocking, they do not preclude powerful abduction. This is also true of small complete tears of the cuff. Arthrograms establish the differential diagnosis.

In some instances, the pain and muscle spasm do not allow the patient to abduct the arm. In such cases it is difficult to determine whether the lesion is a complete massive tear or an incomplete tear. In these instances, the injection of 10 ml. of a 1 percent solution of procaine into the suspected area of injury will relieve pain and muscle spasm sufficiently to allow the patient to abduct the arm, provided that the continuity of the cuff is intact. If the patient cannot abduct the arm or if abduction cannot be maintained against resistance, then it must be assumed that the lesion is a mas-

sive tear of the cuff. Again, the arthrograms establish the differential diagnosis.

## Management

Most incomplete tears respond to the conservative treatment described for the supraspinatus syndrome. However, if after 6 weeks severe pain and disability still persist, the shoulder should be explored, the incomplete tear visualized and the defective portion of the cuff excised. This surgical procedure is described on page 223.

### COMPLETE TEARS OF THE ROTATOR CUFF

Complete tears of the rotator cuff implicate the entire thickness of the cuff so that there is direct communication between the joint cavity and the subacromial bursa. As reported previously, these lesions may exist in people after the fourth decade without clinical manifestations or loss of abduction. They represent an advanced stage of the degenerative changes that normally occur with aging in the rotator cuff. Of the 96 shoulders investigated, 9.3 percent had complete tears of varying size, ranging from 1 centimeter to massive separation of the cuff from the humeral head (*see* p. 114).

It becomes apparent that in the face of severe degeneration of the cuff, excessive stress imposed on the rotator unit may cause a tearing away of a degenerated but intact cuff from its insertion or may extend an existing complete tear. The amount of force necessary to produce these lesions varies greatly. In general, the more profound the alterations the less is the force required to disrupt the cuff. Indeed, in some instances, extensive lesions may occur without any injury.

### Types of Complete Tears

Clinically, the cuff may exhibit four types of tears: (1) the pure transverse tear, (2)

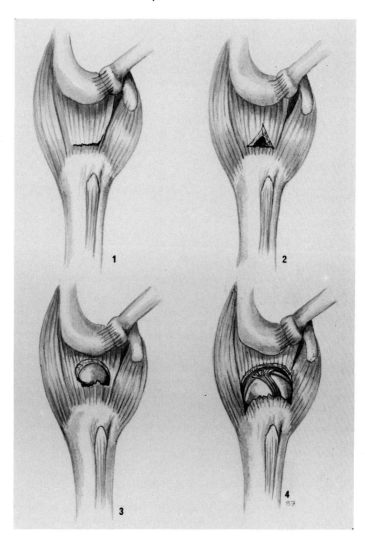

FIG. 11-5. Types of Tears: (1) pure transverse tear; (2) pure vertical tear; (3) tears with retraction; (4) massive avulsion of the cuff.

pure vertical tears or rents, (3) tears with retraction and (4) massive avulsion of the cuff (Fig. 11-5).

## Pure Transverse Tears

These are not common lesions. Transverse tears occur in the cuff fibers just proximal to their line of insertion into the tuberosity. The torn tendon retracts very little if at all, because the edges of the defect are continuous with the adjacent intact cuff. Interestingly, in a study I made of shoulders of autopsy or cadaver specimens, I found no pure transverse tears.

The small complete tears were irregular, circular defects in the cuff, some of which exhibited a longitudinal extension of varying length, starting from the anterior margin of the defect. The large tears were either triangular or crescentic. From these findings it is logical to assume that the pure transverse tear found at operation is the direct result of injury, usually in the form of excessive stress, superimposed upon a weakened and degenerated cuff.

Also, it is reasonable to assume that many pure transverse tears do not cause serious disability, that many heal spontaneously, just as incomplete tears do, and

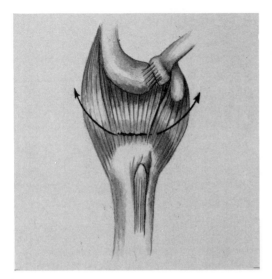 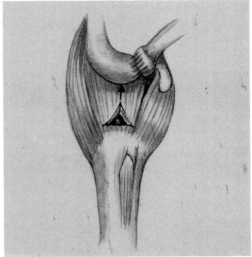

(*Left*) FIG. 11-6. One concept of the evolution of a complete tear with retraction (Jones). A rupture of the cuff at a point just proximal to the insertion of the supraspinatus tendon. Divergent forces produced by the rotator muscles cause extension of the defect.

(*Right*) FIG. 11-7. Another concept of the evolution of complete tears with retraction. The primary tear is transverse; its edges are anchored by the adjacent intact cuff; the final defect is caused by the pull of the supraspinatus in a proximal direction.

that very few require surgical exploration and repair.

### Pure Vertical or Longitudinal Rents

These are the lesions usually sustained by young persons. Great force is required to produce them; often they are concomitant with fractures and dislocations of the humeral head. As a rule, the rents run parallel with the cuff fibers through the fibers of the coracohumeral ligament which occupies the interval between the supraspinatus and the subscapularis. Once the tear occurs its edges are kept separated by the opposing forces of the external rotators and the internal rotator (subscapularis). This mechanism prevents healing and favors extension of the tear.

I found no complete longitudinal tears, as described above, in the cuffs of cadaver or autopsy specimens. This leads me to conclude that such lesions invariably result from violent injury inflicted on strong, healthy musculotendinous cuffs of young persons. These cuffs are capable of resisting tearing of their fibers from their bony insertions.

In large tears the humeral head may subluxate into an anteroinferior position. In these instances, the intact, strong subscapularis pulls the head inferiorly and anteriorly.

Small longitudinal tears may give rise to no disability and most likely heal spontaneously. However, large rents cause marked dysfunction and require surgical repair. When the tear is in proximity to the biceps tendon, simple side-to-side repair may alter the gliding mechanism of the biceps tendon, causing bicipital tenosynovitis. In these instances, it is wise to anchor the biceps tendon in its groove and hence preclude the above complication.

### Tears with Retraction

At operation, the lesion presents as a triangular or crescentic defect in the cuff. There is considerable disagreement as to the mechanism producing this configuration of the defect. Some believe that as the result of repeated minor trauma or of a severe single trauma some fibers of the cuff are pulled off their insertions where the cuff exhibits the greatest amount of degeneration. This point is just proximal to the facet in the greater tuberosity into which the supraspinatus tendon inserts. The defect is thus subjected to forces pulling in opposite directions; the supraspinatus pulls directly upward, the infraspinatus and teres minor backward and the subscapularis forward and downward. This mechanism prevents healing and favors extension of the defect (Fig. 11-6).

Some workers are of the opinion that the primary tear is transverse; its edges are anchored by the adjacent intact cuff and the final defect in the cuff is caused by the pull of the supraspinatus in a proximal direction (Fig. 11-7). Others are of the opinion that excessive strains on a degenerated cuff produce a transverse tear. Repeated minor stresses cause a longitudinal split in the cuff, starting at the anterior end of the transverse tear and extending proximally. Further traumas, minor or severe, increase the size of the lesion along both the transverse and the longitudinal axis of the cuff fibers. In addition, divergent forces act on the longitudinal limb of the defect. The subscapularis pulls the anterior margin of the tear forward and the external rotators pull the posterior margin backward. The resulting defect is triangular or crescentic (Fig. 11.8).

In old lesions further degeneration of the cuff occurs. Also, a smooth, hypertrophied margin forms around the entire defect on its synovial side. This is Nature's frustrated attempt to repair the defect by a proliferative process in the synovialis just proximal to the torn cuff fibers. Codman referred to this thickened synovial margin as the "falciform ligament." At this point, a distinct transverse and longitudinal rent is no longer demonstrable, and the existing lesion can readily be misinterpreted as a transverse tear with retraction of the supraspinatus.

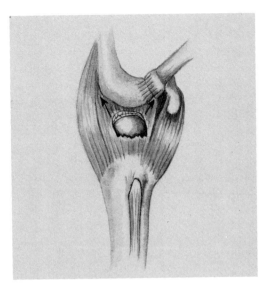

Fig. 11-8. Another concept of the evolution of complete tears with retraction. First a transverse tear occurs, then repeated stress produces a longitudinal split in the cuff; further traumas increase the size of the defect, and divergent forces act on the longitudinal limb of the defect, producing a triangular or crescentic defect (McLaughlin).

It may seem that the preceding discussion is purely academic and historical and has no bearing on the management of this lesion. This is not true. Understanding the evolution of the tear with retraction is necessary in order to evolve an operation that will correct the forces responsible for the lesion. I am in agreement with McLaughlin that the triangular or crescentic defect in the cuff is caused by divergent forces acting on a transverse tear with a longitudinal extension. Also, the repair he designed is a logical one, for by first doing a side-to-side repair the size of the defect is reduced and pull of the divergent forces is decreased.

## Massive Avulsion of the Cuff

The characteristic features of these lesions are massive avulsion and retraction of the cuff. Usually the greater portion of the cuff comprising the external rotators is involved. The longitudinal tear occurs, in most instances, between the supraspinatus and the subscapularis. But, in some instances, it runs through the very substance of the subscapularis muscle. Not infrequently the cuff slips between the glenoid and the humeral head. In a few instances, all four components of the cuff tear away from the head of the humerus and then retract. Most of these lesions occur in elderly people, but occasionally they occur in young persons who have sustained a violent injury. They are often concomitant with anterior dislocations, and often they are responsible for chronic subluxation of the shoulder.

**Clinical Features.** The pertinent clinical features are related to age, occupation, history of injury, pain, impaired function and local clinical findings.

AGE. Such lesions usually occur past middle life—a period during which there is indisputable evidence of attritional changes in the musculotendinous cuff. When complete tears occur in young people there is always a history of severe trauma.

OCCUPATION. In general, the lesions occur in people who perform strenuous work. These persons not only suffer minor trauma to the cuff constantly, which enhances the degenerative process, but also, by the very nature of their work, are vulnerable to trauma that may precipitate a complete tear.

HISTORY OF INJURY. Most patients give a history of injury, usually a fall on the outstretched arm. Next in frequency is a history of sudden abduction of the arm while grasping a heavy object. Occasionally the injury is so minor and insignificant that it is difficult to correlate it with the resulting cuff lesion. However, in the face of severe alterations in the cuff even minor trauma may produce severe cuff tears.

PAIN. A constant and characteristic feature is sudden, sharp pain localized to the tip of the shoulder. Also, the pain is referred to the insertion of the deltoid muscle. Not infrequently the patient feels a snapping or tearing sensation in the shoulder. Within a few hours the pain subsides only to recur with greater intensity in the next 6 to 12 hours. For the next 4 to 7 days, the pain becomes even more severe and then gradually diminishes. This return and increase of pain after a short period of relief is caused by hemorrhage which distends the affected tissues. Then, with cessation of bleeding and absorption of the blood, the pain subsides. During this painful period, muscle spasm may be so pronounced that an adequate examination of the shoulder is impossible. Later the pain becomes less intense but it is constant and any movements of the shoulder make it worse.

IMPAIRED FUNCTION. Impaired function may result either from disruption of the normal mechanics of the joint or from muscle spasm and pain. Muscle spasm and pain are always present in the acute stage in instances of severe cuff lesions. However, this may also be true when the cuff lesion is a trivial one. On the other hand, in some instances of minor cuff tears severe pain occurs only when the torn portion of the cuff squeezes under the acromion or the coracoacromial ligament during abduction of the arm. After the injured cuff passes beneath these structures the patient experiences immediate relief. The painful arc of movement is between 80 and 120°. When the arm is lowered to the side, pain is again felt at 120° and disappears at 80°. In patients with this painful arc syndrome, if the pain factor is eliminated, free, painless abduction is possible. The injection of 10 ml. of a 1 percent solution of procaine into the painful area readily demonstrates this point. This test has great significance, for, if the patient is now able to abduct the arm 150 to 160° and can maintain this abduction, most likely the tear is a small one and should respond to conservative measures. This is true even if an arthrogram shows direct communication between the joint cavity and the subacromial bursa.

On the other hand, in the acute stage, if

the procaine test eliminates pain and muscle spasm but the patient still is unable to abduct the arm in any of the humeral arcs or cannot maintain abduction against slight resistance, then it must be assumed that a severe cuff lesion exists and surgical repair may be necessary. In these instances, the arthrogram not only shows direct communication between the joint and subacromial bursa but also shows rapid filling of the bursa.

In my opinion, most suspected complete tears should be given a "cooling-off period" of several weeks before any surgery is performed. The exceptions to this are those patients who, after the area has been infiltrated with procaine, exhibit a total loss of abduction in all the humeral arcs and whose arthrograms show rapid filling of the subacromial bursa. In these instances, it must be assumed that a massive avulsion of the cuff is present and requires surgical repair. There are no advantages in delaying surgery in these patients.

On the other hand, if, after pain and muscle spasm are eliminated, the patient has some power of abduction, a delay of two or three weeks is justified. As previously pointed out, the presence or its extent of a complete tear—except in massive avulsions of the cuff—does not preclude good function. If what remains of the cuff is still capable of fixing the head of the humerus in the glenoid cavity and of balancing the pull of the deltoid, the patient will be able to abduct the arm. Whether this balance between the rotator muscles and the deltoid will be established can only be determined by time.

A wait of two or three weeks allows pain and muscle spasm to subside; also, the patient will be more cooperative and less apprehensive. The patient may show a steady increase in the power and range of abduction so that in 6 to 8 weeks he has almost normal function. On the other hand, if abduction is still very weak or if the patient is unable to maintain 90° of abduction against slight resistance, the cuff tear is of

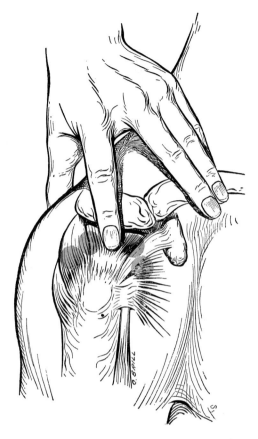

FIG. 11-9. The tip of the forefinger is in position to locate site of maximum tenderness in ruptures of the supraspinatus region of the cuff. The finger drops into the sulcus and the eminence may be palpated just external to the sulcus.

such severity that the cuff cannot stabilize the humeral head against the pull of the deltoid. These shoulders should be explored and the cuff tear repaired.

A good example of the delicate balance between the rotator cuff and the deltoid is found in linear complete tears of the cuff in athletes, especially baseball pitchers. These men have powerful deltoids so that the slightest weakness in the rotator muscles affects the balance. Although these athletes have a normal range of motion and good abduction of the arm, the arm gives out after a few innings of pitching. Also, careful evaluation of the abduction

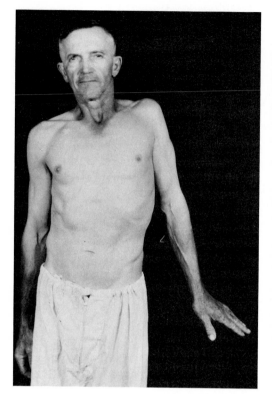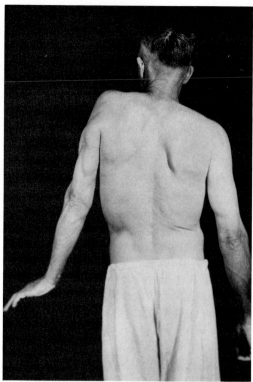

FIG. 11-10. Patient with a massive tear of the cuff. Note that in attempting to abduct the arm he shrugs the shoulder; the normal scapulohumeral rhythm is completely disrupted. (*Left*) Front view. (*Right*) Posterior view.

power invariably reveals some loss of strength. The same lesion in a person with a less powerful deltoid would, most likely, produce no dysfunction.

The same reasoning applies to complete tears with or without retraction. This provides an explanation for the marked impairment of function we all observe clinically and at the operating table in patients with strong, powerful deltoids who sustain only small or moderate tears, and for the good function in elderly persons with extensive tears of the cuff but with small and relatively less powerful deltoids.

LOCAL CLINICAL FINDINGS. *Tenderness.* In the acute stage, tenderness can always be elicited over the site of rupture of the cuff. When the supraspinatus alone is involved, the tenderness is directly over the tip of the greater tuberosity. When the tear ex-

tends into the infraspinatus region, point tenderness can also be elicited just below and lateral to the tip of the tuberosity. Another point of marked tenderness lies at the insertion of the deltoid. The sensitivity of these areas diminishes with time and in long-standing instances it is not very significant.

*Jog and Soft Crepitus.* To demonstrate these clinical signs the patient must be able to abduct the arm above the horizontal plane. Clearly, in the acute stage, pain and muscle spasm would preclude abduction; however, the pain and muscle spasm can be eliminated by local infiltration of procaine.

Later, when the acute pain has subsided, and if the patient can abduct the arm, the examiner can feel a characteristic jog and soft crepitus between his fingers and the humeral head as the arm abducts above the horizontal. They are produced when the torn portion of the cuff and the tuberosity pass under the acromion or the coracoacromial ligament. When the arm is lowered, both jog and crepitus again appear as the torn cuff and tuberosity slip from under the coracoacromial arch. It should be remembered that these signs are no more than presumptive evidence of a complete tear of the cuff because they also occur in other shoulder derangements.

*Atrophy of the Spinati Muscles.* After two or three weeks atrophy of the spinati is a constant finding; it is more pronounced in the infraspinatus. The degree of atrophy increases with time, and in lesions of long standing the teres minor and trapezius also show considerable atrophy.

On the other hand, the deltoid may disclose apparent or real hypertrophy; there is reason for this appearance of the deltoid. When the torn rotator cuff fails to provide an adequate fulcrum the deltoid performs powerful contractions with each attempt to elevate or abduct the arm. This overactivity certainly prevents atrophy of the deltoid and, in some instances, results in hypertrophy.

*Eminence and Sulcus.* Tears extensive enough to give rise to impaired function often can be detected by the presence of an eminence and a sulcus. The sulcus is a palpable defect at the site of rupture in the musculotendinous cuff. The eminence is the normal prominence of the greater tuberosity to which may still be attached some remnants of the insertion of the cuff. This eminence can be felt just anterior to the edge of the acromion when the arm is in backward extension. The jog and crepitus are caused by the passing of the eminence and sulcus under the coracoacromial arch (Fig. 11-9).

*Unrestricted Passive Motion.* This is a very significant feature of complete tears of the cuff, for it rules out other lesions that cause pain and disability of the shoulder. Patients with complete tears allow the ex-

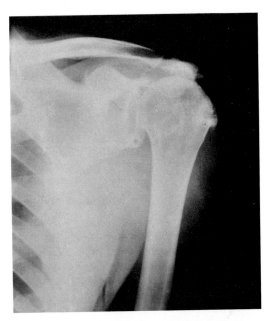

Fig. 11-11. Roentgenogram of a shoulder with a massive tear of the cuff. Note that the head rides high in relation to the glenoid; the tuberosities have receded somewhat, and the greater tuberosity shows small cystic areas and small areas of sclerosis; also note the sclerosis of the end of the acromion.

aminer to put the arm through a complete range of motion. Even in the acute stage unrestricted motion can be demonstrated by having the patient stoop to the horizontal position, with the knees extended and the arms hanging loosely towards the floor. In this position, all muscles around the shoulder girdle, including the deltoid, are relaxed, and the patient requires little effort to swing the arm into a position of complete elevation.

*Faulty Scapulohumeral Rhythm.* With a massive tear of the cuff, the patient is unable to raise the arm; instead, when he attempts abduction, he shrugs his shoulder. This is caused by the inability of the rotator muscles to hold the humeral head on its fulcrum in order to permit normal abduction. Now, when the deltoid contracts, it brings the arm upward along the vertical axis of the humerus and forces the scapula to rise

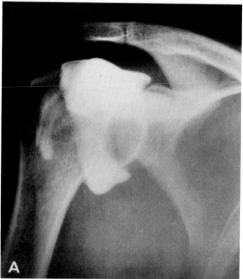

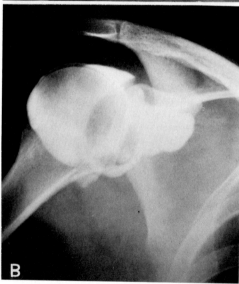

FIG. 11-12. Arthrogram of a normal Shoulder. (*Top*) External rotation. (*Bottom*) Internal rotation. (Courtesy of R. H. Freiberger)

and to rotate on the chest wall. In short, the normal scapulohumeral rhythm is completely disrupted (Fig. 11-10).

In all patients with weak abduction the normal scapulohumeral rhythm is altered. When these individuals raise the arm all movement occurs in the scapulothoracic joint while the glenohumeral joint maintains a fixed flexion position. This continues until the arm reaches the horizontal position, then elevation is completed by motion entirely in the glenohumeral joint.

When the arm is lowered the movements are reversed. As the arm descends the relationship between the scapula and humerus remains unchanged until the arm reaches the horizontal position. All motion up to this point takes place in the scapulothoracic joint. From the horizontal the arm drops suddenly to the side. In this phase all motion occurs in the glenohumeral joint.

It should be understood that a faulty scapulohumeral rhythm is not pathognomonic of tears of the cuff. It occurs in other disorders of the shoulder, such as calcific tendinitis and frozen shoulder.

**X-Ray Examination.** Unless the osseous elements are involved—for example, a fracture through one of the tuberosities—radiographic examination, as a rule, reveals no significant observations. However, the absence of a calcific deposit does eliminate this entity as the source of pain and impaired function. In the acute stage, if marked muscle spasm is present, the humeral head may ride high in the glenoid cavity.

Long-standing lesions may reveal some changes in the region of the greater tuberosity; the tip of the tuberosity may show some spur formations and its cortical surface some irregularity; cystic areas or small areas of sclerosis may be scattered throughout the greater tuberosity. When the lesion is a massive avulsion of the cuff and is of long standing, the tuberosities may seem to recede or undergo resorption and the outer and upper end of the humeral shaft may show hypertrophic, irregular bone formation (Fig. 11-11).

**Arthrography.** This is a most useful diagnostic tool. It establishes the diagnosis of a complete tear by showing direct communication between the joint cavity and the subacromial bursa. In some instances, it may even indicate the size of the tear. For example, if the dye rapidly fills up the subacromial bursa, it can be assumed that the

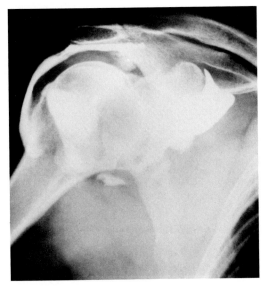 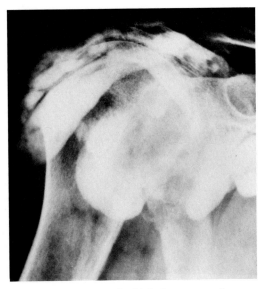

FIG. 11-13. Arthrogram of a complete tear of the rotator cuff. (*Left*) Arthrogram of a small tear; the dye just trickles into the bursa. (*Right*) Arthrogram of a large tear; the dye rapidly fills the subacromial bursa. (Courtesy of R. H. Freiberger)

defect in the cuff is relatively large. On the other hand, if the dye slowly trickles into the bursa, the tear most likely is small.

This test clearly shows the thickness of the normal cuff, the size and configuration of the joint cavity and the synovial sheath of the biceps tendon (Fig. 11-12). Disorders affecting the cuff, capsule or biceps tendon and its sheath alter the normal configuration of the arthrogram in the respective areas. Thus, in addition to showing complete and incomplete cuff tears, arthrograms also reveal rupture of the biceps tendon, changes in the bicipital groove, adhesive capsulitis and the large anterior capsular pouch in anterior recurrent dislocations.

The diagnosis of partial rupture of the cuff by arthrography may be difficult; only tears on the inner side of the cuff are demonstrable. The defect of the partial tears may fill with dye only after the arm is exercised. This is an important point to remember (Fig. 11-13).

TECHNIQUE OF ARTHROGRAPHY. Place the patient in the supine position, with a sandbag under the elbow and the arm in slight rotation. This position relaxes the tissues on the anterior aspect of the shoulder. Next, pick a point just inferior and lateral to the coracoid process, it lies in line with the acromioclavicular joint. Infiltrate both the deep and the superficial tissues in this area with 1 percent procaine. Through the selected point, push straight into the joint a no. 20 spinal needle 3 inches long. The point of the needle can be felt to pierce the capsule and drop into the joint.

Inject into the joint 12 to 15 ml. of one of the contrast media. I use 17.5 percent Diodrast. Watch the flow of the dye. In large complete lesions the dye flows freely and swiftly into the subacromial bursa. The average normal joint cavity accepts 12 to 15 ml. of fluid; then the capsule becomes distended and, if intact, offers resistance to the injection of more fluid. If the joint cavity accepts more than 20 ml. of fluid, assume that there is a leak through the capsule. Most likely a complete cuff tear exists. However, it also leaves the joint

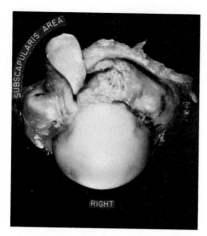

FIG. 11-14. In this specimen, looking at the humeral side of the joint, note that the tuberosities have receded, and the intracapsular portion of the biceps tendon has slipped out of the groove and lies on the edge of the subscapularis tendon.

cavity when the subscapularis bursa ruptures or if there is a tear in the inferior capsular region or in the sheath of the biceps tendon.

After the injection is completed and the needle removed, exercise the arm several times through all the arcs of motion; then take roentgenograms of the shoulder. These should include anteroposterior views, with the arm in varying degrees of internal and external rotation, and axillary views.

### Conservative Treatment of Complete Tears

As stated previously, all shoulders with complete tears, except those with massive avulsions of the cuff, should be observed for 2 to 3 weeks before considering surgical intervention. The managment of this group is the same as that described for incomplete tears of the cuff. At the end of this period, the shoulder should be carefully reexamined and its further management decided. Many patients at this time show an increase in the power and range of abduction. These patients should be main-

tained on a conservative regimen for 6 to 8 weeks more. During this period the rotator apparatus may develop sufficient power to balance the action of the deltoid. When this occurs, the rotators will hold the fulcrum and permit free and strong abduction of the arm. If the residual disability is not acceptable, then surgical intervention is indicated. The operative technique to repair complete tears of the rotator cuff is described on page 229.

### BICIPITAL TENOSYNOVITIS AND FROZEN SHOULDER

My clinical and surgical experience and my investigations on several hundred shoulder joints convince me that bicipital tenosynovitis is a specific clinical entity. Yet, there are some surgeons who do not recognize it as such and believe it is always secondary to some other lesion of the shoulder joint. In Chapter 8 it was noted that pain and stiffness in the shoulder may be the result of acute strains of the biceps tendon. Repeated strains of the tendon, such as are caused by overhand or underhand throwing, may produce an inflammatory process of the tendon and its sheath in the bicipital groove. If not treated adequately, the acute syndrome may become chronic in nature and may seriously impair the performance of the athlete.

Primary bicipital tenosynovitis also occurs after the age of 40 years; however, other basic etiological factors come into play and these must be given serious consideration. In this age group, in addition to trauma, single or repetitive, degenerative alterations in the biceps tendon associated with aging and physiological wear and tear play a major role in the evolution of the bicipital syndrome. These changes are recorded in Chapter 6. To recapitulate briefly, with aging the biceps tendon shows progressive alterations in the form of fraying, thickening and shredding of its fibers. The abnormalities are always associated with degenerative changes in the rotator

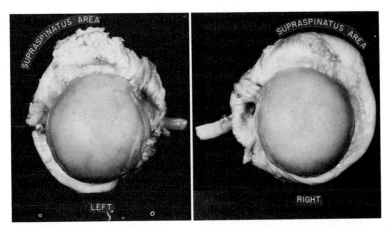

Fig. 11-15. In both of these specimens the intracapsular portion of the biceps tendons has been resorbed and the tendons have gained attachment to the shaft of the humerus. The patient who provided these specimens related that approximately 12 to 15 years prior to his last hospital admission he had developed pain and stiffness, first in one shoulder and then in the other. The symptom complex described was consistent with that of frozen shoulders.

cuff. The latter changes tend to enhance the alterations in the tendon, for, as the cuff becomes weaker, the humeral head tends to ride higher in the glenoid. Now, on abduction of the arm the tuberosities impinge on the acromion and exert abnormal pressure on the subacromial structures. Not infrequently bony excrescences form on the tuberosities and in the bicipital groove. The resulting roughening, irregularity and narrowing of the groove interfere with the gliding mechanism of the tendon and its sheath which in turn become inflamed and thickened. Also, adhesions form, binding the tendon to the groove, and, at the point where the tendon leaves the joint, it may become adherent to the fibrous capsule. It becomes apparent that trauma, in any form, may accentuate the pathological process in and about the biceps tendon and cause a painful and stiff shoulder; on the other hand, the degenerative changes alone may be responsible.

In the later decades, as a result of constant impingement of the tuberosities against the acromion, the tuberosities may wear away, obliterating the intertubercular sulcus. In these instances, the intra-articular portion of the tendon may slip out of the groove and lay on a sling made by the tendon of the subscapularis, or it may disappear and the extra-articular end becomes attached to the shaft of the humerus (Figs. 11-14 and 11-15). Finally, congenital abnormalities of the bicipital groove may interfere with the normal gliding mechanism of the tendon. Of the shoulders studied, 9 percent revealed a supratubercular ridge which narrowed the depth of the groove and predisposed to subluxation of the tendon. Also, in approximately 22 percent the obliquity of the medial wall of the bicipital groove was 45° or less, and in 50 percent it was 60° or less. This, too, predisposes to subluxation of the tendon (see Fig. 4-23).

Functional demands on the shoulder play a role in the development of bicipital tenosynovitis. In a great many human endeavors the arm must perform in varying degrees of forward flexion and internal rotation. This position places the biceps tendon on the medial wall of the bicipital groove and forces the tendon to perform at a great mechanical disadvantage.

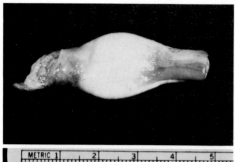

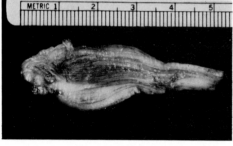

FIG. 11-16. Specimens of the intra-capsular portions of biceps tendons removed at surgery. (*Top*) Note the marked swelling of the tendon. (*Bottom*) Note the thickening, widening and shredding of the tendon.

There is considerable disagreement on the role that bicipital tenosynovitis plays in the evolution of the frozen shoulder. Also, if it does play a role, is it a primary or secondary one? This is like trying to decipher the riddle of the chicken and the egg—which came first? We must admit that we do not know the basic pathological processes responsible for frozen shoulder. On the other hand, certain clinical and surgical findings are constant and cannot be disregarded: for example, many frozen shoulders develop after injuries to tissues at some distance from the shoulder and in patients who had no pain or stiffness in the shoulder prior to the injury. Many patients whose activity has been reduced or who have been confined to bed by long chronic illness—e. g., tuberculosis, cardiac disease, or mental disorders—frequently develop a frozen shoulder. The only common denominator in these groups is reduction of activity of the arm. I have yet to see at the operating table a true frozen shoulder without an inflammatory process of the biceps tendon and its sheath.

It must be remembered that the cardinal features of bicipital tenosynovitis are pain, muscle spasm and restricted motion. These reduce the over-all activity of the arm. Whether this loss of motion, in some instances of bicipital tenosynovitis, initiates the inflammatory process, producing a frozen shoulder, or whether the bicipital tenosynovitis per se is secondary to the pathology in the periarticular structures are the controversial points.

Bicipital tenosynovitis is the most common cause of pain and limitation of motion in the shoulder; also, it is the main source of pain in an established frozen shoulder. This conclusion is based on clinical experience—that is, in the first group, once the gliding mechanism of the biceps tendon is eliminated the patients experience relief of pain and regain motion of the shoulder; in the second group, the same procedure markedly reduces the intensity of the pain; this sets the stage for resumption of motion.

I have come to the following conclusions: Both before and after the age of 40 years, primary bicipital tenosynovitis is a definite clinical entity. However, after age 40, the degenerative processes in the tendon render it more vulnerable to trauma and over-activity (Fig. 11-16). For this reason, there is a higher incidence of bicipital tenosynovitis in the older age group. In my series of 100 consecutive cases, 28 were under 40 and 72 over 40 years of age; the highest incidence was between the ages of 45 and 55 years. The lesion was bilateral in 7 cases.

Although all these patients have pain, muscle spasm and restricted motion, they have a relatively free, painless range of passive internal and external motion of the glenohumeral joint when the arm is at the side and the elbow flexed. This indicates that the periarticular structures, especially the capsule, are not implicated; this is the most characteristic feature of primary bicipital tenosynovitis.

In frozen shoulder, the structure involved primarily is the fibrous capsule of the joint. The pathological process is an inflammation, producing fibrosis and contraction of the capsule. The surrounding soft tissues become secondarily involved, the spinati muscles atrophy and shorten, the biceps muscle lies in a mesh of inflammatory tissue that often binds the tendon to its sheath and the sheath to the bicipital groove and capsule, and the subacromial bursa may be obliterated by adhesions.

Inactivity of the arm is the single constant finding prior to the development of frozen shoulder, and primary bicipital tenosynovitis reduces the activity of the arm. But even in the presence of inactivity not all shoulders become frozen. Therefore, there must be some other predisposing or constitutional factor which, when present and coupled with inactivity, triggers the mechanism producing frozen shoulder. This factor is most prevalent in persons between the ages of 40 and 60 years. A true frozen shoulder in a person under 30 years of age is indeed rare.

## Clinical Picture of Bicipital Tenosynovitis (After the Age of 40 Years)

In most instances, some form of trauma, minor or severe, precipitates the syndrome. Not infrequently symptoms follow a fall on the point of the shoulder or the flexed elbow, forcing the humerus upward against the acromion. Strenuous exercises such as tennis or shoveling snow may initiate the symptoms. In some instances, there is no trauma and the onset is insidious.

The chief clinical symptom is pain in the anterolateral aspect of the shoulder. It is often referred to the insertion of the deltoid and the muscle belly of the biceps and even into the flexor surface of the forearm. In severe forms, the pain radiates posteriorly to the region of the scapula and to the cervical region. Pain may be more pronounced at night and may interfere with sleep. Upon lying on the affected side, pressure on the point of the shoulder accentuates the pain. Some restriction of motion is present in all directions, but a certain free range of painless motion always exists. If the arcs of this range are exceeded, the pain is accentuated.

The most constant physical finding, and a very significant one, is exquisite tenderness on pressure over the bicipital groove and over the tendon. Maneuvers that stretch the biceps tendon actively or passively produce pain: abduction and external rotation of the arm, backward flexion and external rotation with the elbow extended, and forward adduction of the arm against resistance with the elbow extended. As previously stated, in an uncomplicated bicipital tenosynovitis, when the arm is at the side and the biceps tendon is not under undue tension, a relatively free, painless arc of internal and external rotation is always present passively. On the other hand, rotatory movements with the tendon under tension cause pain. Depending upon the severity of the pain, spasm of the muscles of the shoulder is present in varying degrees. The muscles affected are, usually, the deltoid, trapezius and the scaleni and, at times, the forearm muscles.

The syndrome may be acute, particularly if an injury occurred, or it may be subacute or chronic in nature. In the latter instances, the pain and dysfunction are usually within the limits of the tolerance of the patient. However, exacerbations of the symptoms are not infrequent with overusage of the arm or minor trauma. The condition may be relatively disabling and protracted, and may not respond to conservative measures and rest. In a few instances, the lesion may progress until the biceps tendon becomes adherent in the groove and to the capsule in the region of the coracohumeral ligament. In this case motion is markedly restricted, but is not a true frozen shoulder. I have demonstrated this pathology many times at the operating table. These are the cases that get complete restoration of painless

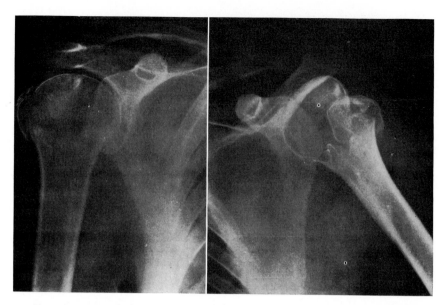

FIG. 11-17. Fractures implicating the bicipital groove, such as these frequently are complicated by bicipital tenosynovitis and then progress to a frozen shoulder. Both of these patients developed frozen shoulders.

function after anchorage of the tendon to the upper end of the humerus. Not infrequently, in these instances, the patient experiences a sudden snap in the shoulder, after which motion dramatically increases. The biceps tendon has ruptured proximal to its exit from the shoulder joint.

## X-Ray and Arthrography

X-ray examination gives no pathognomonic information that might establish a diagnosis of bicipital tenosynovitis. However, in some instances, irregularity of the groove caused by bony spurs or the presence of some abnormality of the tuberosities may be suggestive of pathology in the tendon. These are best seen in axial views of the shoulder. On the other hand, an arthrogram may show distortion or obliteration of the sheath of the biceps tendon. This is positive evidence that the tendon and its sheath are implicated in some inflammatory process.

The possible implication of the biceps tendon in shoulder dislocations and in

fractures of the greater tuberosity which occur in young people were examined in Chapter 9. Many fractures and fracture-dislocations in older persons also involve the bicipital groove—for example, fractures through the tuberosities, depressed or comminuted fractures of the humeral head and fractures through the anatomical neck of the humerus (Fig. 11-17). In these instances, the biceps tendon may be injured primarily at the time of the injury or it may be involved secondarily because of changes in the configuration of the bicipital groove. The outcome is unpredictable. In my experience, not all persons who develop bicipital tenosynovitis after fractures of the upper end of the humerus also develop frozen shoulder. On the other hand, a great many do, particularly those between the ages of 40 and 60 years, whose arms have been immobilized too long and whose general health is below normal. In these patients, there must be some other predisposing or constitutional factor that is activated by the enforced reduction of activity of the limb after injury.

## Management of Primary Bicipital Tenosynovitis

The greater number of uncomplicated lesions respond to conservative measures. The most essential features are rest of the limb, and restriction of motion to the painless arcs. Physical therapy in the form of wet hot packs to the shoulder helps to reduce the inflammatory process. All movements that put the biceps tendon on stretch must be avoided. All exercises must be within the patient's tolerance. For the subacute and chronic forms of bicipital tenosynovitis the injection of one of the corticoids may be very effective.

In some instances, conservative measures fail regardless of the thoroughness of the treatment. The great majority of these patients can be cured by surgical treatment. In the uncomplicated form, deletion of the gliding mechanism of the biceps tendon produces the desired favorable results. The procedure of my choice is excision of the intracapsular portion of the tendon and anchoring of the stump of the extracapsular portion to the shaft of the humerus. The operation is described on page 467.

When fractures and fracture-dislocations of the upper end of the humerus in which the bicipital groove is violated or the tendon is dislocated are treated surgically, the tendon should in all cases be anchored to the upper end of the humerus and its intraarticular portion should be excised. If these lesions are treated conservatively and subsequently a recalcitrant bicipital tenosynovitis develops, the tendon should be treated in a similar manner.

## FROZEN SHOULDER

### Historical Considerations

For a discussion of "frozen shoulder" a clear understanding of what this term designates is needed. This is most important, for many physicians and surgeons use the term too loosely and apply it to many lesions that cause a painful and stiff shoulder. In this discussion, the term *frozen shoulder* is restricted to the shoulder that, without evidence of intrinsic pathology, develops pain and restriction of motion insidiously. The disorder runs a specific clinical course: Pain and stiffness increase slowly but steadily to a certain level of intensity; then, after an unpredictable number of months, the pain subsides gradually, motion returns slowly, and ultimately full recovery is attained. There are exceptions to this general description of frozen shoulder; these will be discussed later.

In spite of the many investigations of this entity, the cause of frozen shoulder still remains an enigma. I am sure that much of the work done by the earlier investigators concerned itself primarily with the frozen shoulder and its many side effects. The first worker to focus his attention on the "painful and stiff" shoulder was Duplay. In 1896 he described the syndrome and incriminated the subacromial bursa as the source of the trouble. He designated the entity "scapulohumeral periarthritis." Unfortunately this term soon came to embody a host of heterogeneous entities all having the common denominator —pain and stiffness in the shoulder. Since this original work, other investigators succeeded in isolating specific entities causing a painful and stiff shoulder and removed them from the all-inclusive designation "scapulohumeral periarthritis." Among these investigators are Baer, Painter, Munford, Codman, Pasteur, Meyer and Gilcrest. More recently, the work of Lippman, Abbott, Saunders, Hitchock and Bechtol, McLaughlin and Neviaser have added considerably to our knowledge of shoulder disorders.

To Meyer must go the credit for being the first to recognize that the biceps tendon plays a significant role in certain derangements of the shoulder. He worked on anatomical specimens. He observed degenerative changes in the biceps tendon in the form of fraying, shredding, fasciculation and tearing of the tendon fibers. Some specimens disclosed partial or complete displacement from the bicipital groove; in others the intra-articular portion of the tendon was absent and the stump of the extra-articular portion had attached itself to the shaft of the humerus. Unfortunately he was unable to evaluate the clinical significance of these findings. Nevertheless, he proposed that the alterations were produced by one of several mechanisms: (1) contact of the tendon with the supra-tubercular ridges (when present), (2) friction between the tendon and excrescences in the floor of the groove, and (3) contact between the tendon and irregular and elevated cartilaginous margins on the head of the humerus or contact with the lesser tuberosity. He believed that these mechanisms came into play when the upper extremity performed in the position of abduction and external rotation. All these findings I confirmed in my investigation made on postmortem shoulder specimens and they are recorded in Chapter 6.

Following Meyer's work, many investigators soon came to recognize and appreciate the role of the biceps tendon in frozen shoulder. Notable among these was Pasteur. He coined the term *teno-bursite,* believing that the biceps tendon was the responsible culprit for frozen shoulder. In 1943, Lippman described what he called *adhesive tenosynovitis;* he, too, believed that the biceps tendon was the chief source of trouble.

On the other hand, Codman in his classic treatise on the shoulder wrote: "Personally I believe the sheath of the biceps tendon is less apt to be involved than are other structures. I have never proved its involvement in a single case. I think that the substance of the supraspinatus tendon is most often involved."* Codman believed that the basic lesion of frozen shoulder was tendonitis of the rotator tendons.

Within the past few decades many frozen

* Codman, E. A.: The Shoulder. Boston, Thomas Todd, 1934.

shoulders have been explored surgically. This has added considerably to our knowledge of the pathology of frozen shoulder; yet, we still know nothing of the process producing the pathological alterations in the soft tissues of the scapulohumeral joint.

**Etiological Considerations**

Although the cause of frozen shoulder is not known, certain circumstances are constantly and intimately associated with this syndrome. In all cases, muscular inactivity and dependency of the limb precede the onset of frozen shoulder. In most instances, the persons affected are over 40 years of age; they usually show signs of emotional instability; often they are under great mental stress caused by prolonged illness, socio-economic pressures or poor nutrition.

A true frozen shoulder rarely develops in persons under the age of 40 years. In all series studied, the greatest number of cases occur in the fourth and fifth decades. It is during this period of life that the soft tissue components of the scapulohumeral joint exhibit frank degenerative changes— changes that are the result of normal wear and tear of the shoulder. This suggests that these degenerative alterations may be a necessary part of the background of frozen shoulder. In their absence a classic frozen shoulder rarely develops.

As previously mentioned, the onset of the syndrome is invariably preceded by muscular inactivity and dependency of the upper extremity. In regard to these conditions, the single most significant cause is pain. Pain in the shoulder is associated with muscle spasm; together, they enforce reduced activity and dependency of the arm. It should be remembered that pain in the shoulder is not always caused by an intrinsic lesion; the cause may be a lesion at some distance from the shoulder— a lesion in the cervical spine, a Pancoast tumor of the lung, a cardiac disorder or a subdiaphragmatic lesion. In these instances the pain can be relieved only by correction

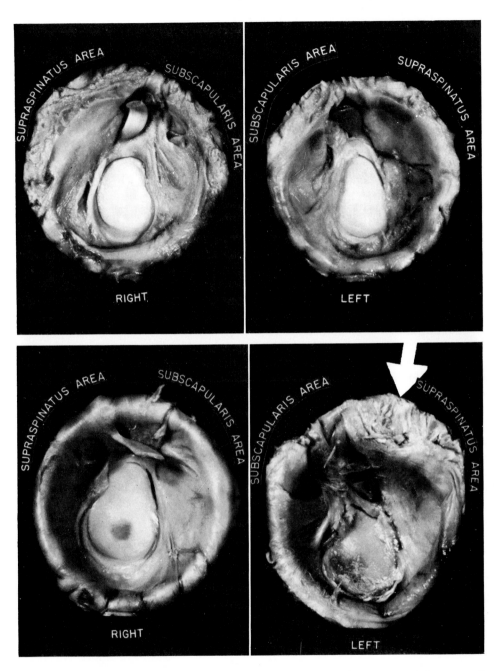

FIG. 11-18. Glenoid side of the glenohumeral joint of 4 shoulders of the second (*top, left*), third (*top, right*), sixth (*bottom, left*) and seventh (*bottom, right*) decades. Note the progressive increase in the degenerative alterations in all components of the joints.

of the primary lesion. Therefore an extensive and thorough physical examination of every patient with a frozen shoulder is essential. Not infrequently frozen shoulder may be aborted by eradication of the primary source of pain.

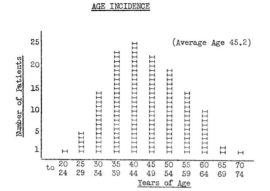

FIG. 11-19. Rise of severity of degenerative changes in the biceps tendon, the musculotendinous cuff and labrum in successive decades.

Reduced muscular activity and dependency of the arm are often forced on the patient when the limb is treated in a sling for a lesion at some distance from the shoulder—for example, fracture of the wrist or the forearm, and fractures about the elbow. The hazards of immobilizing the arm to the side, in a middle aged or elderly person for prolonged periods of time, regardless of the reasons, are well known to all of us.

Frequently, pain, muscular inactivity and dependency present with no manifestations of a primary extrinsic cause, and, many investigators believe that, in these instances, there is no intrinsic cause for the pain. I am not in agreement with this premise; rather it is my belief that the source of the pain in most of these instances is bicipital tenosynovitis. Also, if these patients are adequately treated, many of them will make a successful recovery. At this point, I wish to emphasize that bicipital tenosynovitis is not the cause of frozen shoulder, but it *is* the cause of pain, dependency and muscular inactivity—the factors that appear to be essential to the initiation of the still unknown process responsible for frozen shoulder.

The most recent studies on the etiology of frozen shoulder point to the fibrous capsule as the site of the primary trouble. However, the true nature of the pathological process—a process that converts an elastic, voluminous capsule to a nonelastic, friable, shrunken structure—is still not clear.

## Clinical Features

I have studied in detail 72 patients with frozen shoulders, 42 of which were explored surgically. Now, I will again record the observations and conclusions I made in this study. No patient with calcareous tendinitis was included in this investigation. An attempt was made to correlate the pathological findings in the shoulders explored surgically with the findings in the earlier study of the aging shoulder in various decades. This correlation led to certain conclusions on the role that the biceps tendon plays in frozen shoulder. The observations made in the study of the frozen shoulder and the conclusions based on them are reviewed and discussed in the following sections.

**Age, Sex and Incidence.** Of the 72 patients with frozen shoulders only one was under the age of 40 years. The incidence was highest in patients between 50 and 60 years of age. More women than men were affected—72 percent of the patients were women—and the left shoulder was involved more often that the right. In 8 percent both shoulders were involved at the time of the initial examination and in 6 percent the contralateral shoulder had been involved prior to the examination.

The period of life in which frozen shoulder is found most frequently corresponds to that period in which severe degenerative changes occur in the shoulder. Figure 11-18 depicts the glenoid side of four shoulders in the third, fourth, sixth and seventh decades of life. Note the progressive increase in intensity of the degenerative alterations in the articular cartilage of the glenoid fossa, synovialis, musculotendinous cuff and biceps tendon. Observe also the severe changes in the labra and the supra- and infraspinatus regions of the cuff in specimens of the sixth and seventh decades. The latter changes are really incomplete tears of the cuff. Figure 11-19 graphically reveals the progressive rise in gradient in each successive decade of the degenerative changes in the labrum, biceps tendon and musculotendinous cuff. Note the sharp rise after the fourth decade.

In the light of these observations it is reasonable to assume that the changes described above must be present before a frozen shoulder can come into being. It is also apparent that in people with metabolic and nutritional disorders and in those with poor health due to cardiac, pulmonary or mental diseases degenerative changes are more severe than in people in good general health. Hence, frozen shoulder is more likely to develop in the former than in the latter group. Clinical experience confirms this point.

**Onset of Syndrome.** In the great majority of the patients the onset is insidious; there is no injury to the extremity. In some, the onset follows an injury—often only a minor injury—to the shoulder or to some other part of the extremity. In my series, 11 patients developed frozen shoulder after a direct injury to the shoulder; in 14 it followed an injury to the elbow, wrist or hand: in 47 there was no injury, and the onset came on insidiously. Regardless of the manner of onset, in all groups there was a common denominator, namely, reduced muscular activity and dependency of the arm. In those with injury, inactivity and dependency were, at first, the products of the treatment; the arm was immobilized at the side; later pain was the responsible agent. Pain on motion of the shoulder was the prime factor for reduced activity in those with an insidious onset.

These observations lead to the conclusion that, in the face of degenerative

alterations of the shoulder, reduced activity of the extremity and dependency are required to trigger the mechanism causing a frozen shoulder.

**Pain and Muscle Spasm.** Pain is the most outstanding symptom of the disease; it is constant and interferes with sleep. Constant pain invariably evokes persistent muscle spasm, which may be either subclinical or apparent. The pain and muscle spasm may be limited to the region of the shoulder, but usually it extends from the occiput to the wrist and occasionally even to the fingers. Also, from the shoulder as a central focus, the pain may radiate posteriorly to the scapular region, anteriorly to the pectoral region, into the region of the triceps, deltoid or the biceps and to the extensor surface of the forearm. With chronic muscle spasm, reduced muscular activity, and dependency, regional vasospasm is the inevitable sequel. Although this is a secondary phenomenon, occasionally it may present with overwhelming rapidity and severity, so much so that it may obscure the primary focus. In such cases it may be difficult to determine whether the vasomotor disturbance is secondary to chronic muscle spasm caused by a primary lesion in the shoulder or whether the shoulder manifestations are secondary to a primary vasomotor disturbance in the hand.

It should be remembered that muscles in chronic spasm become painful and tender. When this secondary phenomenon predominates in different anatomical areas, confusing clinical pictures evolve. Implication of the pectoral muscles suggests cardiac disorders; involvement of the trapezius draws attention to the cervical spine as the source of trouble, as does pain in the deltoid and extensor muscles of the forearm, whereas pain in the latissimus implicates the chest or the axilla.

When the syndrome suggests neurological implications, a careful neurological examination must be done to establish the

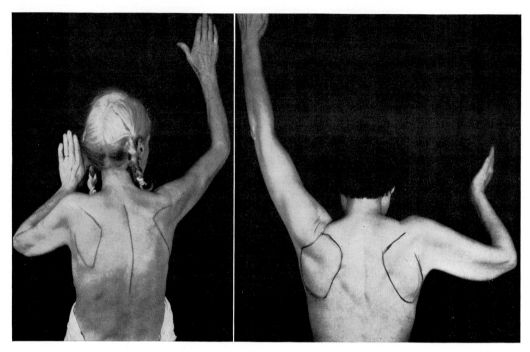

FIG. 11-20. Both patients show the characteristic features of a frozen shoulder. (*Left*) This patient's general health is poor. Note the relationship of the axis of the shaft of the humerus to that of the spine of the scapula, forming approximately a right angle. This relationship is maintained during all movements of the arm and is clearly discernible in roentgenograms taken during different stages of elevation. (*Right*) This patient shows the same features as those pointed out in the patient shown on the left, except that the patient's general health is better.

site of the primary lesion. It is helpful to remember that radiating pain caused by irritation of a nerve root is sharp and lancinating and exhibits a specific regional pattern consistent with the areas supplied by the affected root. On the other hand, radiating pain caused by irritation of mesodermal tissue, such as occurs in chronic muscle spasm, is vague and ill defined and does not follow a radicular pattern. Also, as a rule, the deep tendon reflexes of muscles in chronic spasm are overactive rather than depressed. Finally, sensory deficits caused by irritation of nerve roots are clearly defined and exhibit a specific anatomical pattern, whereas those caused by vasospasm and chronic muscle spasm are diffuse and inconstant. Remember that lesions of the cervical spine and of the thoracic viscera may produce, secondarily, pain, chronic

muscle spasm and vasomotor disturbances in the shoulder and arm. Also, the primary cause of frozen shoulder must be established before appropriate treatment can be instituted.

**Objective Features.** As a rule, the patient with frozen shoulder is apprehensive and often emotionally disturbed, below par physically and fearful of being hurt. The patient holds the arm at the side and if asked to perform actively movements of the shoulder, she performs them slowly and guardedly. Muscle spasm, especially of the trapezius, may be apparent and in well established syndromes the spinati and deltoid exhibit varying degrees of atrophy; in some instances, the atrophy may be profound.

Invariably, pressure over the intertubercular sulcus elicits severe pain, as does

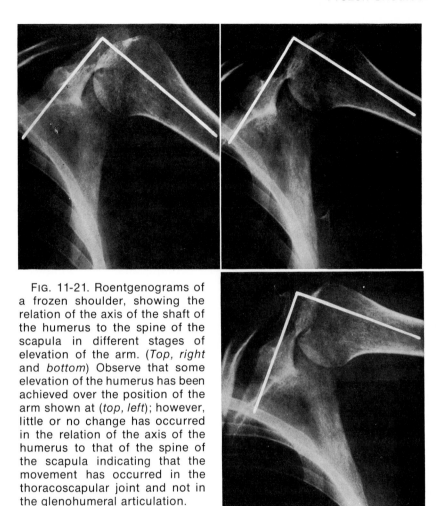

Fig. 11-21. Roentgenograms of a frozen shoulder, showing the relation of the axis of the shaft of the humerus to the spine of the scapula in different stages of elevation of the arm. (*Top, right* and *bottom*) Observe that some elevation of the humerus has been achieved over the position of the arm shown at (*top, left*); however, little or no change has occurred in the relation of the axis of the humerus to that of the spine of the scapula indicating that the movement has occurred in the thoracoscapular joint and not in the glenohumeral articulation.

rolling the biceps tendon under the thumb. This constant finding implicates the biceps tendon as the chief source of pain. This is further substantiated by placing the limb in positions that put the tendon on tension which markedly accentuates the pain. The positions are abduction and external rotation of the arm, backward flexion and external rotation with the elbow extended, and forward adduction against resistance with the elbow extended.

The amount of restriction of motion varies greatly from patient to patient and depends upon the phase of the disease at the time of the examination. In the early phase, because pain may still be tolerable, motion in the scapulohumeral joint may not be diminished. But, even in these patients, a certain amount of restriction of internal and external rotation of the humerus can be demonstrated. In testing for scapulohumeral motion the scapula must be grasped firmly in order to prevent any scapulothoracic motion. Now the amount of total elevation and the amount of scapulohumeral elevation can be estimated. Also, invariably these patients find difficulty in raising the arm to the top of the head and women are unable to hook their brassieres. To me this indicates that in addition to implication of the biceps tendon, the fibrous capsule is involved and is becoming adherent to the tendon at its site of exit from the joint. As a result, internal and external rotation of the humerus is restricted and painful.

In the later phases of the disorder, motion in the scapulohumeral joint diminishes until little or no motion is present. Usually, even in the most rigid joints a few degrees of motion remains in the sagittal plane. At this stage, the limb hangs at the side in internal rotation; all motions are guarded and painful and atrophy of the spinati and deltoid is pronounced. On the other hand, I have seen instances of completely stiff shoulders with little or no pain. In these people, it appears that the disease process has burnt itself out and left in its wake only a rigid shoulder. All patients with this disorder, regardless of the phase, show faulty scapulohumeral rhythm in the affected limb. But, remember that this phenomenon, though significant, is not pathognomonic of frozen shoulder (Fig. 11-20 and 11-21).

**Vasomotor Disturbances.** In some instances, particularly those with severe pain and pronounced muscle spasm, the arm shows evidence of vasospasm. The hand is slightly puffy and cool, and the wrist and joints of the hand and fingers are stiff and painful. In a very few, all the clinical manifestations of reflex dystropy (shoulder-arm-hand syndrome) may be present.

### Course of the Disease

The syndrome shows great variations in both the intensity of the pain and the degree of restriction of motion. Some have little restriction and much pain; others have practically no motion and little or no pain. Between these extremes there are many combinations of degrees of stiffness and intensity of pain. In general, this clinical entity can be divided into three phases: (1) the initial or freezing phase, (2) the intermediate or frozen phase, and (3) the final or thawing phase.

The characteristic features of the initial phase are discomfort and a catching sensation when the arm is placed in certain positions, usually those positions that stretch the biceps tendon. During this period the pain is localized in the anterolateral aspect of the shoulder but it may extend to the insertion of the deltoid. Gradually, the shoulder becomes stiffer and more painful and slowly enters the intermediate or frozen phase.

During the frozen phase pain is more or less constant. It is worse at night and the patient is unable to sleep. Attempts to use the arm cause more pain and muscle spasm. Usually it is during this phase that the patient seeks medical aid. Now, the degree of fixation of the scapulohumeral joint reaches it peak and, in some instances, the side effects of prolonged vasospasm and constant muscle spasm become apparent. After an unpredictable period — weeks, months or even years — the pain slowly begins to subside; the syndrome is entering the final or thawing phase.

Throughout the final phase the constant pain becomes less intense and the shoulder slowly but progressively loosens up and gains more and more mobility.

From the above description of the syndrome it becomes apparent that the clinical course is uncertain but not totally unpredictable. In almost all patients the disease terminates spontaneously; in some this may occur within a few weeks or months, but in some it may remain static for many months before the pain subsides and motion returns. In my series three patients had had frozen shoulders for 3, 6, and 8 years respectively, with no evidence of improvement. Such cases are indeed rare and exceptional, and occur in patients suffering from some chronic disease; they are poorly nourished, asthenic and under great emotional stress. Such was the case in my three patients.

In any given case, with or without treatment, it is difficult to arrive at the exact

length of time required to attain full recovery. Recovery is always so gradual that
even the patient is unable to state exactly
when the shoulder attained a full range of
painless motion. It is my opinion that very
few patients with a true frozen shoulder,
regardless of how mild the syndrome might
be, recover fully in less than 6 to 9 months
that is, have a full range of painless motion,
have no twinge on certain movements of
the arm and use the shoulder fully and without restraint.

As noted previously, frozen shoulder may
occur simultaneously in both shoulders, or
first in one and then the other shoulder.
I have never seen a recurrence in a shoulder
previously affected and cured. This is also
the experience of other observers.

The patients in my series fell into two
groups: (1) those who recovered spontaneously relatively early in the disease and (2)
those who pursued a long protracted course.
In general, the patients in the first group
were able to maintain a fair range of shoulder
motion because the pain factor was not so
severe as to enforce total immobility and
dependency of the arm. Also, in this group,
the patients were in relatively good general
health and muscular development was good.
On the other hand, the patients in the second
category were severely disabled, pain was
constant and profound and general health
and nutrition were poor. It appears that
muscular activity, if maintained, can reverse the process of frozen shoulder. But
this is not possible until the pain becomes
tolerable or eliminated. The question that
arises naturally is: what is the cause of the
pain and why does it disappear early in
some patients and late in others? It is my
belief that the biceps tendon provides the
answer to this question. This will be discussed in the following section.

### Pathology of the Frozen Shoulder

In an earlier report I recorded the observations made on 42 frozen shoulders
explored surgically. In most of these shoul-

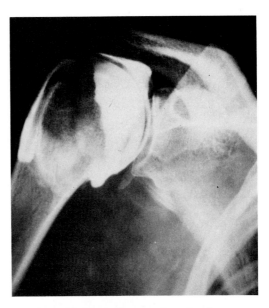

Fig. 11-22. Arthrography of a frozen
shoulder. Note that the volume of the
joint is reduced and the capsule retracted. (Courtesy of R. H. Freiberger)

ders the disease was long and protracted.
I have explored many shoulders in the earlier phases of the disease, and these have
added considerably to my knowledge of
the pathology of the frozen shoulder. All
these shoulders were studied macro-
scopically and microscopically. Many observers hold that one or another particular
area in the shoulder was responsible for
the disease. Duplay implicated the subacromial bursa, Pasteur and Lippman the
biceps tendon, Codman the supraspinatus
tendon, Aufranc and others the rotator
cuff and Neviaser the inferior aspect of
the capsule. My explorations lead me to
believe that the central focus of the pathological process is in the fibrous capsule.
Once the essential ingredients—muscular
inactivity, dependency and degenerative
changes in the cuff—are added to the so-
called X, or constitutional factor, the inflammatory process is set in motion.
With time all the soft tissue elements become involved in the process: capsule,
synovialis, fascial coverings, musculoten-

dinous cuff, biceps tendon and its sheath, and the subacromial bursa.

That the capsule is the first and primary focus of involvement is readily demonstrated in the early cases. In all those instances, arthrography shows reduction of the volume of the joint and retraction of the capsule (Fig. 11-22). Exploration of these shoulders reveals retraction of the fibrous capsule and obliteration of the inferior nictating capsular folds. The other tissues appear relatively normal except for some filmy adhesions between the biceps tendon and its sheath.

In the late phase of the disease the picture is entirely different. In addition to severe retraction of the capsule, most or all of the other structures are implicated. In general, the process comprises degeneration of the collagenous fibers, increased fibrosis of the affected tissues, areas of increased vascularity, and thickening and fibrosis of the synovial membrane. The tissues lose their elasticity and are shortened and fibrotic; in some instances, the tissues are extremely friable and tear readily when the humerus is abducted or rotated.

In these advanced lesions the pathological findings in specific areas are significant. The coracohumeral ligament invariably is converted into a thick, contracted cord between the tuberosities and the coracoid process. Together with the subscapularis tendon, it then functions as a powerful check rein to external rotation of the humerus.

In the specimens studied, the different portions of the musculotendinous cuff, particularly the supra- and infraspinatus and the subscapularis regions of the cuff, also were short, tight, fibrotic and friable. They held the head tightly against the glenoid fossa and restricted rotation in all directions. The fibrous capsule and synovialis showed the same inflammatory changes; as previously noted, the capsule is thickened, fibrotic and contracted around the humeral head. The synovial membrane also is thickened and loses its luster; the synovial recesses, superior and inferior subscapularis recesses, are occluded. The folds in the capsule and synovial membrane along the inferior aspect of the humeral neck are obliterated. The capsule and synovialis adhere firmly to the bone so that, when the arm is abducted, they tear and together peel off the bone.

The walls of the synovial bursa are usually thickened and the bursa obliterated by adhesions binding the rotator cuff to the undersurface of the acromion; however, in a few cases, the bursal walls were atrophic and contracted with very few adhesions.

In all the shoulders explored there was some implication of the biceps tendon and its sheath. The most profound and varied pathology was noted in the advanced frozen shoulders. In some shoulders of the latter group, the biceps tendon lay in a mesh of filmy, hemorrhagic adhesions, in others it was firmly anchored to the bicipital groove and to the under surface of the capsule in the region of the intertubercular sulcus. In 7 shoulders, the tendon was so adherent to the floor of the groove that it required sharp dissection to free it; in 2 shoulders the tendon had a bony attachment to the floor of the groove. It appeared as if, in the natural course of the disease, the objective of the process was to obliterate the gliding mechanism of the biceps tendon by anchoring the tendon to the shaft of the humerus and, thereby, relieve pain. Once the patient is free of severe pain he can begin to move the arm, increase muscular activity and slowly restore scapulohumeral motion.

The following case history is an excellent example of the sequence of events related above. The patient, a 73-year-old man, was examined three months prior to death. At this time no clinical evidence of shoulder dysfunction was found in either shoulder, and the patient was unaware of any disability in either extremity. However, his past medical history revealed that 15 to 17 years prior to this examination he experienced a severe episode of pain and loss of motion, first in the right shoulder and then in the left. After an indefinite period—2 to 3 years—the pain subsided and motion returned slowly in both shoulders. From his history, I concluded that the shoulder disorders were frozen shoulders.

This patient died of causes unrelated to the shoulders. Both scapulohumeral joints with the musculotendinous cuff intact were removed at autopsy. In both biceps tendons the intracapsular portion was absent, and the extracapsular portion had attained a bony insertion just below the tuberosities (see Fig. 11-15). In this instance, a cure had been effected by deleting the gliding mechanism of the biceps tendon.

Between the shoulder with minimal pathology as seen in the early phase of the disease and the shoulder with profound changes observed in the late phases, there are great variations in the severity of the pathology and the areas affected. Hence, the observations of one surgeon are seldom the same as those of another. Herein lies the reason for the great discrepancies in the literature in regard to the specific structure or structures responsible for frozen shoulder. If the reader keeps in mind that once the process starts in the capsule, if the disease lasts long enough, (1) all soft tissue elements surrounding the capsule eventually become involved; (2) the process progresses very slowly so that not all tissues are affected to the same degree simultaneously, and (3) the process may spontaneously reverse itself before all elements of the joint are implicated, he can appreciate fully the reason for the conflicting pathological findings recorded by different surgeons.

## Treatment

The first consideration in the management of frozen shoulder is to establish the diagnosis beyond any doubt. Remember that incomplete tears of the cuff, calcareous tendinitis and bicipital tenosynovitis also produce a stiff and painful shoulder. Having established the diagnosis, the consideration of next importance is to give the patient assurance that the disorder is self limited and in time pain will subside and motion will return. These apprehensive patients need their confidence restored. Next, determine by the history and the physical examination the phase of the disorder.

This is most important, for, in the early phase when some scapulohumeral motion still remains and the pain is still tolerable, much can be done by simple measures to reverse the process. However, in the late phase, especially if the patient has already passed through the therapeutic mill, more radical measures are indicated. Regardless of the phase of the disease the patient's general health and nutrition must be improved. Also, adequate sedation should be prescribed, to relieve the patient's restless, emotional state.

### Early Phase

During this period, pain and muscle spasm are chiefly responsible for the loss of shoulder motion. At this stage, I prefer to put the patient to bed for 7 to 10 days. Prescribe enough sedation to reduce restlessness and relieve pain and apply continuous hot packs to the shoulder region. Encourage the patient to exercise the arm at regular intervals in the supine position. All exercises are performed within the painless arcs of motion. I find the injection of the cervical sympathetic ganglia with 10 ml. of a 1 percent solution of procaine a valuable adjunct for relief of pain and muscle spasm. Also, one or two injections of $\frac{1}{2}$ ml. of one of the corticosteroids directly into the bicipital sheath may reduce the intensity of the pain.

After the period of bedrest, support the arm in a sling, but institute gravity-free exercises on a regulated schedule. Each exercise is performed 10 to 12 times every hour, and always performed within the painless arcs of motion. Usually with this program, within a few days, the pain subsides sufficiently to discard the sling. Now add antigravity exercises such as wall crawling, and using the pully and wheel. Within 6 to 8 weeks many patients have little or no pain and a fair range of scapulohumeral motion. However, in most instances, many months (6 to 9 months) must pass before the shoulder achieves total restoration of motion.

Many patients refuse to go to bed; the treatment prescribed for these ambulatory patients is the same as that described above. In my series, 19 of 28 patients in the early phase of the disease responded favorably to the conservative measures. However, 9 patients did not improve and progressed to the late phase of frozen shoulder.

When a patient, in the early phase of the disease, fails to respond to adequate conservative management either institute another form of treatment, or advise the patient to accept the natural course of the disease. The choices of treatment remaining are (1) manipulation, and (2) surgical mobilization.

**Manipulation.** Many years ago I was convinced that manipulation of the shoulder was a futile and dangerous procedure. My opinion was based, primarily, on the number of poor results I encountered following manipulation and, also, on the observations I made on a group of frozen shoulders manipulated under vision. The latter group comprised 11 patients whose shoulders were explored surgically and then manipulated. In all instances, the arm was put through a full range of motion. To achieve this in some shoulders considerable force was required.

In all instances, when the arm was externally rotated, regardless of how gently the maneuver was performed tears of varying sizes occurred in the subscapularis tendon and its lower muscle fibers. In 2 shoulders the tendon tore completely away from the lesser tuberosity. Abduction of the arm invariably produced transverse tears in the inferior portion of the fibrous capsule. In 3 shoulders the inferior capsule peeled off the humeral neck, exposing the articular surface of the head of the humerus. Rupture of the biceps tendon occurred in 3 shoulders and in another the surgical neck of the humerus fractured.

TECHNIQUE OF MANIPULATION OF THE SHOULDER JOINT. The mutilation of the soft tissue structures of the joint by manipulation is indeed frightening, and it has been observed by other surgeons as well. Yet I have observed some excellent results following manipulation of the shoulder. Also, this method has a number of strong supporters. After much thought and speculation it occurred to me that the method of manipulation employed might solve the enigma, and, since the prime goal of any treatment is to relieve pain so that muscular activity can be restored, the ideal manipulative maneuver would be one that would obliterate the gliding mechanism of the biceps tendon with minimal disruption of the other joint structures. In these instances, this implies rupture of the tendon.

The maneuver that achieves this is elevation of the arm from the side in the sagittal plane until it reaches the hyperextended position. The procedure is performed slowly; the internal condyle of the humerus always faces forward, the humerus is never rotated and the maneuver is never repeated. As the arm is elevated a soft crepitus is heard and felt in the axilla; this is produced by the capsule as it peels off the inferior neck of the humerus. Then a sharp snap occurs, followed by sudden release of the humeral head; now, the arm readily reaches the point of maximum elevation. Considerable force may be necessary to elevate the arm to the hyperextended position, for not only the retracted capsule and rotators resist the movement but also the shortened, strong muscles comprising the anterior and posterior axillary folds.

Before manipulating the shoulder, I inject into the joint 10 ml. of 1 percent Xylocaine. Then I distend the capsule with normal saline. The capsule is distended when, upon release of the thumb pressure on the plunger of the syringe, the plunger rises out of the barrel of the syringe. This usually requires 10 to 15 ml. of solution. More saline is forced, under pressure, into the joint until, suddenly, a free flow is established. This indicates that the capsule has ruptured at some point. As seen by arthrograms the point of rupture may be through the subscapularis bursa, the bicipital sheath or the inferior portion of the capsule. During the procedure the patient may experience considerable discomfort, but as yet I have never had to resort to general anesthesia.

After the manipulation the wrist is tied to the top of the bed, holding the arm in the elevated position. Four or five times every day the wrist is released and the patient moves the arm actively in all directions. After the third day the patient becomes ambulatory, supporting the arm in a sling; now he does pendulum exercises every hour. The range of the exercises must never exceed the patient's tolerance of pain. Within a few days the patient starts antigravity exercises using the pulley and wheel and wall crawling.

All the patients whom I have treated in the manner described above attained considerable relief of pain, so much so that after a few days they were able to exercise the shoulder with relative ease. In some, motion in the scapulohumeral joint returned rapidly; in others, it returned slowly. I am unable to say how much, if any, the total period of the disease was shortened in any of these patients, since the natural course of the disease varies considerably. Moreover, I seriously doubt that the patients themselves are able to pinpoint the exact time at which complete free, painless motion was obtained. In any case, these patients were now free of pain and, except for some discomfort and twinges on certain motions of the shoulder, they were able to return to their normal activities.

**Tenodesis of the Biceps Tendon.** The alternative to manipulation is tenodesis of the biceps tendon. Anchoring the biceps tendon to the upper end of the humerus, in my hands, also is followed by relief of pain in frozen shoulders. I now reserve this procedure for those patients who are in the early phase of the disease and are not responding to conservative treatment and in whom, in my judgment, the biceps tendon has not as yet attained firm fixation to the humerus.

### Late Phase

Some patients are first seen when the late phase of the disease is well established. Many of these already have had the shoulder manipulated without success. If, in my judgment, the previous conservative treatment prescribed was inadequate or if no definitive treatment had even been given, I institute the course of conservative therapy. Although few in number, some of these patients will respond to conservative measures. If they do not respond, my first choice is manipulation of the arm and my second is tenodesis of the biceps tendon.

OPERATIVE TECHNIQUE (TENODESIS OF THE BICEPS TENDON). Expose the anterior aspect of the shoulder by an anterior incision in line with the axillary crease. It begins just medial to the acromioclavicular joint and extends downward on the anterior aspect of the shoulder for 3 to 3½ inches. Expose the medial margin of the deltoid and develop the deltopectoral interval; do not injure the cephalic vein, which lies in the interval. Retract the vein and the pectoralis major medially and the deltoid laterally; this exposes the coracoid process. By rotating the humerus internally and externally the intertubercular groove spanned by the transverse humeral ligament comes into view.

Divide the transverse humeral ligament longitudinally and identify the biceps tendon in the intertubercular groove. Extend

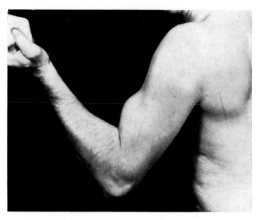

FIG. 11-23. Rupture of the long head of the biceps tendon; the rupture occurred at the supraglenoid tubercle. Note that when the supinated forearm is flexed against resistance, the biceps muscle forms a bulge in the lower part of the arm.

the incision proximally for 5 centimeters through the fibers of the coracohumeral ligament; this exposes the intracapsular portion of the biceps tendon. Next, sever the tendon close to its insertion into the apex of the glenoid fossa and withdraw it from the joint and excise the intracapsular portion of the tendon.

With a sharp curette scarify the floor of the intertubercular groove down to bleeding bone. Place the tendon in the groove and anchor it in the groove with interrupted sutures passing through the transverse humeral ligament. Occasionally, I use a staple to anchor the tendon in the groove. Close the split in the coracohumeral ligament with a few interrupted sutures.

POSTOPERATIVE MANAGEMENT. Place the arm in a sling and institute pendulum exercises on the first postoperative day. The exercises must be performed a prescribed number of times three or four times each day. After the fifth day the patient discards the sling and increases progressively the range of motion during the exercise periods. The range of motion must not exceed the patient's tolerance of pain. After 3 weeks encourage the patient to use the arm in all daily activities. Optimum

function returns slowly—the time varies from 3 to 4 months; however, during this period the patients are relatively free of pain.

## RUPTURE OF THE BICEPS TENDON

### General Considerations

Rupture of a normal biceps tendon rarely occurs. In young athletes, rupture occasionally follows unguarded, forceful contraction of the biceps muscle. As a rule, the lesion occurs in people past middle life when varying degrees of degeneration are present in the tendon. As recorded in Chapter 6 degeneration of the tendon is common and progresses from decade to decade. Hypertrophic bony changes in the tuberosities and in the intertubercular groove are partially responsible for the fraying, shredding and, finally, partial or complete rupture of the tendon fibers.

Spontaneous rupture is not an infrequent occurrence in shoulders with advanced dengerative abnormalities in the rotator cuff and head of the humerus. In some of these shoulders, before rupture occurs, the extracapsular portion of the tendon adheres by a bony attachment to the shaft of the humerus just below the lesser tuberosity. Also, in the face of these extensive changes, forceful contraction of the biceps may produce a rupture of the tendon.

Many occupations require the arm to work in abduction and internal rotation. Now, the tendon lies directly on the lesser tuberosity. This position not only favors subluxation of the tendon but also increases the friction between the tendon and the bone. This accentuates the degenerative alterations in the tendon. Abnormal stress applied to the weakened tendon is capable of rupturing it. An indirect force, such as forceful contraction of the biceps, causes most of the ruptures. Only a few ruptures result from a direct blow or a fall on the shoulder.

## Site of Rupture

The weakest portion of the tendon is the segment lying just distal to its exit from the joint cavity. Most ruptures occur at this site. The intracapsular portion of the tendon lies free in the joint cavity while the extra-articular portion is pulled distally. Less frequently the rupture occurs (1) at the supraglenoid tuberosity, or (2) at the musculotendinous juncture or within the muscle mass.

Usually the rupture is complete; occasionally it is partial. In the former instance, the tendon usually lies curled up at varying distances below the intertubercular sulcus; or it may bend upon itself like a jack-knife. When the rupture is partial, the torn fibers may reattach themselves to the bicipital groove.

## Clinical Features

When the rupture occurs in a normal tendon or one with minimal degenerative changes, usually the history records a sudden, forceful contracture of the biceps against resistance. A sharp, audible snap follows, accompanied by lancinating pain in the shoulder. The pain radiates, extending to the anterior aspect of the upper arm. On the other hand, in a severely degenerated tendon, as a rule, there is no sudden onset. Rather, these individuals give a history of some vague discomfort and weakness in the shoulder. Often they are under treatment for bursitis, tendinitis or sprains.

If the rupture is complete, the muscle mass contracts distally, forming a soft swelling in the lower third of the arm. This is particularly noticeable when the arm is extended. Upon flexing the arm, the bulge of the biceps is less firm than that on the normal side (Fig. 11-23) and the interval between the biceps and the deltoid is increased. When the rupture occurs at the lower musculotendinous juncture, the muscle mass draws upward in the upper third

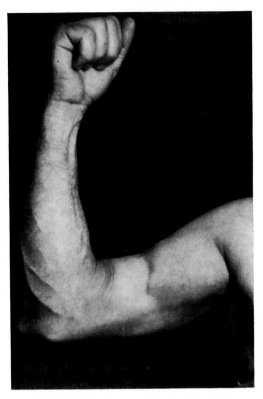

FIG. 11-24. Rupture of the biceps muscle at the lower musculotendinous junction. When the muscle is contracted the muscle mass moves proximally. Note the flattened area in the lower part of the arm below the bulging muscle.

of the arm while the lower third appears flat (Fig. 11-24).

In partial ruptures the position and size of the muscle mass depend upon the extent of the tear and the distance the muscle belly draws away from the site of rupture. A rupture through the substance of the muscle belly results in a hiatus between the two ends, and its size depends on the number of muscle fibers torn. In complete tears a wide gap forms when the forearm is flexed against resistance, whereas in incomplete tears only a small sulcus appears.

If the rupture occurs through the avascular portion of the tendon, no ecchymosis follows; but when the tear occurs through the musculotendinous junction or through the muscle belly, often a large hematoma and discoloration form on the anterior and inner aspects of the arm. Also, in recent ruptures pressure over the bicipital groove and over the muscle, depending on the site of rupture, elicits tenderness. This subsides slowly until only some soreness remains. Tenderness can also be elicited in old ruptures or when the rupture was a gradual one in a degenerated tendon. Many tests have been devised for a rupture of the biceps tendon — Yergaron's, Ludington's and Hueter's — none of which is very reliable.

Impairment of function depends on the extent and location of the rupture and the cause. In acute traumatic rupture of the tendon or the muscle belly, immediate pain and severe impairment of function ensue. After the acute symptoms subside, weakness of the arm and discomfort may persist for a long time. On the other hand, especially when the rupture occurs slowly in a degenerated tendon, the disability may be insignificant except, perhaps, for some stiffness and soreness.

## Treatment

In the young, especially athletes, it is most essential to provide the distal end of the ruptured tendon with a bony point of fixation. All patients with rupture of the biceps tendon have some weakness of the arm. It should be remembered that the biceps is a powerful supinator of the forearm. Loss of this muscle power in young people can be a great handicap. On the other hand, in middle aged persons and especially the elderly this impairment is of little or no significance. It does not interfere with their normal daily activities. Clearly surgical repair in the young is a "must," whereas in the older age group repair is indicated only if pain and pronounced dysfunction persist. This is indeed rare.

Many types of repair of rupture of the tendon have been described. I now prefer to anchor the tendon to the floor of the bicipital groove. The technique is described on page 467. Recent ruptures through the muscle belly or the musculotendinous junctions are best repaired by deep interrupted sutures. If the suture line appears weak, it can be reinforced by a piece of fascia lata. Old ruptures may require excision of considerable scar tissue. In these instances, the suture line should always be reinforced with a fascial transplant.

## TRAUMATIC DISLOCATION OF THE BICEPS TENDON

As noted in Chapter 6, in advanced degenerative change of the rotator cuff often the biceps tendon subluxates or dislocates from the intertubercular groove. This is usually the result of tearing away of some of the upper fibers of the tendon of the subscapularis from the anterior lip of the intertubercular sulcus. Also, the displacement may be enhanced by a supratubercular ridge in the sulcus, but these lesions differ from acute traumatic displacement of the tendon. However, the supratubercular ridge facilitates dislocation of the tendon when the lesion is produced by trauma.

### Clinical Features

The usual mechanism of dislocation of the tendon, particularly in the young, is forceful abduction and external rotation of the arm. In the presence of congenital anomalies of the intertubercular sulcus, displacement may occur with little or no force. Following an acute dislocation the patient experiences severe pain in the shoulder which travels to the anterior aspect of the arm. All movements are painful, especially external rotation and abduction and forward flexion and abduction. An audible snap in the shoulder occurs at the time of dislocation of the tendon. The patient can reproduce this by bringing the externally rotated arm down from the elevated position in the coronal plane. As the arm passes the horizontal, the tendon slips mesially over the lesser tuberosity, producing the snap.

Following the initial dislocation, recurrences occur relatively frequently. As the result of repeated dislocations, bicipital tenosynovitis develops, causing a painful and stiff shoulder.

## Treatment

There is only one cure for this lesion. The tendon must be anchored to the upper end of the shaft of the humerus. In addition, I always excise the intracapsular portion of the tendon. The surgical technique is described on page 467.

## CALCAREOUS TENDINITIS

Calcific deposits in the tendons of the rotator cuff are frequent causes of painful and stiff shoulders. Calcareous tendinitis is second in frequency only to bicipital tenosynovitis. The entity is often described under such designations as subacromial or subdeltoid bursitis with calcification. These are misnomers, for the primary lesion is not in the subacromial bursa but rather in the tendons of the rotator cuff. The bursa is involved secondarily. Calcific deposits occur in other sites; in fact, they may occur in any tendon or ligament in the body. Next to the rotator tendons the most common sites are tendons attached to the greater trochanter, radiohumeral joint, tendo Achillis and the flexor tendons of the fingers. I studied in detail 136 patients with calcareous tendinitis of the shoulder. The data presented in the following sections are derived largely from this study.

## Epidemiology

**Site.** Calcific deposits can occur in practically every tendon in the environs of the shoulder. There may be single or multiple lesions. Some people have a constitutional predisposition to form calcific deposits. In

the shoulder, the lesion occurs most frequently in the supraspinatus tendon. In my series the lesion occurred in the supraspinatus tendon in 90 percent of the shoulders. In 52 percent the lesion was a single deposit in the supraspinatus tendon, and in 22 percent multiple deposits in the same structures. Thus, 74 percent of the shoulders exhibited implication of the supraspinatus tendon alone. In 16 percent the lesion occurred simultaneously in the supraspinatus area and some other area of the cuff. In the remaining 10 percent the supraspinatus area was not involved; rather, the lesion appeared in some other region of the shoulder. One lesion occurred in the tendon of the teres major and one in the tendon of the subscapularis. Also, in cases not included in this study, I have encountered calcific deposits in the tendon of the pectoralis major, the conjoined tendon arising from the coracoid process, and the biceps tendon.

**Age and Sex of Patient, and Unilateral vs. Bilateral Involvement.** Generally, calcareous tendinitis of the rotator tendons occurs most commonly in the fourth and fifth decades, but occasionally it is seen in the third decade. Rarely does it occur after the sixth decade. In my series, the age of the patients ranged from 24 to 72 years. Only 5 percent of the patients were from 24 to 30 years of age and 8 percent from 60 to 72 years. The greatest number (36%) were between 40 and 50 years of age. The average age was 45.2 years.

In most series reported in the literature the sexes are about equally divided. In my series there was a predominance of females; 60.3 percent were females and 39.7 were males. The right shoulder was involved in 57 percent and the left in 43 percent. Fourteen percent of the patients had bilateral involvement. These data differ from other series which report approximately 50 percent bilateral involvement. The discrepancy might be explained by the failure on my part to take x-rays of both shoulders in patients with unilateral symptoms. The opposite shoulder may have a silent lesion. Not infrequently, a patient presents with a symptomatic deposit in one shoulder and then several months later develops symptoms in the opposite shoulder.

**Occupation.** Forty-one percent of the patients were housewives, 10 percent were secretaries and 10 percent were laborers. The remainder were engaged in wholly sedentary work. Whereas ruptures of the cuff occur in persons doing laborious work, the above data indicate that calcareous tendinitis occurs in people who perform light work in which the arm is used, in slight abduction for many hours at a time. This position tends to accentuate any existing attritional abnormalities in the cuff.

**Trauma.** The use of the arm in the slightly abducted and internally rotated position can reasonably be considered a form of repeated minor trauma. The cumulative effect of this type of trauma has a definitely deleterious effect on the degenerative cuff. Sudden, severe trauma also aggravates the degenerative changes in the cuff. However, it appears that a considerable interval must elapse between the initial trauma and radiographic evidence of calcification in the cuff. Rarely is a calcific deposit demonstrable by radiograms taken immediately after an injury, and I have never seen one at that time. However, I have seen several develop within 6 to 9 months after the injury, although radiograms failed to show a calcific deposit when the injury occurred. Many quiescent deposits, not giving rise to symptoms, may suddenly flare up after a bout of overactivity or acute, severe trauma, producing an acute syndrome.

**Infection and Constitutional Diseases.** Infection as a local or distant focus plays no part in the causation of calcareous tendinitis. Cultures and smears of the calcareous material removed at operation never exhibit a responsible organism. Moreover, patients with proved foci of infection respond to therapy regardless of whether the focus is treated or not.

Likewise, there is no evidence that constitutional diseases are in any way related to this entity.

## Pathogenesis and Pathology

Many concepts of the formation of amorphous calcium deposits in tendons have appeared from time to time in the literature. As yet, the process is not clear. However, there must be some abnormal local, biochemical process concerned with calcium metabolism that is responsible for the formation of calcific deposits. Also, we know that these deposits form in degenerated tendon fibers. In the case of the rotator cuff the deposits originate, most often, in that portion of the cuff which endures the greatest amount of stress and most frequently undergoes extensive degneration— the supraspinatus tendon. Codman designated the region of greatest stress in the supraspinatus the "critical zone"; it lies just proximal to the insertion of the tendon into the greater tuberosity. This is the area in which calcific deposits most frequently form.

The process begins with degeneration of the central tendon fibers and, at first, is in no way related to the joint cavity or the subacromial bursa. I have confirmed this many times in autopsy specimens. Small degenerated areas within the substance of the supraspinatus tendon are frequent findings in the cuffs of persons past middle life. These areas do not communicate with the joint cavity or the subacromial bursa. These are the foci in which calcific deposits form.

The nature of the pathological changes in the bursal walls and the cuff fibers immediately surrounding a calcific deposit depends upon the severity of the inflammatory reaction around the deposit. When the deposits are small and discrete, lie deep in the tendon fibers and do not irritate the floor of the bursa, they give rise to no symptoms. In this state they are quiescent and may remain so for many years. Frequently

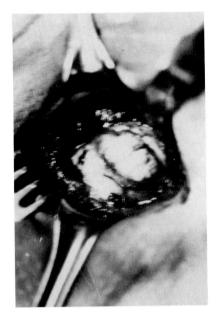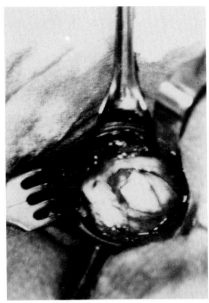

FIG. 11-25. Characteristic appearance of a calcareous deposit producing an acute syndrome. In this instance, there are two large deposits under much tension; they are greyish white in appearance, and the floor of the bursa is tightly stretched over the swelling.

they are discovered accidentally by radiologists.

Some deposits slowly increase in size until they contact the floor of the bursa. They may then cause pain by impinging against the edge of the coracoacromial arch when the arm is abducted, elevated or rotated. This frictional trauma may produce a low-grade inflammatory reaction in the floor of the bursa and the surrounding tissues. At this stage, the deposit becomes a well defined swelling with a white center, but it is not under tension. The floor of the bursa may become thickened and even may be covered with small synovial villi.

Incision of such a tumefaction discloses a whitish, gritty material incorporated within the degenerated tendon fibers. It can be removed only by curettage or excision of the entire area, leaving a fair-sized cavity. These lesions, as a rule, do not cause acute symptoms, but they do cause some discomfort in the shoulder. However, the lesions are potential sources of trouble.

Continued frictional trauma or sudden strains may increase the inflammatory process around the deposit and produce subacute or acute symptoms.

The character of the deposit depends upon the intensity of the inflammatory reaction around it which in turn governs the severity of the symptoms. Lesions producing a subacute syndrome lie directly under the floor of the bursa which is stretched tightly over the calcareous mound. The swelling has a whitish or yellow center and is surrounded by a circular bluish zone of congested synovial membrane. The bursal wall is thickened and slightly edematous. The size of the deposits vary greatly, from a few millimeters to five or six centimeters in length; the average size is 1½ to 2 centimeters. When such a deposit is incised, a whitish or yellow material, which has the consistency of tooth paste, escapes. In some instances, the material contains hard, gritty particles.

In longstanding cases, the deposit may

show different features. The calcareous material may be so enmeshed in the tendon fibers that it does not flow freely when the deposit is incised. Often, bits of degenerated tendon fibers intermingle within the calcareous material.

Lesions causing acute symptoms do not differ greatly from those producing a subacute syndrome except that the inflammatory reaction in all the tissues surrounding the deposits is more pronounced. The calcareous mound is under much pressure; its center is grayish-white, around which is a zone of congestion, deep red or violet in color. The floor of the bursa is tightly stretched over the swelling and is very thin; the remaining portion of the bursal floor is thick and edematous (Fig. 11-25). If the top of the tumefaction is nicked with a scalpel, a milky fluid escapes. It appears that the acuteness of the syndrome parallels the consistency of the calcareous material: the more acute the symptoms, the more fluid the calcareous material. This milky, amorphous material is found also in the subacromial bursa when the mound ruptures spontaneously.

It is apparent from the pathology of calcareous tendinitis that the subacromial bursa becomes involved secondarily. Also, the intensity of the symptoms depends upon the severity of the inflammatory reaction around the calcific deposit and the amount of tension within the deposit. When the deposit ruptures, as it often does, and the pressure within it is reduced, the patient experiences great relief of pain.

## Clinical Features

Depending on the nature of the pathology, the entity presents three distinct variations: the chronic, the subacute and the acute syndrome. But this clinical classification does not apply to all instances; many are borderline in character, and others present all three stages at different times.

**Chronic Syndrome.** Mildness of the symptoms is the characterisitc feature of the chronic syndrome. The only complaint may be a "catch" or a slight twinge of pain on internal rotation or elevation of the arm. Muscle spasm is absent and shoulder motion is not restricted. The twinge of pain results from impingement of the calcific deposit against the falciform edge of the coracoacromial arch when the arm is elevated or rotated. This condition may persist for years without disability. However, these shoulders are vulnerable, and, at any time, excessive use or acute strains may precipitate subacute or acute syndromes.

**Subacute Syndrome.** Most patients with calcific deposits disclose subacute clinical manifestations. Usually, the onset is insidious; the patient feels a catch or twinge in the shoulder on certain motions of the arm. As in the chronic syndrome, the pain is caused by impingement of the calcareous mass against the edge of the coracoacromial arch. After the mass passes under the arch the pain disappears. For this reason, many patients sleep with the arm abducted and the hand behind the head.

The pain becomes progressively more severe. When this occurs, the patient avoids movements that produce the pain and uses the arm only within painless arcs of motion. Not infrequently, this pattern of the syndrome may remain static for many months and then disappear. On the other hand, pain in the shoulder may become constant and excruciating when the mass abuts against the coracoacromial arch. In severe forms, the pain always radiates, traveling to the insertion of the deltoid and, at times, to the inferior angle of the scapula, to the cervical and suboccipital regions and even to the back of the forearm and fingers, particularly the thumb and the index finger. Occasionally the dorsum of the hand becomes puffy and the fingers swollen and painful. Generally, the pain is more severe at night; the patient is unable to find a comfortable position for the arm and spends many restless nights.

Examination invariably elicits marked tenderness when pressure is made over the inflamed bursa and over the insertion of the deltoid. At times, a small, tender mass which rotates with the humerus can be felt just proximal to the greater tuberosity. In the early stages, spasm of the rotator muscles may or may not be present, but later muscle spacm is constant and pronounced. Motion in the scapulohumeral joint decreases progressively until abduction and elevation are barely possible to the horizontal and take place entirely in the scapulothoracic joint. In addition, the spinati and deltoid reveal advanced atrophy; now the clinical picture is one of frozen shoulder. In some patients, as the range of scapulohumeral motion decreases, the patient experiences less pain; some have no motion and no pain.

It is apparent that calcareous tendinitis, like bicipital tenosynovitis, may initiate in the capsule of the joint the pathological process producing frozen shoulder. However, this process is never permanent, for, with the disappearance of the calcific deposit, the entire process reverses itself and painless, free motion returns.

Fortunately, most instances of the subacute syndrome do not run such a violent course. Generally, the course is more clement and complete recovery occurs in a relatively short period, provided that treatment is adequate.

In some instances, the outstanding features are restricted scapulohumeral motion and little pain. In these, spasm and restriction of motion are predominant features from the very onset of the syndrome. In other instances, from the onset and throughout the course of the disease, motion is relatively free but pain is intense and constant.

**Acute Syndrome.** The acute syndrome comes on suddenly and pursues a brief and fulminating course. Not infrequently, the patient is unaware of any shoulder disorder prior to its onset, but, in some instances, a subacute or chronic syndrome antedates the acute attack. As a rule, overactivity or trauma precipitates the acute syndrome.

The characteristic clinical features are sudden, severe pain in the anterior aspect of the shoulder which is markedly accentuated by the slightest motion. Also, the rotator muscles are in pronounced spasm and even light pressure in the subacromial region elicits severe tenderness.

Frequently, the pain radiates, involving the insertion of the deltoid, the forearm and even the fingers. The agonizing pain may appear suddenly during the night. It is so severe that the commonly used sedatives fail to give relief, and the patient puts in many sleepless nights.

In untreated cases, such symptoms may persist for a week or two and then subside. Subsequently, the muscle spasm decreases and motion returns slowly. In other instances, some muscle spasm or impairment of motion may persist for many months. Although the duration of the syndrome and its sequelae are unpredictable, full recovery is the rule.

What is the cause of the sudden onset of pain and why, in some instances, does it subside as suddenly? Comprehension of the pathology of the lesion provides the answer to these questions. The sudden and severe pain is caused by the acute inflammatory reaction of the tissues surrounding the calcareous deposit. The deposit enlarges and the sensitive floor of the bursa is subjected to great tension. As long as the tension is maintained, and pain is severe, the rotator muscles stay in spasm and motion is restricted.

Should the floor of the bursa rupture, the milky fluid escapes from the lesion into the bursa; the calcareous mound and surrounding tissues are decompressed and the pain subsides. Once evacuated into the bursa, the calcareous material is readily absorbed. If absorption of the calcific substance is complete, the affected tissues heal readily and no recurrence is likely. However, if some material remains in the tissues there is always the possibility of another acute attack or the lesion may pursue a subacute or chronic course.

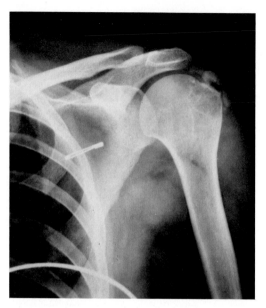

FIG. 11-26. Typical amorphous calcific deposit in the rotator cuff found in the acute syndrome. Note that it is crescent shaped and parallels the fibers of the cuff; also in this instance the deposit has ruptured through the bursa and is seen in the bursal sac.

## Roentgenographic Features

Roentgenographically, the calcareous deposits present two patterns: In one pattern the deposit is amorphous and exhibits a fluffy, fleecy appearance. Often its periphery is poorly defined and the mass is spotty, conforming to the long axis of the cuff. Its length varies from a few millimeters to five or six centimeters. Occasionally a thin crescent or amorphous streak or globular mass in continuity with the main mass appears in the subacromial bursa (Figs. 11-26, 11-27, 11-28, 11-29 and 11-30). This indicates that the deposit has ruptured through the bursal floor. The above lesions occur in the acute forms of the disease. The second pattern discloses discrete, homogeneous deposits. The density may be uniform throughout the mass or it may be spotty. As a rule, the borders are well defined and parallel the long axis of the cuff. This type occurs in subacute and

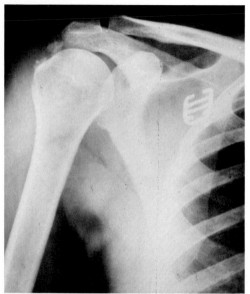

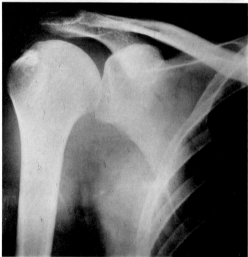

(Top) FIG. 11-27. Radiographic appearance of multiple amorphous calcific deposits in the cuff.

(Bottom) FIG. 11-28. An unusual location of a large amorphous calcific deposit. It lies in the tendon of the pectoralis major.

chronic forms of the entity (Figs. 11-31 and 11-32).

Roentgenographic visualization and precise localization of the deposits may be difficult. Routinely, films should be taken in different positions of internal and external rotation. As noted above, there is some

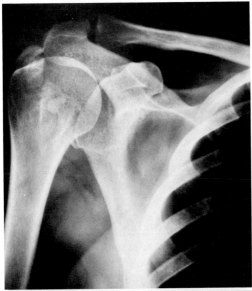

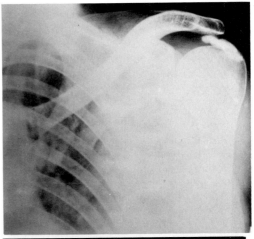

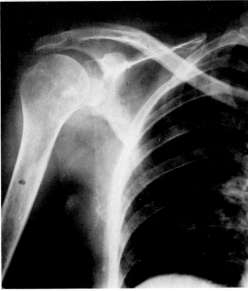

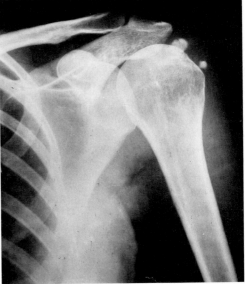

(*Top*) FIG. 11-29. Multiple irregular amorphous calcific deposits. They involved both the supraspinatus and subscapularis tendons.

(*Bottom*) FIG. 11-30. Large amorphous calcific deposits in the subscapularis tendon.

(*Top*) FIG. 11-31. Typical calcific deposit found in chronic forms of calcific tendinitis. The deposit is discrete, well defined and homogenous. It parallels the long axis of the cuff.

(*Bottom*) FIG. 11-32. Multiple, discrete calcific deposits; one lies in the teres minor tendon.

correlation between the configuration and density of the deposit and the nature of the clinical syndrome. However, the size of a calcific deposit, as seen in roentgenograms, does not always indicate the nature of the syndrome that the patient presents. Small deposits may produce severe acute symptoms, whereas large deposits may produce only mild or no symptoms. Also, routine roentgenograms may fail to depict the true size of the lesion. Often, however, an elusive deposit can be localized and its size determined by fluoroscopic examination and the taking of spot films of the lesion.

## Treatment

All calcareous deposits, regardless of the stage of the syndrome, should first be treated by conservative measures. The goal of this treatment is to induce absorption of the calcareous material, and this can best be achieved by multiple puncture of the calcific deposit. The severe pain in the acute stage often ends abruptly, indicating that the deposit has ruptured spontaneously into the bursa. These patients need no further treatment. However, if the material is not completely absorbed the syndrome may recur. Failure to respond to conservative measures justifies surgical excision of the calcific deposit.

**Aspiration and Needling of the Deposit.** This is more or less a blind procedure, and, if more than one deposit is present, this method may fail to rupture all of them. Inject a few ml. of a 1 percent solution of procaine into the skin immediately over the point of maximum tenderness. Use a large gauge needle to infiltrate the subcutaneous tissue, muscle and the roof of the bursa. Now, insert an 18 gauge needle on a syringe partially filled with 1 percent procaine into the deposit and withdraw the plunger of the syringe. This maneuver may suck up into the syringe some fine, flaky material. Continue the barbotage in different areas and levels of the deposit until all accessible material is withdrawn. This is indicated by the return of clear fluid into the syringe. When the calcific deposit is firm and discrete or is firmly emmeshed in tendon fibers, it may not be possible to aspirate any calcareous material.

Following the barbotage perforate the entire area by multiple punctures, using the same needle. The object of this step is to produce an active hyperemia which enhances dissolution and absorption of any remaining calcific material. Next, inject 1 ml. of one of the corticosteroids into the area.

AFTER TREATMENT. For the first 24 to 48 hours after the procedure described above, give adequate sedation to control the pain. Also apply continuous hot packs to the shoulder. Encourage the patient to move the arm through a normal range of motion several times a day. When the pain subsides institute a program, first, of pendulum exercises and then of antigravity exercises – wall crawling, and using the pulley and wheel. Motion should always be within the patient's tolerance of pain. As the pain subsides, the arcs of motion increase. Radiant heat and gentle massage add to the patient's comfort.

Other methods are occasionally employed in the treatment of calcareous tendinitis; they are x-ray and manipulation. In my opinion, x-ray therapy has no place in the treatment of this entity. Those instances of acute calcareous tendinitis that respond dramatically to x-ray therapy do so because the deposit ruptured. I am sure that rupture occurred spontaneously and was not caused by the therapy. Often this method accentuates the pain and, in many instances, weeks and even months of treatment are given before recovery. In this latter group the disease is pursuing its natural course.

The object of manipulation is to rupture the deposit. This is most difficult to achieve by manipulative maneuvers which may do more harm than good to the soft tissues of the shoulder joint.

**Surgical Management.** Operative intervention in calcareous tendinitis has some advantages: (1) Relief from pain is prompt and certain, (2) restoration of normal motion is more rapid than in other methods, and (3) recurrences are indeed rare. I have never seen a recurrence.

SURGICAL TECHNIQUE. An anterior deltoid-splitting incision is simple and provides adequate exposure of the subacromial bursa. The patient is placed on the table in a sitting position, with a sandbag under the affected shoulder and another under the corresponding hip. By drawing the patient close to the edge of the table, the elbow may be dropped below table level, thereby making the tuberosity more prominent. The hand and the forearm on the affected side are draped so that the arm may be maneuvered freely during the operation.

The skin incision begins immediately below the acromioclavicular joint and extends distally on the anterior aspect of the arm for from 2½ to 3 inches. The incision is deepened through the full thickness of the anterior portion of the deltoid by blunt dissection, exposing the roof of the bursa. While the forearm is held vertical to the table, the roof of the bursa is incised, the opening being directly over the bicipital groove. All regions of the bursa can be visualized readily merely by rotating the arm. No difficulty is encountered in locating the calcareous deposit if it is beneath the floor of the bursa in the supraspinatus region of the cuff.

Visualization of the mass may be slightly more difficult if it lies in the subscapularis region or in the extreme end of the infraspinatus, or in the teres minor regions. The tumefaction is incised parallel with the cuff fibers, and its contents are evacuated with a curette. Occasionally, the necrotic walls of the remaining cavity are excised by elliptical incision parallel with the axis of the tendon fibers. The cavity is irrigated thoroughly with normal saline solution. If the defect is extensive, it is closed by side-to-side sutures.

A thorough search for the presence of any other deposits should be made, and any suspicious areas should be nicked with the point of the scalpel to determine the existence of hidden calcareous masses. Multiple punctures of the cuff adjacent to the lesion ensure an active hyperemia, which favors absorption of any remaining calcareous material. To facilitate free excursion of the humeral head under the coracoacromial arch, the coracoacromial ligament is divided routinely at its insertion into the medial edge of the acromion.

For the first 24 hours following operation the arm is suspended to an overhead frame, with lateral traction. On the second day gravity-free pendulum exercises are

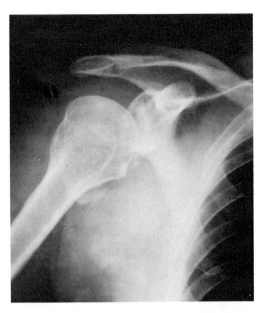

FIG. 11-33. Intraosseous deposit; note some flakes of calcific material in the fibers of the overlying tendon.

started on a schedule of every 3 hours, for from 3 to 5 minutes. The range of motion is at all times maintained within the patient's tolerance of pain. As the acute symptoms subside, exercises are done every hour, and wall-crawling and pulley exercises are added.

Physical therapy should supplement this regimen. Application of radiant heat and gentle massage to the shoulder girdle and the upper arm add to the comfort of the patient. In most instances full restoration of painless motion is attained in 3 weeks, although a few cases (complicated with pronounced fixation of the glenohumeral joint prior to operation) may require from 6 to 8 weeks. As with other therapeutic measures, the more acute the syndrome prior to operation the sooner will recovery take place.

## Complications of Calcareous Tendinitis

Three complications may occur in this entity: (1) intraosseous calcific deposit, (2) bicipital tenosynovitis, and (3) frozen shoulder.

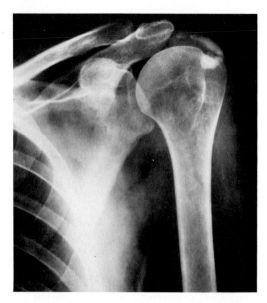

FIG. 11-34. A large crescentic calcific mass lies in the cuff but some of the calcareous material has burrowed into the head of the humerus just proximal to the insertion of the cuff. Note that the intraosseous deposit is discrete and sharply delineated from the surrounding bone.

**Intraosseous Calcific Deposit.** Occasionally the deposit burrows into the humeral head to occupy an intraosseous site. Usually, the point of penetration is in the sulcus along the line of insertion of the cuff into the head of the humerus. When this occurs, roentgenograms show the deposit lying below the ridge of the greater tuberosity, and the overlying bone more or less obscures the deposit (Fig. 11-33). This lesion invariably produces a protracted syndrome which is resistant to any form of treatment except surgical removal. In the series studied, 8 of the 136 patients showed intraosseous deposits. Six of the eight were available for final evaluation; five of these had been treated surgically and one had been treated by needling. The 5 patients treated surgically all attained a satisfactory result; the one treated conservatively had a poor result.

Generally, patients with intraosseous lesions present a chronic syndrome. However, the lesion may flare up into an acute syndrome; this occurred in one patient in the group discussed above.

The roentgenographic features of the deposits are relatively constant. A ring of increased density sharply delineates the defect in the humeral head. The calcareous material within the defect has a density greater than that of the surrounding bone. Occasionally, small areas less dense than the surrounding bone are seen in the defect; these may be new areas of bone absorption (Fig. 11-34). As a rule, the intraosseous material is continuous with streaks or flakes of calcareous matter or even with large deposits in the overlying cuff. In very old lesions, little or no calcareous matter is seen in the cuff and the upper rim of the defect may produce irregular reactive bone (Fig. 11-33).

**Bicipital Tenosynovitis.** If the calcific deposit is close to the bicipital groove, the biceps tendon and its sheath may be secondarily involved in the inflammatory reaction surrounding the deposit. The patient then presents clinical manifestations of bicipital tenosynovitis. It is reasonable to assume that, in many instances, after the inflammatory process subsides, the biceps tendon returns to normal. In my series, bicipital tenosynovitis occurred in 16 of the 136 patients. It so happened that 13 of the 16 patients were treated by surgical excision of the calcific deposit. Six of the 13 showed severe involvement of the biceps tendon; the tendons were emmeshed in an acute inflammatory process that obliterated the interval between the tendon and the groove. In these six patients, in addition to evacuating the calcific deposit, the biceps tendon was surgically anchored to the floor of the groove. All made an excellent recovery.

In the remaining seven patients the tendon was not severely implicated, and, therefore, was not disturbed surgically.

These patients also attained a good result. Therefore, we must assume that once the focus of irritation (the calcific deposit) was removed the inflammation in the biceps tendon and its sheath subsided.

From the above data, it appears that bicipital tenosynovitis as a concomitant lesion of calcareous tendinitis occurs more frequently then is generally realized. The clinical manifestations of calcareous tendinitis may obscure the involvement of the biceps tendon unless special care is taken to elicit the syndrome. At operation, a decision must be made concerning the disposition of the implicated biceps tendon. This is a rather delicate matter and lies entirely within the judgment of the surgeon.

**Frozen Shoulder.** Frozen shoulder may complicate calcareous tendinitis. Although in longstanding instances muscle spasm plays a role in the loss of scapulohumeral motion, changes in the fibrous capsule play even a greater role. This was demonstrated in patients with calcareous tendinitis complicated by frozen shoulder who were treated surgically. When the patient was under anesthesia and all muscle spasm was eliminated, marked restriction of motion in the scapulohumeral joint still persisted. In this study there were six such patients. In three, because the biceps tendon was severely involved in addition to excision of the deposit, the tendon was fixed to the floor of the bicipital groove; in the remaining three it was not disturbed. All these patients regained a painless, full range of motion.

## Result of Treatment

The significance of concomitant lesions associated with calcareous tendinitis is reflected in the period of convalescence. As a rule, uncomplicated cases recover promptly, whereas those with complications may require many weeks of intensive aftercare before maximum level of painless function returns. The best immediate results are attained in patients treated conservatively; in this series 84 percent were cured in 1 to 4 weeks. However, in this group, one patient required 12 weeks and another 26 weeks to attain a good result. Both these patients developed frozen shoulders after needling of the calcific deposit. Also, in the group treated conservatively there were two other shoulders with complications; the associated lesion in one was bicipital tenosynovitis and in the other frozen shoulder. Both were treated conservatively for 12 weeks before a satisfactory result was achieved.

Surgical management invariably cures calcareous tendinitis. In this series, of the 53 patients treated surgically, at the final evaluation results were rated good in 51 patients (96%) and fair in 2 patients (4%). What is more impressive is that none of the patients treated surgically had a recurrence. However, the convalescence following surgical treatment is different, by far, from that following conservative treatment. Eighty-three percent of the patients were fully recovered 2 to 10 weeks after surgery; but 11 patients required over 10 weeks postoperative care. One shoulder was treated for 24 weeks and another for 30 weeks; both of these patients developed frozen shoulders after the surgery.

The postoperative course is even more protracted if the calcareous tendinitis is complicated by bicipital tenosynovitis or frozen shoulder before surgery. Those complicated by bicipital tenosynovitis, in this series, recovered in 3 to 14 weeks; those complicated by frozen shoulder recovered in 6 weeks to 8 months.

These observations reveal that long-term results of surgical treatment are better than those of conservative treatment of both the uncomplicated and the complicated forms of calcareous tendinitis. However, the period of convalescence is much greater in patients treated surgically than in those treated conservatively, and complicating lesions prolong this period even more.

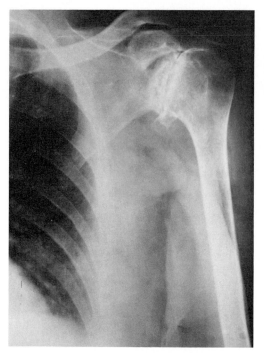

FIG. 11-35. Osteoarthritis of the left shoulder joint; note the thin joint space, and the subchondral sclerosis and marginal osteophytes on both the glenoid and the humeral head.

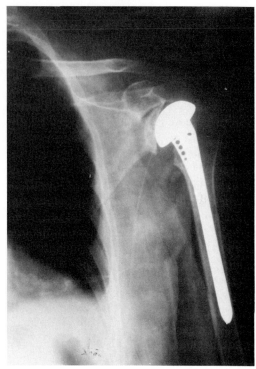

FIG. 11-36. Same shoulder depicted in Figure 11-35, after the insertion of a Neer prosthesis.

## DEGENERATIVE LESIONS OF THE ARTICULAR SURFACES OF THE GLENOHUMERAL JOINT

The articular surfaces of the glenohumeral joint may be the seat of many local, metabolic or systemic diseases. Comprehension of the nature of these disorders is essential in order to institute appropriate treatment. The disorder most commonly affecting this articulation is primary degeneration of the articular cartilage associated with aging. I shall discuss this entity first.

### Degeneration of the Articular Surfaces Associated with Aging

Although the glenohumeral joint is not a weight-bearing joint, the normal mechanics of this articulation subject its articular surfaces to enormous pressures. For the humeral head to attain a fulcrum, the articular

surfaces are subjected to pressures up to 10 times the weight of the limb when the arm is abducted 90°. In addition, the weight of the limb, through the capsule, makes constant traction on the attachment of the fibrous capsule to the rim of the glenoid fossa. Finally, when the arm is externally rotated, the glenohumeral ligaments also exert traction on the bony attachment of the capsule. Yet, in spite of all these stresses, the joint is not a frequent source of pain.

In Chapter 6 it was pointed out that with aging degenerative changes occur in the articular surfaces of the joint. These begin as early as the second decade. On the glenoid side of the joint the greatest alterations occur in the lower half of the glenoid fossa (the head of the comma). The alterations consist of fibrillation, loss of elasticity and scalloping of the articular cartilage. The

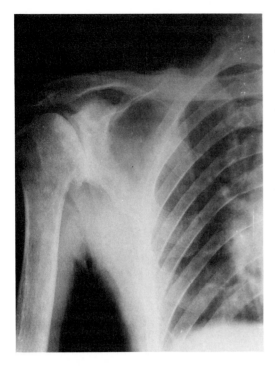

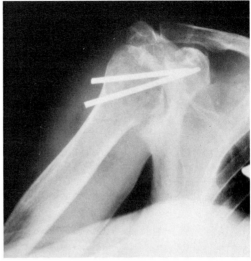

FIG. 11-37. (*Left*) Advanced osteoarthritis of the glenohumeral joint. (*Right*) Fusion of the glenohumeral joint depicted at left; this patient had a massive avulsion of the cuff.

changes reach their greatest intensity in the sixth decade, but they are never so severe as to involve large areas of subchondral bone. In general, the alterations surpass those on the articular surface of the head of the humerus. The explanation for this discrepancy is that contact area on the glenoid fossa is far greater than that on the humeral head and is subjected to more constant pressures.

Marginal proliferation of bone and cartilage occur along the rim of the glenoid fossa, especially on the inferior and anterior portions. These alterations are more pronounced in the late decades of life. They are not the result of pressure but are caused by traction stresses applied through the fibrous capsule (*see* Fig. 6-1).

The cartilage of the humeral head reveals the same changes found in the glenoid fossa, but they are always less in severity and never extensive, except in very few shoulders, even in the late decades of life. Along the periphery of the articular cartilage, bony spurs and excrescences are frequent findings in the late decades. Some

shoulders reveal great incongruity of the articular surfaces; but it should be noted that these same findings are often seen in patients without symptoms.

It should be remembered that the primary degenerative changes in the articular surfaces do not parallel those in the rotator cuff; therefore, minimal involvement of the cartilage and bone components of the joint does not indicate minimal implication of the cuff, for the cuff may show profound degeneration.

Occasionally a patient presents with constant, disabling pain in the shoulder. The syndrome may follow excessive activity or some trivial trauma, or it may occur spontaneously. Usually the patient is an elderly male whose activities are already reduced. If the cause of the disorder is primary degeneration of the articular surfaces, some restriction of motion, especially of abduction, is invariably present. Active and passive movements, particularly rotatory movements, may elicit coarse crepitus and even a grinding sensation. Some atrophy of the spinati and deltoid, owing to reduced ac-

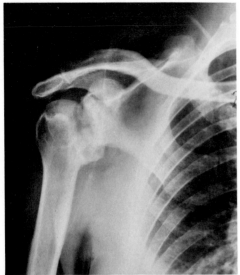

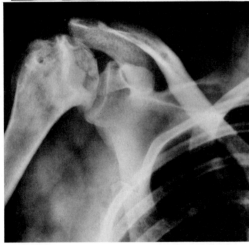

(*Top*) FIG. 11-38. Severe comminution of the humeral head, causing
marked incongruity of the articular
surfaces of the glenohumeral joint.

(*Bottom*) FIG. 11-39. Segmental necrosis of the head of the humerus, following a fracture through the neck of
the humerus.

tivity, is usually present. Pressure over
the anterior and superior areas of the shoulder produces tenderness. The roentgenograms may show all the characteristics of
primary degeneration of the articular surfaces: narrowed joint space, subchondral
sclerosis in some areas of the humeral
head, perhaps some cystic areas in the
head and greater tuberosity, and marginal

osteophytes on the humeral head and the
rim of the glenoid fossa (Fig. 11-35).

However, because primary osteoarthritis
is rarely the cause of pain and great disability, a careful study of the patient must
be made in order to exclude all other causes
capable of producing a similar clinical picture. Among the local causes that may be
responsible in this age group are tendinitis
of the rotator muscles, partial or complete
tears of the cuff, bicipital tenosynovitis,
calcareous tendinitis and lesions of the
acromioclavicular joint.

**Treatment.** Most instances of primary
degenerative osteoarthritis of the glenohumeral joint respond to conservative measures. These comprise rest of the arm,
elimination of painful arcs of motion, mild
exercises within painless arcs of motion,
anti-inflammatory drugs (phenylbutazone derivatives) and injections of one of
the corticosteroids into the articulation.
Injections must be performed under meticulously sterile techniques. I have seen
six disastrous pyogenic infections following injection therapy.

Conservative measures should be continued as long as there is clinical evidence
of improvement. If after several months of
treatment pain and disability still persist,
surgical intervention is justified. The only
surgical procedure that will relieve pain
and restore function is replacement of the
head of the humerus with a Neer prosthesis,
provided that the rotator cuff is intact and
capable of normal function (Fig. 11-36).
This is a very gratifying operation and is
most effective in primary degenerative
osteoarthritis of the glenohumeral joint.
The surgical technique is described on
page 203. In some instances, fusion of the
shoulder is indicated—for example, when
the rotator cuff is inadequate because of a
massive complete tear (Fig. 11-37).

### Incongruity of the Glenohumeral Joint
### Caused by Trauma

Malunion of fractures through the surgical neck, anatomical neck and tuberosities

of the humerus may produce pronounced incongruity of the articular surfaces of the joint (Fig. 11-38). This is also true of some segmental fractures of the head of the humerus and defects in the head produced by primary or recurrent dislocations of the shoulder. In some fractures of the upper end of the humerus the blood supply to the head may be severely compromised, resulting in segmental necrosis of the head of the humerus (Figs. 11-39 and 11-40). Not infrequently degeneration of the articular surfaces rapidly follows these injuries, thereby increasing the existing incongruity and disturbing further the mechanics of the joint.

In some instances, the pain is not relieved and the disability is not decreased by conservative measures. Many of these patients are in the most productive period of their lives; therefore, every attempt must be made to restore to the patient a useful limb. Replacement of the humeral head with a Neer prosthesis achieves this goal in many instances. If the nature of the lesion is such that a prosthetic replacement is contraindicated, an arthrodesis of the shoulder is justified.

## Rheumatoid Arthritis

During the active stage, the diagnosis of rheumatoid arthritis is readily made. However, in the "burned-out" phase of the disease secondary degenerative changes occur in the articular cartilage; the process is not unlike primary osteoarthritis of the joint. Any reconstructive operation on the shoulder in the active stage of the disease invariably fails. However, although not the best material for arthroplasties, some of these shoulders can be mobilized by replacement of the humeral head with a Neer prosthesis (Fig. 11-41).

## Infections

Pyogenic infections of the glenohumeral joint occasionally follow injection of the joint; however, these patients rarely pre-

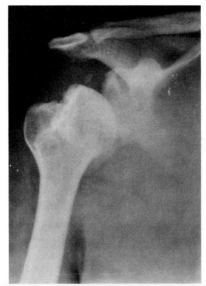

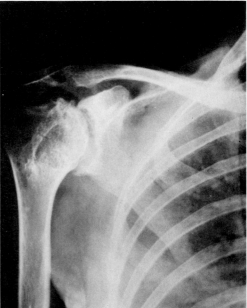

(*Top*) Fig. 11-40. Large defect in the humeral head and secondary osteoarthritic changes in the glenohumeral joint in a recurrent dislocating shoulder.

(*Bottom*) Fig. 11-41. Rheumatoid arthritis, with secondary changes in the glenohumeral joint.

sent the clinical picture of an acute pyogenic arthritis. Undoubtedly, the corticosteroid and antibiotics change the nature

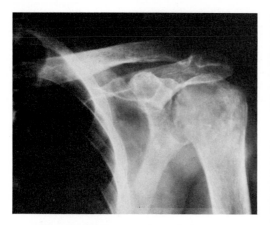

FIG. 11-42. Destruction of the gleno-humeral joint by a pyogenic infection which followed injection of a corti-costeroid into the joint.

of the pathological process. Nevertheless, the joint invariably goes on to complete destruction. The articular cartilage of both the humeral head and the glenoid fossa disintegrates completely, and, in all cases I have encountered, the subchondral bone

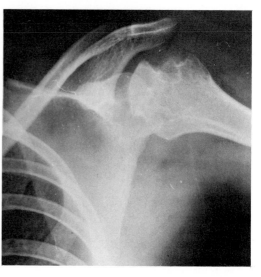

FIG. 11-43. Shoulder of a 19-year-old female, showing destruction of the humeral head and glenoid caused by tuberculosis. This is a case of tuberculosis sicca. This patient attained an excellent functioning shoulder, following a long period of immobilization and antitubercular therapy.

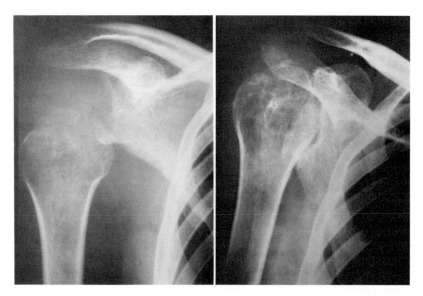

FIG. 11-44. (Left) Tuberculosis of the glenohumeral joint, with inferior subluxation of the humeral head in a patient 33 years old. (Right) Same shoulder shown at left, after 8 months of immobilization and antitubercular therapy. Note that the articular surface of the head and glenoid are destroyed completely. This shoulder was painful and eventually was fused.

is also involved. Even after the infection is controlled these joints do not lend themselves to successful arthroplasties. If any surgical procedure is considered it should be an arthrodesis of the joint (Fig. 11-42).

Today, tuberculosis of the glenohumeral joint is rarely seen. When tuberculosis sicca occurs, the process produces large, scalloped-out erosions of the articular cartilage and the underlying bone. The patient may have no constitutional manifestations of the disease, for the lesion is a very slow, chronic process, involving only one joint. I have seen several such lesions, one being in a young lady 19 years old (Fig. 11-43). With appropriate antituberculosis therapy the disease can be cured, but it leaves in its wake marked destruction of the articular cartilage and a joint with considerable incongruity of its articular surfaces.

After the disease is cured, secondary degenerative changes develop in both the joint destroyed by a pyogenic infection and in that destroyed by tuberculosis. The tubercular joint, as the pyogenic joint, does not lend itself to arthroplasties and, if painful, should be fused (Fig. 11-44).

## Neurotrophic and Neurotrophic-like Joints

Neurotrophic joints associated with nervous disorders pose no problem of diagnosis in the late stages of joint involvement: There is profound disintegration and dissolution of both sides of the articulation (Fig. 11-45). This is not true in the early stages of the disease; the joint may show nothing more than some thinning of the joint space and irregular spotty areas of increased bone density. The roentgenographic picture in this early stage may simulate that of primary degenerative osteoarthritis (Fig. 11-46). Although most of these joints are painless, occasionally considerable pain and muscle spasm is present. This confuses the clinical picture even more.

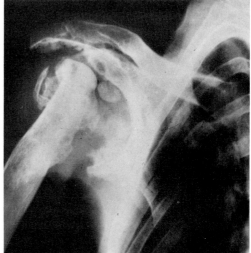

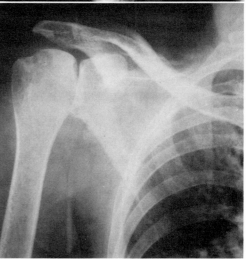

(*Top*) FIG. 11-45. Advanced primary neurotrophic disorder of the glenohumeral joint. The joint is completely destroyed; this joint was painless and freely movable.

(*Bottom*) FIG. 11-46. Primary neurotrophic joint in the early stages. The roentgenographic features are not unlike those of primary degenerative arthritis. Later this joint underwent complete disintegration.

Neurotrophic-like joints may occur after long administration of intra-articular corticosteroids. These joints too present roentgenographic pictures similar to primary degenerative osteoarthritis. Since, in most

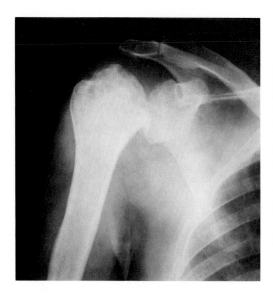

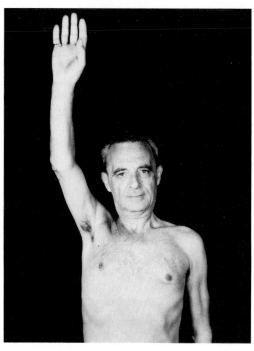

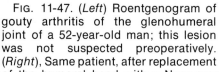

FIG. 11-47. (*Left*) Roentgenogram of gouty arthritis of the glenohumeral joint of a 52-year-old man; this lesion was not suspected preoperatively. (*Right*), Same patient, after replacement of the humeral head with a Neer prosthesis; he attained a normal range of motion.

instances, the corticosteroids were given for pain associated with osteoarthritis, it may be difficult to distinguish primary from superimposed, secondary pathology, or the latter may not be recognized. Fortunately, these joints exhibit abnormal passive mobility and the movements elicit little or no pain. These clinical features, together with the history, should suggest a neurotrophic-like joint.

**Metabolic and Hereditary Diseases**

Many of these diseases cause changes in the glenohumeral joint not unlike those of primary degenerative osteoarthritis. When these changes occur in young people, probably some disease other than degenerative arthritis is at work; when the joint changes occur in older persons, it is more difficult to establish the true diagnosis.

The diagnosis of gouty arthritis is readily made in a person with a known history of gout and with an elevated serum uric acid. However, no such history may be available and the serum uric acid may be within nor-

mal limits. The patient may have a crippling, low grade arthritic process in the shoulder that does not respond to the conservative measures. The roentgenograms appear not unlike those of primary degenerative arthritis. Such was the clinical picture of the patient whose shoulder is depicted in Figure 11-47 (*left*). In addition, this patient had been given several injections into the joint which were followed by an acute inflammatory process. I suspected a pyogenic infection and explored the joint. At operation the diagnosis became clear: The entire articular cartilage of the humeral head was a free sequestrum in the joint; the raw bony surface of the head presented multiple punched-out areas containing granulation tissue; the cartilage and the raw bone were studded with calcium urate crystals. I removed the humeral head and replaced it with a Neer prosthesis. The patient attained an excellent result (Fig. 11-47, *right*).

Ochronosis is another metabolic disease that destroys articular cartilage. When the shoulder of a young person is affected with a process similar to degenerative arthritis, ochronosis should be considered. In these instances, the test for homogentisic acid in the urine confirms the diagnosis. If the pain and shoulder disability are great, replacement of the humeral head with a prosthesis may give a very serviceable joint.

Other diseases that can produce joint lesions simulating degenerative arthritis are sickle cell anemia, Gaucher's disease, caisson disease and hemophilia. As a rule, operative intervention on joints affected by these diseases is not justified (Fig. 11-48 and 11-49).

## Degenerative Arthritis of the Acromioclavicular Joint

Pain and stiffness in the shoulder caused by primary degenerative arthritis of the acromioclavicular joint is more frequent than is generally realized. The incidence of this lesion is underestimated and often goes unrecognized. The acromioclavicular joint is not a very stable joint and its articular surfaces are small and normally incongruous. Movements at the joint are such that they subject the articular surfaces to constant shearing stresses. The interarticular disc undergoes rapid deterioration and offers the articular surfaces no protection.

The above circumstances explain the rapid degeneration of the joint so that in middle life most joints exhibit advanced degenerative arthritis. The acromioclavicular joint is the most exposed articulation of the shoulder complex and hence it is often the recipient of direct and indirect trauma. Yet, in most persons, even in the face of these extensive alterations, the joint is capable of functioning without pain or disability.

Overuse, laborious work or trauma may produce pain and disability in the joint. Usually abduction and adduction of the arm are restricted and cause pain. Active and passive motion often elicits crepitus and pressure over the joint produces tenderness. Occasionally, on palpation the joint margins feel irregular, and the cap-

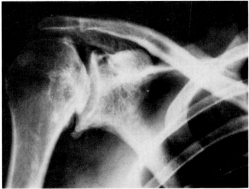

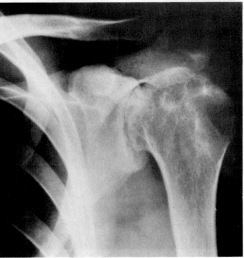

(*Top*) Fig. 11-48. Degenerative changes in the glenohumeral joint in a patient with sickle cell anemia.

(*Bottom*) Fig. 11-49. Advanced degenerative changes in the glenohumeral joint in a patient with hemophilia. This shoulder was the site of many episodes of intra-articular hemorrhage.

sule and ligaments swollen. Roentgenograms may show some irregularity of the joint surfaces and marginal lipping; however, these roentgenographic findings are not always present.

Secondary degenerative arthritis may follow severe trauma or subluxation of the joint. These findings are relatively common in athletes.

**Treatment.** Most instances of primary degenerative arthritis respond to conservative measures such as rest and elimination of painful arcs of motion, together with anti-inflammatory drugs and injection of one of the corticosteroid derivatives. If after several months of conservative therapy the pain and disability persist, surgical intervention is justified. The best operative procedure is excision of the outer ½ inch of the clavicle.

## BIBLIOGRAPHY

Abbott, L. C., and Saunders, L. B. deC. M.: Acute traumatic dislocations of the tendon of the long head of the biceps brachii; a report of six cases with operative findings. Surgery, 6:817, 1939.

Baer, W. S.: Operative treatment of subdeltoid bursitis. Bull. Johns Hopkins Hosp., 18:282, 1907.

Bosworth, B. M.: An analysis of 28 consecutive cases of incapacitating shoulder lesions radically explored and repaired. J. Bone & Joint Surg., 22:369, 1940.

_____: Calcium deposits in the shoulder and subacromial bursitis; a survey of 12,122 shoulders. JAMA, 116:2477, 1941.

_____: Examination of shoulders for calcium deposits. J. Bone & Joint Surg., 23:567, 1941.

Boyd, H. B.: Affections of Muscles, Tendons and Tendon Sheaths; Campbell's Operative Orthopedics. pp. 1212-1262. St. Louis, C. V. Mosby, 1949.

Breckner, W. M.: Prevalent fallacies concerning subacromial bursitis; its pathogenesis and rational operative treatment. Am. J. Med. Sci. 149:351, 1915.

Bruns, P. V.: A System of Practical Surgery. Vol. 1. p. 119. Philadelphia, Lea & Febiger, 1904.

Codman, E. A.: The Shoulder. Boston, Thomas Todd, 1934.

Cooper, W.: Calcareous tendinitis in metacarpophalangeal region. J. Bone & Joint Surg., 24:114, 1942.

Cotton, F.: Subluxation of shoulder, downwards. Boston Med. Surg. J., 185:405, 1921.

DePalma, A. F.: Calcareous deposits in soft tissues about the proximal interphalangeal joint of the index finger. J. Bone & Joint Surg., 29:808, 1947.

_____: Surgery of the Shoulder. Ed. 1. Philadelphia, J. B. Lippincott, 1950.

_____: Frozen shoulder. Instructional Course Lectures of the American Academy of Orthopaedic Surgeons, 1952.

_____: Loss of scapulohumeral motion (frozen shoulder). Ann. Surg. 135:193, 1952.

DePalma, A. F., and Kruper, J. S.: Long-term study of shoulder joints afflicted with and treated for calcific tendinitis. Clin. Orthop., 20:61, 1961.

DePalma, A. F., Bennett, G., and Callery, G.: Variational anatomy and degenerative lesions of the shoulder joint. Instructional Course Lectures of the American Academy of Orthopaedic Surgeons, 1949.

DePalma, A. F., White, J. B., and Callery, G.: Degenerative lesions of the shoulder joint at various age groups which are compatible with good function. Instructional Course Lectures of the American Academy of Orthopaedic Surgeons, 1950.

DeQuervain: Ueber eine Form von chronischer Tendovaginitis. Corr.-Blatt. Schweiz. Aerzte 25:339, 1895.

Dickson, J. A., and Crosby, E. H.: Periarthritis of the shoulder; analysis of two hundred cases. JAMA, 99:2252, 1932.

Duplay, S.: De la périarthrite scapulo-humerale. Rev. frat. trav. méd., 53:226, 1896. (Tr., M. Week, 4:253, 1896; M. Press, 59:571, 1900)

Duchenne, C. B.: Physiologie des mouvements. Paris, Baillière, 1867, pp. 7-17.

Elmorilie, R. C.: Calcareous deposits in supraspinatus tendon. Brit. J. Surg., 20:190, 1932.

Fairbank, T. S.: Fracture-subluxations of the shoulder. J. Bone & Joint Surg., 30-B454, 1948.

Freykman, G.: Shoulder-hand finger syndrome. Acta orthop. scand. Supp. 108. pp. 116-127. 1967.

Gilcreest, E. L.: Rupture of muscles and tendons. JAMA, 84:1819, 1925.

_____: Spontaneous rupture of long head of biceps flexor cubiti. Surg. Clin. N. Am., 6:547, 1926.

_____: Common syndrome of rupture, dislocation and elongation of long head of biceps brachii; analysis of one hundred cases. Surg., Gynec. Obstet., 58:322, 1934.

_____: Dislocations and elongation of long head of biceps brachii. Ann. Surg., 104:118, 1936.

Gilcreest, E. L., and Albi, P.: Unusual lesions of muscles and tendons of shoulder girdle and upper arm. Surg., Gynec. Obstet., 68:903, 1939.

Goldenberg, R. R., and Leventhal, G. C.: Supratrochanteric calcification. J. Bone & Joint Surg., 18:205, 1936.

Harrison, S. H.: Painful shoulder (x-ray changes in upper end of humerus). J. Bone & Joint Surg., 31-B418, 1949.

Hitchcock, H. H., and Bechtol, C. O.: Painful shoulder; observations of the role of the tendon of the long head of the biceps brachii in its causation. J. Bone & Joint Surg., *30-A*: 263, 1948.

Howland, V.: Etiology and pathogenesis of rickets. Medicine, *2*:349, 1923.

Howorth, M. B.: Calcification of tendon cuff of shoulder. Surg., Gynec. Obstet., *80*:337, 1945.

Hueter, C.: Arch. klin. Chir., *5*:321, 1864.

Inman, V. T., Saunders, J. B. deC. M., and Abbott, L. C.: The function of the shoulder joint. J. Bone & Joint Surg., *26*:1, 1944.

Jones, L.: The shoulder joint; observation on the anatomy and physiology, with an analysis of a reconstructive operation following extensive injury. Surg., Gynec. Obstet., *75*:433, 1942.

Key, L. A.: Calcium deposits in the vicinity of the shoulder and other joints. Ann. Surg., *129*:737, 1949.

King, J. M., Jr., and Holmes, G. W.: Diagnosis and treatment of 450 painful shoulders. JAMA, *89*:1956, 1927.

Lans: Beitr. klin. Chir., *29*:410, 1901.

Lapidus, P. W.: Infiltration therapy of acute tendinitis. Surg., Gynec. Obstet., *76*:715, 1943.

Lattmann, I.: Treatment of subacromial bursitis by roentgen irradiation. Am. J. Roentgenol., *36*:55, 1936.

Leddenhose: Zur Frage der Rupture des Biceps brachii. Deutsche Z. Chir., *101*:126, 1909.

Lippman, R. K.: Frozen shoulder; periarthritis, bicipital tenosynovitis. Arch. Surg., *47*:283, 1943.

_____:Bicipital tenosynovitis. Arch. Surg., *47*: 283, 1943.

_____: Bicipital tenosynovitis. N. Y. State J. Med., *44*:2235, 1944.

Ludington, N. A.: Rupture of long head of biceps flexor cubiti muscle. Am. J. Surg., *77*: 358, 1923.

McLaughlin, H. L.: Muscular and Tendinous Defects at Shoulder and Their Repair. Am. Acad. Orthop. Surg., Reconstruction Surgery of the Extremities, Ann Arbor, Edwards, 1944.

_____: Lesions of the musculotendinous cuff of the shoulder. J. Bone & Joint Surg., *26*:31, 1944.

_____: Muscular and tendinous defects at the shoulder and their repair. Instructional Courses 1944, Ann Arbor, Edwards, 1945.

_____: Lesions of the musculotendinous cuff of the shoulder; observations on the pathology, course, and treatment of calcific deposits. Ann. Surg, *124*:354, 1946.

Meyer, A. W.: Unrecognized occupational de-

struction of the tendon of the long head of the biceps brachii. Arch. Surg., *2*:130, 1921.

_____: Spontaneous dislocations of the long head of biceps brachii. Arch. Surg., *13*:109, 1926.

_____: Chronic functional lesions of the shoulder. Arch. Surg., *35*:646, 1937.

_____: Spontaneous dislocation and destruction of the tendon of the long head of biceps brachii. Arch. Surg., *17*:493, 1928.

_____: Quoted by Abbott & Saunders, surgery, 6:6, 199, 812, 1939.

Mosely, H. F.: Rupture of supraspinatus tendon. Canad. M. A. J., *41*:280, 1939.

_____: Shoulder Lesions. Springfield, Ill., Charles C Thomas, 1945.

Mumford, E. B., and Martin, F. S.: Calcified deposits in the subdeltoid bursa. JAMA, *97*: 690, 1931.

Neviaser, J. S.: Adhesive capsulitis of the shoulder. J. Bone & Joint Surg., *27*:211, 1946.

Nichols, E. H., and Richardson, F. L.: Arthritis Deformans. J. Med. Res., *21*:149, 1909.

Outland, T. A. M., and Shephard, W. F.: Tears of the supraspinatus tendon, résumé of twelve operated cases. Ann. Surg., *107*:116, 1938.

Painter, C. F.: Subdeltoid bursitis. Boston M. J., *156*:345, 1907.

Parker, F., Keefer, C. S., Myer, W. F., and Irwin, R. L.: Histologic changes in knee joint with advancing age. Arch. Path., *17*:516, 1934.

Pasteur, F.: La teno-bursite bicipitale. J. radiol. électrol., *16*:419, 1932.

_____: Ténobursite bicipitale. Presse méd., *41*:142, 1933.

_____: La teno-bursite de la longue portion du biceps. Gas. hop., *107*:477, 1934.

_____: Sur une forme nouvelle de périarthralgie et d'ankylose de l'épaule. J. radiol électrol., *18*:327, 1934.

Patterson, R. L., Jr., and Darrach, W.: Treatment of acute bursitis by needle irrigation. J. Bone & Joint Surg., *19*:993, 1937.

Pendergrass, E. P., and Hodes, P. J.: Roentgen irradiation in the treatment of inflammation. Am. J. Roentgenol., *45*:74, 1941.

Sandstrom, C.: Peritendinitis calcarea; a common disease of middle life; its diagnosis, pathology and treatment. Am. J. Roentgenol., *40*:1, 1938.

Schrager, V. L.: Tenosynovitis of the long head of the biceps humeri. Surg., Gynec. Obstet., *66*:785, 1938.

Stevens, J. H.: The action of the short rotators on the normal abduction of the arm, with a consideration of their action in some cases of subacromial bursitis and allied conditions. Am. J. Med. Sci. *138*:870, 1909.

Tarsy, J. M.: Bicipital syndromes and their treatment. N. Y. State J. Med., 46:996, 1946.

Wells, H. G.: Calcification and Ossification. Harvey Lectures, New York, 1910-11, p. 102.

———: Calcification and ossification. Arch. Int. Med., 7:721, 1911.

Wilson, C. L.: Lesions of supraspinatus tendon; degeneration, rupture and calcification. Arch. Surg., 46:307, 1943.

Wilson, P. D.: Complete rupture of the supraspinatus tendon. JAMA, 96:433, 1931.

———: The painful shoulder, Brit. M. J., 21:1261, 1939.

Yergason, R. M.: Supination sign. J. Bone & Joint Surg., 13:160, 1931.

# 12

# Shoulder-Arm-Hand Pain of Mesodermal, Neurogenic and Vascular Origin, and Obstetrical Paralysis

Pain in the upper extremity may arise from sources at a distance from the shoulder such as the cervical spine, the root of the neck and the thorax. A host of disorders in these regions are capable of producing pain, which, depending on its source, has specific characteristics; it may arise from irritation of neural elements or vascular elements or a combination of both the neural and the vascular elements. In many instances, the clinical manifestations produced by these different disorders are similar so that it may be very difficult to identify the causative locus. But, in general, individual features of each lesion are also present and aid in localizing the specific disorder. In order to appreciate the pathophysiology of these lesions it is essential to know the normal and variational anatomy of the root of the neck. This is the region that harbors the structures capable of producing the many neurovascular disorders affecting the upper extremity.

## ANATOMY OF THE ROOT OF THE NECK

The root of the neck lies at the junction of two very mobile parts, the cervical spine and the shoulder. At this point, the great vessels and the major nerves of the brachial plexus converge, regroup and then pass through the isthmus, the "thoracic outlet," to enter the axilla. The clavicle divides the entire region into three anatomical and functional areas—supraclavicular, infraclavicular and retroclavicular; also each region is identified with specific disorders having individual characteristics.

The upper end of the thorax terminates in a crescent-shaped opening enclosed by the first rib laterally, the vertebral column, the trachea and the esophagus medially and the sternoclavicular area anteriorly. The first rib from its vertebral to its sternal end is approximately only three inches long in the adult. The dome of the pleura (pleural cupola) pushes upward $1\frac{1}{2}$ inches above the sternal end of the first rib into this space. This relatively small space is traversed by a number of important structures. Through it pass the great vessels, the phrenic and vagus nerves, the sympathetic trunk and the thoracic duct. The space is sealed by the deep fascia that stretches from the cervical muscles, trachea, esophagus and great vessels to the first rib. Just above the pleural cupola lies the supraclavicular region.

### Supraclavicular Region (Posterior Triangle of the Neck)

The posterior wall and floor of the supraclavicular space comprises the posterior and medius scaleni as they stream downward and outward from the cervical spine to their insertions into the first and second

493

ribs (see Fig. 4-15). The anterior scalenus forms the anterior wall of the triangular space; it is separated from the scalenus medius by a distinct cleft through which pass the roots of the brachial plexus and the subclavian artery. This muscle arises from the transverse processes of the third, fourth, fifth and sixth cervical vertebrae and inserts into the tubercle of the first rib. The floor of the space is covered by a dense fascia—the prevertebral fascia (see Fig. 4-14).

In order to understand the mechanisms of the different syndromes that can occur in the supraclavicular region, it is necessary to grasp the intimate relationships between the important structures in this region. The second portion of the subclavian artery lies entirely behind the scalenus anterior which also separates this part of the subclavian artery from the subclavian vein. The subclavian vein just barely rises above the superior border of the clavicle and lies in front of the scalenus anterior. More inferiorly, the subclavian vein comes to lie slightly below and in front of the artery (see Fig. 4-15).

In the upper region of the supraclavicular area the nerve roots composed of the anterior division of the fifth, sixth, seventh and eighth cervical and the first thoracic spinal nerves and a few fibers from the second thoracic proceed downward and laterally in the cleft between the scalenus medius and scalenus anterior. In the lower region of the area the roots lie on the scalenus medius; here they regroup to form the upper, middle and lower trunks, each dividing into an anterior and a posterior division. Immediately under the clavicle the divisions also regroup, forming the lateral, posterior and medial cords. The cords continue distally and, under the pectoralis minor and slightly beyond, their components rearrange themselves to form the radial, median, ulnar musculocutaneous and anxillary nerves. Finally, the brachial plexus enters the axilla and then proceeds down the arm. In the lower region of the space the neural elements are in close re-

lation to the great vessels; the plexus occupies a lateral position and the subclavian vein a medial position, and the artery lies between the plexus and the vein but slightly above and behind the vein. These structures maintain these positions as they pass beneath the clavicle and the pectoralis minor. Under the clavicle the subclavius is the only soft tissue structure between the clavicle and the subclavian vessels (see Fig 4-15).

On the left side, the subclavian artery arises from the arch of the aorta inside the thorax. It runs vertically upward, then it makes a sharp turn laterally over the pleural cupola and continues behind the scalenus anterior and across the first rib (see Fig. 4-7). On the right side, the artery branches off the innominate just behind the sterno-clavicular joint; then it curves over the pleural cupola and continues on behind the scalenus anterior and over the first rib (see Fig. 4-7). Because the root of the neck lies at the junction of the mobile cervical spine and the mobile shoulder, the relationship of the clavicle to the neurovascular structures is subject to change. For example, when the shoulder is elevated the supraclavicular area is depressed and the subclavian artery is then well behind the clavicle. Depression of the shoulder reverses this relationship: the artery rises in relation to the clavicle and is more exposed.

From the preceding description of the anatomical relationships of the structures within the supraclavicular region, it is clear that in the upper region of the space only neural elements can be involved in pathophysiological disturbances. Such lesions may involve any segment of the neural elements from the spinal cord to just above the clavicle. This includes lesions of the spinal cord (tumors), pressure on a cervical root by extruded intervertebral disc material, compression of the root by hypertrophic changes in the intervertebral foramina and injuries to the proximal elements of the brachial plexus.

On the other hand, disorders affecting the structures just above the clavicle may

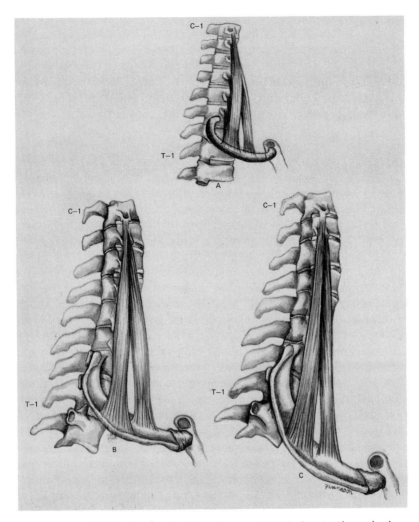

FIG. 12-1. The descent of the sternum in relation to the spinal column from birth to maturity. At birth the sternum is on the same plane as the top of the first thoracic vertebra (A); at maturity it is on a plane with the lower border of the second thoracic vertebra in the male (B) and of the lower border of the third thoracic vertebra in the female (C).

implicate both neural and vascular elements. In this group are the syndromes produced by a cervical rib, abnormal development of the first rib and hypertrophy or spasm of the scalenus anterior.

## Retroclavicular Region

The space between the undersurface of the clavicle and the first rib is a very critical zone. Any alteration of its bony boundaries that reduces or distorts the configuration of the space may compress the neurovascular structures as they pass through to reach the arm. The clavicle has two distinct curves; both the convexity of the medial curve and the concavity of the lateral curve face forward. Also, the medial portion of the clavicle is a rigid tube whereas its lateral portion is flattened. On the undersurface of the clavicle lies the subclavius muscle, the only buffer between the clavicle and the neurovascular structures (see Fig. 4-9).

The first rib presents a flat superior surface the central portion of which is traversed by two grooves; the subclavian artery runs through the posterior groove and the subclavian vein through the anterior groove. The scalenus tubercle, into which the scalenus anterior inserts, lies between the grooves.

Many pathological disorders may compromise the space between the clavicle and the first rib; these should be considered as costoclavicular disorders in contrast to those entities causing compression at the level of the coracoid process and the pectoralis minor. The important costoclavicular entities are acute fractures of the clavicle with displacement, malunion of comminuted fractures of the clavicle, tumors of the clavicle and first rib, and congenital malformations of the cervical spine and first rib.

It should be remembered that with maturation and aging the relationship of the cervical spine, the upper thorax and the shoulder changes. These changes may decrease the capacity of the costoclavicular space and render the neurovascular structures more vulnerable to compression as they pass through the canal. At birth, the upper border of the sternum and the body of the first thoracic vertebra are on the same plane. This relationship permits the clavicle to hold the shoulder up, out and backward; the thoracic outlet is short and wide and the cleft between the scalenus medius and scalenus anterior is also broad. With growth, the anterior portion of the thorax descends slowly and progressively, so that, when adulthood arrives, the upper border of the sternum has descended to the level of the lower border of the second thoracic vertebra in the male and the third thoracic in the female. The anterior thoracic cage follows the sternum in its downward course, thereby pulling the shoulder girdle forward, downward and close to the lateral chest walls. These developmental alterations lengthen the canal but also narrow it; also the interscalenus interval is narrowed (Fig. 12-1).

Congenital anomalies of the brachial plexus may also be contributory factors to the development of costoclavicular syndromes. This is especially true if abnormalities of the thoracic rib are also present. The most common variations of the plexus are the prefixed plexus and the postfixed plexus. The prefixed plexus includes the primary ramus of the fourth cervical nerve in its formation, but it receives few fibers from the first thoracic nerve. The postfixed plexus lies at a lower level; it receives a large contribution from the second thoracic nerve, no fibers from the fourth cervical and only a few from the fifth. Because of the low position of the plexus, the first and second thoracic nerves must arch higher over the first thoracic rib to join the higher root (Fig. 12-2).

Besides anatomical, developmental, congenital and traumatic factors, posture and occupational causes may contribute to development of costoclavicular disorders. Chronic diseases associated with generalized loss of muscle tone may cause the shoulder girdle to droop; poor posture, and as may be seen in people with long necks, forward drooping of the shoulders and an increased dorsal curve may contribute to narrowing of the costoclavicular canal. The carrying of heavy loads or packs by persons with poor muscular development may also produce compression of the neurovascular elements beneath the clavicle.

### Infraclavicular Region

The anatomy of the infraclavicular region is such that compression of the neurovascular structures can readily occur in the region extending from beneath the clavicle to the lower border of the pectoralis minor and on into the axilla. After the neurovascular bundle emerges from under the subclavius muscle and clavicle it lies, at first, directly under the clavipectoral fascia and then under the pectoralis minor. It must be remembered that immediately below the clavicle the upper extremity joins the trunk, so that this area is a point of motion be-

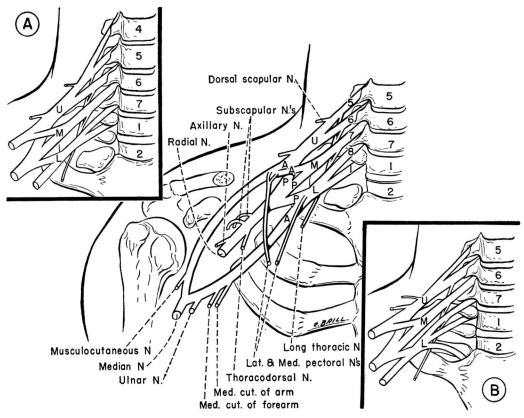

Fig. 12-2. Brachial plexus and the most common variations. (A) Prefixed plexus. (B) Postfixed plexus. (Haymaker and Woodhall, Peripheral Nerve Injuries, Philadelphia, Saunders, p. 129. Redrawn with supplementations.)

tween the mobile arm and the less mobile segment of the cervical spine. It follows that there is a great differential between the mobility of the segment of the neurovascular bundle in the arm and the mobility of the segment at the base of the cervical spine. Some movements that change the relationship of the scapula to the arm, such as abduction and external rotation, place great traction stress on the pectoralis minor at its insertion into the coracoid process. This in turn is capable of compressing the neurovascular structures against the coracoid process. In some instances, simple hypertrophy of the pectoralis minor produces the same result. The syndromes resulting from the mechanisms described above can be grouped in one category — the clavipectoral compression syndromes.

The initiating causes of these syndromes vary; they may be functional, structural or postural.

## MESODERMAL, NEURAL AND VASCULAR PAIN

It is generally known that referred pain in the upper extremity may have its origin in many structures: the neck, the shoulder, the thorax and the neural and vascular elements in the root of the neck. This poses many diagnostic problems that must be carefully evaluated in every detail before a particular structure can be indicted as the locus of origin of the pain. Clinical and investigative evidence reveals that irritation of somatic structures, such as ligaments, fascia, deep muscles, anulus fibrosus, capsular tissues of the cervical spine and even the viscera of the thorax, tends to produce referred pain in the limb that has a definitive segmental distribution. For example, irritation of the anulus fibrosus of more than one intervertebral disc may reproduce one specific pattern of referred pain. Also the same pattern is reproduced by irritating the longus colli muscle.

When referred pain is present, isolated areas such as the rhomboid muscles, trapezius and semispinalis frequently become very painful and tender. Irritation of these areas by injection of normal saline greatly accentuates the referred pain. The injection of a local anesthetic agent into these tender areas relieves both the local and the referred pain. Much research, both clinical and basic, needs to be done before we can attain a clear understanding of those phenomena. The study by Hollinshead is pertinent. He pointed out that the arrangement of the muscles of the spinal column is very complex. With the exception of the interspinales and intertransversarii, the muscle groups have multiple origins and insertions. The complexity is further compounded by the arrangement of the muscle fiber bundles; the fiber bundles from one origin do not proceed to one insertion but diverge to several insertions. Likewise, each insertion comprises fiber bundles from several origins. Finally, the nerve supply to these muscle groups comes from more than one segmental level.

Although there are many gaps in our knowledge of the origin of referred pain in the upper extremity, the character and nature of the pain do indicate the tissues involved. On this basis we can recognize referred pain arising from irritation of somatic, neural, and vascular elements. Recognition of the type of pain is not difficult when only one element is involved; often, however, more than one is implicated, the clinical picture becomes confused, and identification of the primary source of trouble may be difficult.

## Pain of Somatic Origin (Scleratogenous Pain)

The source of this pain is stimulation of the sensory nerve endings in the structural soft tissues of the cervical spine. Characteristic of the pain is the absence of any objective features implicating the nerve roots or spinal cord; there are no sensory, motor or reflex changes. The earliest subjective manifestations are pain and stiffness in the neck, on the top of the shoulders and in the region of the scapulae. Then, gradually the pain projects to the upper arms but rarely descends below the elbows. It is diffuse and deep in nature and is poorly localized by the patient. Although the pain has a segmental distribution it has no definitive pattern, nor does it have the lancinating quality observed in true radicular pain. It is not accentuated by coughing and sneezing; it is relieved by rest and intensified by stress. Certain movements of the neck may increase the pain. Not infrequently muscles in the path of reference become tender and spastic: the rhomboids, trapezius and semispinalis are most frequently involved.

Although the pain is constant, its intensity varies, depending on the character of the stimulation and the structure affected. The pain has no cutaneous distribution and is confined to the deep structures. It progresses to the mesodermal elements connected to the skeleton; these elements are of the same embryonic origin as the mesodermal tissues initially stimulated. The area of radiation is designated the sclerotome, in contrast to the cutaneous area of pain distribution called a dermatome which follows irritation of a nerve root. Not infrequently, when the tissues are severely stimulated, a vasovagal response occurs, characterized by nausea, decreased blood pressure and even collapse.

After the initial stimulation, radiation of pain does not occur immediately and may be delayed, sometimes for hours. From

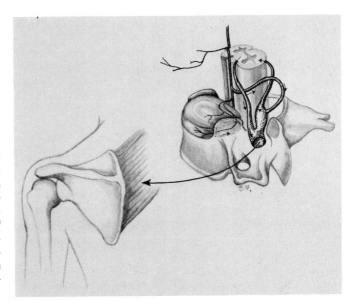

FIG. 12-3. Origin, course and distribution of the sinuvertebral nerve. Deep pain and muscle spasm (reflex phenomena) may occur in the posterior structures following stimulation of the endings of the sinuvertebral nerve; the impulses produced take the pathways shown diagrammatically in this illustration.

the point of origin it radiates distally without a break in continuity; the extent and spread of the pain is in direct proportion to the intensity of the initial stimulation at the site of origin. The clinical picture just described is seen today with increasing frequency in acceleration and deceleration injuries of the cervical spine.

Although the complex structural arrangement of the muscles of the spinal column and the exact innervation of these structures is not clear, nevertheless, the mechanism whereby pain is referred to distant points has been deciphered. The soft tissue elements of the spine are innervated by the sinuvertebral nerves and the posterior primary divisions of the spinal nerves. Both these nerves contain sympathetic and sensory fibers. Many of the fibers are myelinated: of these the smaller fibers are, in all probability, pain fibers, whereas the larger ones are proprioceptive fibers. The sinuvertebral nerve takes origin near the spinal ganglion one or two segments above the foramen it enters to regain access to the spinal canal. Here it divides into ascending and descending branches. These proceed toward the disc above and the disc

below and supply the peripheral layers of the anulus fibrosus. Other branches innervate the dura mater, the vascular elements, the posterior longitudinal ligament and the periosteum. In the spinal canal, filaments of adjacent nerves anastomose with each other, and some fibers even cross the midline (Fig 12-3).

The posterior rami amply supply the skin and muscles of the dorsal spinal column and also distribute sensory fibers to the fascia, the ligaments, the periosteum and the posterior intervertebral joints. The areas of distribution of the posterior rami overlap considerably.

The referred pain is initiated by stimulation of the sensory receptors of the sinuvertebral nerve located in the deep soft tissues of the cervical spine—anulus fibrosus, posterior and anterior longitudinal ligaments, pretracheal fascia etc. The impulses are conveyed by the sinuvertebral nerve to the posterior nerve root and through the spinal cord. Then they emerge through the anterior root and motor nerve to the muscles of the neck, scapula and arm (Fig. 12-3). The muscles develop varying gradations of spasm which are responsible for the local pain. Of the mechanisms that produce referred pain in the upper extremity this is undoubtedly the most common, for it can be initiated by myriad disorders affecting the soft tissue elements of the spine.

### Neural Pain

This pain is more readily understood. It is produced by direct stimulation of the neural elements anywhere from the spinal cord to the termination of the brachial plexus below the clavicle. Characteristic of this pain is the constant pattern of cutaneous distribution which is determined by the specific nerve elements involved. Stimulation of a nerve root may produce two types of cutaneous or dermatogenous pain—"fast," and "slow." Fast pain is sharp and lancinating and is clearly localized to a specific cutaneous area—the dermatome. Stimulation evokes an immediate response, and appreciation of the pain disappears as soon as stimulation ceases. On the other hand, slow pain is vague, dull aching, with no clear localization. The response to stimulation is delayed and adaptation is poor. The pain spreads to a wide skin area that is poorly defined. Stimulation of a nerve root by contact, traction or pressure may produce both fast and slow pain. However, the predominant type depends on the nature and duration of the stimulus. In both types the longitudinal extension of pain is in direct proportion to the amount of pressure on the nerve root. This explains the great variation in the longitudinal extent to which a dermatome may be involved in patients with a cervical disc protrusion. Extrusions making only minimal contact with a nerve root produce pain that radiates only a short distance along the dermatome, whereas those exerting great pressure produce pain which extends the entire length of the dermatome of the affected root.

An irritated nerve root becomes hypersensitive so that any movement or maneuver that stretches it or exerts more pressure on it accentuates the pain. In cervical disorders produced by neural irritation, such as an extruded cervical disc, the pain is aggravated by coughing, sneezing, jarring and certain movements of the neck. Continued irritation of the neural elements causes loss of neural function, and motor, reflex and sensory deficits follow.

After the nerve roots leave the intervertebral foramen they divide and intermingle to form the brachial plexus. Irritation of the neural elements beyond the foraminal level does not produce radiating pain conforming to any specific dermatome. It produces an entirely different pattern of cutaneous pain distribution—that of a peripheral nerve.

### Vascular Pain

The great vessels lie at the junction of the mobile shoulder and the trunk; hence, motion of the shoulder is continuously transmitted to the vessels. In this area the vessels may be subjected to traction, compression or both. Irritation of the vessels produces a characteristic type of pain, discomfort and parasthesia at the periphery. The distribution of the pain is ill defined and is not localized to any one specific area. There is a sensation of fullness, numbness and tingling. Swelling of the hand and fingers may be present, and there also may be pallor, rubor and cyanosis. The hand may be cool and moist. Characteristic of this pain is the inconstant appreciation; also, in many instances, it is influenced by certain movements and postures of the extremity.

The mechanism producing vascular pain has not been clearly defined, but there is clinical and experimental evidence that the prime culprit is vasoconstriction. Pressure and traction on the vessels initiate vasoconstriction which itself produces peripheral pain. This in turn causes an upset of the normal metabolic processes at the periphery. The altered metabolic processes together with the ischemia caused by the vasoconstriction of the vessel irritate the sensory nerve endings and sympathetic system, thereby producing peripheral pain and sympathetic disturbances. In some instances the pain is intermittent and resembles intermittent claudication.

The diffuse nature of the pain is an outstanding feature of vascular pain and is in marked contrast to the peripheral distribution of neural pain. If the vasoconstriction persists, secondary changes based on ischemia occur, such as blanching, diminished sensation and ulceration. Fortunately, these severe vascular changes rarely occur in vascular compression syndromes at the root of the neck.

The great veins also may be subjected to compression; the resulting obstruction to the flow of venous blood results in dilation of the peripheral veins.

## Simultaneous Neural and Vascular Pain

Although not a common occurrence, there are syndromes in which both the neural and the vascular elements are involved. The resulting clinical picture may be very confusing, for it may be difficult to differentiate between true neural and true vascular components of the syndrome. As a rule, the vascular components dominate in the early stage because the vascular elements are more sensitive and respond more readily to traction and pressure than the neural elements. With time, the clinical picture may reverse itself, for, when the neural elements do respond, their clinical manifestations eventually outweigh the vascular.

## SUPRACLAVICULAR SYNDROME

### Acute Soft Tissue Injury of the Cervical Spine

Acute injuries to the soft tissues of the cervical spine are frequently causes of pain in the neck, shoulder and arm. Most of the injuries are caused by rear-end collisions. The mechanism of injury is, essentially, stretching and hyperextension of the neck.

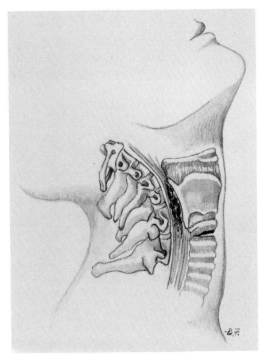

FIG. 12-4. Hyperextension and prolongation of the cervical spine may stretch and even tear the muscular strata of the esophagus; the trachea may be injured.

During the phase of hyperextension the soft tissues sustain injuries of varying gradation, depending upon the intensity of the forces applied to the cervical structures. In the simple form of rear-end collision no passive force is applied to the head, so that disruption of the osseous elements rarely occurs.

**Pathology.** When the anterior muscles of the neck are caught off guard and are severely hyperextended, they may be severely stretched and some of their fibers even torn. This is particularly true of the sternocleidomastoid, scaleni and longus colli. This accounts for the severe muscle spasm and limitation of motion that the patient frequently presents with, 12 to 48 hours after the accident. It also accounts for the pain and tenderness at the root of the neck. If one side of the neck is involved more than the other, the patient may exhibit the typical features of torticollis.

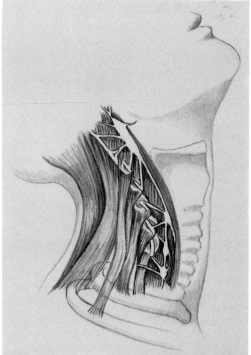

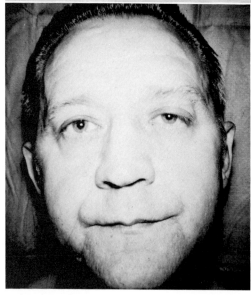

(*Top*) Fig. 12-5. Hyperextension and prolongation of the cervical spine may severely stretch or even tear the longus colli muscles and the sympathetic chains which intimately relate to the muscles.

(*Bottom*) Fig. 12-6. Note the dilatation of the right pupil; this followed an acceleration injury of the cervical spine.

Stretching and tearing of the muscle strata of the esophagus may occur, producing hemorrhage and edema in the retropharyngeal space. Also, the trachea may be injured (Fig. 12-4). This pathology readily explains the symptoms of dysphagia and hoarseness, which are frequently present.

It should be remembered that the sympathetic chain runs over the longus colli. Injuries capable of stretching and tearing this muscle also implicate the sympathetic chains. Also, the hemorrhage and edema that invariably follow further involve the sympathetic nerve fibers. This explains the many bizarre signs and symptoms with which the patients frequently present, such as nausea, blurring of vision, dizziness, nystagmus, deafness, tinnitus and occasionally dilatation of the pupil (Figs. 12-5 and 12-6).

If the hyperextension forces are severe, the intervertebral discs may be injured. The disc may be crushed and the longitudinal ligament attenuated or even torn. This invariably results in disintegration of the disc and secondary osteoarthritic changes which may implicate the foramen and at times the cervical nerve roots.

Even more profound injuries may occur to the discs. With rupture of the anterior longitudinal ligament the discs may be avulsed from either the caudal or the cephalic vertebra. Unfortunately, roentgenograms do not reveal this lesion, but as time passes the disc spaces show some diminution in height. Occasionally, the separation can be visualized in roentgenograms taken with the head in acute flexion and extension. I have made this radiological diagnosis in four patients immediately after injury. With wide disruption of the attachments of the cervical discs, hemorrhage and edema inevitably implicate the soft tissue elements surrounding the intervertebral foramina, causing compression of the nerve root and the vertebral artery which lies in close proximity to the foramina. Thus, in such severe injuries the patient may experience pain from irritation of both the mesodermal tissues and the nerve root — both scleratogenous and neural pain.

**Clinical Manifestations.** Immediately after the injury the patient is usually unaware of its magnitude. However, after 12 to 24 hours he begins to realize that something is radically wrong. He experiences pain in the root of the neck both posteriorly and anteriorly; motion in any direction elicits pain and he holds his head in a guarded position. If the esophagus and trachea are involved, he experiences difficulty in swallowing and his voice is hoarse. If the sympathetic nerves are injured, nausea, dizziness, visual disturbances, tinnitus and even precordial pain may be present.

During this early phase of the cervical syndrome, the objective findings are fairly constant. The patient holds the head slightly flexed, guarding against any motion in any arc. Occasionally, spasm of one of the sternocleidomastoid muscles produces torticollis. The anterior and posterior muscles of the neck and one or both of the trapezius muscles are in spasm. All movements of the neck, active and passive, are restricted and painful. Pressure over the base of the neck elicits tenderness. Generally, the neurological examination is negative; however, I have observed dilatation of one pupil in several patients. As a rule, radiological examination at this time provides no information.

In patients without involvement of the neural elements, the acute symptoms begin to subside 7 to 10 days after the injury, and a clearer clinical pattern evolves. The severe spasm of the cervical muscles decreases and motion increases. However, in some instances, hyperextension and rotation to one or the other side may be restricted and painful for many months. The pain becomes diffuse, more like a dull ache in the neck and the interscapular and the suprascapular regions. There may be pain in the region of the occiput, the pectoralis region and in the shoulder and arm as far as the elbow. The sympathetic symp-

toms such as dizziness, blurring of vision and tinnitus may or may not persist. Certain movements of the neck may aggravate the pain, and in cases of long duration certain areas about the shoulder and arm become painful and tender on pressure — over the biceps tendon, the insertion of the deltoid and the epicondyles of the humerus. The patient finds some relief if the neck is slightly flexed, especially while sleeping.

Objectively, pressure over the sore muscles of the neck and scapular regions always elicits tenderness and often increases the referred pain to the shoulder and arm. If a local anesthetic is injected into these areas, the local pain and spasm disappear and the referred pain may decrease substantially. In a few instances, symptoms of vascular origin, such as faintness, giddiness and drop attacks, are present, indicating irritation and spasm of the vertebral artery. In most instances, the pain is not constant and varies in intensity and, no doubt, is influenced by the patient's activity and emotional state.

As time passes the patients become more and more apprehensive, nervous and frustrated. This aspect of the syndrome may become so pronounced as to dominate the clinical picture.

In patients with implication of the cervical roots, the clinical manifestations are the same as those described above except that radicular pain, with its motor and sensory characteristics, is the most prominent aspect of the syndrome. The features of neural cervical root involvement are discussed under cervical disc lesions.

## Chronic Cervical Syndrome

In some instances, with or without treatment, the injury may be followed by months or even years of pain and disability. One must assume in these patients that, following the acute injury, a reparative process is at work characterized by scar tissue and degeneration of the disc. The process may involve the sympathetic chains, the verte-

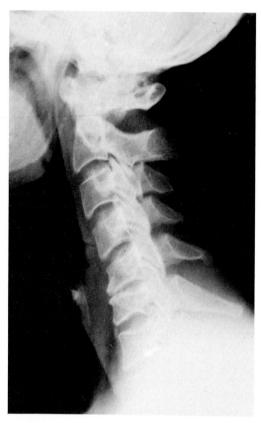

FIG. 12-7. The disc (C5-C6) has degenerated completely following a hyperextension injury. Note the thinness of the disc space and the formation of peripheral osteophytes on the adjacent surfaces of the fifth and sixth cervical vertebrae.

bral arteries and the nerve roots. Osteoarthritic changes occur in the posterior articulations; osteophytes form in a circumferential configuration along the peripheries of the involved vertebral bodies which involve the joints of Luschka; and the lumen of the intervertebral foramina diminishes in size. Inadequate healing of the supporting structures of the disc may result in excessive mobility of the involved vertebra; this in itself is cause for protracted disability. If the injury occurs in a normal spine, the changes described are usually limited to one and occasionally two segments; the remaining cervical column appears normal (Fig. 12-7).

It should be remembered that osteo-arthritic changes in the cervical spine are common findings in people over 40 years of age. In fact, the most frequent cause of pain in the neck and arm in patients in this age group is osteoarthritis. There may or may not be a neck injury in the past history. The segments usually involved are C4-C5, C5-C6 and C6-C7. As a rule, the changes are bilateral; the disc degenerates and initiates hypertrophic bone formation along the peripheries of the adjacent vertebrae; the intervertebral space decreases in height; similar changes occur in the apophyseal joints which may subluxate; the joints of Luschka show similar changes, and the intervertebral canal containing the nerve root becomes studded with bony excrescences which encroach upon its lumen. Fortunately, narrowing of the intervertebral foramina does not, in most instances, compromise the nerve root. In some instances, the nerve is constricted or some degenerated disc material may extrude into the canal and compress the nerve root (Fig. 12-8).

Often the clinical manifestations follow some mild trauma superimposed on the degenerative changes, or a bout of overactivity or a sudden twisting movement of the neck may be the initiating factors. In some instances, however, the symptoms come on spontaneously without a previous history of injury. The clinical picture varies considerably; pain may be localized to the neck or may be referred to the arm, stiffness of the neck is always present, and the referred pain tends to be segmental but usually is distributed over several segments. The common sites of reference are the suprascapular region, the interscapular region, the occiput, the area behind the ear, the retro-orbital areas, the deltoid insertion, the back of the elbow and the epicondylar areas. Usually the pain is bilateral but it may be more intense in one extremity than the other. The intensity of pain varies but is never excruciating; rather it is a dull ache more pronounced in the neck than in the arm. It is aggravated locally, but not to the points of reference, by

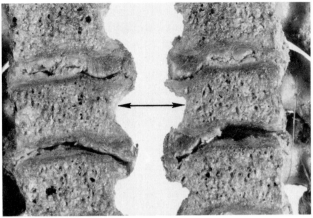

Fig. 12-8. Specimen of a cervical spine of an elderly person, sectioned in the midsagittal plane. Note the advanced degeneration of the discs and the formation of peripheral osteophytes on the surfaces of the adjacent cervical vertebrae. Also note the extension of the osteophytes into the intervertebral foramina.

certain movements of the neck, especially extension of the spine, and by coughing and sneezing.

When a cervical nerve root is irritated either by some extruded disc material or by narrowing of the intervertebral foramina, neural type of pain is superimposed on the pain pattern described above. Indeed, the radicular pain may be so intense that it dominates the clinical picture. Now, the pain is referred specifically to definite dermatomes, depending on the root involved.

The objective findings are fairly constant. Pressure over the muscles of the neck and over the suprascapular and interscapular regions produce tenderness. Some spasm is always present in the neck muscles, especially the trapezius. Motion of the cervical spine accentuates both the local neck pain and the pain in the arm and other reference points. Unless a cervical root is implicated there are no motor, sensory or reflex changes.

**Management of Acute Injuries of the Soft Tissues.** The greater majority of patients with acute injuries to the soft tissues of the spine respond to conservative measures. However, for the treatment to be effective, the patient's apprehensiveness and emotional instability must be controlled. To achieve this it is necessary to gain the patient's confidence and to explain to him the natural course of the disorder and the reason for the long course of therapy. Sedatives and tranquilizers should be ad-

ministered as required to control the patient's emotional state. The most important facet of the local treatment is rest to the cervical spine. This is best achieved by some form of immobilization such as collars, braces, bedrest and traction. In severe injuries, treatment immediately following injury should be bedrest with the neck in a cervical collar. Usually after a period of 7 to 10 days of bedrest the acute symptoms subside sufficiently to allow the patient to be ambulatory. In these acute cases, I do not use traction, for this modality stretches the injured soft tissues and often increases the pain.

After the symptoms have subsided the use of a simple felt collar provides adequate immobilization of the cervical spine. The collar should hold the neck in the slightly flexed position and it should be worn day and night. During sleep, the head rests on two pillows, so that the neck is always in the neutral or slightly flexed position regardless of the position the patient assumes during the night. Maintain this type of immobilization for 2 to 3 weeks in order to allow the soft tissues to progress well into the healing process. Within the next two or three weeks, gradually wean the patient from the collar and institute a regimen of graduated isometric exercises to strengthen the musculature of the cervical spine. Complete healing of the soft tissues requires 6 to 8 weeks.

During the period of treatment injections

of 5 to 10 ml. of 1 percent procaine into the tender area often produce dramatic relief of both local and referred pain. The relief attained may last for days or even weeks. Also, physical therapy in the form of hot packs, radiant heat and gentle massage adds considerably to the patient's comfort. Some patients, in spite of good treatment, continue to have local and referred pain. If a nerve root has been injured, they may have typical radicular pain. Others reach a certain level of improvement and progress no further. These patients often have recurrent acute attacks of pain. When the above circumstances present, the patient must be carefully re-evaluated and considered for surgical intervention.

**Management of the Chronic Cervical Syndrome.** The treatment for this group of patients is the same as for patients with acute soft tissue injuries. Most of these patients respond to conservative measures: immobilization with a felt collar, sedation, anti-inflammatory drugs and muscle relaxants. Local injections of tender areas with an anesthetic agent relieves both local and referred pain. In this group, intermittent cervical traction applied daily may be beneficial. Analgesics and sedatives are necessary to control discomfort and the anxiety associated with the disorder.

Many patients reach a level of improvement at which the residual discomfort is tolerable, and these patients learn to live within the limitations of the disease. Some patients do not respond to treatment, especially those that have a clear-cut superimposed radicular distribution of pain owing to implication of a cervical disc. As in the acute syndromes, these patients must be carefully re-evaluated and considered for surgical intervention.

## CERVICAL ROOT DISORDERS

In general, the pain produced by irritation of the cervical roots is characterized by a distinct pattern of radiation involving the upper extremity, by motor, sensory and reflex changes and by implication of the neck. By far the most frequent cause of irritation is pressure on the roots owing to changes in the intervertebral foramen following disc degeneration. The next most frequent cause is pressure on the roots by extruded disc material; it occurs in 4 to 5 percent of the patients with cervical root syndromes and is encountered more frequently in men than in women; the ratio in different series of cases varies from 4 to 1 to 10 to 1. The left side is involved more frequently than the right. Compression of the root caused by intraforaminal lesions or extruded disc substance occurs most frequently at the C5-C6 and C4-C5 levels.

At the onset of the syndrome, pain is localized to the neck and shoulder region but soon it radiates, following a specific dermatome of the upper extremity. The pain is sharp and lancinating in quality and is associated with parasthesias in the fingers and occasionally in the forearm.

Certain movements of the neck, as well as jarring, accentuate both the local and the radicular pain. Also, increased intra-abdominal and intrathoracic pressure (e.g., from coughing and sneezing) increases the intensity of the pain. Although neck and shoulder pain persists, the radicular pain and paresthesias (numbness and tingling in the fingers) become the dominant features of the syndrome.

Often local areas of tenderness appear in the shoulder and arm which may detract from the clearness of the clinical picture; also, if two roots are involved or if there is a bilateral lesion at the same level, the resulting clinical picture may be confusing. Fortunately, usually only one root is involved. With involvement of the sixth cervical root there may be numbness in the thumb, weakness of elbow flexion and a decreased biceps reflex; involvement of the seventh root may present as numbness in the index and long fingers, weakness of elbow extension and a reduced triceps reflex; implication of the eighth root may produce numbness along the ulnar border

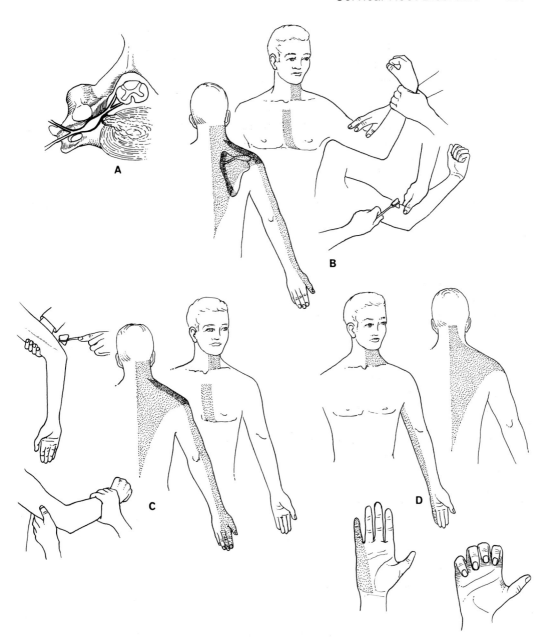

FIG. 12-9. (A) Compression of the nerve root by nuclear tissue at its site of exit from the spinal canal. (B) Involvement of the C6 nerve root. (C) Involvement of the C7 nerve root. (D) Involvement of the C8 nerve root.

of the hand and the little finger, some intrinsic muscle weakness in the hand and no reflex changes (Fig. 12-9).

As a rule, neck motion is restricted, especially hyperextension and lateral rotation. In fact, most patients experience consid-

erable pain when maneuvers of hyperextension are performed. Paravertebral muscle spasm is a frequent finding. There are two types of tenderness in this syndrome. One is more or less diffuse over a broad area of the paravertebral muscles and is

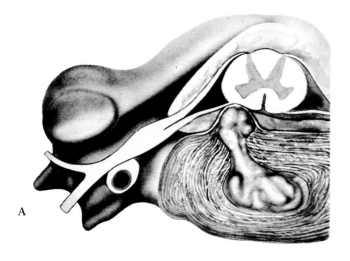

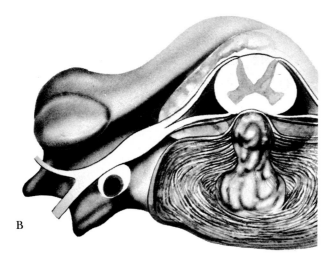

FIG. 12-10. (A) Ventro-lateral lesion encroaching on the nerve root and lateral part of the cord. (B) Midline lesion encroaching on the central anterior portion of the cord. (DePalma, A. F., and Rothman, R. H.: The Intervertebral Disc. Phila-delphia, W. B. Saunders, 1970)

readily elicited by compression of the para-vertebral muscles. The other is more spe-cific and is localized to certain areas such as the nerve root at its exit from the fora-mina and over the spinous processes of the involved vertebrae. Pressure in these areas usually reproduces both neck and radicular pain.

Sudden pressure applied to the vertex of the head transmits stress to the disc and may reproduce the neck and arm pain. When the maneuver is performed with the neck hyperextended or flexed laterally, the pain may be excruciating.

It should be remembered that often in the cervical syndrome the sympathetic chain is also implicated. Stimulation of the sympathetic nerves may produce inequality of the size of the pupils.

Radiological studies are of little signifi-cance in spines with widespread degenera-tion. Many such spines are asymptomatic. However, when only a single unit shows degenerative changes of the disc and en-croachment of the foramina by secondary osteoarthritic changes, the findings are very significant in localizing the level of the cervical root involved, especially if the clinical picture corresponds to the segment of the spine showing the degenerative alterations.

Myelography, in my experience, has not

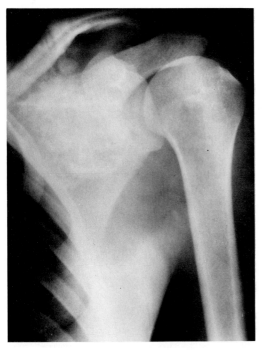 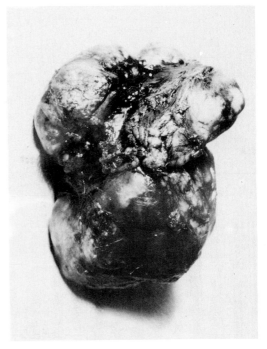

FIG. 12-11. (*Left*) A large tumor occupying the entire infraclavicular area. (*Right*) Gross specimen of the tumor depicted at left. This proved to be a benign fibromatous tumor, well encapsulated and easily shelled out of its bed overlying the brachial plexus.

proved helpful in localizing the disc responsible for the disorder. Changes in the spinal canal associated with disc degeneration produce a myelographic defect similar to that produced by extruded disc material. However, when the cervical spine shows only minimal changes, or none, a positive myelogram does have diagnostic value in localizing the lesion. The evaluation given here in regard to the usefulness of myelography is also true of discography. The only test that has given me helpful information in a large number of cervical disc disorders is the cervical disc distention test. By distending the cervical disc under local anesthesia, it is frequently possible to reproduce the local and radicular pain.

**Management.** Most cervical root disorders respond to conservative treatment along the lines described for chronic disc disorders. When these measures fail, the patient must be carefully re-evaluated and then considered for surgical intervention.

## VENTROLATERAL AND MIDLINE CERVICAL DISC LESIONS

When extruded disc material compresses the nerve root at its site of exit from the spinal canal, a typical clinical picture, as described above, of neck and shoulder pain and radicular pain in the upper extremity evolves. However, the extrusion may occur in relation to the ventrolateral portions of the cord or in the midline (Fig. 12-10). The lesions cause cervical myelopathy, and the character and severity of the syndrome they evoke depends upon their size, location and duration.

Ventrolateral lesions encroach upon the root and the lateral aspect of the cord adjacent to it. They produce all the manifestations of nerve root compression, but pain is not a significant symptom. The chief radicular motor signs are weakness and loss of tone and power of the muscles of the upper extremity, particularly the del-

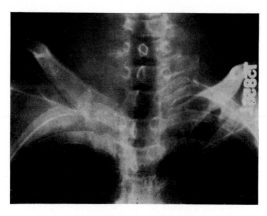

FIG. 12-12. Pancoast tumor occupying the right lower cervical and upper thoracic regions. Note the erosion of the first and second thoracic ribs and transverse process of the seventh cervical vertebra.

toid, triceps and beceps. There may be atrophy of the muscles of the hand; usually there are no sensory disturbances. Larger lesions implicate the cord and produce pyramidal tract signs and spasticity or even an incomplete Brown-Sequard syndrome. The disorder mimics intrinsic diseases of the spinal cord, especially amyotrophic lateral sclerosis. The diagnosis is difficult to make, and all available diagnostic aids should be employed; in these instances, myelography provides valuable information.

Midline lesions intrude upon the central region of the anterior portion of the spinal cord. They cause no compression of the nerve root and, hence, no radicular pain. Both lower extremities exhibit prime involvement, although there may be some involvement of both upper extremities also.

## TUMORS

Tumors, although they are not common, may involve the cervical nerve roots and the spinal cord, producing pain in the neck, shoulder and arm. These lesions should be suspected when pain is deep and boring, is not relieved by rest and is accompanied by extensive motor and sensory manifestations. They may encroach on the neural elements in the foramen or lie in an extradural or intradural location. The tumor most commonly found in the intervertebral canal of the root is the neurofibroma. Characteristic of lesions of the cord is extension of the motor and sensory findings beyond the upper extremities and often involvement of the pyramidal tracts.

Single neurofibromas occasionally arise from nerves of the brachial plexus and may be demonstrable by palpation of the cervical, supraclavicular or axillary regions. Generalized neurofibromatosis may implicate the entire brachial plexus (Fig. 12-11).

The superior pulmonary sulcus may be the site of a Pancoast tumor. Its characteristic features are pain, referred only to the shoulder at the onset but later radiating, extending to the axilla and down the ulnar aspect of the arm; atrophy and weakness of the muscles of the hand, particularly the interossei and the hypothenar muscles; and Horner's syndrome and roentgenographic evidence of a mass in the apex of the lung, with erosion of the upper ribs, the transverse processes and, in some instances, the vertebral bodies (Fig. 12-12). The tumor usually occurs in the sixth decade of life and rarely occurs in women. Its course is rapid and the pain is intractable. It is not clear whether the Horner's syndrome is caused by pressure on the sympathetic fibers of the common trunk of the eighth cervical and first thoracic nerve root or from involvement of the stellate ganglion.

Other primary bronchogenic tumors and tumors metastatic to the apices of the lungs may implicate the neurovascular structures in the supraclavicular and cervial regions by direct extension. Not infrequently breast cancer invades the brachial plexus. Lymphosarcoma and Hodgkins disease involving the lymph nodes in the supraclavicular and cervical regions may invade the brachial plexus and produce the syndrome of neurovascular involvement.

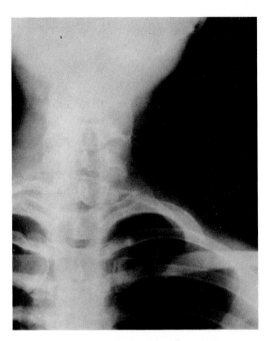

FIG. 12-13. Bilateral cervical ribs. In this 22-year-old female only the cervical rib on the left side produced symptoms.

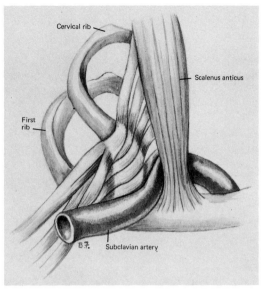

FIG. 12-14. Drawing of an anatomical specimen, showing compression of the subclavian artery and brachial plexus between the scalenus anticus and a well formed cervical rib.

## INJURIES TO THE NEURAL ELEMENTS

Certain nerve injuries cause neck, shoulder and arm pain and dysfunction of the shoulder. Among these are injury of the accessory nerve (causing paralysis of the trapezius), injury to the axillary nerve (causing paralysis of the deltoid), injuries to the brachial plexus and injury to the musculocutaneous nerve. These lesions have been described in Chapter 8.

## SUPRACLAVICULAR LESIONS WITH NEURAL AND VASCULAR PAIN

Just above the clavicle the neural and vascular elements are in close proximity so that disorders in this region usually affect both elements. Now, the clinical picture is more complex because it is colored by neural and vascular pain. Whereas in lesions well above the clavicle neural involvement is restricted to the cervical roots, in disorders immediately above the clavicle

the neural structures affected are the cords or trunks of the brachial plexus. The neural pain does not have a clearly defined dermatome distribution; it is more diffuse and widespread. The medial cord or the inferior trunk is involved more frequently; the pain follows the distribution of the ulnar nerve.

The vascular component of the syndrome is characterized by a sense of numbness and tingling in the entire hand and in the fingers, especially in the third and fourth fingers. Movements of the neck and shoulder influence the nature of the pain.

It should be remembered that the neural structures in the region under discussion are joined by the sympathetic nerves; therefore, the syndrome may exhibit sympathetic disturbances. The disorders encountered most frequently in this region are the cervical rib syndrome and the scaleni syndrome.

### Cervical Rib Syndrome

Congenital anomalies of the cervical spine and the thoracic cage at the root of

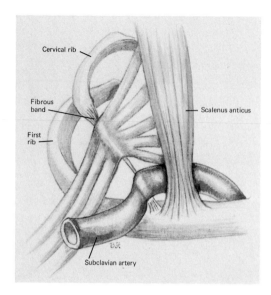

Cervical rib

Fibrous band

First rib

Scalenus anticus

Subclavian artery

FIG. 12-15. A fibrous band extends from the cervical rib to the first thoracic rib; it makes upward pressure on the brachial plexus and subclavian artery from below.

the neck occur relatively frequently. These are often associated with aberrations of the brachial plexus and occasionally with anomalies of the subclavian artery or vein. During evolution, man lost the cervical ribs which date back to fishes and reptiles, but rudimentary or malformed cervical ribs still occasionally appear in the cervicothoracic region of man. Overton found either rudimentary or complete ribs in 0.5 percent of all persons. Fortunately, cervical ribs produce symptoms in very few persons.

Aberrant ribs exhibit considerable variation in length, shape and direction. They may appear as small processes, projecting just beyond the transverse processes or they may form complete ribs, joining the first thoracic rib anteriorly. There are many variations between these two types. Most often they occur unilaterally but they may occur bilaterally. Bilateral ribs are not symmetrical; the difference between the two, in regard to length and shape, may be considerable. The rib most likely to cause symptoms arises from the seventh cervical

vertebra, but ribs from any cervical vertebra may produce symptoms (Figs. 12-13 and 12-14). Often a tense fibrous band stretches from the end of the cervical rib to the first thoracic rib. Such a band may be present without a cervical rib. In these instances, it extends from the transverse process of the seventh cervical vertebra to the first rib (Fig. 12-15). A rib more than 5 centimeters long tends to elevate the neurovascular structures. Usually the subclavian artery, as it proceeds distally, lies over the top of the rib and, in this position, it is vulnerable to compression from the rib below. The neural structures usually affected are the components of C7, C8 and T1.

Cervical rib syndromes rarely occur in persons under 30 years of age. It seems that some other predisposing factors play a role in the initiation of the symptom complex. Sagging of the shoulder girdle may be a predisposing factor, as also may be congenitally high fixation of the sternum and ribs, a high first thoracic rib, a low brachial plexus and hypertrophy of the scalenus anterior muscle.

**Clinical Picture.** The syndrome occurs most frequently in the fourth decade, but I have seen a full blown syndrome in a young lady 19 years of age. Women are affected more frequently than men. The right side is involved more often than the left; also, involvement is greater on the right side, even in bilateral lesions. The cardinal features are pain, discomfort and stiffness in the neck, and pain in the shoulder, usually radiating, progressing to the elbow and ulnar side of the forearm, hand and the fourth and fifth fingers. The pain worsens during the day and with activity and is relieved with rest. Paresthesias, such as tingling and numbness, extend along the area of pain distribution. They tend to subside or even disappear on elevation of the arm, but increase in intensity when the arm is pulled downward. The sensory phenomena point to implication of the lower nerve trunks, but at times all three trunks may be involved.

The character of the pain is variable. It may be deep, boring and continuous, or sharp and lancinating. It may be reproduced or accentuated by depressing the shoulder and relieved by elevating the shoulder. The patient often holds the head tilted toward the affected side; this position reduces the tension on the neurovascular structures and relieves pain.

In some instances, vascular involvement may be severe; the hand and fingers exhibit recurrent swelling, coldness, pallor, cyanosis and tingling. In extreme instances, gangrene of the finger tips may occur; this complication is indeed rare. The exact mechanism of vascular involvement must vary with local circumstances because not all syndromes exhibit the same manifestations. The subclavian artery may be compressed by changes in position of the arm, producing transient obliteration of an otherwise normal radial pulse. In these instances, the recurrent vascular changes noted above occur in the hand and fingers, but these manifestations may be associated with increased pulsation and bruit over the subclavian artery above the clavicle. Surgical exploration of these patients often reveals a patent aneurysmal dilatation of the third part of the subclavian artery. Finally, ischemic changes in the limb and emboli in the fingers indicate a complete or partial obliteration of the aneurysmal dilatation of the subclavian artery by atheromatous degeneration.

Some degree of sympathetic involvement is present in most of the cervical rib disorders. When both the vascular and the sympathetic manifestations are well established it may be difficult and even impossible to distinguish one from the other. I have seen two patients with a Horner's syndrome associated with cervical rib disorders. Objectively there is always tenderness on pressure over the root of the neck. Some restriction of motion of the cervical spine is usually present. Forceful rotation or tilting the neck away from the affected side and pressure over a cervical rib reproduces local and referred pain. Some fullness of the pulse—at times, excessive—is demonstrable in the supraclavicular area. Also, palpation in this area invariably reveals a tender mass, and occasionally a bruit is heard over the subclavian artery.

The various maneuvers described in the literature to obliterate the radial pulse have proved to be of little value in establishing a definitive diagnosis. These maneuvers obliterate the pulse in many normal individuals. Also, compression of the subclavian vessels can be produced by several disorders, so that obliteration of the pulse does not indict any one disorder as the cause.

Objective motor findings do not occur frequently; when motor phenomena are present the syndrome is usually far advanced. There may be weakness, atrophy and fasciculations of the intrinsic muscles of the hand and forearm. When the components of the ulnar nerve are involved, hyperesthesia of the fourth and fifth fingers may be present. Also, atrophy of the interossei, the hypothenar muscles and the adductor of the thumb points to implication of the ulnar nerve. But, occasionally the median nerve is also involved; now, the above changes appear in the hyperthenar muscle. Changes in the deep reflexes of the biceps and triceps and the radioperiosteal reflex seldom if every occur.

**X-Ray.** Radiograms of the cervical spine and thorax readily show the presence of a cervical rib; also they clearly reveal its size, shape and relationship to the clavicle and first rib and they exhibit any bony abnormalities at the root of the neck. However, a cervical rib syndrome may be caused by a fibrous band from the transverse process of the seventh cervical vertebra to the first rib. The fibrous band may not be demonstrable on the radiogram. In these instances, by angiography; compression of the subclavian artery can be identified and located, this is a valuable diagnostic tool and should be used more often.

**Management.** All cervical rib syndromes should first be treated by conservative measures. In many instances, these suffice

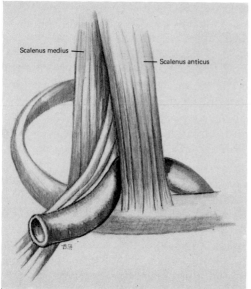

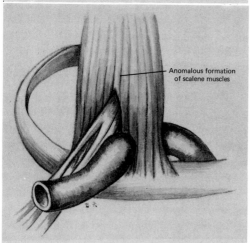

(*Top*) FIG. 12-16. The neurovascular bundle may be constricted by a hypertrophied scalenus anticus without the presence of a cervical rib.

(*Bottom*) FIG. 12-17. The neurovascular structures may be constricted by an anomalous formation of the scaleni muscles.

to relieve the symptoms. Essentially they consists of (1) exercises that elevate sagging shoulders, to improve the general posture, (2) exercises that improve the tone and power of the suspensory muscles of the shoulder girdle and (3) changes in the patient's working and sleeping habits so

that at no time he assumes a slumped posture.

If these measures fail and objective evidence of neural and vascular compression persists, surgical intervention is justified. Some workers advocate simple division of the scalenus anterior at its insertion into the first rib. Theoretically, this procedure allows the first rib to retract, thereby relieving the pressure on the neurovascular structures. However, in my hands, this procedure alone does not produce the desired results in most instances. A significantly greater number of patients are cured if the scalenotomy is combined with resection of a portion or all of the cervical rib. The surgical techniques for this operation are described on page 264.

### Anterior Scalene Syndrome

This syndrome is related to the transit of the neurovascular bundle through the scalene cleft. It should be recalled that under normal circumstances a triangular interval exists between scalenus medius and scalenus anterior; the base of the interval is the first rib. Compression of the subclavian artery and trunk of the brachial plexus produces the so-called scalene syndrome (Fig. 12-16). The compression may be the result of some alterations in the size of the interval owing to congenital abnormalities of the components of the space. In these instances, the syndrome is a primary entity. Occasionally the bellies of scalenus medius and scalenus anticus fuse into one mass through which the trunks of the brachial plexus traverse (Fig. 12-17); again, the trunks may split the fibers of the scalenus anticus instead of passing through the cleft. Also, the interval may be narrowed by hypertrophy of the scalenus anticus. Finally, the insertion of the scalenus anticus may be located too far laterally, thereby constricting the cleft.

Besides those mentioned above, there are other developmental anomalies responsible for hypertrophy of the scalenus anticus. This muscle is innervated by the brachial plexus. The plexus may be irritated by an abnormally situated first rib; such irritation causes spasm and hypertrophy of the muscle. Also, a low shoulder, a high sternum, a high first rib and a low-placed postfixed brachial plexus may produce irritation of the plexus. In these instances, the lower elements of the plexus are stretched tightly as they pass over the first rib. When these circumstances prevail, any condition capable of causing the shoulders to sag may initiate the syndrome. In this group are muscular atonia such as occurs in debilitating diseases, nervous disorders, occupations tending to depress the shoulders and trauma applied to the top of the shoulder that forces it downward.

In most patients presenting a scalenus syndrome the hypertrophy and spasticity of the scalenus anticus is secondary to some other disease — most commonly, osteoarthritis of the cervical spine; other lesions are injuries to vertebrae, ligaments and discs of the cervical spine, extrusion of a cervical disc and rheumatoid arthritis.

**Clinical Picture.** When only the subclavian artery is compressed the resulting pain has a vascular quality. The onset may be sudden or insidious, the pain has more the character of an ache or discomfort, starting in the neck and radiating, including the hand and fingers. Numbness and tingling in the hand and fingers become the predominant feature of the syndrome. The patient has difficulty in localizing the distribution of the pain, for it does not have the clear-cut pattern of distribution seen in cervical nerve root lesions or in cervical rib disorders. The pain is accentuated by certain movements of the cervical spine. Extension, a maneuver that tends to reduce the size of the scalene cleft, aggravates the pain, whereas flexion relieves it. Traction on the arm, dragging the shoulder downward, also increases the discomfort.

This pattern of pain changes when the neural elements are involved, and this usually occurs in lesions of longstanding.

Usually the lower trunk of the plexus is compressed. Now the pain is sharper and radiates, progressing to the medial side of the forearm and the fourth and fifth fingers. The syndrome resulting from compression of both the vascular and neural elements is similar to the syndrome produced by cervical rib disorders, and even cervical root lesions, but it rarely is as severe. It may be impossible to make a correct diagnosis in the face of these circumstances.

The scalene syndrome usually occurs in the middle period of life. It is commoner in women than men and affects the right side more than the left. Not infrequently the patients exhibit sagging shoulders and poor muscular development of the shoulder girdles. The patient may hold the head tilted toward the affected side; this relieves the tension of the scalenus anticus. Palpation in the supraclavicular fossa usually reveals a tense and tender scalenus anticus, and pressure over the muscle elicits severe local and radiating pain. Extension of the neck invariably aggravates or reproduces the pain. Not infrequently, the hand is hyperesthetic and cool. As a rule, motor and sensory deficits and reflex changes are absent. The muscles of the forearm and hand show no atrophy or weakness. In rare instances, the sympathetic system is implicated. I have encountered two patients with a typical Horner's syndrome. Local injection of an anesthetic agent relieves the spastic element of the scalenus anticus and produces relief of symptoms. In some instances the relief is permanent.

X-ray examination may give valuable information in regard to the existence of bony malformations in the root of the neck, such as the presence of a cervical rib or an abnormal first rib. But more important is angiography; the site of any compression of the subclavian artery can be located by this method.

**Management.** Most patients respond to conservative measures. Since many of these people are apprehensive and nervous, this facet of the syndrome needs careful consideration; tranquilizers should be given in sufficient quantities to control the unstable emotional state.

Frequently injections of a local anesthetic agent directly into the scalenus anticus produce dramatic relief which may be permanent. Physical therapy in the form of gentle massage and radiant heat is beneficial. But most important is a program designed to improve the patient's posture and working and sleeping habits. The shoulders should be held up and extension movements of the neck avoided. The program includes a regimen of postural exercises to improve power and tone of the supporting muscles of the shoulder girdle.

Since the syndrome is often secondary to some other disorder of the cervical spine, a careful differential study of every case on an individual basis is mandatory. When the primary etiologic factor is uncovered, it should be dealt with first.

Surgical intervention is justified when all conservative measures have failed and the symptoms are intolerable. In my opinion surgery for a scalene syndrome is always exploratory in nature, particularly when roentgenologic studies fail to find any abnormalities of the cervical spine and the thoracic outlet. Anomalies of the muscles, the neural elements and the subclavian artery can be identified only by exploration of the region. In most instances, combined operations are necessary, such as scalenotomy and excision of a cervical rib, or scalenotomy and excision of the first rib. Scalenotomy alone should be performed only when a careful exploration of the region fails to uncover any abnormality of the thoracic outlet or of the root of the neck. The operative procedures are described on page 264.

## RETROCLAVICULAR LESIONS

Changes in the configuration and size of the interval between the clavicle and the first rib may cause compression or irritation of the neurovascular bundle as it courses over the first rib. The causative factors may be congenital, developmental or traumatic. The disorders encountered in this region are the costoclavicular syndromes. These should be considered separately from the clavipectoral syndromes which arise from disturbances in the infraclavicular region at the level of the coracoid process.

An increase in the convexity of the medial portion of the clavicle narrows the costoclavicular interval. Also, many abnormalities of the first rib may occur which alter the configuration and size of the retroclavicular space. It should be remembered that during embryonic development the neural elements form before the skeletal structures and, therefore, influence the development and the relationship of the costal elements at the root of the neck. When the neural structures occupy a cephalic position in relation to the segments of the spinal column, the costal element articulates with the seventh cervical vertebra, forming a cervical rib of varying size and shape. However, the elements may occupy an inferior position, so that the first thoracic nerve is required to make a long loop over the first rib in order to join the eighth cervical. The course of the first thoracic nerve may vary; it may ascend in front of the neck of the first rib and run along its upper border to reach the other elements of the plexus. In this position, the nerve is vulnerable to compression when the arm is pulled downward.

Normally, the first thoracic rib points downward and forward, but variations of this axis may occur. It may occupy a horizontal position or it may even be directed upward. In this position, the rib may make pressure on the overlying neurovascular bundle; downward traction on the arm or sagging shoulders can readily compress these structures. The thoracic outlet may be distorted by congenital abnormalities of the cervicothoracic region, such as cervicothoracic scoliosis and congenital hemivertebra. In these deformities the rib is pushed upward, making traction on the nerves and vessels.

These altered relationships of the osseous and neural and vascular elements at the root of the neck do not, per se, necessarily give rise to symptoms. However, these elements are thus made vulnerable to irritation and compression by many mechanisms. These mechanisms usually are at work during the middle period of life when body adaptations are complete. Certain positions of the shoulder and neck tend to reduce the size of the thoracic outlet. Forcing of the extended shoulder backward and hyperextension of the neck may narrow the costoclavicular space sufficiently to compromise the neurovascular structures. This may occur in people with no radiographic evidence of abnormalities at the root of the neck. Occupations requiring the person to work with the arms elevated above the head and the neck in the hyperextended position may be contributing factors in the development of costoclavicular syndromes. Debilitating diseases and long chronic illnesses that result in atrophy and loss of tone of the supporting muscles of the shoulder girdle may also be contributory factors.

Fractures of the clavicle and first rib that heal with excess callus or in malposition may compromise the costoclavicular space. Acute comminuted fractures of the clavicle, with the displacement of the fragments, may compress or even lacerate the neurovascular structure.

Much has been written about the so-called *first thoracic rib syndrome,* but I do not consider this a distinct entity. Syndromes related to the first rib are really disorders of the costoclavicular space, for their clinical manifestations do not differ from those caused by distortion of the space on the clavicular side of the interval. Hypertrophy of the subclavius muscle may produce the same symdrome.

**Clinical Manifestations.** The onset may be sudden or gradual. Pain and discomfort are felt in the neck and shoulder and radiating discomfort, tingling and numbness in the entire arm. At first, the symptoms are caused by vascular compression; the whole hand aches intermittently; the hand may be swollen, cold, dry and cyanotic; the radial pulse may be decreased. Later, symptoms of neural compression appear, particularly along the medial aspect of the foream and hand. Numbness and tingling through the entire arm can be aggravated, or reproduced, by pushing the extended shoulder backward and at the same time hyperextending the neck. Occasionally, this maneuver produces distention of the veins of the upper chest and arm. In some instances, the maneuver decreases or even obliterates the radial pulse, but this is not a reliable test; the same phenomenon may occur in people without symptoms. The symptoms are relieved by lowering the arm and flexing the neck. Motor deficits rarely occur. Swelling of the hand, coldness, dryness and cyanosis can be produced by vascular compression or irritation of the sympathetic nerve fibers; which of the two is the culprit is not clear.

From the clinical picture it is apparent that it may not be possible to distinguish a cervical rib syndrome or a scalene syndrome from costoclavicular syndromes, on the clinical evidence alone. All diagnostic aids must be employed to arrive at the correct diagnosis. The most important of these are roentgenograms of the entire cervical and upper thoracic spine and angiography.

**Management.** In general, except for acute injuries to the neurovascular bundle resulting from fracture of the clavicle, retroclavicular syndromes respond to conservative measures. These are the same measures as those described for the conservative treatment of the scalene syndrome.

When the conservative treatment fails and the severity of the symptoms and the disability are unacceptable to the patient, the area should be explored. The operation that produces the highest incidence of good results is the combined procedure of scalenotomy and resection of the first rib. See page 264 for the description of this procedure.

## TRAUMA

### Acute Fracture of the Clavicle

Acute traumatic compression of the thoracic outlet may cause severe injuries to the contents of the costoclavicular space. The most common of these injuries is a comminuted fracture of the clavicle produced by direct trauma to the top of the clavicle. The fragments are actually driven downward into the space, where they may impale, lacerate or crush the neurovascular structures. If the force continues downward, the nerve trunks and vessels may be stretched, torn or lacerated.

These lesions pose no diagnostic problem; a history of violent injury is always present. The subsequent weakness and paralysis of muscle groups in the arm, sensory deficits and reflex changes point to the cervical roots or brachial plexus as the site of damage. The rapid formation of a large hematoma in the supraclavicular region, the axilla and the upper chest wall, and a deficiency in the arterial supply of the upper extremity indicate rupture or laceration of the subclavian artery.

When the subclavian vein is lacerated, the swelling is more gradual and the veins in the anterior chest wall and arm become distended. Eventually the hematoma compresses the artery and the nerves.

Penetrating wounds of the subclavian artery and vein may produce an arteriovenous aneurysm. Immediately after the injury there may be no evidence of injury to the vessels. However, within a few days or weeks — or, sometimes, months — an ache develops in the arm and hand; also numbness and tingling in the hand and fingers and swelling of the hand appear. In some instances, the neural elements are severely compressed so that the pain is excruciating.

The treatment of acute lesions is surgical; these are surgical emergencies. Because repair of the vessels may be necessary, a vascular surgeon should participate in the operation. The exposure must be adequate so that the structures above, behind and below the clavicle are readily accessible. The bony fragments must be elevated carefully to prevent further injury to the nerves and vessels. After the vascular lesions are identified, the necessary repair of the vessels is performed.

### Old Fractures of the Clavicle

Occasionally fractures of the clavicle heal with great displacement of the fragments. This, together with excessive callus formation, may compress the structures in the costoclavicular space. The syndrome develops slowly; first, clinical manifestations of compression of the subclavian vessels and, later those of pressure on the neural structures appear.

Usually, surgery is required to decompress the interval and to relieve the symptoms. This entails removal of the exuberant callus or resection of a portion of the clavicle.

### Acute Fracture of the First Rib

This is not a common injury; it may occur as the result of extreme muscular effort. Often the diagnosis is not made until roentgenograms show callus formation around a fine, translucent area in the rib. The lesion is comparable to a fatigue fracture.

No treatment other than rest of the extremity for several weeks is required; for this, a sling is adequate.

## INFRACLAVICULAR SYNDROMES (CLAVIPECTORAL SYNDROMES)

As previously pointed out, the neurovascular bundle may be compressed as it runs beneath the coracoid process. Also, the anatomy of the subcoracoid region and the predisposing causes and mechanism of compression of the neurovascular structure have been discussed. The vascular elements chiefly are involved in the clavipectoral syndromes, but in syndromes of long standing the neural components of the neurovascular bundle may also be implicated. The syndromes fall into two categories: (1) those related to function, and (2) those related to posture.

## Hyperabduction Syndromes

Wright, in 1945, directed attention to compression of the neurovascular structures in normal persons when the arm is hyperabducted. By this maneuver he was able to obliterate the radial pulse in the great majority of the individuals studied. When the arm is hyperabducted, the neurovascular bundle is pulled tightly around and beneath the coracoid process and, at the same time, is compressed by the pectoralis minor. The greatest amount of torsion occurs at the point of transition between the subclavian and the axillary artery and vein. These phenomena are readily demonstrated in anatomical specimens and at the operating table. Under normal conditions, hyperabduction of the arm causes no symptoms, but, in the presence of structural, functional or postural changes in the relationship of the clavicle and coracoid process, or because of thickening of the pectoralis minor or the costocoracoid membrane, hyperabduction of the arm may produce severe compression of the bundle, sufficient to initiate a painful syndrome (Fig. 12-18).

The hyperabduction syndrome usually occurs in young, muscular men. Short, stocky persons with a short, thick neck are the usual victims of this disorder. As a rule, the symptoms are first noted while working. Generally, the work requires using the arms above the horizontal, with the neck hyperextended. The clinical manifestations are a sense of fullness in the hand and fingers and numbness and tingling in the forearm and fingers. The symptoms are, undoubtedly, the result of repetitive injuries to the subclavian artery over a long period. Evidence of neural irritation is rarely found,

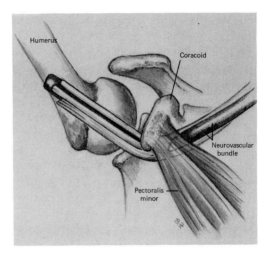

FIG. 12-18. Mechanism of the hyperabduction syndrome. With the arm hyperabducted, the neurovascular structures are pulled tightly around and beneath the coracoid process and compressed by the pectoralis minor.

and ischemic changes due to constant vascular irritation are indeed rare.

Objectively, the only significant and constant observation is tenderness over the pectoralis minor just below the coracoid process. Pressure over this area increases the local discomfort and reproduces the symptoms in the forearm, hand and fingers. In most instances, hyperabduction of the shoulder obliterates the radial pulse, although this also may occur in the normal extremity. However, there is a difference; the "marginal position" is reached sooner on the affected side than on the normal side. The marginal position is the level of abduction just below the level at which obliteration of the pulse is produced. Not infrequently, the patient is aware of the exact level of abduction at which the symptoms occur.

**Management.** Most patients are relieved by changing their work and their postural habits. They should be advised to avoid using the arms in positions above the horizontal and the neck in hyperextension. In a few instances, the syndrome is not relieved by these measures and is of sufficient intensity to justify surgical intervention.

Division of the insertion of the pectoralis minor into the coracoid process is the procedure of choice.

## Postural Disturbances

This comprises the larger group of clavipectoral syndromes. Many names have been given to these disorders, such as sleep dysesthesias, nocturnal dysesthesias and nocturnal palsy. The symptoms are directly related to the position the arm assumes during sleep. The universal complaint is numbness of the upper extremity, especially the forearm and hand, upon awakening; the arm is "asleep." The patient soon learns that the symptoms are alleviated by changing the position of the arm or by getting up from the recumbent position and shaking the arm. The syndromes are not progressive and rarely is there evidence of trophic or ischemic changes. However, Wright did report a case of gangrene of the fingertips in a patient who was in the habit of sleeping with his arms elevated and abducted over his head; this position always produced numbness and tingling in the hands and arms. As a rule, the syndrome is unilateral.

Management. These syndromes respond to the same measures employed in the hyperabduction syndromes. The most important facet in the treatment is changing the position of the arm that causes compression of the vascular structures. This brings instant and complete relief. Surgical intervention is rarely indicated. However, if the patient is not relieved by conservative measures, the pectoralis minor muscle should be divided at its insertion into the coracoid process.

## SHOULDER-HAND-FINGER SYNDROME

The complexity of this syndrome was first recorded by Mitchell, Morehead and Keen in 1864. It has appeared in the literature under such designations as: épaule-main, adhesive capsulitis, painful stiff shoulder, frozen shoulder and post-traumatic reflex dystrophy. There are two components to the syndrome: the shoulder and the hand. Although the full syndrome is not encountered frequently, the early phase of the shoulder or the hand component are relatively common. A maze of mystery enshrouds the etiology, pathogenesis and pathology of this entity. Yet, within the past two decades, beginning with Moberg in 1951, two theories of the pathogenesis of the disease have emerged. Before considering these theories I shall first discuss the clinical picture of the disorder and its variations.

Clinical Picture. The total picture presents three stages. In the first stage, following an injury to the upper extremity or during the course of some constitutional disease, a feeling of discomfort or a burning sensation develops in the shoulder. Within a short period of time, the hand and fingers become swollen and painful. In some instances, the hand symptoms appear without implication of the shoulder. At this stage the patient tends to hold the extremity in a dependent position; he moves the shoulder in progressively smaller arcs of motion; the skin folds of the hand and fingers disappear; flexion of the fingers is limited and painful, and passive motion of the fingers elicits pain. Osteoporosis of the bones of the wrist and hand is a common finding in this stage. The duration of the first stage is 3 to 6 months.

During the second stage, the scapulohumeral joint becomes fixed but pain free. Also, the swelling in the hand and fingers decreases, but the pain in the fingers may increase and finger motion is further decreased. The skin of the hand and fingers is smooth and cold, and may even exhibit dystrophic changes. Occasionally the palmar fascia becomes thickened and contracted, presenting the clinical features of Dupuytren's contracture. As these tissue changes progress the syndrome enters the third stage.

In the third stage the patient presents a severely disabled extremity; the shoulder is "frozen," the hand is stiff and deformed and the skin is thin and atrophic. Yet, both the shoulder and hand are free of pain. The final deformity of the hand depends upon the balance of muscle power between the long flexors and extensors, and the intrinsic muscles of the hand. Hence, one of two forms may develop: the "intrinsic minus" hand and the "intrinsic plus" hand. The former is the more common type. In the "intrinsic minus" hand the metacarpophalangeal joints freeze in extension and the interphalangeal joints in flexion. In the "intrinsic plus" hand some flexion power at the metacarpophalangeal joints remains while the interphalangeal joints stiffen in extension.

Not all patients present equal involvement of both the shoulder and the hand components. In fact, in the early stages, generally only one component is affected; in the later phases of the disease this may emerge as the dominant clinical component. Clinically, the two components are intimately interrelated, forming a chain of circumstances characteristic of this disabling disorder.

**Etiology.** Usually this entity develops after some trauma to the upper extremity, but in some cases there may have been no trauma. In these instances, generally the patient is afflicted by some internal or constitutional disease—heart disease, rheumatoid arthritis or cerebral injury. Most of the patients exhibit emotional instability and are anxious, hypersensitive persons. What role the psychological factors play in the etiology of this entity is not clear; however, clinical evidence indicates that they do tend to aggravate and even maintain the condition.

Age and sex are important considerations in the development of the disease. It rarely occurs in persons under the age of 40 years and the highest incidence is over the age of 50 years. Females are affected more often than males.

**Pathogenesis.** Two theories of pathogenesis have emerged from the clinical and experimental investigations of this disorder, each of which has its supporters. According to one of the theories the syndrome can be explained on the basis of a reflex mechanism caused by a disturbance of the autonomic nervous system. From a peripheral focus, pain stimuli travel up afferent pathways to reach the spinal centers; then, after being dispersed through the internuncial pools, they reach the efferent sympathetic pathways. The internuncial pools are cells in the gray matter of the spinal cord, forming an intricate network of interconnected neurons. Impulses finding their way to these pools can be dispersed to the anterior or lateral parts of the spinal cord and to different segments of the cord.

The second theory takes an entirely different tack. According to this theory, the basic pathophysiology of the disease is the altered circulation of the extremity caused by a defective pumping mechanism which results in edema of the tissues of the hand and shoulder. Whereas the maintenance of the normal arterial supply depends upon the blood pressure, on the venous side, where the pressure is low, the normal flow of blood and lymph away from the extremity can be maintained only by active muscle function of the entire limb. The shoulder and the hand are the chief contributors to the pumping action of the arm. Clearly, when function of the shoulder or the hand, singly or concurrently, is impaired, the normal return of blood and lymph from the hand and shoulder is seriously impaired. The resulting edema of the tissues of the hand and shoulder is responsible for the viciousness of this syndrome.

The starting point may be in the shoulder or in the hand. Any circumstance that causes muscular inactivity of the shoulder favors dependency of the arm. The circumstances may be an injury to the extremity, debility caused by constitutional disease, or even psychogenic disorders. The pumping mechanism of the shoulder is impaired and the return of venous blood and lymph from the extremity is deterred. The next link in the chain of events is swelling of the hand; it appears first in the dorsal region and later in the palm and fingers. The fingers become stiff and painful; this reduces the muscular activity and the pumping action of the hand.

The sequential links in the chain of events may occur in the reverse order. The starting point may be in the hand. Following injury or paralysis that causes muscular inactivity and the loss of the pumping action of the hand, the resulting edema produces stiffness and pain in the hand and fingers. This causes dependency of the arm and eventual loss of muscular activity in the shoulder.

The edema is responsible for the crippling changes in the hand. If the syndrome is not reversed and muscular activity restored, the edema induces the formation of fibrosis and scar tissue formation in all tissues, particualrly in the subcutis. The longer the edema persists the more severe are the residual deformities of the hand. From this process emerges the "intrinsic minus" and "intrinsic plus" hands.

As noted previously, the frozen shoulder is a self-limited disease and eventually, with or without treatment, the outcome is a painless shoulder with good function. Also, many frozen shoulders do not develop the hand-finger component of the shoulder-hand-finger syndrome. Of the two components, the hand component is the most vicious, for, once it is involved, few patients escape without some permanent impairment of hand function. The incidence may be as high as 65 percent of the affected hands.

**Treatment.** Treatment of this disorder should be guided by the surgeon's concept of its pathogenesis. I myself believe that the syndrome is the result of a disturbance of the pumping mechanism of the shoulder and hand. Further, in my experience, very few patients with a true shoulder-hand-finger syndrome failed to exhibit some evidence of involvement of the sympathetic nervous system. For this reason I direct treatment to both the autonomic nervous system and to the defective pumping mechanism of the shoulder and hand.

First in the order of treatment attention should be directed toward the patient's general and mental health, and defects in these areas should be corrected. Next, the pain factor should be minimized; give enough sedation to attain the desired effect.

Most important is prevention of the syndrome in patients with injuries—regardless of how trivial—to the upper extremity or in patients with debilitating diseases that reduce muscular activity of the arm and favor dependency of the limb. Whenever possible, slings, splints and immobilizing gear should be avoided, particularly in patients over 40 years of age, and the patient must be encouraged to move actively the shoulder and all joints of the hand and fingers. To attain the best results the exercises should be performed on a regulated program and, if necessary, under supervision. The syndrome frequently follows fractures about the wrist and hand in elderly persons. In these instances the only safeguard against development of the syndrome is active shoulder and finger motion. Avoid the use of a sling.

When the syndrome is established, the process must be reversed if great disability is to be avoided. This means restoring the pumping action of the shoulder and hand by active exercises, administration of anti-inflammatory drugs such as phenylbutazone derivatives and repeated blocks of the stellate cervical ganglion. I have found the use of dynamic finger splints very helpful in preventing and correcting finger deformities and restoring meaningful power in the muscles of the hand and fingers. The earlier treatment is instituted the better is the prognosis. Early treatment, however, depends on the making of an early diagnosis. It behooves the surgeon always to be on the alert for the first manifestations of the disorder and to institute the corrective measures promptly.

## OBSTETRICAL PARALYSIS

During birth, the brachial plexus may be injured; also the shoulder joint may be injured at the same time. Immediately after birth the extremity exhibits a flaccid paralysis; as time passes, some muscles regain varying degrees of power and, depending upon the type of muscle imbalance present, the extremity assumes characteristic deformities. With the development of contractures, the deformities become fixed.

Since the report of Smellie (1764), in which he described paralysis of both arms following a difficult delivery, many contributions to our knowledge of the pathology and pathogenesis of this disorder have been made. Among the chief contributors are Erb, Duchenne, Klumpke, Seeligmuller and Schoemaker. To Clark, Taylor and Prout must go the credit for our first knowledge of the disruption of neural and other soft tissue that is produced by traction on the brachial plexus. To Gravellona we are indebted for his contribution showing severe damage to the spinal cord and brachial plexus following a difficult delivery. More recently, Wickstrom and Adler and Patterson, through their studies of long-term results of the treatment of birth palsies, have given us a clearer understanding of the course, prognosis and residual deformities of these disorders.

The incidence of obstetrical palsies has decreased significantly within the past few decades. This reduction is due to the improved diagnostic methods used to recognize cephalopelvic disproportion and the new methods of management of this complication.

It should be remembered that during birth the skeletal elements of the shoulder may be injured without an injury to the plexus. In such instances, because of pain,

the infant presents a flaccid extremity. As the pain subsides, the infant begins to move the arm and the extremity shows no motor or sensory deficits. On the other hand, both lesions — injuries to the plexus and injuries to the skeletal elements of the shoulder — may occur at the same time. The commonest deformity following injury to the shoulder is posterior subluxation of the humeral head. If this deformity is not recognized and corrected early, secondary developmental alterations occur in the head of the humerus and the glenoid.

At birth, the proximal growth center of the humerus is not visible in roentgenograms; therefore, injuries involving the epiphysis or the epiphyseal plate cannot be recognized immediately after birth. After several weeks, the appearance of callus and bone is clear evidence of injury to the upper end of the humerus; and after a period of 4 to 6 months, the nature of the injury and the changes in position and configuration of the proximal humeral epiphysis are demonstrable by roentgenograms.

Separation of the proximal humeral epiphysis may occur proximal to the epiphyseal plate; the injury may occur with or without injury to the brachial plexus. As growth proceeds at the metaphysis, the epiphysis is displaced backward. The posterior displacement may be sufficient to produce posterior subluxation of the joint. Such a humeral head may show some alteration in its size and shape. These deformities may also occur if the blood supply to the epiphysis is disturbed. However, posterior subluxation of the humeral head may be secondary to the position of the arm and to contracture of the intrinsic rotators. In these instances, contracture of the internal rotators is such that the arm is constantly held in fixed internal rotation. Also, this position forces the child to elevate the arm in flexion rather than abduction. Both these factors force the humeral head to first impinge on

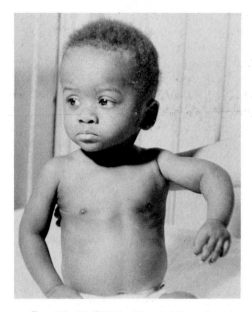

Fig. 12-19. Child with a birth palsy of the Erb-Duchenne type. The arm is held in internal rotation, owing to contractures of the internal rotators; the forearm is flexed and pronated; also an abduction contracture of the shoulder is present. In addition, this child had a posterior subluxation of the glenohumeral joint.

and finally slip by the posterior lip of the glenoid fossa.

Depending upon the degree of involvement of the brachial plexus, three classic types of brachial palsy have evolved. However, it must be remembered that this classification provides nothing more than a general idea of the location and severity of the injuries to the brachial plexus. Frequently, it is indeed difficult to determine the exact location of the injury because of the overlap of innervation of muscles by different trunks of the brachial plexus. This results in incomplete paralysis of the muscles innervated in this manner.

### Upper Arm or Erb-Duchenne Type

Of the three types, the upper arm palsy is the commonest. It involves the fifth and sixth cervical nerve roots, producing paralysis of the deltoid, the biceps, the brachialis and the supinator longus. Sometimes paralysis also occurs in the supraspinatus, infraspinatus, subscapularis, supinator brevis and the extensors of the wrist and fingers. As a rule, the lesion is produced by spreading of the interval between the head and shoulder, such as occurs when traction is made on the head at birth, or by forcing the shoulder downward and backward.

In this group, the return of motor power indicates that only minimal nerve damage has occurred; apparently, transmission of nerve impulses is not seriously impaired. Most likely, the injury causes epineural hemorrhage and edema of the nerve trunks. With resolution of the acute pathology, perineural adhesions form and the nerve trunks are enmeshed in scar tissue.

The limb assumes a characteristic attitude; both the arm and the forearm are adducted and internally rotated; the forearm is slightly flexed and pronated. Lesions of long duration exhibit profound atrophy of the deltoid, the biceps, the brachialis and the supinators. There is loss of abduction and external rotation of the arm and loss of flexion and supination of the forearm (Fig. 12-19).

Characteristic of this type is the lack of sensory disturbances, except for a small patch of loss of sensation over the posterolateral aspect of the shoulder. Generally, with correct management the prognosis for partial or complete recovery is favorable.

### Lower Arm or Klumpke Type

This lesion is indeed rare. It implicates the lower roots of the brachial plexus—eighth cervical and first thoracic roots—and the cervical ganglia. The muscles affected are the intrinsic muscles of the hand and the flexors of the forearm. Because of involvement of the sympathetic nerve fibers there may be inequality of the pupils (the pupil on the affected side is smaller).

The lesion is produced by the forcing of

the extremity upward and, hence, making tension on the lower roots of the plexus, such as is caused by traction made in breech presentations with the arms extended. Atrophy of the paralyzed muscles occurs. The child is unable to close the hand completely and exhibits a sensory deficit in the dermatome distributions of the eighth cervical and first thoracic nerve roots.

## Whole Arm Type

In this lesion the entire brachial plexus is severely injured. The result is flaccid paralysis of the entire limb and complete sensory paralysis. Many gradations of paralysis occur between the upper arm and the whole arm types, depending on the number of roots affected. Both extremities may be involved.

## Diagnosis and Prognosis

The diagnosis of a brachial plexus injury is not difficult to make immediately after birth. Usually there is a history of a difficult delivery or a breech presentation. The newborn does not actively move one extremity, yet the range of passive motion in the affected limb is equal to that of the uninvolved extremity. When active and passive motions are equally restricted, an injury to the upper end of the humerus, particularly the proximal humeral epiphysis, should be suspected.

Immediately after birth, it is impossible to prognosticate the extent of motor recovery. The incidence of full recovery varies from 7 percent to 13.4 percent. Evidence of implication of the sympathetic nerves, such as a Horner's syndrome, carries a poor prognosis insofar as recovery of motor power is concerned. The same is true of paralysis of the thoracoscapular muscles owing to lesions of the anterior thoracic and the dorsal scapular nerves, and profound sensory deficits. In general, the infants showing an early return of motor power (2 to 3 months) have less damage to

the brachial plexus than those who exhibit little improvement after a much longer period (18 months or more). In the latter group, many have marked sensory impairment and sympathetic involvement. Finally, children with involvement of the lower plexus or of the whole plexus have a more protracted and incomplete return of motor power than those with involvement of the upper roots.

## Residual Deformities

The great majority of patients exhibit some degree of residual deformity and impaired function with or without treatment, and regardless of the type of neonatal care. Of the residual soft-tissue deformities the commonest is weak abduction and restricted external rotation of the arm. The overactive, unopposed internal rotators cause secondary changes in the bony elements of the shoulder joint; the scapula rotates forward and laterally and the humerus rotates medially so that the insertion of the deltoid assumes more of an anterior position than a lateral one. Likewise, the overactive coracobrachialis and the short head of the biceps produce a curved elongation of the coracoid process. The acromion is usually elongated and bent forward in front of the head of the humerus.

Many children exhibit varying degrees of abduction contractures of the shoulder. Although the deformity is influenced by the type of initial treatment, it also may occur in patients who have had no treatment. A factor that may influence the development of this deformity is the constant overactivity of the abductor muscles in opposing the shortened internal rotators during elevation of the arm so that the hand can reach the face.

In a small number of patients the humeral head subluxates posteriorly. As noted earlier, this deformity is, most likely, the result of the arm being held constantly in internal rotation, a position forcing the arm to elevate in forward flexion rather than abduction. Hence, the humeral head first tends to abut against the posterior lip of the glenoid fossa and then slips beyond it. Also, the subluxation may be the result of injury to the proximal epiphysis sustained at the same time the brachial plexus was injured.

After the age of three the shaft of the humerus may show varying degrees of medial torsion, owing to the overactive internal rotators. In some instances, in older children, the humeral epiphysis is underdeveloped and misshapen and the glenoid fossa is flattened.

Mention must be made of the residual deformities of the elbow in obstetrical palsies. Approximately 40 percent of the patients show some form of elbow deformity and dysfunction of the elbow joint. The deformity most commonly found is a flexion contracture of the elbow caused by either overactivity of the flexors or osseous changes related to the original trauma or to bracing. Next in order of frequency is posterior dislocation of the radial head which may occur in the first few months after birth. In older children, posterior dislocation of the radial head is associated with bowing of the ulna. Finally, the elbow joint, in a few instances, may disintegrate completely. The radial head dislocates posteriorly and the ulna dislocates posteriorly and medially, owing to flattening of the trochlea. The lesion is progressive and does not respond to conservative or surgical measures. In very few instances the radial head dislocates anteriorly, but this is more like a deformity present at birth rather than one developing after birth.

As a rule, posterior dislocation of the radial head is encountered in patients with extensive paralysis. In infants, the only indication of the lesion is clubbing of the proximal radial metaphysis and progressive bowing of the ulna. By the time the child is from five to eight years of age the posterior dislocation is complete and the opposing part of the capitellum is flattened. Radiographic evidence of the proximal radial epiphysis, which appears between the eighth and the fourteenth year, shows it to be underdeveloped and flattened.

As noted previously, the most likely causes of the elbow deformities are muscle imbalance and prolonged bracing in an abnormal position. The deformities may be minimized, when they are developing or after they are present, by proper bracing. As recommended by Aitken, the best position of the extremity when immobilized is moderate abduction and complete external rotation of the shoulder, and extension of the elbow beyond 90° (120°), with the forearm in the neutral position. Of course, the bracing must be supplemented by an intensive program of passive and active exercises, putting all joints through full ranges of motion.

During the growth period, excision of the radial head does not improve either the motion of the elbow or supination of the forearm. If excision is contemplated, it should be performed after the growth period and should be combined with an osteotomy of the ulna through its proximal third. However, even this procedure may be very disappointing.

**Early Management**

There is general agreement that early and adequate treatment reduces the incidence and severity of the residual deformities of the shoulder and elbow. Contractures occur early and it is easier to prevent them than to correct them after they are established. With inadequate treatment, residual deformities may occur and impair function even when there is complete return of motor power.

There is some disagreement as to the advisability of immobilizing the extremity in abduction and external rotation. Some observers contend that immobilization favors the development of abduction contractures of the shoulder and osseous deformities about the elbow. Other observers believe the use of braces is necessary to prevent internal rotation and adduction deformities of the shoulder. Both points of view have merit. If abduction braces are applied for too long a period of time, and if the shoulder, elbow and hand are not passively exercised repeatedly through a full range of motion, contractures about the shoulder and elbow inevitably occur. On the other hand, proper bracing, supplemented by diligent and gentle passive exercises putting all the joints of the extremity through a full range of motion, is the most effective form of early management of obstetrical palsy. It prevents contractures and facilitates any reconstructive procedures that may have to be performed at a later date to improve function. When such a program cannot be instituted, passive bracing favors the development of abduction contractures and alterations in the osseous elements of the shoulder and elbow.

With the preceding comments in mind, I prefer the following course of early treatment: Immediately after birth the paralyzed arm is protected by tying the sleeve of the gown to the head of the crib. For the first few days after birth no other treatment is necessary and any form of massage, exercises or stretching at this time is prohibited. It should be remembered that the brachial plexus has suffered an acute traumatic injury, and during this active stage the tissues should not be subjected to any further trauma. Later, an abduction splint is applied. I prefer the splint modified by Wickstrom; it holds the arm in 70° of abduction, complete external rotation, and 45° of forward flexion and the elbow in 120° of flexion and the forearm in the neutral position. For the first 6 to 8 weeks the splint is worn day and night, but during this period all the joints of the extremity are put through a full range of motion several times each day. This passive exercising is performed on a regulated regimen and must be closely supervised. Parents should be impressed with the importance of the program in achieving the maximum return of

motor power with minimal residual deformity of the extremity, if any.

When the child begins to move the arm actively the splint is removed during the day but is worn at night for two or three months. Again, during this entire period, passive and actively assisted exercises are continued on a regulated program. The return of muscle tone or active movements of the arm usually occurs within 2 to 3 months in children with minimal injury to the brachial plexus; but, in more severe injuries, return of motor power may be delayed as long as 6 to 18 months.

Just as soon as the child is able to cooperate in the active exercises, the intensity of the program is increased and the child should be encouraged to use the affected arm in all daily activities. In older children with fixed deformities the same program is instituted. In this group, I do not prescribe the use of a splint, for I do not believe it is effective in correcting internal contractures of the shoulder. In fact, in this group, even carefully supervised exercise programs have little bearing on the deformities.

## Surgical Management

I have never been convinced that the amount of functional improvement obtained following exploration of the brachial plexus justified the procedure. However, some surgeons believe that exploration of the plexus should be done when, after 3 months, the return of motor power is only slight, particularly in the whole plexus type of obstetrical palsy. The advocates of this line of treatment contend that if the nerve trunks are emmeshed in scar tissue, neurolysis enhances return of nerve function; however, if there is disruption of the nerve roots and neurorrhaphy is required, the expectation for improvement of function is indeed slim.

The most common of the deformities of the shoulder are contractures of the internal rotators which restrict external rotation, and abduction and adduction contractures. The functional improvement of the extremity following any type of surgery to correct these deformities is greatly influenced by the bony configuration of the glenohumeral joint. In fact, if the humeral head is subluxated or deformed, these alterations are decisive factors in choosing the appropriate operation. In general, better results are obtained when the glenohumeral joint is within normal limits and the deformities can be corrected by soft tissue surgery alone then when surgery on the bony elements is necessary to correct the deformities.

Five operations to correct the deformities of the shoulder are currently used; each has its specific indications and limitations.

**Sever Operation.** This procedure is indicated when the configuration of the glenohumeral joint is normal, the external rotators and abductors can still function and the chief deforming factor is contracture of the internal rotators. In this procedure the entire pectoralis major tendon and the subscapularis tendon are divided; when contracted, the coracobrachialis and short head of the biceps are released; and, if the coracoid and acromion processes interfere with function, these are divided.

This operation is a modification of the operation devised by Fairbank in 1913. It differs from the Fairbank procedure in that Fairbank did not completely sever the tendon of the pectoralis major; he divided the anterior capsule in addition to the subscapularis tendon; and, if necessary, he divided the coracoid process, the coracohumeral ligament and the supraspinatus tendon.

Studies of long-term results reveal that the Sever operation falls far short of its goal. The operation does not improve the strength of the shoulder and, in most instances, the internal rotation contracture recurs. Far better results are obtained when this operation is combined with transfer of the latissimus dorsi and teres major

to the lateral aspect of the humerus, thereby converting them into external rotators of the shoulder. This is the operation of L'Episcopo.

**L'Episcopo Operation (Zachary Modification).** Steindler pointed out that contractures of the latissimus dorsi and the teres major restricted abduction of the shoulder. He recommended dividing these muscles when Sever's operation was performed. L'Episcopo utilized these muscles by transferring them to the lateral aspect of the humerus so that they functioned as active external rotators of the shoulder. In addition, he divided the anterior capsule of the joint to further overcome any internal rotation contractures. The end results of this procedure are by far superior to those of the Sever operation. Later, Zachary simplified the procedure by utilizing a posterior approach to transfer the latissimus dorsi and the teres major to the lateral aspect of the humerus.

**Fairbank Operation (Modified).** In addition to the internal contractures and restricted external rotation and abduction, the head of the humerus may be subluxated posteriorly. In those cases with a normal or nearly normal humeral head without retroversion, the subluxation can be reduced by the Fairbank operation. After reduction, the corrected position is maintained by transfixing the humeral head and the glenoid with pins. If the pectoralis major tendon is lengthened instead of divided, internal rotation power can be preserved.

**Sever Operation and Osteotomy of the Humerus.** Deformity of the upper end of the humerus may be secondary to the obstetrical palsy or to birth injury to the upper proximal epiphysis, or to both lesions. In these instances, a complex deformity evolves. The humeral head is subluxated or dislocated posteriorly; in addition, the humeral head is retroverted in relation to the shaft, and the arm is held in internal rotation and adduction by muscle contractures. The posterior displace-

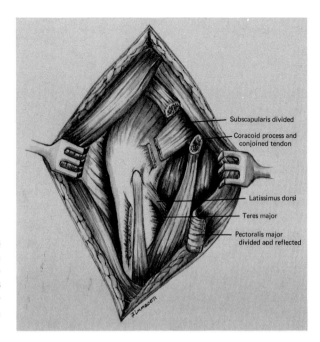

Subscapularis divided

Coracoid process and
conjoined tendon

Latissimus dorsi

Teres major

Pectoralis major
divided and reflected

FIG. 12-20. Sever operation. The subscapularis and pectoralis major tendons are divided completely. The coracoid process is resected just proximal to the insertion of the conjoined tendon. The capsule is not opened.

ment of the humeral head can be corrected by the Sever operation, but now the arm is in extreme external rotation. To prevent redisplacement of the head, an osteotomy of the humerus is performed above the level of the insertion of the deltoid, and the lower fragment is internally rotated. This corrects the retroversion of the humeral head.

**Osteotomy of the Humerus.** A severe internal rotation deformity may exist in association with a flat, misshapen humeral head. In these patients the internal rotation deformity can be corrected by an osteotomy of the humerus. This procedure does not increase the amount of rotation of the glenohumeral joint; but, by placing the arm in a more advantageous position of function, abduction power of the shoulder is improved in many patients, and in all the over-all performance of the extremity is definitely enhanced.

## Surgical Techniques

**Sever's Operation.** Perform the operation through an anterior incision. The skin incision extends from just lateral to the acromioclavicular joint straight downward over the anterior third of the deltoid to a point distal to the insertion of the pectoralis major. Divide the tendon parallel to the humerus. Develop the interval between the deltoid and the pectoralis major; do not injure the cephalic vein. Retract the deltoid laterally and the pectoralis major medially, exposing the coracoid process. Usually the coracoid is elongated and beaked; if so, identify the conjoined tendon of the coracobrachialis, the short head of the biceps and the pectoralis minor and resect the distal end of the coracoid process just proximal to the common tendon insertion. This step increases the range of external rotation and abduction of the arm. Now, with the arm rotated externally, find the lower edge of the tendon of the subscapularis at its insertion into the humerus. With a groove director elevate the entire tendon from the capsule and divide it; do not cut into the capsule. Abduction and external rotation of the shoulder should now be almost normal.

The acromion process may be elongated

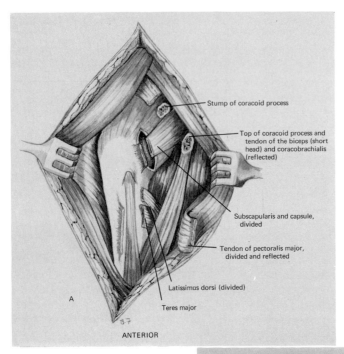

Stump of coracoid process

Top of coracoid process and
tendon of the biceps (short
head) and coracobrachialis
(reflected)

Subscapularis and capsule,
divided

Tendon of pectoralis major,
divided and reflected

Latissimus dorsi (divided)

Teres major

A

ANTERIOR

FIG. 12-21. L'Episcopo operation (Zachary modification). (A) The subscapularis and pectoralis major tendons are divided completely; also the anterior portion of the capsule is divided. The coracoid process is resected proximal to the insertion of the conjoined tendon, and, finally, the tendons of the latissimus dorsi and teres major are freed.

FIG. 12-21 (Continued). (B) First, the interval between the long and lateral heads of the triceps is developed and the radial nerve and artery are identified in the triangular space. Next, the tendons of the latissimus dorsi and teres major are passed through a slit in the proximal portion of the lateral head of the triceps and anchored to the posterolateral aspect of the humerus.

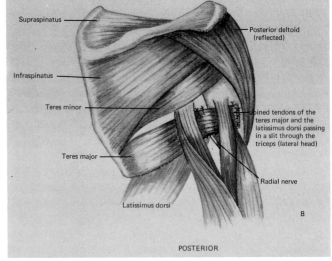

Supraspinatus

Posterior deltoid
(reflected)

Infraspinatus

Teres minor

Joined tendons of the
teres major and the
latissimus dorsi passing
in a slit through the
triceps (lateral head)

Teres major

Radial nerve

Latissimus dorsi

B

POSTERIOR

and hooked over the head so that it interferes with abduction. If such is the case, expose the tip of the acromion subperiosteally and resect enough of it to permit complete abduction; or divide the acromion and elevate the distal portion (Fig. 12-20).

POSTOPERATIVE MANAGEMENT. Apply a shoulder spica plaster cast holding the arm in 120 degrees of abduction and complete external rotation, the elbow flexed 90 degrees, the forearm supinated and the wrist extended. After two weeks remove the spica and apply a brace holding the same position. The brace should be removed three or four times daily and all the joints passively and actively exercised. Discard the brace after four weeks but continue the program of active exercises for several months.

L'Episcopo Operation (Zachary Modifica-

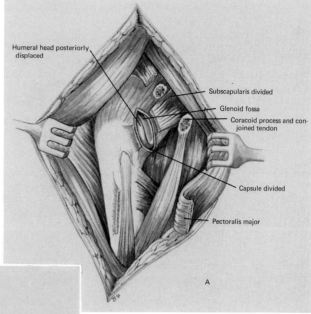

Humeral head posteriorly
displaced

Subscapularis divided

Glenoid fossa

Coracoid process and con-
joined tendon

Capsule divided

Pectoralis major

A

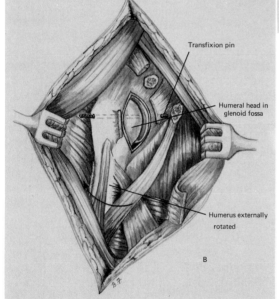

Transfixion pin

Humeral head in
glenoid fossa

Humerus externally
rotated

B

FIG. 12-22. Fairbank operation (modified). (A) The subscapularis and pectoralis major tendons are divided completely; also the anterior capsule is divided, exposing the posterior subluxation of the humeral head. The coracoid process is resected proximal to the insertion of the conjoined tendon. (B) By external rotation of the arm the posterior subluxation is reduced, and the position is maintained by a transfixion wire passing through the humeral head into the glenoid.

tion). The first part of the operation is essentially the Sever operation. In addition, divide the anterior capsule completely, to gain the maximum amount of external rotation. Also, retract the coracobrachialis and short head of the biceps medially and isolate and divide the tendons of the latissimus dorsi and the teres major at their insertions into the humerus (Fig. 12-21A).

The second part of the operation is the transfer of the tendons of the latissimus dorsi and the teres major to the postero-

lateral aspect of the humerus. Make a curved longitudinal skin incision over the upper posterior third of the arm. Develop the interval along the posterior border of the deltoid and retract the deltoid anteriorly to expose the triceps muscle. Identify the long and lateral heads of the triceps and develop the space between them, exposing the radial nerve and the deep radial artery in the triangular space (Fig. 12-21B). Make a slit through the proximal portion of the lateral head of the triceps and pass through

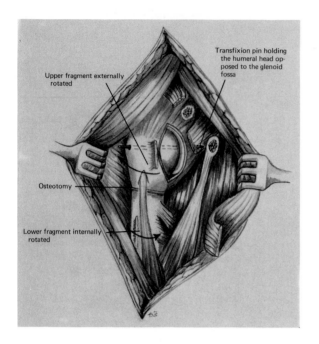

Upper fragment externally rotated

Transfixion pin holding the humeral head opposed to the glenoid fossa

Osteotomy

Lower fragment internally rotated

FIG. 12-23. Sever operation and osteotomy of the humerus. First a Sever operation is performed; then the anterior capsule is divided, the humerus is externally rotated and the position is maintained by a transfixion wire passing through the humeral head into the glenoid. An osteotomy is performed through the surgical neck of the humerus and the lower fragment is rotated internally.

it the tendons of the latissimus dorsi and teres major. With the arm in complete external rotation anchor the tendons under an osteoperiosteal flap on the posterolateral aspect of the humerus. (On several occasions I have used a staple to anchor the tendons to the humerus.)

POSTOPERATIVE MANAGEMENT. Apply a shoulder spica plaster cast holding the arm in complete external rotation, slight abduction and 45 to 60° of forward flexion. Remove the cast after 4 weeks and institute a program of active exercises to develop the external rotation power in the latissimus dorsi and teres major.

**Fairbank Operation (Modified).** Expose the anterior aspect of the joint in the same manner as that described for the Sever operation. Divide completely the tendon of the pectoralis major. After the subscapularis tendon is divided, divide the anterior capsule also. Now reduce the posterior displacement of the humeral head by externally rotating the arm and elevating the head into the glenoid fossa. To maintain the corrected position of the head, pass a wire transversely through the head into the glenoid (Fig. 12-22).

POSTOPERATIVE MANAGEMENT. Apply a shoulder spica plaster cast holding the arm in the new position. Remove the cast and transfixion wire after 4 to 5 weeks and institute a program of active exercises to improve external rotation of the shoulder and prevent internal rotation contractures.

**Sever Operation and Osteotomy of the Humerus.** I perform this operation in one stage. First perform the Sever operation as described above and reduce the retroverted humeral head by external rotation of the arm and elevation of the head into the glenoid fossa. If the anterior capsule is shortened and interferes with reduction of the humeral head, divide it. To hold the corrected position pass a stout threaded wire or pin transversely through the head and into the glenoid (Fig. 12-23).

Next expose the shaft of the humerus above the insertion of the deltoid by subperiosteal dissection. Do an osteotomy through the surgical neck and internally rotate the distal fragment. This step corrects the retroversion of the head in relation to the shaft (Fig. 12-23).

POSTOPERATIVE MANAGEMENT. Apply a shoulder spica plaster cast holding the arm in the corrected position. After 4 to 5 weeks remove the pin and the spica and start a program of active exercises to restore mobility in the shoulder joint.

**Osteotomy of the Humerus.** Make a skin incision on the upper anterior aspect of the arm between the deltoid and the pectoralis major. Develop the interval between these two muscles and by subperiosteal dissection expose the surgical neck of the humerus. With the arm abducted, divide the bone approximately 2 inches below the joint. Now externally rotate the distal fragment 90°. Fix the fragments with a small compression plate. This eliminates the use of a plaster shoulder spica and permits immediate motion of the shoulder. If it is impossible to apply a compression plate, apply a plaster spica to hold the corrected position (Fig. 12-24).

Postoperative Management. When a compression plate is used, start immediately to mobilize the shoulder. When a shoulder spica is used, it should hold the shoulder abducted 90°, the elbow flexed 90°, and the forearm supinated.

Remove the cast at the end of 6 to 8 weeks and start active exercises to mobilize the shoulder.

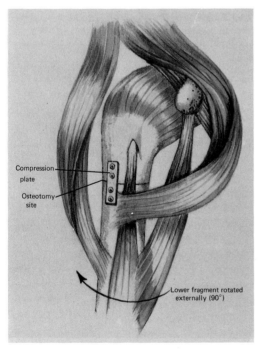

Fig. 12-24. Osteotomy of the humerus. An osteotomy is performed through the surgical neck of the humerus and the lower fragment is rotated externally about 90°. The corrected position of the fragments is held by a small compression plate.

## BIBLIOGRAPHY

Adson, A. W.: Surgical treatment for symptoms produced by cervical ribs and the scalenus anticus muscle. Surg. Gynec. Obstet., *85*:687, 1947.

⸺: Cervical ribs; symptoms, differential diagnosis for section of the insertion of the scalenus anticus muscle. J. Internat. Coll. Surg., *16*:546, 1951.

Adson, A. W., and Coffey, J. R.: Cervical rib: a method of anterior approach for relief of symptoms by division of the scalenus anticus. Ann. Surg., *85*:839, 1927.

Ahone, I.: The scalenus anticus syndrome and the results of operative treatment. Ann. Chir. Gynaec. Fenn., *51*(Fasc 2):211, 1962.

Aitken, J.: Deformity of the elbow joint as a sequel to Erb's obstetrical paralysis. J. Bone & Joint Surg., *34-B*:352, 1952.

Ansart, Bastos: Quoted by Erlacher.

Anson, B., and Maddock, W. G.: Callanders Surgical Anatomy. Philadelphia, W. B. Saunders, 1952.

Armstrong, J. R.: Lumbar Disc Lesions; Pathogenesis and Treatment of Low-Back Pain and Sciatica. ed. 3. Baltimore, Williams & Wilkins, 1965.

Ashkenazy, M.: Severe unilateral face pains as a presenting symptom of cervical spine lesions. Texas J. Med., *58*:633, 1962.

Atkins, H. J. B.: Sympathectomy by axillary approach. Lancet, *1*:538, 1954.

Barr, J. S.: Personal communications.

Bateman, J. E.: The shoulder and Environs. St. Louis, C. V. Mosby, 1955.

⸺: Neurovascular syndromes about the shoulder. Instructional Course Lectures. Vol. 18. C. V. Mosby, 1961.

⸺: Trauma to Nerves in Limbs. Philadelphia, W. B. Saunders, 1962.

⸺: Neurovascular syndromes related to the clavicle. Clin. Orthop., *58*:75, 1968.

Bettmann, E. H., *et al.*: Cervical disc pathology resulting in dysphagia in an adolescent boy. N. Y. J. Med., *60*:2465, 1960.

Bonney, G. L. W.: Prognosis in traction lesions of the brachial plexus. J. Bone & Joint Surg., *41-B*:4, 1959.

Bovill, E. G., Jr., and Drazek, J. A.: An anatomic study of the cervical spine based on a clinical-roentgenologic concept of the etiology of trachialgia. Univ. Mich. Med. Bull., *16*:387, 1950.

Boyer, G. F.: The complete histo-pathological examination of the nervous system of an unusual case of obstetrical paralysis 41 years after birth, and a review of the pathology. Proc. Roy. Soc. Med. (Neurol. Sect.), *5*:31, 1911.

Boyes, J. H.: Bunnell's Surgery of the Hand. ed. 5. Philadelphia, J. B. Lippincott, 1970.

Bradshaw, P.: Pain caused by cervical spondylosis. Rheumatism, *17*:2, 1961.

Brain, L.: Some unsolved problems of cervical spondylosis. Brit. Med. J., *5333*:771, 1963.

Brannon, E. W.: Cervical rib syndrome: an analysis of nineteen cases and twenty-four operations. J. Bone Jt. Surg., *45-A*:977, 1963.

Buonocore, E., *et al.*: Cineradiograms of cervical spine in diagnosis of soft tissue injuries. JAMA, *198*:143, 1966.

Burr, C. R.: Spinal birth palsies; a study of 9 cases of "obstetric paralysis." Boston M. & S. J., *127*:235, 1892.

Burrows, E. H.: The sagittal diameter of the spinal canal in cervical spondylosis. Clin. Radiol., *14*:77, 1963.

Camera, R.: Alterazioni del guoieto nelle paralisi obstetriche dell'arto niperiare. Minerva Orthop., *6*:303, 1955.

Charnley, J.: Orthopaedic signs in diagnosis of disc protrusion, with special reference to straight-leg-raising test. Lancet, *1*:186, 1951.

Clagett, O. T.: Presidential Address: Research and prosearch. J. Thorac. Cardiovasc. Surg., *44*:153, 1962.

Clark, L. P. Taylor, A., and Prout, T. P.: A study on brachial birth palsy. Am J. Med. Sci., *130*:670, 1965.

Cloward, R. B.: The anterior approach for removal of ruptured cervical disks. J. Neurosurg., *15*:602, 1958.

————: New method of diagnosis and treatment of cervical disc disease. Clin. Neurosurg., *8*:93, 1962.

Costanzo, D.: Sul trattamento chirurgico degli esti di paralisis obstetrica. Orthop. e traumatol., *22*:447, 1954.

Déjerine-Klumpke, A.: Des polynévrites en général et des paralysies et atrophies saturnines en particulier. Étude clinique et anatomo-pathologique. Paris, Ancienne Librairie Germer Baillière et Cie, 1889.

DePalma, A. F.: Surgery of the Shoulder. Ed. 1. Philadelphia, J. B. Lippincott, 1950.

————: Study of the cervical syndrome. Clin. Orthop., *38*:135, 1965.

DePalma, A. F., and Rothman, R. H.: The Intervertebral Disc. Philadelphia, W. B. Saunders, 1970.

Deterling, R. A.: Vascular Disorders of the Hand.

Duchenne, G. B.: De l électrisation localisée, et de son application à la pathologie et à la thérapeutique. Ed. 3, 357-362. Paris, J. B. Baillière et Fils, 1872.

————: Physiology of motion demonstrated by means of electrical stimulation and clinical observation and applied to the study of paralysis and deformities. (Translated and edited by Emanuel B. Kaplan) Philadelphia, J. B. Lippincott, 1949.

Dupont, C., Cloutier, G. E., Prevost, Y., and Dion, M. A.: Ulnar-tunnel syndrome of the wrist; a report of four cases. J. Bone & Joint Surg., *47-A*:757, 1965.

Eaton, L. M.: Neurologic causes of pain in the upper extremities. Surg. Clin. N. Am., *26*:810, 1946.

El-Sallab, R. A., *et al.*: Oesophageal and tracheal pseudo-tumors due to anterior cervical osteophytes. Brit. J. Radiol., *38*:682, 1965.

Erb, W. H.: Ueber eine eigenthümliche Localisation von Lähmungen im Plexus brachialis. Verhandl. Naturhist. Med. Heidelberg, N.F. *2*:130, 1874.

Erlacher, E. B.: Die Technik des orthopaedischen Eingriffes: Plastik nach Bastos Ansart. Vienna, Julius Springer, 1928.

Facer, J. C.: Osteophytes of the cervical spine causing dysphagia. Arch. Otolaryng., *86*:341, 1967.

Fairbank, H. A. T.: Birth palsy: subluxation of the shoulder joint in infants and young children. Lancet, *1*:1217, 1913.

Falconer, M. A., and Li, F. W. P.: Resection of first rib in costoclavicular compression of the brachial plexus. Lancet, *1*:59, 1962.

Falconer, M. A., and Weddell, G.: Costoclavicular compression of the subclavian artery and vein; relation to scalenus syndrome. Lancet, *2*:539, 1943.

Falconer, M. A., *et al.*: Observations on the cause and mechanism of symptom-production in sciatica and low-back pain. J. Neurol. Neurosurg. Psychiat., *11*:13, 1948.

Fielding, J. W.: Cineroentgenography of the normal cervical spine. J. Bone & Joint Surg., *39-A*:1280, 1957.

Fieux: De la pathogénie des paralysies brachialles chez le nouveau-né; paralysies obstétricales. Ann. gynec., *47*:52, 1897.

Fineman, S., Barrelli, F. J., Rubinstein, B. M., Epstein, H., and Jacobson, H. G.: The cervical spine: transformation of the normal lordotic pattern into a linear pattern in the neutral posture. J. Bone & Joint Surg., *45-A*: 1179, 1963.

Flynn, J. E.: Hand Surgery. Baltimore, Williams & Wilkins, 1966.

Friedenberg, Z. B., and Miller, W. T.: Degenerative disc disease of the cervical spine; a comparative study of asymptomatic and symptomatic patients. J. Bone & Joint Surg., *45-A*:1171, 1963.

Gasser, H. S.: Pain-producing impulses in peripheral nerves. Asso. Res. Nerv. Ment. Dis. Proc. (1942), *23*:44, 1943.

Geza, D. E. Takats: Vascular Surgery. Philadelphia, W. B. Saunders, 1959.

Gortuai, P.: Insufficiency of vertebral artery treated by decompression of its cervical part. Brit. Med. J., *5403*:233, 1964.

Gravellona: Thèse de Paris, No. 654, July, 1900.

Hadley, L. A.: Constriction of the intervertebral foramen. JAMA, *140*:473, 1949.

Hanflig, S. S.: Pain in the shoulder girdle, arm and precordium due to cervical arthritis. JAMA, *106*:523, 1936.

Hirsch, C. Brachalgia: a panel discussion. Internat. Congress Orthop. and Traum., Paris, France, Sept., 1966.

Hollinshead, W. H.: Anatomy of the spine: points of interest to orthopaedic surgeons. J. Bone & Joint Surg., *47-A*:209, 1965.

Horwitz, T.: Degenerative lesions in the cervical portion of the spine. Arch. Intern. Med., *65*: 1178, 1940.

Hutchinson, E. C., and Yates, P. O.: Cervical portion of vertebral artery: Clinico-pathological study. Brain, *79*:319, 1956.

Inman, V. T., and Saunders, J. B. deC. M.: Anatomicophysiological aspects of injuries to intervertebral disc. J. Bone & Joint Surg., *29*:461, 1947.

Jackson, R.: The Cervical Syndrome. Springfield, Illinois, Charles C Thomas, 1956.

Jackson, R.: Headaches associated with disorders of the cervical spine. Headache, *6*:175, 1967.

Kaplan, E.: Surgical Approaches to the Neck, Cervical Spine and Upper Extremity. Philadelphia, W. B. Saunders, 1966.

Kaplan, E. B. (see Duchenne).

Kapoor, S. C., and Tiwary, P. K.: Cervical spondylosis simulating cardiac pain. Indian J. Chest Dis. (Delhi), *8*:25, 1966.

Kast, H.: Über einen Fall von Muskel-plastik bei Ausfall der Humerusaussen-rotation. Chirurg., *11*:111, 1939.

Keggi, K. J., *et al.*: Vertebral artery insufficiency secondary to trauma and osteoarthritis of the cervical spine. Yale J. Biol. Med., *38*:471, 1966.

Kendrick, J. I.: Changes in the upper humeral epiphysis following operations for obstetrical paralysis. J. Bone & Joint Surg., *19*:473, 1937.

Kennedy, R.: Suture of the brachial plexus in birth paralysis of the upper extremity. Brit. Med. J. *1*:298, 1903.

Kirtley, J. A., Riddell, D. H., Stoney, W. S., and Wright, J. K.: Cervicothoracic sympathectomy in the treatment of neurovascular abnormalities of the upper extremity; experiences in 76 patients. (In press)

Kleinberg, S.: Reattachment of the capsule and external rotators of the shoulder for obstetric paralysis. JAMA, *98*:294, 1932.

Kleinert, H. E., Cook, F. W., and Kutz, J. E.: Neurovascular disorders of the upper extremity. Arch. Surg., *90*:612, 1965.

Kleinsasser, L. T.: "Effort" thrombosis of the axillary and subclavian veins. Arch. Surg., *59*:258, 1949.

Klumpke, A.: Contribution à l'étude des paralysies radiculaires du plexus brachial. Paralysies radiculaires totales, paralysies radiculaires inférieures. De la participation des filets sympathiques oculo-pupillaires dans ces paralysies. Étude clinique et expérimentale, Rev. Méd., pp. 591, 763, 1885. (Mémoire couronné par l'Académie de Medecine, prix Godard, 1886)

Kustner; *In*: Muller, H. von P.: Handbuch der Geburtshilfe. vol. 3. p. 307. Stuttgart, F. Enke, 1889.

L'Episcopo, J. B.: Tendon transplantation in obstetrical paralysis. Am. J. Surg., *25*:122, 1934.

————: Restoration of muscle balance in the treatment of obstetrical paralysis. N. Y. J. Med., *39*:357, 1939.

Lewis, T., Sir: Pain. New York, Macmillan, 1942.

Liebolt, F. L., and Furry, J. G.: Obstetrical paralysis with dislocation of the shoulder. J. Bone & Joint Surg., *35-A*:227, 1953.

Lombard, P.: La paralysie dite obstetricale du membre superieur. Rev. orthop., *33*:235, 1947.

Lovett, R.: The surgical aspect of the paralysis of newborn children. Boston M. & S. J., *127*:8, 1892.

Lyon, E.: Uncovertebral osteophytes and osteochondrosis of the cervical spine. J. Bone & Joint Surg., *27*:248, 1945.

Martorell, F., and Fabre, J.: El sindrome de obliteration de los traucos supra-aorticos. Angiology, *5*:39, 1954.

Mastandrea, G.: Il traplanto del muscolo tricitite brachiale sul bicipite negli esiti della paralisi obstetrica. Orthop. e traumatol., 23:953, 1955.

McBurney, R. P., and Howard, H.: Resection of first rib for thoracic outlet compression. Am. Surg., 32:165, 1966.

McCleery, R. S., Kesterson, J. E., Kirtley, J. A., and Love, R. B.: Subclavius and anterior scalenus muscle compression as a cause of intermittent obstruction of the subclavian vein. Ann. Surg., 133:588, 1951.

Meyer, R. R.: Cervical discography. A help or hindrance in evaluating neck, shoulder, arm pain? Am. J. Roentgenol., 90:1208, 1963.

Michelsen, J. J., and Mixter, W. J.: Pain and disability of the shoulder and arm due to herniation of the nucleus pulposus of cervical intervertebral disks. New Eng. J. Med., 231:279, 1944.

Milgram, J. E.: Discussion of L'Episcopo's presentation. N. Y. J. Med., 39:357, 1939.

Moore, B. H.: A new operative procedure for brachial birth palsy—Erb's paralysis. Surg., Gynec. & Obstet., 61:832, 1935.

———: Brachial birth palsy. Am. J. Surg., 43:388, 1939.

Moore, J. R.: Bone block to prevent posterior dislocation of the shoulder. (personal communication)

Morton, D. E.: A comparative anatomicoroentgenological study of the cervical spine of twenty cadavers. Am. J. Roentgenol., 63:523, 1950.

Murphey, R., and Simmons, J. C.: Ruptured cervical disc. Experience with 250 cases. Am. Surg., 32:83, 1966.

Nichols, H. M.: Anatomic structures of the thoracic outlet. Clin. Orthop., 51:17, 1967.

Ochsner, A., Gage, M., and DeBakey, M.: Scalenus anticus (Naffziser) syndrome. Am. J. Surg., 28:669, 1935.

O'Connell, J. E. A.: Sciatica and mechanism of production of clinical syndrome in protrusions of lumbar intervertebral discs. Brit. J. Surg., 30:315, 1943.

Oppenheimer, A.: Narrowing of the intervertebral foramina as a cause of pseudorheumatic pain. Ann. Surg., 106:428, 1937.

Overton, L. M.: Degenerative changes in the cervical spine as a common cause of shoulder and arm pain. South. Surgeon, 16:599, 1950.

———: Cervical spine nerve root pain. Am. Surg., 17:343, 1951.

———: Chronic rheumatic diseases of the cervical spine as a cause of shoulder girdle and arm pain. Rheumatism (London), 7:68, 1951.

———: The local use of hydrocortisone acetate in the treatment of painful shoulders. Clin. Orthop., 4:115, 1954.

———: The causes of pain in the upper extremities: a differential diagnosis study. Clin. Orthop., 51:27, 1967.

Palumbo, L. T., and Lulu, D. J.: Anterior transthoracic upper dorsal sympathectomy. Arch. Surg., 92:247, 1966.

Payne, E. E., and Spillane, J. D.: The cervical spine: an anatomico-pathological study of 70 specimens. Brain, 80:571, 1957.

Perrone, J. A.: Dysphagia due to massive cervical exostoses. Arch. Otolaryng., 86:346, 1967.

Platt, H.: Opening remarks on birth paralysis. J. Orthop. Surg., 2:272, 1920.

Ray, B. S.: Tumors at the apex of the chest. Surg. Gynec. Obstet., 67:577, 1938.

Riddell, D. H.: Thoracic outlet compression: the role of anterior scalenotomy. J. Miss. Med. Assn., 11:284, 1961.

———: Thoracic outlet syndrome: thoracic and vascular aspects. Clin. Orthop., 51:53, 1967.

Riddell, D. H., Kirtley, J. A., Moore, J. L., and Goduco, R. S.: Scalenus anticus symptoms; evaluation and surgical treatment. Surgery, 47:115, 1960.

Rob, C. G., and Standeven, A.: Arterial occlusion complicating thoracic outlet compression syndrome. Brit. Med. J., 2:709, 1958.

Robbins, H.: Anatomical study of the median nerve in the carpal tunnel and etiologies of the carpal-tunnel syndrome. J. Bone & Joint Surg., 45-A:953, 1963.

Robinson, R. A.: Brachalgia: a panel discussion. Internat. Congress Orthop. and Traum., Paris, France, Sept., 1966.

Robinson, R. A., and Smith, G. W.: Anterolateral cervical disc removal and interbody fusion for cervical disc syndrome. Bull. Johns Hopkins Hosp., 96:223, 1955.

Robinson, R. A., Walker, E. E., Ferlic, D. C., and Wiecking, D. K.: The results of anterior interbody fusion of the cervical spine. J. Bone & Joint Surg., 44-A:1569, 1962.

Robinson, R. A., et al.: Surgical approaches to the cervical spine. Instruc. Lect. Am. Acad. Orthop. Surg., 17:299, 1960.

Rogers, M. H.: An operation for the correction of the deformity due to "obstetrical paralysis." Boston M. & S. J., 174:163, 1916.

Roos, D. B.: Transaxillary approach for first rib resection to relieve thoracic outlet syndrome. Ann. Surg., 163:354, 1966.

Roos, D. B., and Owens, C. J.: Thoracic outlet syndrome. Arch. Surg., 93:71, 1966.

Rosati, L. M., and Lord, J. W.: Neurovascular compression syndrome of the shoulder. Modern Surgical Monographs. New York, Grune & Stratton, 1961.

Rosenberg, J. C.: Arteriographic demonstration of compression syndromes of the thoracic outlet. Southern Med. J., 59:400, 1966.

Sa, A.: Aparelho orthopédico para a paralisia obstetrica do membro superior. Acta ortop. traumatol. iber., 31:38, 1955.

Scaglietti, O.: Lesioni ostetriche della spalla. Chir. org. movimento, 22:183, 1936.

————: The obstetrical shoulder trauma. Surg., Gynec. Obstet., 66:868, 1938.

Schoemaker, J.: Ueber die Aetiologie der Entbindungslahmunge, speciell de Oberarmparalysen. Z. Geburtsh. Gynäk., 41:33, 1899.

Von Schroetter, L.: Erkrankungen der Gefasse. Nothnagel Handbuch der Pathologie und Therapie. Vienna, Holder, 1884.

Seeligmuller, A.: Ueber Lähmungen welche Kinder inter Partum Acquiren. Berlin klin. Wschr., 11:500, 517, 1974.

————: Zur Pathologie des Sympathias. Deutsch Archiv. klin. Med., 20:101, 1877.

Semmes, R. E., and Murphey, F.: The syndrome of unilateral rupture of the sixth cervical intervertebral disk. JAMA, 121:1209, 1943.

Sever, J. W.: Obstetric paralysis. Am. J. Dis. Child., 12:541, 1916.

————: The results of a new operation for obstetrical paralysis. Am. J. Orthop. Surg., 16:248, 1918.

————: Obstetric paralysis. JAMA, 85:1862, 1925.

Sheehan, S., et al.: Vertebral artery compression in cervical spondylosis. Arteriographic demonstration during life of vertebral artery insufficiency due to rotation and extension of the neck. Neurology, 10:968, 1960.

Sjöqvest, O.: The mechanism and origin of Laseque's sign. Acta psych. neurol., Supp. 46:290, 1947.

Slomann, H. C.: Kobenhavns Med. Selskabs Forhandl., 1916-17, p. 95. Quoted by Toft, G.: On obstetrical paralysis of the upper extremities. Acta orthop. scand., 13:218, 1942.

Smellie, W.: Collection of Preternatural Cases and Observations in Midwifery, Completing the Design of Illustrating His First Volume on That Subject. vol. 3. pp. 504-505. London, Wilson & Durham, 1764.

Smith, G. W., and Robinson, R. A.: The treatment of certain cervical spine disorders by anterior removal of the intervertebral disc and interbody fusion. J. Bone & Joint Surg., 40-A:607, 1958.

Smyth, M. J., et al.: Sciatica and the intervertebral disc. An experimental study. J. Bone & Joint Surg., 40-A:1401, 1958.

Spillane, J. D., and Lloyd, G. H. T.: The diagnosis of lesions of the spinal cord in association with "osteoarthritic" disease of the cervical spine. Brain, 75:177, 1952.

Spurling, R. G.: Rupture of the cervical intervertebral disks. J. Int. Coll. Surg., 10:502, 1947.

Stein, A. H.: The relation of median nerve compression to Sudeck's syndrome, Surg. Gynec. Obstet., 144:713, 1962.

Stevens: Quoted by Bunnell. In: Surgery of the Hand, ed. 3. pp. 311-415 and 642. Philadelphia, J. B. Lippincott, 1956.

Stofford, J. S. B.: Compression of the lower trunk of the brachial plexus by a first dorsal rib. Brit. J. Surg., 7:168, 1919-1920.

Stookey, B.: Compression of spinal cord and nerve roots by herniation of nucleus pulposus in cervical region. Arch. Surg., 40:417, 1940.

Stransky, E.: Ueber Entbindungslähmungen der oberen Extremität beim Kinde. Centralbl. Grenzgeb. M. Chir., 5:497, 1902.

Sulas, V.: La pasizione de deratazione esterna abbinate all abduzione dell'arto superiore mella cura della paralisi obstetrica nei primi mesi di vita. Rass. ital. chir. med., 3:53, 1954.

Takayasu, M.: Acta Soc. Ophth. Jap., 12:554, 1908.

Taylor, A. S.: Results from surgical treatment of brachial birth palsy. JAMA, 48:96, 1907.

————: Brachial birth palsy and injuries of similar type in adults. Surg., Gynec. Obstet., 30:494, 1920.

Thomas, T. T.: Laceration of the axillary portion of the capsule of the shoulder joint as a factor in the etiology of traumatic combined paralysis of the upper extremity. Ann. Surg., 53:77, 1911.

————: Traumatic brachial paralysis with flail shoulder joint. Ann. Surg., 66:532, 1917.

————: Brachial birth palsy: a pseudoparalysis of shoulder joint origin. Am. J. Med. Sci., 159:207, 1920.

Thorek, P.: Anatomy in Surgery. ed. 2. Philadelphia, J. B. Lippincott, 1962.

Todd, T. W.: Quoted by Walshe et al.

Toft, G.: On obstetrical paralysis of the upper extremities. Acta orthop. scand., 13:218, 1942.

Toumey, J. W.: Occurence and management of reflex sympathetic dystrophy (causalgia of the extremities). J. Bone & Joint Surg., 30-A:883, 1948.

Walshe, F. M. R., Jackson, H., and Wyburn-Mason, R.: On some pressure effects associated with cervical and with rudimentary and "normal" first ribs, and the factors entering into their causation. Brain, 67:141, 1944.

White, J. C., Poppel, M. H., and Adams, R.: Congenital malformations of the first thoracic rib. Surg. Gynec. Obstet., *81*:643, 1945.

Whiteleather, J. E.: Roentgen demonstration of cervical nerve root avulsion. Am. J. Roentgenol., *72*:1017, 1954.

Wickstrom, J.: Birth injuries of the brachial plexus—treatment of defects in the shoulder. Clin. Orthop., *23*:187, 1962.

Wickstrom, J., Haslam, E. D., and Hutchinson, R. H.: The surgical management of residual deformities of the shoulder following birth injuries of the brachial plexus. J. Bone & Joint Surg., *37-A*:27, 1955.

Williams, A. F.: The role of the first rib in the scalenus anterior syndrome. J. Bone & Joint Surg., *34-B*:200, 1952.

Willshire, W. H.: Supernumerary first rib, clinical records. Lancet, *2*:633, 1860.

Wolf, B. S., *et al.*: Sagittal diameter of bony cervical spinal canal and its significance in cervical spondylosis. J. Mt. Sinai Hosp., *23*:283, 1956.

Wolman, B.: Erb's palsy. Arch. Dis. Child., *23*:129, 1948.

Woodhall, B., and Beebe, G. W.: Peripheral Nerve Regeneration. Washington, D.C., U.S. Government Printing Office, 1956.

Woodhall, B., *et al.*: The Well-leg-raising test of Fajersztajn in the diagnosis of ruptured lumbar intervertebral disc. J. Bone & Joint Surg., *32-A*:786, 1950.

Wright, I. S.: Neurovascular syndrome produced by hyperabduction of the arms. Am. Heart J., *29*:119, 1945.

———: Vascular Diseases in Clinical Practice. Chicago, Year Book Publishers, 1948.

Zachary, R. B.: Transplantation of teres major and latissimus dorsi for loss of external rotation at shoulder. Lancet, *2*:757, 1947.

# Index

*Numerals in italics indicate a figure connecting the subject.*

539

Artery(ies) — (*Continued*)
  in interscapulothoracic amputation, 179, *181*
  subclavian, in supraclavicular region of neck, 494
  suprascapular, course of, 147-148, *57, 58*
Arthritis, degenerative, of acromioclavicular joint,
    489-490
  gouty, in glenohumeral joint, 488, *488*
  rheumatoid, 485, *485*
Arthrodesis of shoulder, indications for, 206
  methods of, 207
  position for, determination of, 206-207
  recommended technique of, 207-210, *208, 209*
    in men, 209-210, *209*
    in women, 210, *209*
Arthrography, technique of, in massive avulsion of
    musculotendinous cuff, 449-450,
Axilla, 75-77
  anterior structures of, 76, *54*
  arch of, abnormality of, 39, *39*
  emergency approach to, technique of, 183-184, *183*
  incision in, in Magnuson-Stack operation, 214, *212*
  nerve of, and deltoid muscle, 144-145, *145*
    injury to, management of, 290
      mechanisms of, 290
    and surgical divisions, 143, *142*
  surgical approach through, technique of, 167-168,
    *166*
  walls of, 76, *74*
    posterior and medial, nerves in relation to, 76-77, *75*

Bankart operation, in recurrent anterior dislocation,
    425
  in recurrent subluxation and dislocation of gleno-
    humeral joint, 417
  technique of, 215, *216, 217*
    anterior incision in, 215, *216*
Baseball, shoulder injuries in, 270-276
Bateman, transfer of trapezius by, 255-258, *258, 259*
Biomechanics of shoulder, 80-99
Birds, evolution of pectoral girdle in, 3
Birth injuries to shoulder joint, 40-41, 523-533
Bone(s), block operations, in recurrent anterior dis-
    locations, 426-427
  chips, cancellous, following resection of bone in
    solitary bone cyst, 198, *197*
  cyst, solitary, cause of, theories of, 195-196
    clinical features of, 196
    roentgenographic features of, 196-198, *196*
    surgical management of, technique of, 198, *197*
  graft(s), in bone block operation for posterior re-
    current dislocations, 222, *224*
    in replacement of bone defect in fibrous dysplasia,
      202-203, *201*
    in replacement of bone defect in giant cell tumor,
      193, *195*
  injuries, of elbow, of young pitchers, 297, *296*
      management of, 297
    of shoulder, of young pitchers, 296, *295*
      management of, 296-297
  loose pieces of, in recurrent dislocation of gleno-
    humeral joint, 411
  resection of, in solitary bone cyst, 198, *197*
Bowling, shoulder injuries in, 273, 277
Brachial plexus, avulsion of, lower roots, 289
  management of, 289-290

  upper roots, 289
  and common variations of, 496, *497*
  injury to, birth. *See* Paralysis, obstetrical
    in sports, 289-290
  posterior cord of, injury to, management of, 290
Bristow operation, in recurrent anterior dislocations,
    426
  technique of, 219-221, *222, 223*
    anterior incision in, 219-220, *222*
Bursa(ae), around shoulder joint, 74-75
  development of, embryonic, 17, *18*
    fetal, 26
  infraserratus, 74-75
  subacromial, 62, *61*
    appearance of, 434, *435*
    degenerative alterations of, 117-118, *113*
    floor of, degenerative alterations of, 118-119, *118,
      119*
    lesions affecting, 435
    location of, 433-434
    motions of, 434
  subscapular, 75
  subscapularis, 74
  supra-acromial, 75
  supracoracoid, 74
Bursitis, 286, *287*
  deltoid, acute, causes of, 275
    symptoms of, 275-276
  subacromial, 435
  subdeltoid, acute, management of, 283

Cervical rib syndrome, aberrant ribs in, 512, *511*
  clinical picture of, 512-513
  fibrous band between ribs in, 512, *512*
  management of, 513-514
  x-ray in diagnosis of, 513
Cervical root disorders. *See* Nerve(s), roots, cervical,
  disorders of
Cervical spine. *See* Spine, cervical
Cervical syndrome, acute, clinical manifestations of,
    503, *502*
  management of, 505-506
  pathology of, 501-503, *501, 502*
  chronic, disc degeneration in, 503-504, *504*
    management of, 506
    objective findings in, 505
    osteoarthritic changes in, 504, *505*
    referred pain in, 504-505
Charley-horse, 279
Chondroblastoma, benign, clinical features of, 187
  histological features of, 187, *189*
  incidence and sites of, 185
  roentgenographic features of, 187-188, *190*
  treatment of, 188
    technique of, 188, *191*
Clavicle(s), abnormalities of, congenital, 33-36, *34,
    35, 36*
  local developmental, 35
  in arm elevation, 87, 88, *87*
  configuration of, 495
  study of, 44-49, *43, 44, 45, 46, 47*
  congenital pseudarthrosis of, incidence of, 211
    repair of, technique of, 213-214, *210, 211*, 311-313,
      *310*